The Person with HIV/AIDS

Nursing Perspectives

FOURTH EDITION

Jerry D. Durham, PhD, RN, FAAN, is Professor of Nursing and Chancellor of Allen College, Waterloo, Iowa. Prior to assuming his current position, he served as Vice-Chancellor of Academic Affairs at the University of Missouri at St. Louis. He has also held leadership positions at Indiana University School of Nursing, Mennonite College of Nursing, and Illinois Wesleyan University. Dr. Durham has earned six university degrees, including three in nursing and a doctorate in higher education administration. In addition to his role as an educator, he has held positions as a staff nurse, clinical manager, private practitioner in mental health nursing, and consultant in education and research. He was among the first researchers to investigate the nature of private practice in psychiatric nursing. He has received two fellowships in ethics from National Endowment for the Humanities. From 2006 through 2008 Dr. Durham cochaired the Emerging and Infectious Diseases Expert Panel of the American Academy of Nursing.

Felissa R. Lashley (formerly Felissa L. Cohen), **PhD, RN, FAAN, FACMG,** is professor emeritus and immediate past dean of the College of Nursing, Rutgers, the State University of New Jersey. Dr. Lashley is also dean emeritus and professor emeritus of the School of Nursing at Southern Illinois University, Edwardsville. She previously served as professor and Head of the Department of Medical-Surgical Nursing at the University of Illinois at Chicago (UIC) College of Nursing; Clinical Chief for Medical-Surgical Nursing at UIC Hospital and Clinics; and associate professor in the Department of Genetics, School of Medicine, UIC. Dr. Lashley received her doctorate in human genetics with a minor in biochemistry from Illinois State University. She is certified as a PhD Medical Geneticist by the American Board of Medical Genetics (the first nurse to be so certified) and is a founding fellow of the American College of Medical Genetics. Dr. Lashley began her practice of genetic evaluation and counseling in 1973. She has authored more than 300 publications. Dr. Lashley was the first nurse to serve on the AIDS Research Review Committee, National Institute of Allergy and Infectious Disease, National Institutes of Health (NIH). She was a member of the HIV Nursing Clinical Advisory Committee of the National AIDS Education and Training Centers, HRSA Bureau of Health Professions. In 2005, she received the "Woman of Excellence" award from the New Jersey Women and AIDS Network.

The Person with HIV/AIDS

Nursing Perspectives

FOURTH EDITION

JERRY D. DURHAM, PhD, RN, FAAN

FELISSA R. LASHLEY, PhD, RN, FAAN, FACMG

EDITORS

SPRINGER PUBLISHING COMPANY
NEW YORK

Springer Publishing Company, LLC
11 West 42nd Street
New York, NY 10036
www.springerpub.com

Acquisitions Editor: Allan Graubard
Project Manager: Judy Worrell
Cover design: TG Design
Composition: Six Red Marbles

Ebook ISBN: 978–0–8261–2138–7

09 10 11 / 5 4 3 2 1

Library of Congress Cataloging-in-Publication Data

The person with HIV/AIDS: nursing perspectives/Felissa R. Lashley, Jerry D. Durham, [editors].—4th ed.
   p. ; cm.
   Includes bibliographical references and index.
   ISBN 978-0-8261-2137-0
   1. AIDS (Disease)—Nursing. I. Lashley, Felissa R., 1941– II. Durham, Jerry D.
   [DNLM: 1. Acquired Immunodeficiency Syndrome—nursing. 2. HIV Infections—nursing. WY 153.5 P467 2009]
   RC606.6.P47 2009
   616.97'920231—dc22

                                                                    2009029810

The authors and the publisher of this Work have made every effort to use sources believed to be reliable to provide information that is accurate and compatible with the standards generally accepted at the time of publication. Because medical science is continually advancing, our knowledge base continues to expand. Therefore, as new information becomes available, changes in procedures become necessary. We recommend that the reader always consult current research and specific institutional policies before performing any clinical procedure. The authors and publisher shall not be liable for any special, consequential, or exemplary damages resulting, in whole or in part, from the readers' use of, or reliance on, the information contained in this book. The publisher has no responsibility for the persistence or accuracy of URLs for external or third-party Internet Web sites referred to in this publication and does not guarantee that any content on such Web sites is, or will remain, accurate or appropriate.

Printed in the United States of America by The Hamilton Printing Company

I dedicate this book to my wife, Kathy, for her enduring love and support throughout our lives together.

—Jerry D. Durham

With love to my wonderful family: Heather Cohen; Neal, Anne, Jacob, and Grace Cohen; Peter, Julie, Ben, Hannah, and Lydia Cohen; and Ruth Lashley. In the time since the first edition of this book, HIV/AIDS has changed from a fatal to a chronic illness. May there be both an effective vaccine and complete cure before the next edition.

—Felissa R. Lashley

Contents

APPENDICES 559

INDEX 611

Contributors

Mary G. Boland, DrPH, CPNP, FAAN
Dean and Professor of Nursing, School
of Nursing and Dental Hygiene
University of Hawaii at Manoa
Honolulu, HI

Joe W. Burrage Jr., PhD, RN, FAAN
Treasurer, Association of Nurses in
AIDS Care
Associate Professor, Nursing
Indiana University
Indianapolis, IN

**Jane Dimmitt Champion, PhD, MA, MSN,
APRN, FAAN**
Professor, School of Nursing
University of Texas Health Science
Center at San Antonio
Director, Center for Community-
Based Health Promotion for
Women and Children
San Antonio, TX

Judith B. Cornelius, PhD, MS, RN
School of Nursing
University of North Carolina
Charlotte, NC

**Donna M. Gallagher, RNC, MS, ANP,
FAAN**
Member, International Nursing
Committee for the Association
of Nurses in AIDS Care
Principal Investigator and Adjunct
Professor
University of Massachusetts Medical
School
Worcester, MA

Susan W. Gaskins, DSN, ACRN, RN
Board Member, HIV/AIDS Nursing
Certification Board of the
Association of Nurses in AIDS Care
Professor of Nursing
Capstone College of Nursing
University of Alabama
Tuscaloosa, AL

Joan S. Grant, DSN, CS, RN
Professor of Nursing
University of Alabama at Birmingham
Birmingham, AL

Deborah Gritzmacher, MSN, RN
Board Member, AID Atlanta
Assistant Professor, Health Care
Management and Nursing
Clayton State University
Morrow, GA

**Sandra "Sande" Gracia Jones, PhD, ARNP,
ACRN, CNS, FAAN**
Associate Professor, Nursing
Florida International University
Miami, FL

Norman L. Keltner, EdD, APRN
Professor of Nursing
University of Alabama at Birmingham
Birmingham, AL

Michael K. Klebert, PhD, APN, RN
Member, Ryan White Title I Planning
Council
Study Coordinator and Research
Instructor
Washington University School of
Medicine
St. Louis, MO

Carl A. Kirton, DNP, RN, ANP-BC, ACRN
President, Association of Nurses in
   AIDS Care
Vice President, Nursing & Nurse
   Practitioner
North General Hospital
Associate Adjunct Professor of Nursing
New York University, College of
   Nursing
New York, NY

Carol A. "Pat" Patsdaughter, PhD, CNE, ACRN, RN
Associate Editor, *Journal of the
   Association of Nurses in AIDS Care*
Professor
Florida International University
Miami, FL

J. Craig Phillips, PhD, LLM, RN, ARNP, PMHCNS-BC, ACRN
Nominations Committee Chair,
   Association of Nurses in AIDS Care
Assistant Professor, Nursing
University of British Columbia
Vancouver, B.C., Canada

James L. Raper, DSN, CRNP, JD, FAANP
Director, 1917 HIV Outpatient,
   Research and Dental Clinics
Associate Professor, Medicine-
   Infectious Disease
Clinical Associate Professor, Nursing
University of Alabama at Birmingham
Birmingham, AL

Elizabeth M. Saewyc, PhD, PHN, RN
Chair, Applied Public Health Research
Canadian Institutes for Health
   Research and Public Health Agency
   of Canada
Senior Scientist, Child Family
   Research Institute
Professor, Nursing
University of British Columbia
Vancouver, Canada

Richard L. Sowell, PhD, RN, FAAN
Professor of Nursing
Kennesaw State University
Kennesaw, GA

David J. Sterken, MN, CNS, CPNP
Chairperson, HIV+ Nurse Committee
   for the Association of Nurses in
   AIDS Care
Clinical Nurse Specialist, Pediatric
   Services
Helen DeVos Children's Hospital
Grand Rapids, MI

Deborah S. Storm, PhD, RN
Director for Research and Evaluation,
   François-Xavier Bagnoud (FXB)
   Center
Clinical Associate Professor, School of
   Nursing
University of Medicine and Dentistry
   of New Jersey, Newark
Newark, NJ

David E. Vance, PhD, MGS
Assistant Professor, School of Nursing
University of Alabama at Birmingham
Birmingham, AL

Ann C. White, MPH
Cochair of HIV/AIDS Task Council of
   Charlotte
Executive Director, Metrolina AIDS
   Project
Charlotte, NC

Jacqueline C. Zalumas, PhD, RN, FNP-BC
Member, Editorial Board, *Journal of
   Correctional Health Care*
Professor of Nursing
Georgia Baptist College of Nursing
Mercer University
Atlanta, GA

Preface

In the almost three decades since 1981, when the first cases of AIDS were reported in the United States, HIV/AIDS has become a pandemic, affecting virtually all people of the world, men and women, young and old. An estimated 33 million people worldwide are now living with HIV. Early in the evolution of this pandemic, a diagnosis of HIV infection or of AIDS was a certain death sentence because scientific knowledge of the disease and the means to treat it were limited. In the 1980s, prior to the development of antiretroviral therapy (ART) and highly active antiretroviral therapy (HAART), patients and practitioners encountered "pervasive institutional and professional resistance to caring for persons with AIDS" (Bayer & Oppenheimer, 2006). This resistance stemmed from multiple causes, including denial, homophobia, AIDS-related stigma, discrimination, and fear of contagion. During the first decade of the HIV/AIDS epidemic, acts of extraordinary courage and compassion on the part of the physicians and nurses caring for AIDS patients were common and bound those in the AIDS movement together as a community who, if they couldn't save those who were infected, could at least bear witness to epidemic.

While our recognition of HIV/AIDS came with its emergence among American gay white men, over the past two decades the epidemic has evolved as a global phenomenon, affecting men and women almost equally in some parts of the world. The epidemiological patterns of HIV/AIDS vary greatly around the globe, with HIV/AIDS now disproportionately affecting the haves and have-nots. For example, in the United States today only a relatively small number of infants are born with an HIV infection because of prenatal testing of their mothers and the availability of ART; however, in some parts of the world, and especially in resource-limited countries, such prenatal testing may not be common, and ART may not be readily available. So in spite of international efforts, hundreds of thousands of HIV-infected children born to infected mothers do not receive the ART they need. (Only about one-third of infected pregnant women receive ART to prevent transmission.) In addition, many of these children are orphaned and at risk of multiple problems in terms of their development, health, and education. In the United States, AIDS has evolved to have a disproportionate impact on minority communities. While ethnic and racial minorities comprised 34% of the U.S. population in 2006, they accounted for 70% of new AIDS cases that year.

While much is now known about HIV infection, its direct and indirect effects continue to challenge patients, families, communities, and caregivers. A new generation of health care providers is now needed to provide care for persons living with HIV/AIDS (PLWH). Unlike earlier professional caregivers whose armamentarium of treatments was extremely limited and whose interventions often included caring for the dying, the new generation of caregivers must understand HIV/AIDS as a chronic condition that PLWH may live with for several decades. These professional caregivers are in short supply in many resource-limited regions of the world and are often hampered in their caregiving efforts by a lack of facilities, money, drugs, and professional colleagues. Even in resource-rich nations like the United States, projected shortages of health care personnel and a sagging economy threaten to cause setbacks in the progress that has been made to date in the care of PLWH.

Prevention remains the best means to control the HIV/AIDS pandemic; however, only a small portion of the people in the world at risk of HIV have access to effective prevention methods such as HIV testing, education, clean needles and syringes, condoms, and mother-to-child transmission prevention programs. Although new biomedical prevention approaches are being tested (e.g., vaccines, preexposure prophylaxis, HSV-2 suppressive therapy, cervical barriers, topical microbicides, male circumcision), none has yet proven to be the "magic bullet" in preventing HIV transmission. Social and cultural factors continue to have an impact on the epidemic. Stigma, poverty, low literacy, sexual exploitation, and the devalued status of women in some parts of the world present formidable challenges to efforts to implement many prevention strategies. Political ideologies and religious dogma have also hampered prevention efforts in some parts of the world, including the United States. Many of the so-called "hard-to-reach," marginalized, at-risk populations of the world (e.g., sex workers and transgender persons) have not received effective prevention interventions tailored to their specific needs. More recently, some prevention leaders have called for "combination HIV prevention," a more long-term approach to reducing HIV risk and vulnerability by addressing both individual and contextual factors (e.g., environmental, political, social, cultural, attitudinal factors). Speaking to the taboos that have thwarted past prevention efforts, Sepkowitz (2006, p. 2414) concluded:

> The prime mover of the epidemic is not inadequate antiretroviral medications, poverty, or bad luck, but our inability to accept the gothic dimensions of a disease that is transmitted sexually. Only when we cease to dodge this fact will effective HIV-control programs be established. Until then, it is no exaggeration to say that our polite behavior is killing us.

In the face of these many challenges, significant progress has been made in efforts to prevent and control the HIV/AIDS pandemic. By the end of 2008, there were about 30 approved drugs (or combination drugs) to treat HIV infection. These drugs have proven remarkable in prolonging the lives of PLWH and in reducing some of the more troublesome symptoms of HIV—at least in those parts of the world where such drugs are available. Even in high-income nations, however, ART and HAART exact a toll on those whose lives depend on this treatment. Toxicity, drug resistance, and side effects commonly occur. In addition, access to treatment may be limited by insurance, income, and a lack of expert providers. Adequate drug treatment and availability of the appropriate medications is necessary for those with HIV infection, especially to interrupt maternal–child transmission.

The crisis that HIV/AIDS wrought in many resource-poor parts of the world resulted in responses aimed at stabilizing those countries or regions. After several failed (or at least less than fully successful) efforts by world bodies, including the World Health Organization (WHO), during the first decade of the HIV/AIDS epidemic, a core of the world's leaders eventually came to understand that failure to deal with the burgeoning pandemic could destabilize some countries and regions. Building on WHO's early Global Program on AIDS, the Joint Programme on HIV/AIDS (UNAIDS) was established in 1996 to coordinate a multisectoral global response to the pandemic. While this new world effort faced a variety of challenges and setbacks, by 2000 additional support from the World Bank, increasing awareness of the impact of AIDS on Africa, greater support by religious groups for condom use and sex-related prevention programs, and the increasing spread of HIV led to an enhanced global response to HIV/AIDS, including a special U.N. session on HIV/ AIDS (2001) and the establishment of the Global Fund to Fight AIDS, Tuberculosis and Malaria. In 2003, the United States established the President's Emergency Plan for AIDS Relief (PEPFAR), which was funded in 2008 for $48 billion for the next five years. These international efforts, as well as new ones supported by foundations and nongovernmental organizations, have resulted in greater numbers of people worldwide having access to HIV prevention and treatment programs. Still, only an estimated 20 to 37% of persons in low- and middle-income countries who need ART receive this treatment, and only about 20% of people in these countries even know they are infected.

Nurses have played key roles in responding to the HIV/AIDS epidemic. They were among the first professional caregivers to work at the bedsides of persons with AIDS; and now, as HIV/AIDS has become a more manageable disease, they work in the homes of PLWH, in specialty clinics, and in hospitals—in every setting where the PLWH needs care. They have formed an organization, the Association of Nurses in AIDS Care, dedicated to supporting nurses with an interest and expertise related to HIV/AIDS. Extensive HIV-related research, conducted by nurse-scholars, is now reported in the *Journal of the Association of Nurses in AIDS Care (JANAC)* and other HIV-related publications. Advanced practice nurses with HIV expertise—and especially nurse practitioners—now collaborate closely with other specialists to manage the day-to-day care of PLWH. Nurses have incorporated HIV/AIDS content into undergraduate nursing programs and established graduate programs in HIV/AIDS nursing. While the HIV pandemic will continue to provide many challenges in the future, nurses will remain a constant source of hope and succor for people struggling with HIV/AIDS throughout the world.

REFERENCES

Bayer, R. & Oppenheimer. (2006). Pioneers in AIDS care—Reflections on the epidemic's early years. *New England Journal of Medicine, 355,* 2273–2275.

Sepkowitz, K. (2006). One disease, two epidemics. *New England Journal of Medicine, 354,* 2411–2414.

The editors of this book wish to acknowledge and sincerely thank Rhonda Gilbert of Allen College for her support throughout this project. Rhonda carefully checked all references and tracked the book's progress. The editors also want to thank Allen College graduate student Tim Doyle who identified many of the resources in the appendices.

HIV Disease: Core Issues

HIV Infection and AIDS: Etiology, Epidemiology, and Transmission

1

FELISSA R. LASHLEY

Almost three decades ago the first observations of rare opportunistic infections, immunodeficiency, and Kaposi's sarcoma (KS) were first made in previously healthy young homosexual men. These observations heralded the beginning of one of the most medically, emotionally, and politically troubling epidemics of this century (Centers for Disease Control [CDC], 1981a, b). In an extremely short period of time, relatively speaking, we have learned more about human immunodeficiency virus (HIV) infection and acquired immunodeficiency syndrome (AIDS) than perhaps any other organism and disease in history, and some of what we have learned has been applied to other diseases such as cancer. As a result of these advances and new treatments, HIV/AIDS is now considered a chronic disease.

DEFINITIONS

Case definitions for both HIV and AIDS have undergone several revisions since the onset of the pandemic. The most recent change, reflecting increased knowledge and advances in diagnostic testing, requires laboratory-confirmed evidence of HIV infection (CDC, 2008e). The 2008 surveillance case definition for HIV infection among adults and adolescents (aged ≥13 years) is only for public health surveillance and not for clinical diagnosis. The 2008 surveillance case definition replaces the HIV infection classification system and the HIV infection and AIDS case definitions (CDC, 1987b, 1992, 1999, 2008d). (See Appendix I.)

3

The 2008 case definition for HIV infection among children aged 18 months to <13 years (CDC, 2008d, p. 5) replaces the 1987 and 1999 definitions (CDC, 1987b, 1999). This case definition is for public health surveillance only and not a guide for clinical diagnosis. This definition also applies to all variants of HIV. Confirmation of HIV infection through the diagnosis of AIDS-defining conditions alone is excluded. Laboratory-confirmed evidence of HIV infection is required in this age group (CDC, 2008d).

The 2008 case definition for HIV infection among children aged <18 months (CDC, 2008d, p. 5) replaces the 1999 definition (CDC, 1999). For surveillance purposes, a child aged <18 months is categorized as definitively or presumptively HIV infected if born to an HIV-infected mother and if the laboratory criterion or at least one of the other criteria is met. The CDC (2008d) states that these categories are for surveillance classification purposes and should not be used to guide clinical practice. Therefore, a child with perinatal HIV exposure should continue to be monitored clinically according to nationally accepted treatment and care guidelines (King, 2004; Public Health Service Task Force, 2008; Working Group on Antiretroviral Therapy and Medical Management of HIV-Infected Children, 2009). (See Appendix I and Chapter 14.)

ETIOLOGY

The etiologic agent of AIDS is the human immunodeficiency virus (HIV). (Also see Chapter 3.) HIV is a retrovirus belonging to the *Lentivirus* genus of the *Retroviridae* family. There are two types, type 1 and type 2, which are commonly written as HIV-1 and HIV-2. HIV-1 has several genetic subtypes or clades which are M (main), O (outlier) and N (non-M, non-O). Group M consists of at least nine subgroups or clades (A through H, J and K) and 15 circulating recombinant forms (CRF). More than 95% of global HIV isolates are in the M group. The A and B subtypes of the M group are responsible for most human infections. HIV-2 is mainly found in West Africa and is infrequently found elsewhere (Knipe & Howley, 2007; Smith et al., 2008). A belief by some persons that HIV does not cause AIDS (commonly referred to as "AIDS denialism") has been refuted by the scientific and medical communities (The Durban Declaration, 2000); however, this belief has delayed early and effective treatment for HIV-infected persons in some parts of the world (e.g., South Africa).

Historical Background

Clues from epidemiological surveillance first suggested that AIDS was caused by a transmissible agent. These clues included the following: (1) The AIDS epidemic was new; (2) it appeared first in limited geographic areas and then spread; (3) the initial groups of people affected (homosexual men and intravenous drug users) and later identified groups (hemophiliacs and blood transfusion recipients) were prone to communicable diseases but were socially, economically, and geographically disparate; and (4) clustering of cases suggested common links and contacts. Early patterns of the distribution of affected persons were reminiscent of hepatitis B (Curran et al., 1985; Gallo, Shaw, & Markham, 1985; Seale, 1984). By 1982 the most probable virus candidates appeared to be cytomegalovirus, Epstein-Barr virus, certain adenoviruses, a human parvovirus, and the retroviruses (Fauci et al., 1984).

Several lines of thinking began to implicate a retrovirus, particularly one similar to human T-cell lymphotropic viruses (HTLV), which are also known as human T-cell leukemia viruses (HTLV-I causes adult T-cell leukemia in humans). These included the knowledge that (1) T-4 lymphocytes were selectively depleted in AIDS, and HTLV had already been shown to have this tropism; (2) HTLV could be transmitted by intimate contact or blood products; (3) HTLV could cause immunosuppression; (4) the retrovirus known as the feline leukemia virus could cause a type of cancer (leukemia) as well as immunosuppression leading to opportunistic infections in cats; and (5) there was a high incidence of AIDS among Haitians and Africans. (Both Haiti and Africa are endemic areas for HTLV-I.) Later assays of AIDS patients showed that they had evidence of exposure to an HTLV-I related virus (Broder & Gallo, 1985; Essex et al., 1985; Fauci et al., 1984; Lane & Fauci, 1985).

By 1983 and 1984, respectively, three groups of researchers had isolated, identified, and characterized the virus that was established as the cause of AIDS. Gallo and his group at the National Cancer Institute named it "HTLV-III"; Montagnier and his associates at the Pasteur Institute in Paris, in cooperation with the CDC, named it "lymphadenopathy-associated virus" (LAV); and Levy and his group in California named it "AIDS-associated retrovirus" (ARV) (Barré-Sinoussi et al., 1983; Gelman et al. 1983; Levy et al., 1984). A task force sponsored by the International Committee on the Taxonomy of Viruses was assembled to reach a decision on a name (Norman, 1985). The name recommended by this committee in May 1986 was "human immunodeficiency virus" (HIV) (Coffin et al.,

1986), a term that continues in use today. The importance of identifying the cause of AIDS included the ability to identify persons infected with HIV; describe the viral characteristics; epidemiologically characterize viral transmission and patterns; describe the natural history of infection; and develop screening and diagnostic tests, approaches to prevention, treatment, and vaccine development. In 2008, Françoise Barré-Sinoussi and Luc Montagnier shared the 2008 Nobel Prize for physiology or medicine for their discovery of HIV (Françoise Barré-Sinoussi and Luc Montagnier share . . . , 2009). Some scientists took issue with the omission of Gallo from also sharing this recognition (Abbadessa et al., 2009).

Human Immunodeficiency Virus Type 2 (HIV-2)

In October, 1985, Clavel, Montagnier, and their colleagues identified a new human immunodeficiency virus in blood samples from persons with AIDS in Portugal who had lived in western Africa. It was also described in asymptomatic West African prostitutes (CDC, 1989; Gallo & Montagnier, 1988). This virus was eventually designated human immunodeficiency virus type 2 (HIV-2). It is closely related to the simian immunodeficiency virus (SIV) (Guerrant, Walker, & Weller, 2006; Wain-Hobson, 1998). HIV-2 has been mainly detected, and is thought to have originated, as a zoonotic disease in western Africa; however, there is a reported decrease in HIV-2 infections in many West African countries concurrently with an increase in HIV-1 infections (Rowland-Jones & Whittle, 2007). The first reported AIDS case in the United States due to HIV-2 was diagnosed in December 1987 in New Jersey in a patient who was originally from western Africa (CDC, 1988). Based on screening for antibody in frozen sera, researchers have concluded that HIV-2 may have been present in western Africa since at least 1966 (Kawamura et al., 1989).

HIV-2 is transmitted in the same ways as HIV-1, but it appears less transmissible sexually and perinatally (Whittle, Ariyoshi, & Rowland-Jones, 1998; World Health Organization [WHO], 2008). Most persons in West Africa with HIV-2 infection exhibit delayed disease progression and are known as long-term nonprogressors (Rowland-Jones & Whittle, 2007), or they are asymptomatic (de Silva, Cotten & Rowland-Jones, 2008). There has been relatively little spread beyond West Africa. Few cases of HIV-2 are detected in the United States; however, in the United States in 2008, there was a report of the emergence of a new strain of HIV-2 in an immunosuppressed person who immigrated to the United States from Sierra Leone (Smith et al., 2008).

Origin of HIV and AIDS

Scientists have remained interested in the origin of HIV for various reasons, including that identifying the origin and how the virus causes disease in other hosts might give clues to control of HIV (Essex & Kanki, 1988; Worobey et al., 2008). Some scientists have postulated that HIV crossed the host–species barrier and spread as a "virgin soil" epidemic. Such an organism may be harmless to its natural host but highly lethal to its new host. For HIV-2, the animal host is considered to be the sooty mangabey monkey (*Cercocebus atys*) (Van Heuverswyn & Peeters, 2007). The common chimpanzee (*Pan troglodytes*) has been implicated as the natural reservoir for HIV-1, although the introduction into human populations appears more complex than the route for HIV-2 (Keele et al., 2006).

Various case reports and retrospective analyses of stored serum samples suggest the presence of AIDS in the United States in 1968, and perhaps even earlier, although it has also been suggested that some positive serological results may have been artifacts due to prolonged storage (Garry et al., 1989). The earliest reported case was in a Norwegian merchant seaman who was infected in 1961 or 1962 with HIV-1 group O in Cameroon. He subsequently transmitted HIV to his wife and daughter. Another early reported case in Africa was that of a female Danish surgeon who contracted the disease while working in Zaire in 1976 and who died in 1977 (Bygbjerg, 1983). Other early cases appear to have occurred in Kinshasha in 1959 (Hooper, 1997; Nahmias et al., 1986).

The World Health Assembly stated in 1987 that HIV is a "naturally occurring retrovirus of undetermined geographic origin" (Mann et al., 1988, p. 82). Despite this pronouncement, the subject of the origin of HIV and AIDS became a political issue. One highly publicized theory was that SIV-contaminated African chimpanzee tissue was used in the culturing of oral polio vaccine leading to an unintended iatrogenic disease (Hooper, 1999; 2001). This theory has not been substantiated (Worobey et al., 2004).

TRANSMISSION

To date, HIV has been isolated from a variety of body fluids, cells, and tissues, including peripheral blood, lymph nodes, brain tissue, cerebrospinal fluid, tears, bone marrow, cell-free plasma, saliva, retina, cornea, ear secretions, bronchial fluid, semen, seminal fluid, breast milk, cervical cells, Langerhans cells of the skin and mucous membranes, synovial fluid, and cervical and vaginal secretions. HIV has not been recovered from sweat (CDC, 1997a,b; Marwick, 1985; Pomerantz et al., 1987; Thiry et al., 1985; Vogt et al., 1986; Withrington et al., 1987; Wofsy et al., 1986). The CDC (2005a), in discussing occupational exposures, has indicated that the following fluids are potentially infected: blood, cerebrospinal fluid, synovial fluid, pleural fluid, peritoneal fluid, pericardial fluid, amniotic fluid, semen, and vaginal secretions, as well as any fluids or tissues containing visible blood. The CDC does not consider feces, nasal secretions, saliva, sputum, sweat, tears, urine, or vomitus to be potentially infectious unless they are visibly bloody (CDC, 2005b). The importance of these fluids, cells, and tissues in transmission varies as does the concentration of HIV within them. Periods of higher infectiousness and transmissibility coincide with higher viral load on the part of the HIV-infected person, certain genetic susceptibility and resistance factors, and increasing immunosuppression. Characteristics of HIV itself such as the viral phenotype, clades and subtypes, its cellular tropism (macrophage or other), and the viral load are also important in degree of transmissibility. Many of the genetic susceptibility and resistance factors (such as HLA type and CCRX variants, and CCL3L1 dose), and characteristics of the virus have been exploited in designing effective tests and therapies, some of which result in specific treatments for specific genotypes but are beyond the scope of this chapter. Transmission efficiency also depends on mode of transmission. For example, transmission by blood transfusion is much more efficient than transmission by oral sex with an infected person.

The CDC has recommended standard precautions be applied for all patient care contact with specific transmission-based precautions applied in addition to standard precautions depending on the particular infectious agent and its mode of transmission. For HIV infection alone, only standard precautions would be used. These precautions replace universal precautions. However, additional precautions may be necessary if coinfection is present. For example, if a person with HIV also has active pulmonary tuberculosis, then airborne precautions would be necessary in addition to standard precautions (Siegel et al., 2007).

The major documented ways that HIV may be transmitted are by intimate sexual contact, both homosexual and heterosexual, with an HIV-infected person; through exposure to contaminated blood or blood products either by direct inoculation, sharing of drug apparatus, transfusion, or other methods; and through passage of the virus from an infected mother to her fetus or newborn in utero, during labor and delivery, or in the early newborn period. The CDC (2005a,b) has delineated levels of risk for HIV transmission. The highest to lowest risks of acquisition of HIV if HIV contamination is present are the following: blood transfusion, needle sharing with injection drug use, receptive anal intercourse, percutaneous needle stick, receptive penile-vaginal intercourse, insertive anal intercourse, insertive penile-vaginal intercourse, with both receptive oral intercourse and insertive oral intercourse between men representing less per-act risk. Bite injury, while another potential route of transmission, is actually a rare route of actual acquisition of HIV.

Sexual Transmission

Initially in the United States, the most common mode of spread was male-to-male sexual transmission. Male-to-male sexual contact is still cumulatively the major transmission category for U.S. adult men, as discussed below (CDC, 2008b). Heterosexual transmission of HIV can occur both from males to females and from females to males. Male-to-female transmission is a more efficient means of transmission (Powers et al., 2008). Heterosexual transmission can occur during both penile-vaginal and penile-anal intercourse and more rarely through oral-genital contact (Vermund, 1997). The estimated male-to-female transmission probability per incident is between 1 in 200 and 1 in 2,000 (De Jong & Geijtenbeek, 2008). Langerhans cells in genital mucosal tissue have been identified as having potential protective functions (de Jong & Geijtenbeek, 2008). HIV transmission due to artificial insemination from an infected donor has been reported. There have also been a limited number of reports of female-to-female sexual transmission (Greenhouse, 1987; Marmor et al., 1986; Monzon & Capellan, 1987), and women who have sex with women may also have other risk factors such as sex with men or injection drug use. The CDC (2006) has reported that in the United States there are no confirmed cases of female-to-female sexual transmission of HIV. Transmission by oral sex has also been described, but the risk is believed to be very low and to result from blood contact (CDC, 1997a,b; Rozenbaum et al., 1988; Spitzer & Weiner, 1989).

The HIV infection epidemic exposed our ignorance of the type and frequency of various sexual practices in the United States. Sex researchers have estimated that about 25% of American women occasionally engage in anal receptive intercourse and that about 10% do so on a regular basis for either pleasure or contraception (Bolling & Voeller, 1987). Acquisition of HIV may be made easier by the presence of genital ulcers, sexually transmitted infections, or trauma, and the presence of inflammation or exudates, which can facilitate virus entry into the cell. Menstruation may facilitate transmission whereas menopause resulting in vaginal dryness may lead to trauma and also facilitate transmission. First sexual experiences may be associated with bleeding, and immature vaginal tissue in young girls may be less resistant to trauma and bleeding. Infectious cells such as lymphocytes or macrophages that enter the genital tract because of the presence of one of the above are believed to increase transmissibility. Lack of circumcision in men is believed to result in higher intraurethral loads of infectious cells that increase transmissibility. Thus sex with an uncircumcised man may be riskier than with one who is circumcised in relation to HIV infection (de Jong & Geijtenbeek, 2008; Vermund, 1997).

In addition to factors mentioned above, sexual transmission of HIV is influenced by the:

- Number of different sexual partners
- Likelihood that the sexual partner is infected (for example, behaviors such as injection drug use)
- Prevalence of HIV infection in the geographic area
- Number of sexual exposures with a HIV-infected person
- Status of rectal and vaginal mucosa (for example, whether it is dry or whether sexually transmitted infections are present)
- Infectiousness of the partner (this may include viral load and use of antiviral drugs)
- Use of barriers during sex (for example, proper use of latex condoms)
- Degree of risky sexual behaviors that are practiced (Vermund, 1997; Vernazza et al., 1999).

Transmission between regular sexual partners, only one of whom is HIV infected (called "HIV discordant couples") has been of particular interest for many reasons, including the potential for prevention of spread. The transmission rate among such discordant couples has varied. Sexual transmission is further discussed below.

Bloodborne Transmission

Transmission of HIV by exposure to HIV-infected blood or blood products occurs mainly through piercing of the skin with a contaminated needle or sharp object; through sharing of needles or other drug-related apparatus, especially among injection drug users; or transfusion from an infected donor to someone requiring blood because of temporary illness, surgery, or chronic illness such as hemophilia or dialysis as well as through transplantation. Injuries from needles and sharp objects to health care workers also falls in this category of transmission, as do using contaminated needles and equipment used for therapeutic purposes. Tattooing has also been implicated in the spread of HIV (Doll, 1988) as has ear and body piercing. Reports of confirmed HIV transmission during bloody fist fights are rare but possible (Ippolitto, Poggio, & Arici, 1994). Concerns about blood-related spread resulted in various precautions during contact sports. For example, Nevada required a mandatory HIV test for boxers, and if positive the fighter was disqualified. Other states with similar rules include New York, New Jersey, Washington, Oregon, and Arizona, as well as Puerto Rico (Feller & Flanagan, 1997). HIV infection after acupuncture has been described (Vittecoq et al., 1989) as it has from receiving transplanted organs from an HIV-infected person (CDC, 1987a). Although rare, transmission through human bite by a HIV-infected person is theoretically possible and has been described (Bartholomew & Jones, 2006; Oladokun et al., 2008). HIV transmission through blood is discussed further below.

Perinatal Transmission

Vertical transmission of HIV from an infected mother to her fetus or child in the perinatal period is the third major transmission mode. This includes the times of pregnancy, delivery, and postpartum. Around the time of delivery, transmission is thought to take place due to contact with infected maternal blood and tissue, and most perinatal transmission is believed to occur close to the time of childbirth. Postdelivery, breastfeeding has been implicated in transmission of HIV, and the virus has been isolated from breast milk, both cell-free and cellular components (CDC, 1998; WHO, 2008).

Major advances have occurred in preventing HIV transmission from a mother to her child, and transmission rates have decreased markedly, especially in developed countries, to lows of under 2% (ACOG, 2008; Fowler et al., 2007). In 1994, the groundbreaking results of the AIDS Clinical Trials Group Study 076 were reported (Connor et al., 1994). This study demonstrated that perinatal transmission of HIV infection could be markedly reduced (nearly 70%) by the administration of zidovudine to HIV-infected women during pregnancy and delivery and to their infant after birth (Connor et al., 1994). Other measures to decrease risk led to changes in obstetric management. Since that time, detailed antiretroviral protocols have been developed to treat HIV-infected pregnant women and their infants. (Also see Chapters 13 and 14.)

The strongest data implicating breast-feeding in transmission originally resulted from case reports of women who acquired HIV from postpartum blood transfusions and whose infants were subsequently infected (LePage et al., 1987; Ziegler et al., 1985). However, there also were studies that indicated HIV-infected mothers did not transmit HIV to their infants while breast-feeding (Lifson, 1988). This argument was resolved with the recovery of HIV-1 DNA from breast milk (Nduati et al., 1995). Currently it is believed that HIV is associated with both the cell-free and cell-associated breast milk components and that the most likely mode of transmission is through infant gut mucosal surfaces. Without drug treatment, transmission can occur at any time during breast-feeding, and the longer the duration, the greater the cumulative risk. However, at least partly because of the acquisition of immune protection via breast milk, it appears that exclusive breast-feeding is associated with lower rates of HIV transmission to the infant than mixed feedings of both breast milk and formula, although formula feedings alone have lower rates (John-Stewart et al., 2004; WHO, 2008). In one study in South Africa of 137 women, by 15 months of age children who had been exclusively breast fed until at least 3 months had a 25% risk of HIV infection; those who were formula-fed, 19%; and those who were breast fed and received other foods, 36% (Coutsoudis et al., 2001). Transmission is also influenced by duration of breast-feeding, with 68% of transmission occurring after six months of breastfeeding (WHO, 2008).

Both maternal and infant factors are associated with an increased risk of HIV transmission via breast-feeding. Maternal factors include:

- Younger maternal age
- Lower parity
- Increased maternal RNA viral load in plasma
- Increased maternal RNA viral load in breast milk
- Breast clinical conditions such as mastitis and cracked nipples
- Suboptimal maternal nutritional status
- Increased duration of breastfeeding (WHO, 2008)

Local immune factors in breast milk may be protective or, if low, may be associated with a higher risk of transmission. Infant factors include

(1) Interrupted integrity of the mucous membranes; (2) oral thrush; (3) immune system dysfunction; and other factors such as milk stasis and altered sucking (WHO, 2008).

In developed countries such as the United States, the standard recommendations for years have been for women to refrain from breast-feeding if they are HIV infected (CDC, 1985; Public Health Service Task Force, 2008). In resource-poor countries where perinatal transmission is more prevalent, restriction on breast-feeding is more complex and can also be a political issue. In many resource-limited countries, formula feeding carries an increased risk for infant morbidity and mortality (but not HIV transmission), while breastfeeding carries a risk for HIV transmission but has less risk for other severe morbidity and mortality (Coovadia & Kindra, 2008). The WHO has issued the following statement on HIV and infant feeding:

> The most appropriate infant feeding option for an HIV-infected mother depends on her individual circumstances, including her health status and the local situation, and should consider the health services available and the counselling and support she is likely to receive. Exclusive breastfeeding is recommended for HIV-infected women for the first six months of life unless replacement feeding is acceptable, feasible, affordable, sustainable, and safe for them and their infants before that time. When replacement feeding is acceptable, feasible, affordable, sustainable and safe, avoidance of all breastfeeding by HIV-infected women is recommended (¶ 2).

The WHO recommends that all "HIV-positive women who need anti-retroviral treatment for their own health should have it, and this is likely to reduce HIV transmission during breastfeeding" (WHO, 2009, ¶ 3).

OCCUPATIONAL TRANSMISSION AND PROPHYLAXIS

Health care workers are exposed to many health and safety hazards in health care settings, especially hospitals. Many of these involve infectious agents such as HIV, hepatitis B, hepatitis C, and others. Thus, nurses and other health care workers need to follow recommended safeguards to protect themselves and need to be assertive in ensuring that such safeguards are available to them. Most of the acquisitions in the occupational arena occur through exposure to blood. HIV seroconversion after an accident in the work setting has been a source of concern for health care workers. Early information relative to this concern came from the CDC Cooperative Needlestick Surveillance group, which consisted of 335 institutions throughout the United States (Marcus and the Cooperative Needlestick Surveillance Group, 1989). The majority of injuries resulted from needlesticks, and information from these studies resulted in recommended modifications for procedures that would increase safety.

According to current estimates, the average risk for occupational HIV transmission is approximately 0.3% and 0.09% for percutaneous and mucous membrane exposure to HIV-infected blood respectively (CDC, 2005b). Various factors increase the risk for HIV acquisition after occupational exposure, including exposure to a larger quantity of blood from the source patient, source patients with terminal illness reflecting factors such as the presence of syncytia-inducing strains, and presence of visible blood on the injury-causing device used to enter the patient's blood vessel (Gerberding, 1997), in addition to other host and agent factors discussed earlier. However, low viral loads in source patients do not rule out the possibility of transmission.

The original postexposure prophylaxis regimens were promulgated in 1996 and updated in 1998, 2001, and 2005 (CDC, 1998; 2001; 2005b). Employers are required to have exposure control plans. It is important that health care workers report any exposure immediately. The current recommendations about testing, evaluation, counseling, and postexposure drug regimen prophylaxis are in Appendix I. They include information about counseling, adherence, provision of expert advice when needed, and more.

NONOCCUPATIONAL POSTEXPOSURE PROPHYLAXIS

In 1998, the CDC first published recommendations for the management of persons who had nonoccupational exposures to HIV. These were updated in 2005 to reflect advances in prophylactic treatment with the appropriate drug regimen. Nonoccupational postexposure prophylaxis is abbreviated as nPEP (CDC, 2005a). The information on evaluation and protocol may be found in Appendix I. While people in various categories of potential exposures might take advantage of nPEP, use of it is particularly encouraged in both males and females who have been raped. Another group who might take advantage of nPEP are sex workers or intravenous drug users (IDUs) who generally practice risk reduction but who have had an exceptional occurrence of high-risk behavior (CDC, 2005a). Children who are sexually abused or assaulted or who are exposed by accident to an HIV-infected person may be candidates for nPEP. (See guidelines from the American Academy of Pediatrics [Havens and Committee on Pediatric AIDS, 2003]). Prophylaxis should not be considered as a "morning-after pill" and not replace prevention of HIV infection. nPEP treatment should begin within 72 hours of actual or potential exposure (CDC, 2005a).

STATISTICS AND PATTERNS IN THE UNITED STATES
HIV Incidence and Prevalence

Incidence refers to new cases of a specified condition within a specific time period, while prevalence is the total number of persons with that condition during a specific time period. Data may also be reported in terms of persons living with HIV (not AIDS), persons living with an AIDS diagnosis, or persons with HIV/AIDS, which can make comparisons confusing. There have also been changes in the number of states reporting, especially in regard to HIV (not AIDS), and in varying methods and definitions used over the years, making comparisons difficult. Early in the epidemic, AIDS was a reportable disease, but HIV infection itself was not. Therefore, statistics on HIV prevalence were somewhat inaccurate and incomplete. In 2008, the CDC published a report stating that the earlier back-calculation methods used to estimate HIV prevalence were no longer deemed valid or reliable (CDC, 2008a). As of April 2008, all 50 states, the District of Columbia, and five dependent areas (American Samoa, Guam, the Northern Mariana Islands, Puerto Rico, and the U.S. Virgin Islands) use the same confidential name-based reporting system to collect HIV and AIDS data. AIDS is reportable by all 50 states and the District of Columbia as well as the U.S. territories (CDC, 2009). A detailed methodological approach using laboratory assays that can differentiate recent HIV infection from older ones and extensive statistical methods, including an extended back-calculation approach, were used (Hall et al., 2008). The results indicate that there were approximately 1,106,400 million U.S. adults and adolescents living with HIV at the end of 2006, with a prevalence rate of 447.8 per 100,000 (CDC, 2008a). Of these, approximately 21% do not know they are infected (CDC, 2008c). Using new estimates, CDC estimates that the annual rate of new HIV infections is approximately 40% higher than previously estimated (Highleyman, 2008) and that there are approximately 112,000 more persons living with HIV in 2006 than there were in 2003 (CDC, 2008c)

Some of the highlights of the CDC's epidemiological data reported in 2008 for the United States include the following: Approximately 75% of all persons living with HIV are male; 48.1% fell into the male-to-male sexual contact transmission category, while overall 27.6% of all HIV cases fell into the category of high-risk heterosexual contact, although 72.4% of women were in this category; 18.5% fell into the category of injection drug use overall as did about 26% of women. In regard to race and ethnicity, approximately 46.1% of all persons living with HIV were African American while the data for whites, Hispanic/Latino, Asian/Pacific Islander, and American Indians/Alaska Natives were 34.6%, 17.5%, 1.4%, and 0.4% respectively. Overall, about 70% of persons living with HIV in the United States are between the ages of 25 years and 49 years, while about 25% are 50 years of age and older (CDC, 2008a,b; Highleyman, 2008). The increase in HIV prevalence is due not only to the increase in HIV incidence but also to successful treatment. One of the important aspects of these data lies in their application to planning and prevention efforts.

Geographic Distribution

AIDS has been reported in all 50 states plus the District of Columbia (CDC, 2009). The highest number of AIDS cases both in 2007 and cumulatively is New York state while North Dakota reports the lowest number of cases. Looking at the estimated rates per 100,000 population for persons living with AIDS in 2007, the highest rate for both adults/adolescents and children is the District of Columbia, followed by New York state for adults/adolescents and Delaware and Florida for children. In regard to reports of cases of HIV infection (not AIDS), six states (California, Florida, New Jersey, New York, North Carolina, Texas) reported about 51% of the 337,590 cumulative cases of HIV infection (not AIDS) (CDC, 2009). Examining AIDS annual incidence rates per 100,000 population for regions for 2006 cases, the highest rates per 100,000 in adults and adolescents for metropolitan statistical areas of >500,000 (large metropolitan area), 50,000 to 499,999 (medium metropolitan area), and below 50,000 (nonmetropolitan area) were found in the south (CDC, 2008a). The geographic region with the highest number of persons living with AIDS in 2007 was the south, followed by the northeast (CDC, 2009).

Distribution by Sex

As of December 31, 2007, the number of adult female cases of AIDS reported to the CDC was 201,205, accounting for 19.7% of all reported adult cases. Females also accounted for 49.1% of reported U.S. pediatric cases. The rates of AIDS in U.S. women have continued to rise. For adult women in the United States, the major transmission category is now high-risk heterosexual contact with a person known to have or to be at high risk for HIV infection, accounting for about 45% of all female cases, followed by injection drug use, accounting for about 35%. When the category of IDU and the subcategory under high-risk heterosexual contact of "sex with IDU" is added, then about 48% of all AIDS cases in women are known to be related to IDU in some way (CDC, 2009). From 2004 to 2007, the estimated number of newly diagnosed HIV/AIDS cases increased approximately 8% among females and 18% among males, and about 77% of persons living with AIDS were male. AIDS continues to have a disproportionate impact on minority women, particularly black women, in relation to their proportions in the general population as compared to women with AIDS. In terms of cumulative prevalence, the percentage of AIDS in adult women is as follows: black, non-Hispanic, 59.7%; white, non-Hispanic, 19.6%; and Hispanic, 19.1%, with the remainder in other groups. Black women have an HIV prevalence rate of about 1,122 per 100,000, while Hispanic/Latina women have an HIV prevalence rate of 263 per 100,000, and white women have an HIV prevalence rate of 63 per 100,000 (CDC, 2008a,c; Highleyman, 2008). As discussed below, the proportion of new cases of AIDS in younger women is increasing. These trends indicate directions for future prevention as discussed in Chapter 5. There is no separate transmission category for women who have sex with women, and there is a paucity of information relating to it. The issues related to lesbians and women who have sex with women are discussed in Chapter 11.

Age Distribution

In regard to age, at the end of 2007, the peak age range for reported U.S. AIDS cases at diagnosis cumulatively is 30 to 39 years of age, with about

41.8% falling in that range. About 82% of AIDS cases are in persons between the ages of 25 and 49 years (CDC, 2008b). HIV prevalence estimates in regard to age are discussed above. The reported number of new cases of AIDS in the United States in those <13 years of age has decreased each year between 2002 and 2007. For 2006, adults/adolescents between 13 and 29 years of age accounted for the largest number of new HIV infections (about 34%) followed by those 30 to 39 years of age (31%), 40 to 49 years of age (25%), and 50 years and older (10%) (CDC, 2009).

Approximately 2.8 million persons 50 years of age and older are reported globally as living with HIV/AIDS (Nguyen & Holodniy, 2008). Persons 60 years of age and older accounted for about 4% of both male and female cases of U.S. persons living with AIDS in 2007 (CDC, 2009). This percentage has been increasing. Reasons for this increase include that the improved survival of persons with AIDS has allowed more HIV-infected persons to enter advanced age groups. Although not often discussed, older persons may engage in risky sexual behaviors such as not using condoms for sexual encounters because of lack of concern about birth control, lack of awareness about HIV risks, and difficulties in manipulating protective devices due to disorders associated with aging such as arthritis; the availability of drugs such as sildenafil to treat erectile dysfunction, thereby allowing for increased sexual activity in older people; age-related diminution of immune function; and other changes such as drying of vaginal mucosa in women. These age-related factors potentially make older people more vulnerable to infection once exposed. Older people may also engage in IDU as a means to address discomfort. Their IDU use may also represent a continuation of earlier drug use. Older persons may also have a higher risk of HIV infection as a result of greater medical needs involving transfusion or transplant (Lashley, 2006a). HIV has been reported in a woman of 89 years of age (Rosenzweig & Fillet, 1992). Nonmonogamous sexual relationships are becoming increasingly common in the elderly, who may not be using safer sex. Health care professionals often do not discuss safer sex or assess injection drug use in elderly patients (Lashley, 2006a).

As discussed earlier, adolescents may be at particular risk for HIV acquisition. Adolescence is a time of risky behavior and exploring, with a high use of alcohol and experimentation with drugs and sex as well as feelings of invincibility. Data pertaining to adolescents from the Youth Behavior Survey are discussed later in this chapter (CDC, 2008f). Adolescents who are first recognizing their sexual orientation may engage in more risky behavior, and adolescents who are alienated may engage in risky sex to get money for living or for drugs.

Racial/Ethnic Distribution

According to data from the 2000 census (U.S. Census Bureau, 2001), the approximate racial composition of the United States is about 70% white, 12% black, 12.5% Hispanic, 3% Asian, and the rest "other." In 2007, in looking at the total number of persons in the United States living with HIV/AIDS, approximately 48% were black non-Hispanic, 33% were white non-Hispanic, 17% were Hispanic/Latino, and less than 1% each were Asian, American Indian/Alaskan Native, or Native Hawaiian/other Pacific Islander. In regard to newly diagnosed HIV/AIDS cases in 2007, the rates per 100,000 were as follows: black/non-Hispanic (47.3); Native Hawaiian/other Pacific Islander (18.3); Hispanic/Latino (15.2); American Indian/Alaska Native (6.9); white population (5.2); and Asian (3.6). Moreover, blacks accounted for 51% of all HIV/AIDS cases diagnosed in 2006 (CDC, 2008a, 2009). This situation has been called a state of emergency for African Americans (Laurencin, Christensen, & Taylor, 2008). For pediatric cases of AIDS, the distribution is as follows: black, non-Hispanic (65.0%), Hispanic (19.3%); and white, non-Hispanic persons (1.4%) (CDC, 2008a); and, again, there are great ethnic differences. Pediatric AIDS is further discussed in Chapter 14. These differences stem more from factors other than race and ethnicity, such as nutritional status, and social and economic conditions, such as access to quality health care. When examined by transmission categories, there is particular disproportion in the category of injection drug use for both men and women who fall into the categories of black non-Hispanic or Hispanic, while for white non-Hispanic about 77% of adult males fall into the male-to-male sexual contact category (CDC, 2009).

TRANSMISSION CATEGORIES FOR AIDS

Terminology to describe epidemiological groupings of AIDS cases in the United States and elsewhere has undergone various changes over the years. For example, with the switch by CDC in March 1989 to a monthly, instead of a weekly, update on AIDS cases, epidemiologic data reporting formerly entitled "transmission categories" became known as "exposure categories." This shift supersedes a previous revision that occurred in August 1986 when the hierarchy of risk factors for AIDS was revised and entitled "transmission categories" instead of "patient groups." Currently the term "transmission category" is again being used by the CDC for the classification of cases that summarize the risk factors most likely responsible for transmission. The transmission categories are still ordered in a hierarchical, mutually exclusive manner-- thus cases with multiple characteristics who belong in more than one transmission category are assigned to the group that is listed first. There is one combination group that combines male-to-male sexual contact and injection drug use. In hierarchical order in adults/adolescents, the transmission categories for men currently are male-to-male sexual contact (formerly "men who have sex with men"); injection drug use; male-to-male sexual contact and injection drug use (this category includes men who practice both behaviors and are thus classified only in this category and not the previous two); hemophilia/coagulation disorder; high-risk heterosexual contact; receipt of blood transfusion, blood components, or tissue; and other/risk factor not reported or identified (CDC, 2009). The distribution of all adult and adolescent (age 13 years and over) cases of AIDS according to these categories is shown in Table 1.1. For females, the first transmission category in the hierarchy is injection drug use followed by hemophilia/coagulation disorder and then the remainder, as discussed above. Transmission categories for pediatric cases are discussed later in this section.

The transmission categories have also undergone various changes over the years. Among the major changes that occurred were the removal of Haitians as a separate group in 1985, the change in terminology for "male homosexual, bisexual contact" to "men who have sex with men," and currently "male-to-male sexual contact"; the addition of the group known now as "high-risk heterosexual contact"; the change from "IV drug use" to "injection drug use"; the inclusion of other coagulation disorders to the group originally designated as "hemophilia A"; and the renaming of the "none of the above" group to "other/undetermined," with that latter group becoming eventually "other/risk factor not reported or identified." The separate category of male homosexual/bisexual contacts who were also intravenous drug abusers was added in August 1986. Later the title was changed to "men who have sex with men and inject drugs" and is presently "male-to-male-sexual contact and injection drug use." For a period of time Haitians were considered to be a distinct high-risk group for the development of AIDS, but this category was dropped. In 1985, when Haitians were removed as a separate risk group, they were placed into the "other/none of the above" group. In August 1986 they were placed into the heterosexual cases category, and eventually they were categorized in the same manner as that for other persons because it did not appear that "being of Haitian extraction by itself, in isolation from

Table 1.1

REPORTED CUMULATIVE UNITED STATES ADULT/ADOLESCENT AIDS CASES BY TRANSMISSION CATEGORY FROM BEGINNING OF EPIDEMIC THROUGH DECEMBER 31, 2007

TRANSMISSION CATEGORY	NO.	%
Male-to-male sexual contact	445,645	44
Injection drug use	235,842	23
Male-to-male sexual contact and injection drug use	67,797	7
Hemophilia/coagulation disorder	5,567	1
High-risk heterosexual contact	142,842	14
Sex with injection drug user	38,766	4
Sex with bisexual male	5,415	1
Sex with person with hemophilia	603	0.06
Sex with HIV-infected transfusion recipient	1,403	0.14
Sex with HIV-infected person, risk factor not specified	96,665	9
Receipt of blood transfusion, blood components, or tissue	9,315	1
Other/risk factor not reported or identified	114,224	11
Total	**1,021,242**	**100**

Source: CDC, 2009, p. 40. Percentages may not add to 100 due to rounding error.

other risk factors, increases the relative risk of being exposed to HTLV-III" (Landesman, Ginzburg, & Weiss, 1985, p. 525). Information about each transmission category is discussed below.

Male-to-Male Sexual Contact (MSM)

AIDS was first identified among homosexual men presenting with Kaposi's sarcoma and *Pneumocystis carinii* pneumonia (CDC, 1981a,b). In 1982, the CDC reported the occurrence of unexplained persistent generalized lymphadenopathy among homosexual males. It was recommended that such individuals be followed periodically (CDC, 1982a). Other clinicians had noted the occurrence of such a syndrome as early as 1977 in some regions and 1979 in others (Abrams et al., 1984; Miller et al., 1984). A cluster of cases of autoimmune thrombocytopenic purpura in homosexual men was diagnosed in New York after November, 1980. These reports suggested that sexually active homosexual men might be developing disorders of immune regulation (Morris et al., 1982).

Why AIDS first surfaced in large numbers among the homosexual population is not known. The first appearance of AIDS in recognizable proportions among this group, however, provoked varying public reactions from lack of interest to condemnation to accusations to feelings that it was deserved. Later in the pandemic, the term "men who have sex with men" was adopted to describe behavior and as part of the efforts to reduce stigmatization related to homosexual, bisexual, transgender, or other males, such as male sex workers, who engage in male-to-male sexual contact. Persons in this exposure category, male-to-male sexual contact (MSM), still comprise the largest percentage of cases of adult AIDS in the United States. As of December 31, 2007, MSM accounted for about 54% of the total cumulative adult male cases of AIDS in the United States and the category of "MSM and injection drug use" for about another 8%, totaling about 62%, and MSM accounted for 44% of all adult AIDS cases, with "MSM and injection drug use" accounting for 7%, for a total of 51% (CDC, 2009).

Studies to identify risk factors for HIV infection identified large numbers of different male sexual partners as the most important risk factor for HIV acquisition. In regard to the sexual practices studied, the ones most frequently associated with increased risk for infection were frequent receptive anal intercourse and "fisting" (a practice involving the insertion of a hand or fist into the rectum) (Vermund, 1997). These studies have provided important information for the development of educational programs and counseling aimed at prevention, as described in Chapter 5. Extensive efforts in education and prevention of HIV infection, especially from within the gay community, had notable success. These have involved changes in behavior including less promiscuity and increased condom use (Martin, 1987). But while initially MSM were demonstrating safer sexual behaviors, by the 1990s younger homosexual men were noted to have higher levels of sexual risk taking (DeWit, 1996). With the success of many HIV prevention efforts, in large part from the gay community, a decrease in the number of cases in the MSM category was seen. But, in the period from 2001 to 2005, the estimated number of U.S. cases of HIV/AIDS among MSM in the 33 states and U.S. dependent areas with confidential named-based HIV reporting increased 13%. In this same time period, there was a tenfold increase in primary and secondary syphilis cases reported, an indicator of increasing frequency of unprotected sex. Other studies among MSM found a reported increase in unprotected or unsafe sex (Jaffe, Valdiserri, & De Cock, 2007). Worldwide there appears to be a greater risk of HIV-infection among MSM from low and middle-income countries (Baral, Sifakis, Cleghorn, & Beyrer, 2007). The CDC reported an increase in the number of newly diagnosed HIV/AIDS cases among MSM in 2007, as had been the case in 2006. There were more new HIV infections in black MSM (13 to 29 years of age) than any other group (CDC, 2008b, 2009). There has even been a troubling trend toward conversion or "bug parties" where uninfected men ("bug chasers"), often young, seek to become HIV infected from HIV-infected men ("gift givers").

Clinically, Kaposi's sarcoma attributed to the human herpes virus (HHV-8) has a far greater prevalence among HIV-infected MSM than in other HIV-infected groups and also appears to occur in HIV-negative MSM (Lanternier et al., 2008).

Injection Drug Use (IDU)

In 1991, the CDC changed its terminology from "intravenous drug use" to "injecting drug use," and presently it is known as "injection drug use," to describe the use of needles for self-injection of drugs not prescribed by a physician (CDC, 2009). These include those who share needles and apparatus, skin pop, and take unprescribed anabolic steroids, vitamins, or other medications by injection. There are approximately 16 million persons who use injection drugs globally, and there is much variation in regard to HIV prevalence (Mathers et al., 2008). However, Mathers and associates (2008) estimate that of the estimated 16 million injection drug users, an estimated 3 million are HIV positive.

At the end of 2007, approximately 23% of all reported U.S. adult cases of AIDS were in the transmission category of injection drug use. In addition, the category of male-to-male sexual contact and injection drug use accounted for another 7% of all cases, while approximately 4% fell under the category of high-risk heterosexual contact in the subcategory of "sex with injection drug user"; thus, approximately 34% of all reported U.S. adult cases of AIDS at the end of 2007 were directly or indirectly associated with IDU (CDC, 2009). For females, approximately 35% of the cumulative cases of adult U.S. cases of AIDS fall into the IDU category, while about 30% of the total cases in the subcategory of high-risk heterosexual contact fall into the subcategory of "sex with injection drug user" (CDC, 2009). AIDS in IDUs appears to have disproportionately affected blacks and Hispanics. In the United States overall, IDU accounted for 16% and 26%, respectively, of men and women living with HIV--19% overall (CDC, 2008b). In the Youth Risk Behavior Study, 2.0% of adolescents surveyed said they had injected illegal drugs in their lifetime, and 7.2% used some form of cocaine (CDC, 2008e).

IDUs represent a heterogenous group of people whose behaviors vary, a fact that influences both seroprevalence rates and the success of intervention strategies. In addition to comprising the second largest exposure category for AIDS, IDUs are considered a bridge to persons through sexual contact, often unprotected or for money or drugs, and to HIV-infected children. Of the cumulative U.S. AIDS cases associated with perinatal transmission reported through 2007, the transmission category of mothers who reported injection drug use or who had sex with an injection drug user accounted for 51% of cases in the transmission category of mother with documented HIV infection or one of the specified risk factors (CDC, 2009).

Preventive activities with injection drug users have been difficult. (See Chapter 5.) Drug users tend to be a less conspicuous group than the other groups at high risk for the development of HIV infection. They tend not to have advocates in the general population, nor do they generally form advocacy and support groups among themselves. Needle sharing may have associations with communal feeling and socialization in the drug subculture (Black et al., 1986). There are also economic motivations for sharing injection equipment. Syringe exchange programs have proliferated in the United States and Europe. Many of these programs offer not only needle and syringe exchange but also other services, such as HIV counseling and testing, TB testing, sexually transmitted infection (STI) screening, and primary health care. IDUs participating in these programs increase the proportion of sterile syringes used for single-use injections, thus decreasing potential transmission. Another approach is to allow purchase of sterile syringes over the counter in pharmacies, as is done in some areas.

Hemophilia/Coagulation Disorder

In July 1982 the CDC first published reports of three cases of *Pneumocystis carinii* pneumonia (PCP) among three hemophiliacs who had no other underlying disease. The first case was identified in January 1982, and the others were found through surveillance of the use of drugs to treat the disease. All were heterosexual without a history of intravenous drug abuse, and all had received factor VIII concentrates (CDC, 1982b). The majority had hemophilia A, while the rest had hemophilia B, von Willebrand disease, or other blood coagulation defects.

Hemophilia A or factor VIII deficiency is a genetic disorder of blood coagulation that is inherited in an X-linked recessive manner and is the classical type of hemophilia. Hemophilia B (Christmas disease) is a genetic disorder due to deficiency of clotting factor IX. It is also inherited in an X-linked recessive manner. It is only about one-fifth as frequent as hemophilia A (Lashley, 2006b). They are indistinguishable clinically. Hemophilia B tends to be somewhat less severe than hemophilia A. Von Willebrand disease is a genetic disorder of coagulation that is usually inherited in an autosomal dominant manner but may also be inherited in other ways. Part of the management of these disorders includes the administration of clotting factors. Pooled plasma was traditionally used in making these clotting factor concentrates, and each vial could contain material from between 2,500 to 25,000 blood or plasma donors (Levine, 1985).

The majority of persons with hemophilia in the United States became HIV positive between 1979 and 1982 and before 1985, when the screening of donated blood was implemented. The prevalence of HIV infection in adults with hemophilia A and hemophilia B was about 80% and 50%, respectively, of those who had been treated with factor concentrates (Rosenberg & Goedert, 1998). Older hemophiliacs have been more likely to be HIV infected. Most of this group became infected with hepatitis C as well. The cloning of the factor VIII gene allowed recombinant factor concentrates and monoclonally purified concentrates to be developed. Recombinant factor IX concentrates have become available.

At the end of 2007, for this transmission category, the cumulative number of reported AIDS cases in U.S. adults was 5,567, approximately 0.5% of all adult cases. In children below 13 years of age at diagnosis, the cumulative total of reported AIDS cases is 229 or approximately 2.4% of reported pediatric cases. In the year 2007, only 46 new AIDS cases in this transmission category in adults were diagnosed; and, in children below 13 years of age, no new cases were identified. (CDC, 2009).

Sexual partners of hemophiliacs were at increased risk for infection through sexual activity in the category of high-risk heterosexual contact. The cumulative number of AIDS cases in U.S. adults at the end of 2007 was 603 in this category, or about 0.6% of all adult cases. In 2007, there were only 14 new cases identified in this transmission subcategory. In children <13 years of age, there were 36 cumulative cases identified whose mother had sexual contact with a person with hemophilia, and no such new cases were identified in 2006 or 2007 (CDC, 2009). Persons with hemophilia are among the older group of persons with HIV infection (Gianotten & Heijnen, 2009). Detailed 25-year outcomes of one of the hemophilia cohorts from 1982 to 2007 have been published (Eyster, 2008).

High-Risk Heterosexual Contact

The "high-risk heterosexual contact" category is the major one for U.S. women with AIDS, accounting for approximately 45% of all cumulative cases in adult women as of the end of 2007. It accounts for about 6% of cumulative AIDS cases in adult men and about 14% of all U.S. cumulative cases of AIDS. The following subcategories have been identified: (1) sex with injection drug user; (2) sex with bisexual male; (3) sex with person with hemophilia; (4) sex with HIV-infected transfusion recipient; (5) sex with HIV-infected person, risk not specified. As of December 31, 2007, the largest subcategories cumulatively for all adults and for females were "sex with HIV infected person, risk not specified" followed by "sex with injection drug user" (CDC, 2009). In terms of those living with HIV, about 28% overall fell into this category, while for males, high-risk heterosexual contact accounted for 13% and 72% of males and females, respectively, living with HIV (CDC, 2008e).

In January 1983 the CDC published two case reports of women with immunodeficiency who were the sexual partners of males with AIDS. One of these men was an intravenous drug abuser, and one was a bisexual. The women themselves had no recognized risk factors (CDC, 1983). Other case reports began appearing in the literature (Harris et al.,

1983). For example, the previously healthy 71-year-old wife of a 74-year-old hemophiliac who developed *Pneumocystis carinii* pneumonia also developed AIDS. Her only apparent risk factor was infrequent sexual contact with her husband when he was asymptomatic (Pitchenik et al., 1984). Varying percentages of regular sexual partners of HIV-infected persons show evidence of HIV infection depending upon the study and factors related to the host (e.g., viral load) and the virus, as well as whether there has been proper and consistent use of protection such as latex condoms.

The category of heterosexual contact is complex. A woman may be exposed through trading sex for drugs, money, or protection or may be unaware of or choose for a variety of reasons to ignore her partner's risky sexual practices such as promiscuity, IDU, or bisexuality (Cohen & Durham, 1995). Men may also be unaware of a partner's risky sexual activities. Men who seek sexual gratification with a commercial sex worker have an increased risk for acquiring HIV infection. Preventive efforts, as discussed in Chapter 5, focus on education, the proper and consistent use of condoms, access to appropriate health care, and women-controlled prevention and empowerment.

Receipt of Blood Transfusion, Blood Components, or Tissue

Today, especially in developed countries, blood transfusion is a relatively infrequent transmission category. At the end of 2007, the reported number of cumulative U.S. adult AIDS cases resulting from transfusion was 9,315, or about 1%, while the number of newly diagnosed cases in adults in 2007 was 109, or 0.3% of new cases (CDC, 2009). The first case of AIDS associated with a blood transfusion was reported by the CDC in December 1982. The white male infant, who was delivered by cesarean section in March 1981, had erythroblastosis fetalis resulting in hyperbilirubinemia. He received exchange transfusions, whole blood, platelets, and packed red cells during his month of hospitalization following birth. These blood and blood products were from 19 different donors and had been irradiated. After 1 month, the infant appeared well and was discharged from the hospital. At 4 months of age he showed splenomegaly. By 7 months he developed opportunistic infections and showed evidence of unexplained cellular immunodeficiency. The infant ultimately died of *Pneumocystis carinii* pneumonia at 20 months of age. His parents were heterosexual, not intravenous drug users, and were not

Haitian. Subsequent investigation of the blood products received by this infant revealed that one of the 19 donors of blood and blood products had been reported to the CDC later as having developed AIDS. This donor died in August of 1982. At the time of this initial report the cause of AIDS was unknown, and thus it gave further support to the idea that AIDS was caused by an infectious agent. The case also suggested that the agent could be present in the blood before causing symptomatic illness and that the incubation period could be a long one (CDC, 1982b).

A major concern early in the epidemic was that of protecting the nation's blood supply. In 1983, as an interim measure to protect transfusion recipients until specific tests were available, the U.S. Public Health Service (USPHS) recommended that blood and/or plasma not be donated by persons with signs and symptoms of AIDS, sexual partners of AIDS patients or of persons at increased risk for AIDS, or by any other members of groups at increased risk for AIDS. The USPHS also recommended that physicians "adhere strictly to the medical indications for transfusion" (p. 103), and they encouraged autologous blood transfusions (CDC, 1983). There was revision of many criteria for administering blood transfusions and more caution in making that decision. Methods were introduced to reduce blood loss during surgery, and more consumers requested autologous blood donation provisions, designated donor programs, or female donors in their efforts to minimize their risk.

In 1985, testing of potential donors by enzyme-linked immunosorbent assay (ELISA) became possible but was also prone to some false-negative and -positive results. For example, the blood of persons who are HIV-infected but who have not yet developed antibody and seroconverted (called the" window period") would not be identified as HIV infected when using ELISA (or a similar test) for screening. Thus, in 1996, the FDA recommended the use of the p24 antigen assay to screen all donated blood in the United States. In 2000, these problems were solved with the introduction of nucleic acid screening tests for HIV RNA. At present, the estimated risk of acquiring transfusion-transmitted HIV in the United States is approximately one case per 2 million transfusions (Alter & Klein, 2009). In resource-limited countries, this risk is higher.

Other/Risk Factor Not Reported or Identified

Until November 1986 the category "other/risk factor not reported or identified" was known as "none of the above." Then this category became "risk not reported or identified." Persons classified in this group are those with no reported HIV exposure through any of the routes listed in the hierarchy of transmission categories. Cases in this category include those that are under investigation by the local health department personnel; persons whose history is missing because they died, refused to be interviewed, or were lost to follow-up; and cases for whom information is complete but no transmission mode was identified (CDC, 2009). As of December 31, 2007, the cumulative number of U.S. cases of AIDS in adults in this transmission category was 114,224, or approximately 11%. There were 10,005 new cases (approximately 26%) in U.S. adults in this category in 2007. On identification of a transmission mode, persons in this category are reclassified into the appropriate one. Failure to reclassify persons into other transmission categories is probably due to nonrecognition of contributing factors, especially heterosexual contacts. For example, an infected person might not know that his or her sexual partner is bisexual or an IDU or that he or she has had contact with a commercial sex worker or has not been monogamous.

Transmission Categories for Children

The current transmission categories for children younger than13 years of age at diagnosis in hierarchical order are as follows:

- Hemophilia/coagulation disorder
- Mother with documented HIV infection or one of the following risk factors:
  - Injection drug use
  - Sex with injection drug user
  - Sex with bisexual male
  - Sex with person with hemophilia
  - Sex with HIV-infected transfusion recipient
  - Sex with HIV-infected person, risk not specified
  - Receipt of blood transfusion, blood components or tissue
  - Has HIV-infection, risk factor not specified
- Receipt of blood transfusion, blood components or tissue
- Other/risk factor not reported or identified.

The cumulative total for all U.S. pediatric AIDS cases at the end of 2007 was 9,590, or less than 1% of all cumulative U.S. AIDS cases. In 2007, there were only 87 newly diagnosed cases of U.S. pediatric AIDS.

The major transmission category is "mother with documented HIV infection or 1 of the following risk factors" accounting for about 92% of all of the cumulative U.S. pediatric AIDS cases and 84% of those newly diagnosed in 2007. These data are shown in Table 1.2. Perinatal transmission has been discussed earlier and is also discussed in Chapter 14.

WORLDWIDE STATISTICS AND PATTERNS

Accurate reporting of people living with HIV and those with AIDS varies greatly across the globe. However, accuracy has improved over the years. As of December 2007 (the most recent data available), approximately 33 million people were living with HIV. Of these the distribution is as follows:

- Adults: 30.8 million (including 15.5 million women)
- Children under 15 years of age: 2 million

The number of people who were reported as newly infected with HIV in 2007 was 2.7 million. In 2007, the Joint United Nations Programme on HIV/AIDS (UNAIDS) reported approximately 2.0 million deaths from AIDS (UNAIDS/WHO, 2008). Worldwide, about 25 million persons have died of AIDS since the beginning of the epidemic. The number of AIDS orphans (children who lost their mother or both parents to AIDS when they were under the age of 15 years) since the beginning of the epidemic is about 15 million, 11.6 million of whom are in sub-Saharan Africa. This issue is discussed in Chapter 14. Worldwide, UNAIDS/WHO (2008) estimates that women account for about half of the people living with AIDS. Women account for nearly 60% of all HIV infections in sub-Saharan Africa (UNAIDS/WHO, 2008). Globally, those in the age group of 15 to 24 years account for about 45% of new HIV infections, and there is a commitment by WHO to reduce this prevalence by 25% (UNAIDS/WHO, 2008).

Some data are difficult to obtain because of social and cultural norms. For example, in Senegal, West Africa, nine men were arrested for "acts against nature," and such homophobia and criminalization of adult consenting behavior are major barriers to surveillance, treatment, and prevention ("UNAIDS and broad coalition . . . ," 2009). Discussion of the global epidemiological patterns of HIV/AIDS is difficult because

Table 1.2

**REPORTED CUMULATIVE U.S. PEDIATRIC AIDS CASES
(<13 YEARS AT DIAGNOSIS) BY TRANSMISSION CATEGORY
FROM BEGINNING OF EPIDEMIC THROUGH DECEMBER 31, 2007**

TRANSMISSION CATEGORY	NO.	%
Hemophilia/coagulation disorder	229	2
Mother with documented HIV infection or one of the following risk factors	8,797	92
Injection drug use	3,348	35
Sex with injection drug user	1,535	16
Sex with bisexual male	214	2
Sex with person with hemophilia	36	0.38
Sex with HIV-infected transfusion recipient	26	0.29
Sex with HIV-infected person, risk factor not specified	1,550	16
Recipient of blood transfusion, blood components, or tissue	152	2
Has HIV infection, risk factor not specified	1,936	20
Recipient of blood transfusion, blood components, or tissue	383	4
Other/risk factor not reported or identified	181	2
Total	**9,590**	**100**

Source: CDC, 2009, p. 40.

different agencies that collect and report data may not use the exact same groupings from year to year, and the nature of subgroups sampled may vary. The number of countries contributing information to the most recent UNAIDS report has increased almost every year, but this information is still incomplete or missing for some countries. Selected regional information will be discussed briefly below. The number of AIDS cases reported is shown in Table 1.3.

Sub-Saharan Africa

Sub-Saharan Africa continues to bear a disproportionate burden in terms of the number of persons living with HIV. The number of persons living with HIV in 2007 in this region was about 22 million, or two-thirds of the total number of persons living with HIV/AIDS worldwide. This region accounted for 75% of all AIDS deaths in 2007. In some countries, HIV prevalence in adults appears to be stabilizing, but there is significant variation. In 2007, UNAIDS/WHO reported that HIV prevalence in adults exceeded 15% in Botswana, Lesotho, Namibia, South Africa, Swaziland, Zambia, and Zimbabwe. However, in Zimbabwe in 2007, it was reported that HIV prevalence in pregnant women decreased from 26% in 2002 to 18% in 2006 (UNAIDS/WHO, 2008). High-risk heterosexual contact is the most important route of transmission in this area, and one result is that the world's largest population of children living with HIV is in this area. UNAIDS/WHO (2008) estimates that the probability that one's sexual partner is HIV infected is 1 in 4 to 1 in 6. Quinn and Overbaugh (2005) note that, by 22 years of age, 1 in 4 women in South Africa is infected with HIV. In some countries, injection drug use is a factor. For example, in the cities of Mombassa and Nairobi in Kenya, approximately half of the injection drug users tested were HIV positive. In addition, unprotected anal sex between men in sub-Saharan Africa is now thought to be more important than formerly thought. As in any region, many cultural and social factors influence HIV acquisition. For example, Halperin and Epstein (2004) describe the custom of concurrent multiple sexual partners that results in "extensive interlocking sexual networks" that act to facilitate HIV spread. These relationships are also known as concurrent sexual partnerships (Beyrer, 2007). In these relationships, condoms may not be used because the relationships are not seen as casual and involve trust as well as issues that relate to inequality of women, poverty, gender power, and more (Lashley, 2006c). These relationships may be especially prevalent among those who travel with their jobs to different locales,

Table 1.3

TABLE 1.3: GLOBAL DISTRIBUTION OF HIV, 2007

REGION	NUMBER OF ADULTS AND CHILDREN LIVING WITH HIV	NEWLY INFECTED IN 2007	ADULT HIV PREVALENCE %
Global Total	33.2 million (100%)	2.5 million	0.8%
Sub-Saharan Africa	22.0 million (67.8%)	1.7 million	92
South and Southeast Asia	4.2 million (12 %)	230,000	35
Latin America	1.7 million (4.8%)	150,000	16
Eastern Europe and Central Asia	1.5 million (4.8%)	100,000	2
North America	1.2 million (3.9%)	46,000	0.38
East Asia	740,000 (2.4%)	92,000	0.29
Western and Central Europe	730,000 (2.3%)	31,000	16
Middle East and North Africa	380,000 (1.1%)	35,000	2
Caribbean	230,000 (0.7%)	17,000	20
Oceania	74,000 (0.2%)	14,000	4

*All data are as of the end of 2007. Data are for persons 15 to 49 years of age.
Data from Joint United Nations Programme on HIV/AIDS (UNAIDS) and World Health Organization (WHO). AIDS Epidemic Update: 2008. Geneva (Switzerland): UNAIDS, 2008, p. 3.

such as long-distance truck drivers. Difficulties in obtaining condoms and gender inequality are other contributing factors (Beyrer, 2007). Another factor is circumcision. While many studies have indicated that this procedure can reduce HIV incidence in men by as much as 50% to

60% (White et al., 2008), UNAIDS/WHO (2008) has recommended the provision of services for circumcision in countries with high HIV prevalence, others have not supported this initiative for cultural, religious, and other reasons.

Southeast, South, and East Asia

WHO reports statistics for Asia for the following regions separately: (1) South and Southeast, and East Asia and (2) Central Asia with Eastern Europe, although country-by-country data are also published. The latter are considered separately below. Asia did not experience a major HIV epidemic until the late 1980s or early 1990s (Ruxrungtham, Brown, & Phanuphak, 2004). Approximately 5 million persons were living with HIV in 2007 in South, Southeast, and East Asia. Recent trends show declines in HIV prevalence in Cambodia, Myanmar, and Thailand but increases in Indonesia, Pakistan, Viet Nam, Bangladesh, and China. In Vietnam, it is estimated that the number of people living with HIV between 2000 and 2005 more than doubled.

Overall, despite the recent upward trends, China is considered a low HIV-prevalence country (about 0.05%) but with geographic pockets of high transmission. There are indications from surveillance data, which now include provincial sentinel surveillance sites, that HIV prevalence is increasing in China among female sex workers and injection drug users. Risk behaviors have also increased in IDUs, such as sharing needles, but in female sex workers, always using condoms has increased while never using condoms has decreased over the past decade. However, with improved surveillance has come the information that HIV appears to be moving from high-risk groups to the general population (Sun et al., 2007). There is an increase in the number of women who are IDUs in China, and many of these also sell sex (Choi, Cheung, & Chen, 2006). IDUs in both China and Vietnam also frequently purchase sex, and only a small percentage use condoms. In Indonesia, HIV transmission is spreading from IDUs to sex work networks (UNAIDS/WHO, 2008). In Malasia, more than two-thirds of HIV infections fall in the category of IDU (Reid, Kamarulzaman, & Sran, 2007). How culture influences transmission is illustrated by the observation that in Afghanistan narcotics were traditionally either inhaled by smoking or vaporization or ingested orally. Now, injection drug use is spreading, and HIV prevalence is also rising (Todd et al., 2007). In India, a "significant" proportion of HIV-infected women were infected through heterosexual contact with their regular partners who paid for sex

(UNAIDS/WHO, 2008). In Vietnam, women are said to be increasingly at risk to acquire HIV, but their risk is underreported and underestimated (Nguyen et al., 2008). Male-to-male sexual contact is underreported in Asia as in other areas of the world. In Vietnam, 1 in 3 male sex workers from Ho Chi Minh City were HIV infected (UNAIDS/WHO, 2008).

Eastern Europe and Central Asia

An estimated 90% of persons with HIV in this region live in either the Russian Federation or Ukraine. About 1.5 million adults and children were estimated to be living with HIV in this region in 2007. In Ukraine, the annual number of new HIV diagnoses has been estimated as more than doubling since 2001 (UNAIDS/WHO, 2008). In the Russian Federation, the distribution is not equal, and in areas such as Uzbekistan the number of new HIV infections is rising. In this geographic region, the major mode of transmission is injection drug use, with about 62% of the new HIV cases in 2006 resulting from this mode. In a national prevalence study, HIV among the IDUs surveyed in the Ukraine rose from 11% in 2001 to 16% in 2006. There is considerable overlap between IDU and sex work in this region. In parts of the Ukraine, the prevalence of HIV in pregnant women exceeds 1%, and in 2006 about 40% of the newly reported cases in Eastern Europe and Central Asia were among women. It is thought that most of these were due to high-risk sexual contact with men who were IDUs; however, overall, it is estimated that about 35% of HIV-infected women are IDUs and about 50% of HIV-infected women acquired HIV through heterosexual contact with an IDU (UNAIDS/WHO, 2008). There is a relatively low prevalence of reported new cases of HIV among men who have unprotected sex with men, about 1%, but this figure is thought to be an underestimate (UNAIDS/WHO, 2008).

Latin America

In 2007, new HIV infections in Latin America were about 140,000, while about 1.7 million persons were living with HIV in this region. Overall levels of HIV infection have remained relatively stable over the last ten years. Transmission of HIV in this region is mainly attributed to male-to-male sexual contact and sex workers and less often to injection drug use. About 57% of the HIV diagnoses in Mexico are attributed to male-to-male-sexual contact. In many of these countries, between one-quarter and one-third of the men who have sex with men also have sex with women. UNAIDS/WHO (2008) has noted that there are "hidden epidemics" of HIV among men who have sex with men in the following Central American countries: Belize, Costa Rica, El Salvador, Guatemala, Mexico, Nicaragua, and Panama. In South America, it is noted that HIV infection prevalence is lower in female sex workers than MSM. In Honduras, condom promotion efforts in female sex workers seem to have resulted in a decline in HIV prevalence among that group. IDU appears to be accounting for a smaller number of new HIV infections. In studies of IDUs in parts of Paraguay and Uruguay, however, 12% and 19% of female sex workers, respectively, were HIV positive. In several South American countries such as Argentina, Brazil, Peru, and Uruguay, high-risk heterosexual contact accounts for an increasing number of women becoming HIV infected. For example, in Uruguay, high-risk heterosexual contact accounts for about two-thirds of newly reported HIV cases (UNAIDS/WHO, 2008).

Caribbean

The Caribbean has the second highest rate of HIV/AIDS in the world, after sub-Saharan Africa (Inciardi, Syvertsen & Surratt, 2005). Approximately 230,000 persons were living with HIV in this area in 2007. About 75% of them resided in the Dominican Republic and Haiti. The major mode of HIV transmission in this region is heterosexual contact. In Haiti, there has been a decline in HIV prevalence among women attending prenatal clinics from 5.9% in 1996 to 3.1% in 2004. Among female sex workers, HIV prevalence rates of 9% in Jamaica and 31% in Guyana have been reported, while in the Dominican Republic data show that HIV prevalence has declined in this group, probably due to the use of barrier protection. In Cuba, male-to-male sexual contact accounted for about 80% of reported HIV cases, and in the Caribbean region generally about 12% of cases occurred via this mode of transmission (UNAIDS/WHO, 2008). Acquisition through IDU is less common overall, except in Bermuda and Puerto Rico. Various sociocultural factors influence patterns here, including lack of accurate epidemiological data about HIV infection, the acceptance of multiple sex partners and frequent sexual contact, machismo, repression of homosexual relations, low condom use, and migration from island to island (Inciardi et al., 2005; UNAIDS/WHO, 2008).

North America and Western and Central Europe

UNAIDS/WHO (2008) considers these regions together because of many shared commonalities in the patterns of HIV infection. In North America, comprising the United States and Canada, approximately 1.2 million adults and children were estimated to be living with HIV in 2007. In Western and Central Europe, there were approximately 730,000 adults and children living with HIV in 2007. Most data pertaining to the United States are considered earlier in this chapter. The main mode of HIV transmission in this region is MSM. In Western Europe, MSM are most at risk of acquiring new HIV infections. For example, in Germany, between 2002 and 2006, the number of new HIV infections rose by 96%. About one-third of new HIV infections in 2006 in the United States and Canada can be attributed to high-risk heterosexual contact. This is also the largest proportion of new HIV diagnoses in Western Europe, accounting for about 42% in 2006. High-risk heterosexual contact is also the main mode of transmission in Central Europe except for Estonia, Latvia, Lithuania, and Poland, where the major mode is IDU. In Croatia, the Czech Republic, Hungary, and Slovenia MSM is the major transmission mode. In many of the European countries, the proportion of cases due to injection drug use both for new cases and existing ones has decreased (UNAIDS/WHO, 2008).

Middle East and North Africa

While an estimated 380,000 people were living with HIV in 2007 in the Middle East and North Africa, there is a paucity of accurate data for this region (UNAIDS/WHO, 2008). While this area is home to 5% of the global population, it has about 1% of people with HIV; thus, overall it is considered a low HIV-prevalence area (Obermeyer, 2006). The major risk factors across the area are through paid sex and injection drug use. However, in the Sudan, high-risk heterosexual contact is the major factor, with an adult HIV prevalence of 1.4%. In many countries women, who are vulnerable because of religious and social customs, become HIV infected as a result of the risky sexual behavior of their husbands (Obermeyer, 2006). IDU is a major factor in Iran, with a prevalence of IDUs in treatment services in Tehran ranging between 15% and 23%, while in countries such as Algeria, Egypt, Lebanon, and Syria, many persons are engaged in both IDU and commercial sex (UNAIDS/WHO, 2008). Information about male-to-male sexual contact is difficult to ascertain because of stigma and official censorship. Reports from 2006 found that in the studies conducted in parts of Egypt and Sudan 6.2% and 9% of MSM, respectively, were HIV infected (UNAIDS/WHO, 2008).

Oceania

The Oceania region includes Australia, New Zealand, Fiji, and Papua New Guinea. In 2007, about 74,000 persons were living with HIV in this region. In Papua New Guinea (PNG), the reported number of new cases has more than doubled in the period between 2002 and 2006. The primary source of HIV transmission in PNG is through unprotected heterosexual intercourse, particularly unprotected paid sex. It should be noted, however, that about 12% of young males indicated that they had had unprotected sex with males In Australia and New Zealand, unprotected sexual contact between males is the primary transmission category.

CONCLUSION

Studies of epidemiological aspects of the AIDS pandemic have contributed enormously to the identification of HIV and its transmission. Findings from these studies have allowed for targeted prevention efforts and for planning of treatment and management of health services. Additional research is needed to define and clarify the role of cofactors and their influence on both the development of AIDS and its progression, the determinants and modifiers of rapid and slow progression, and effective methods of education for prevention, coupled with enduring behavior change.

REFERENCES

Abbadessa, G., Accolla, R., Aiuti, F., Albini, A., Aldovini, A., Alfano, M., et al. (2009). Unsung hero Robert C. Gallo. *Science, 323,* 206–207.

Abrams, D. L., Lewis, B. J., Beckstead, J. H., Casavant, C. A., & Drew, W. L. (1984). Persistent diffuse lymphadenopathy in homosexual men: Endpoint or prodrome? *Annals of Internal Medicine, 100,* 801–808.

ACOG Committee Opinion. (2008, September). Prenatal and perinatal human immunodeficiency virus testing: Expanded recommendations. *Obstetrics & Gynecology, 112,* 739–742.

Alter, H. J., & Klein, H. G. (2009). The hazards of blood transfusion in historical perspective. *Blood, 112,* 2617–2626.

Baral, S., Sifakis, F., Cleghorn, F., & Beyrer, C. (2007). Elevated risk for HIV infection among men who have sex with men in low-and middle-income countries 2000–2006: A systematic review. *PloS Medicine, 4*(12), e339–e349.

Barré-Sinoussi, F., Chermann, J., Rey, F., Nugeyre, M. T., Chamaret, S., Gruest, J., et al. (1983). Isolation of a T-lymphotropic retrovirus from a patient at risk for acquired immune deficiency syndrome (AIDS). *Science, 220,* 868–871.

Bartholomew, C. F., & Jones, A. M. (2006). Human bites: A rare risk factor for HIV transmission. *AIDS, 20,* 631–632.

Beyrer, C. (2007). HIV epidemiology update and transmission factors: Risks and risk contexts—16th International AIDS Conference epidemiology plenary. *Clinical Infectious Diseases, 44,* 981–987.

Black, J. L., Dolan, M. P., Deford, H. A., Rubenstein, J. A., Penk, W. E., Robinowitz, R., et al. (1986). Sharing of needles among users of intravenous drugs. *New England Journal of Medicine, 314,* 445–447.

Bolling, D. R., & Voeller, B. (1987). AIDS and heterosexual anal intercourse. *Journal of the American Medical Association, 258,* 474.

Broder, S., & Gallo, R. C. (1985). Human T-cell leukemia viruses (HTLV): A unique family of pathogenic retroviruses. *Annual Review of Immunology, 3,* 321–336.

Bygbjerg, L. (1983). AIDS in a Danish surgeon. *Lancet, 1*(8330), 925.

Centers for Disease Control. (1981a). Kaposi's sarcoma and pneumocystis pneumonia among homosexual men—New York and California. *Morbidity and Mortality Weekly Report, 31,* 507–515.

Centers for Disease Control. (1981b). Pneumocystis pneumonia—Los Angeles. *Morbidity and Mortality Weekly Report, 30,* 250–252.

Centers for Disease Control. (1982a). Pneumocystis carinii pneumonia among persons with hemophilia. *Morbidity and Mortality Weekly Report, 31,* 365–367.

Centers for Disease Control. (1982b). Possible transfusion-associated acquired immune deficiency syndrome. (AIDS). California. *Morbidity and Mortality Weekly Report, 31,* 652–655.

Centers for Disease Control. (1983). Prevention of acquired immune deficiency syndrome (AIDS): Report of inter-agency recommendations. *Morbidity and Mortality Weekly Report 32,* 101–103.

Centers for Disease Control. (1985). Recomnmendations for assisting in the prevention of perinatal transmission of human T-lymphotropic virus type III/lymphadenopathy-associated virus and acquired immuno-deficiency syndrome. *Morbidity and Mortality Weekly Report, 34,* 721–732.

Centers for Disease Control. (1987a). Human immunodeficiency virus infection transmitted from an organ donor screened for HIV anti-body–North Carolina. *Morbidity and Mortality Weekly Report, 36,* 306–308.

Centers for Disease Control. (1987b). Revision of the CDC surveillance case definition for acquired immunodeficiency syndrome. *Morbidity and Mortality Weekly Report, 36*(Suppl. 1), 1S–15S.

Centers for Disease Control. (1988). AIDS due to HIV-2 infection—New Jersey. *Morbidity and Mortality Weekly Report, 37,* 33–35.

Centers for Disease Control. (1989). Current Trends Update: HIV-2 Infection—United States. *Morbidity and Mortality Weekly Report, 38,* 572–574, 579–580.

Centers for Disease Control and Prevention. (1992). 1993 revised clas-sification system for HIV infection and expanded surveillance case definition for AIDS among adolescents and adults. *Morbidity and Mortality Weekly Report, 41* (No. RR-17), 1–19.

Centers for Disease Control and Prevention. (1997a, July). The human immunodeficiency virus and its transmission. *HIV/AIDS Prevention,* 1–4.

Centers for Disease Control and Prevention. (1997b). Transmission of HIV possibly associated with exposure of mucous membrane to contaminated blood. *Morbidity and Mortality Weekly Report, 46*(27), 620–623.

Centers for Disease Control and Prevention. (1998). Public Health Service Task Force recommendations for the use of antiretroviral drugs in pregnant women infected with HIV-1 for maternal health and for reducing perinatal HIV-1 transmission in the United States. *Morbidity and Mortality Weekly Report, 47*(RR-2), 1–31.

Centers for Disease Control and Prevention. (1999). Guidelines for national human immunodeficiency virus case surveillance, including monitoring for human immunodeficiency virus infection and acquired immunodeficiency syndrome. *Morbidity and Mortality Weekly Report, 48*(RR-13), 1–32.

Centers for Disease Control and Prevention. (2001). Updated U. S. Public Health Service guidelines for the management of occupational expo-sures to HBV, HCV and HIV and recommendations for postexposure prophylaxis. *Morbidity and Mortality Weekly Report, 50*(RR-11), 1–42.

Centers for Disease Control and Prevention. (2005a). Antiretroviral post-exposure prophylaxis after sexual, injection-drug use or other nonoc-cupational exposure to HIV in the United States: Recommendations from the U.S. Department of Health and Human Services. *Morbidity and Mortality Weekly Report, 54*(RR2), 1–20.

Centers for Disease Control and Prevention. (2005b). Updated U.S. public health service guidelines for the management of occupational exposures to HIV and recommendations for postexposure prophy-laxis. *Morbidity and Mortality Weekly Report, 54*(RR9), 1–17.

Centers for Disease Control and Prevention. (2006). HIV/AIDS among women who have sex with women. CDC *HIV/AIDS Fact Sheet*. Retrieved March 20, 2009, from www.cdc.gov/hiv/topics/women/resources/factsheets/pdf/wsw.pdf.

Centers for Disease Control and Prevention. (2008a). HIV prevalence estimates—United States, 2006. *Morbidity and Mortality Weekly Report, 57*, 1073–1076.

Centers for Disease Control and Prevention. (2008b). *HIV/AIDS surveil-lance report, 2006*. Vol. 18, 1–55.

Centers for Disease Control and Prevention. (2008c, September). MMWR analysis provides new details on HIV incidence in U. S. Populations. *CDC HIV/AIDS Facts*.

Centers for Disease Control and Prevention. (2008d, October 2). *Questions and answers: HIV prevalence estimates—United States, 2006*. Retrieved March 1, 2009, from www.cdc.gov/hiv/topics/surveillance/resources/qa/prevalence.htm.

Centers for Disease Control and Prevention. (2008e). Revised surveil-lance case definition for HIV infection among adults, adolescents, and children aged <18 months and for HIV infection and AIDS among children aged 18 months to <13 years—United States, 2008. *Morbidity and Mortality Weekly Report 57*(RR10), 1–8.

Centers for Disease Control and Prevention. (2008f). Youth risk behavior surveillance —United States, 2007. *Morbidity and Mortality Weekly Report, 57*(No. SS-4), 1–131.

Centers for Disease Control and Prevention. (2009). *HIV/AIDS surveil-lance report, 2007*. Vol. 19, 1-63. Atlanta: CDC. Retrieved March 20, 2009 from www.cdc.gov/hiv/topics/surveillance/resources/reports/2007report/default.htm.

Choi, S. Y. P., Cheung, Y. W., & Chen, K. (2006). Gender and HIV risk behavior among intravenous drug users in Sichuan province, China. *Social Science and Medicine, 62*(7), 1672–1684.

Coffin, J., Haase, A., Levy, J. A., Montagnier, L., Oroszlan, S., Teich, N., et al. (1986). Human immunodeficiency viruses. *Science, 232,* 697.

Cohen, F. L., & Durham, J. D. (Eds.). (1995). *Women, children and HIV/AIDS.* New York: Springer.

Connor, E. M., Sperling, R. S., Gelber, R., Kiselev, P., Scott, G., O'Sullivan, M. J., et al. (1994). Reduction of maternal-infant transmission of human immunodeficiency virus type 1 with zidovudine treatment. Pediatric AIDS Clinical Trials. *New England Journal of Medicine, 331,* 1173–1180.

Coovadia, H., & Kindra, G. (2008). Breastfeeding to prevent HIV transmission in infants: Balancing pros and cons. *Current Opinion in Infectious Disease, 21,* 11–15.

Coutsoudis, A., Pillay, K., Kuhn, L., Spooner, E., Tsai, W. Y., Coovadia, H. M., et al. (2001). Method of feeding and transmission of HIV-1 from mothers to children by 15 months of age: Prospective cohort study from Durban, South Africa. *AIDS, 15,* 379–387.

Curran, J. W., Morgan, W. M., Hardy, A. M., Jaffe, H. W., Darrow, W. W., & Dowdle, W. R. (1985). The epidemiology of AIDS: Current status and future prospects. *Science, 229,* 1352–1357.

De Jong, M. A. W. P., & Geijtenbeek, T. B. H. (2008). Human immunodeficiency virus-1 acquisition in genital mucosa: Langerhans cells as key-players. *Journal of Internal Medicine, 265,* 18–28.

de Silva, T. I., Cotten, M., & Rowland-Jones, S. L. (2008). HIV-2: The forgotten AIDS virus. *Trends in Microbiology, 16,* 588–595.

DeWit, J. (1996). The epidemic of HIV among young homosexual men. *AIDS, 10* (Suppl. 3), S21–S25.

Doll, D. C. (1988). Tattooing in prison and HIV infection. *Lancet, 1* (8575–76), 66–67.

The Durban Declaration. (2000). *Nature, 406,* 15–16.

Essex, M., Allan, J., Kanki, P., McLane, M. F., Malone, G., Kitchen, L., et al. (1985). Antigens of human T-lymphotropic virus type III/lymphadenopathy-associated virus. *Annals of Internal Medicine, 103,* 700–703.

Essex, M., & Kanki, P. J. (1988). The origins of the AIDS virus. *Scientific American, 259,* 64–71.

Eyster, M. E. (2008).Coping with the HIV epidemic 1982–2007: 25-year outcomes of the Hershey Haemophilia Cohort. *Haemophilia, 14,* 697–702.

Fauci, A. S., Macher, A., Longo, D. L., Lane, H. C., Rook, A. H., Masur, H., et al. (1984). Acquired immunodeficiency syndrome: Epidemiologic, clinical, immunologic, and therapeutic Considerations. *Annals of Internal Medicine, 100,* 92–106.

Feller, A., & Flanigan, T. P. (1997). HIV-infected competitive athletes. *Journal of General Internal Medicine, 12,* 243–246.

Fowler, M. G., Lampe, M. A., Jamieson, D. J., Kourtis, A. P., & Rogers, M. F. (2007). Reducing the risk of mother-to-child human immuno-deficiency virus transmission: Past successes, current progress and challenges, and future directions. *American Journal of Obstetrics and Gynecology, 197* (Suppl. 3), S3–S9.

Françoise Barré-Sinoussi and Luc Montagnier share the 2008 Nobel Prize for Physiology and Medicine for their discovery of the human immunodeficiency virus (HIV). (2009). *AIDS, 23,* 1.

Gallo, R. C., & Montagnier, L. (1988). AIDS in 1988. *Scientific American, 259*(4), 40–48.

Gallo, R. C., Shaw, G. M., & Markham, P. D. (1985). The etiology of AIDS. In V. T. DeVita Jr., S. Hellman, & S. A. Rosenberg (Eds.). *AIDS: Etiology, diagnosis, treatment, and prevention* (pp. 31–54). Philadelphia: Lippincott.

Garry, R. F., Witte, M. H., Gottlieb, A. A., Elvin-Lewis, M., Gotlieb, M. S., Witte, C. L., et al. (1989). HIV infection in 1968. *Journal of the American Medical Association, 261,* 2199.

Gelman, E. D., Popovic, M., Blayney, D., Masur, H., Sidhu, G., Stahl, R. E., et al. (1983). Proviral DNA of a retrovirus, human T-cell leukemia virus, in two patients with AIDS. *Science, 220,* 862–865.

Gerberding, J. L. (1997). Occupational HIV infection. *AIDS, 11* (Suppl. A), S57–S60.

Gianotten, W. L., & Heijnen, L. (2009). Haemophilia, aging and sexuality. *Haemophilia, 15,* 55–62.

Greenhouse, P. (1987). Female-to-female transmission of HIV. *Lancet, 2,* 401–402.

Guerrant, R. L., Walker, D. H., & Weller, P. F. (Eds.). (2006). *Tropical Infectious Diseases. Principles, Pathogens, & Practice* (2nd ed.). Philadelphia: Churchill Livingstone Elsevier.

Hall, H. I., Song, R., Rhodes, P., Prejean, J., An, Q., Lee, L M., et al. (2008). Estimation of HIV incidence in the United States. *Journal of the American Medical Association, 300,* 520–529.

Halperin, D. T., & Epstein, H. (2004). Concurrent sexual partnerships help to explain Africa's high prevalence: Implications for prevention. *Lancet, 364,* 4–6.

Harris, C., Small, C. B., Klein, R. S., Friedland, G. H., Moll, B., Emeson, E. E., et al. (1983). Immunodeficiency syndrome. *New England Journal of Medicine, 308,* 1181–1184.

Havens, P. L., and Committee on Pediatric AIDS. (2003). Postexposure prophylaxis in children and adolescents for nonoccupational exposure to human immunodeficiency virus. *Pediatrics, 111,* 1475–1489.

Highleyman, L. (October 7, 2008). CDC updates estimates of HIV prevalence in the United States. Retrieved March 1, 2009, from www.hivandhepatitis.com/recent/2008/100708_a.html.

Hooper, E. (1997). Sailors and starbursts, and the arrival of HIV. *British Medical Journal, 315,* 1689–1691.

Hooper, E. (1999). *The river: A journey back to the source of HIV and AIDS.* London/Boston: Allen Lane-Penguin Press/Little Brown Co.

Hooper, E. (2001). Experimental oral polio vaccines and acquired immune deficiency syndrome. *Philosophical Transactions of the Royal Society of London B: Biological Sciences, 356,* 803–814.

Inciardi, J. A., Syvertsen, J. L., & Surratt, H. L. (2005).HIV/AIDS in the Caribbean basin. *AIDS Care, 17* (Suppl. 1), S9–S25.

Ippolito, G., Poggio, P., & Arici, G. (1994). Transmission of zidovudine-resistant HIV during a blood fight. *Journal of the American Medical Association, 272,* 433–434.

Jaffe, H. W., Valdiserri, R. O., & De Cock, K. M. (2007). The reemerging HIV/AIDS epidemic in men who have sex with men. *Journal of the American Medical Association, 298,* 2412–2414.

John-Stewart, G., Mbori-Ngacha, D., Ekpini, R., Janoff, E. N., Nkengasong, J., Read, J. S., et al. (2004). Breast-feeding and transmission of HIV-1. *Journal of Acquired Immune Deficiency Syndrome, 35,* 196–202.

Kawamura, M., Yamazaki, S., Ishikawa, K., Kwofie, T. V., Tsujimoto, H., & Hayami, M. (1989). HIV-2 in West Africa in 1966. *Lancet, 1,* 385.

Keele, B. F., Van Heuverswyn, F., Li, Y., Bailes, E., Takehisa, J., Santiago, M. L., et al. (2006). Chimpanzee reservoirs of pandemic and nonpandemic HIV-1. *Science, 313,* 523–526.

King, S. M., American Academy of Pediatrics Committee on Pediatric Aids, American Academy of Pediatrics Infectious Diseases and Immunization Committee. (2004). Evaluation and treatment of the human immunodeficiency virus-1-exposed infant. *Pediatrics, 114,* 497–505.

Knipe, D. M., & Howley, P. M. (Eds.). (2007). *Fields virology* (5th ed.). Philadelphia: Wolters Kluwer.

Landesman, S. H., Ginzburg, H. M., & Weiss, S. H. (1985). The AIDS epidemic. *New England Journal of Medicine, 312,* 521–525.

Lane, H. C., & Fauci, A. S. (1985). Immunologic abnormalities in the acquired immunodeficiency syndrome. *Annual Review of Immunology, 3,* 477–500.

Lanternier, F., Lebbé, C., Schartz, N., Farhi, D., Marcelin, A. G., Kérob, D., et al. (2008). Kaposi's sarcoma in HIV-negative men having sex with men. *AIDS, 22,* 1163–1168.

Lashley, F. R. (2006a). AIDS/HIV. In R.Schulz, L. S. Noelker, K. Rockwood, & R. L. Sprott (Eds.). *The Encyclopedia of Aging: A Comprehensive Resource in Gerontology and Geriatrics* (4th ed., pp. 48–52). New York: Springer Publishing Co.

Lashley, F. R. (2006b). *Clinical genetics in nursing practice* (3rd ed.). New York: Springer Publishing Co.

Lashley, F. R. (2006c). Transmission and epidemiology of HIV/AIDS: A global view. *Nursing Clinics of North America, 41*(3), 339–354.

Laurencin, C. T., Christensen, D. M., & Taylor, E. D. (2008). HIV/AIDS and the African-American community: A state of emergency. *Journal of the American Medical Association, 100,* 35-43.

LePage, P., Van de Perre, P., Carael, M., Nsengumuremyi, F., Nkurunziza, J., Butzler, J., et al. (1987). Postnatal transmission of HIV from mother to child. *Lancet, 2,* 400.

Levine, P. H. (1985). The acquired immunodeficiency syndrome in persons with hemophilia. *Annals of Internal Medicine, 103,* 723-726.

Levy, J. A., Hoffman, A, D., Kramer, S. M., Landis, J. A., Shimabukuro, J. M., & Oshiro, L. S. (1984). Isolation of lymphocytopathic retrovirus from San Francisco patients with AIDS. *Science, 225,* 840-842.

Lifson, A. R. (1988). Do alternate modes for transmission of human immunodeficiency virus exist? *Journal of the American Medical Association, 259,* 1353-1356.

Mann, J. M., Chin, J., Piot, P., & Quinn, T. (1988). The international epidemiology of AIDS. *Scientific American, 259,* 82-89.

Marcus, R., & the Cooperative Needlestick Surveillance Group. (1989, June 4–9). *Healthcare workers exposed to patients infected with human immunodeficiency virus (HIV)—United States.* Paper presented at the Fifth International Conference on AIDS. Montreal.

Marmor, M., Weiss, L. R., Lyden, M., Weiss, S. H., Sacinger, W. C., Spira, T. J., et al. (1986). Possible female-to-female transmission of human immunodeficiency virus. *Annals of Internal Medicine, 103,* 909.

Martin, J. L. (1987). The impact of AIDS on gay male sexual behavior patterns in New York City. *American Journal of Public Health, 77,* 578–581.

Marwick, C. (1985). AIDS-associated virus yields data to intensifying scientific study. *Journal of the American Medical Association, 254,* 2865–2868, 2870.

Mathers, B. M., Degenhardt, L., Phillips, B., Wiessing, L., Hickman, M., Strathlee, S. A., et al. (2008). Global epidemiology of injecting drug use and HIV among people who inject drugs: A systematic review. *Lancet, 372,* 1733–1745.

Miller, B., Stansfield, S., Zack, M., Curran, J., Kaplan, J., & Schonberger, L. (1984). The syndrome of unexplained generalized lymphadenopathy in young men in New York City. *Journal of the American Medical Association, 251,* 242–246.

Monzon, O. T., & Capellan, J. M. (1987). Female-to-female transmission of HIV. *Lancet, 2,* 40–41.

Morris, L., Distenfeld, A., Amorosi, E., & Karpatkin, S. (1982). Autoimmune thrombocytopenic purpura in homosexual men. *Annals of Internal Medicine, 96,* 714–717.

Nahmias, A. J., Weiss, J., Yao, X., Lee, F., Kodsi, R., Schanfield, M., et al. (1986). Evidence for human infection with an HTLV III/LAV-like virus in Central Africa, 1959. *Lancet, 1*(8492), 1279–1280.

Nduati, R. W., John, G. C., Richardson, B. A., Overbaugh, J., Welch, M., Ndinya-Achola, J., et al. (1995). Human immunodeficiency virus type 1-infected cells in breast milk: Association with immunosuppression and vitamin A deficiency. *Journal of Infectious Diseases, 172,* 1461–1468.

Nguyen, N., & Holodniy, H. (2008). HIV infection in the elderly. *Clinical Interventions in Aging, 3*(3), 453–472.

Nguyen, T. A., Oosterhoff, P., Hardon, A., Tran, H. N., Coutinho, R. A., & Wright, P. (2008). A hidden HIV epidemic among women in Vietnam. *BMC Public Health, 8,* 37–48.

Norman, C. (1985). What's in a name. *Science, 230,* 641.

Obermeyer, C. M. (2006). HIV in the Middle East. *British Medical Journal, 333,* 851–854.

Oladokun, R., Brown, B. J., Osinusi, K., Akingbola, T. S., Ajayi, S. O., & Omigbodun, O. O. (2008). A case of human bite by an 11-year old HIV positive girl in a paediatrics ward. *African Journal of Medicine and Medical Sciences, 37,* 81–85.

Pitchenik, A. E., Shafron, R. D., Glasser, R. M., & Spira, T. J. (1984). The acquired immunodeficiency syndrome in the wife of a hemophiliac. *Annals of Internal Medicine, 100,* 62–65.

Pomerantz, R. J., Kurtzke, D., de la Monte, S. M., Rota, T. R., Baker, A. S., Albert, D., et al. (1987). Infection of the retina by human immunodeficiency virus type 1. *New England Journal of Medicine, 317,* 1643–1647.

Powers, K., Poole, C., Pettifor, A., & Cohen, M. (2008, July 31–August 2). Rethinking the heterosexual infectivity of HIV-1: A systematic review and meta-analysis [Abstract No. 14]. *3rd international Workshop on HIV Transmission: Principles of Intervention*, Mexico City, Mexico.

Public Health Service Task Force. (2008). *Recommendations for use of antiretroviral drugs in pregnant HIV-infected women for maternal health and interventions to reduce perinatal HIV transmission in the United States.* Accessed March 1, 2009, from http://AIDSinfo.nih.gov.

Quinn, T. C., & Overbaugh, J. (2005). HIV/AIDS in women: An expanding epidemic. *Science, 308,* 1582–1583.

Reid, G., Kamarulzaman, A., & Sran, S. K. (2007). Malasia and harm reduction: The challenges and responses. *International Journal of Drug Policy, 18,* 136–140.

Rosenberg, P. S., & Goedert, J. J. (1998). Estimating the cumulative incidence of HIV infection among persons with haemophilia in the United States of America. *Statistics in Medicine, 17*(2), 155–168.

Rosenzweig, R., & Fillet, H. (1992). Probable heterosexual transmission of AIDS in an aged woman. *Journal of the American Geriatric Society, 40,* 1261–1264.

Rowland-Jones, S. L., & Whittle, H. C. (2007). Out of Africa: what can we learn from HIV-2 about protective immunity to HIV-1? *Nature Immunology, 8,* 329–331.

Rozenbaum, W., Gharakhanian, S., Cardon, B., Duval, E., & Couland, J. P. (1988). HIV transmission by oral sex. *Lancet, 1,* 1395.

Ruxrungtham, K., Brown, T., & Phanuphak, P. (2004). HIV/AIDS in Asia. *Lancet, 364*(9428), 69–82.

Seale, J. R. (1984). AIDS and hepatitis B cannot be venereal diseases. *Canadian Medical Association Journal, 130,* 1109–1110.

Siegel, J. D., Rhinehart, E., Jackson, M., Chiarello, L., Health Care Infection Control Practices Advisory Committee. (2007). 2007 guidelines for isolation precautions: Preventing transmission of infectious agents in health care settings. *American Journal of Infection Control, 35*(10 Suppl. 2), S65–S164.

Smith, S. M., Christian, D., de Lame, V., Shah, U., Austin, L., Gautam, R., et al. (2008). Isolation of a new HIV-2 subgroup in the US. *Retrovirology, 5,* 103–105.

Spitzer, P. G., & Weiner, N. J. (1989). Transmission of HIV infection from a woman to a man by oral sex. *New England Journal of Medicine, 320,* 251.

Sun, X., Wang, N., Li, D., Zheng, X., Qu, S., Wang, L., et al. (2007). The development of HIV/AIDS surveillance in China. *AIDS, 21*(Suppl. 8), S33–S38.

Thiry, L., Sprecher-Goldberger, S., Jonckheer, T., Levy, J., Van de Perre, P., Henri-vaux, P., et al. (1985). Isolation of AIDS virus from cell-free breast milk of three health virus carriers. *Lancet, 2,* 891–892.

Todd, C. S., Abed, A. M. S., Strathdee, S. A., Scott, P. T., Botros, B. A., Safi, N., et al. (2007). HIV, hepatitis C and hepatitis B infections and associated risk behavior in injection drug users, Kabul, Afghanistan. *Emerging Infectious Diseases, 13,* 1327–1331.

UNAIDS/WHO (2008). *2008 Report on the global AIDS epidemic.* Retrieved March 20, 2009, from www.unaids.org/en/KnowledgeCentre/ HIVData/GlobalReport/2008/2008_Global_report.asp.

UNAIDS and broad coalition working towards the release of nine men who have sex with men in Senegal who have been convicted and imprisoned. (2009). Retrieved March 20, 2009, from www. unaids.org/en/KnowledgeCentre/Resources/PressCentre/Press Releases/2009/20090115_senegal.asp.

United States Census Bureau. (2001). Population by Race. Retrieved March 20, 2009 from www.censusscope.org/us/chart_race.html.

Van Heuverswyn, F., & Peeters, M. (2007). The origins of HIV and implications for the global epidemic. *Current Infectious Diseases Reports, 9,* 338–346.

Vermund, S. H. (1997). Transmission of HIV-1 among adolescents and adults. In V. T. DeVita Jr., S. Hellman, & S. A. Rosenberg. *AIDS: Etiology, diagnosis, treatment and prevention* (pp. 147–165). Philadelphia: Lippincott Raven.

Vernazza, P. L., Eron, J. J., Fiscus, S. A., & Cohen, M. S. (1999). Sexual transmission of HIV: Infectiousness and prevention. *AIDS, 13,* 155–166.

Vittecoq, D., Mettetal, J. F., Rouzioux, C., Bach, J. F., & Bouchon, J. P. (1989). Acute HIV infection after acupuncture treatments. *New England Journal of Medicine, 320,* 250–251.

Vogt, M. W., Witt, D. J., Craven, D. E., Byington, R., Crawford, D. F., Schooley, R., et al. (1986). Isolation of HTLV-III/LAV from cervical secretions of women at risk for AIDS. *Lancet, 1,* 525–527.

Wain-Hobson, S. (1998). More ado about HIV's origins. *Nature Medicine, 4,* 1001–1002.

White, R. G., Glynn, J. R., Orroth, K. K., Freeman, E. E., Bakker, R., Weiss, H. A., et al. (2008). Male circumcision for HIV prevention in sub-Saharan Africa: Who, what and when? *AIDS, 22,* 1841–1850.

Whittle, H. C., Ariyoshi, K., & Rowland-Jones, S. (1998). HIV-2 and T cell recognition. *Current Opinion in Immunology, 10*(4), 382–387.

Withrington, R. H., Cornes, P., Harris, J. R. W., Seifert, M. H., Berrie, E., Taylor-Robinson, D., et al. (1987). Isolation of human immunodeficiency virus from synovial fluid of a patient with reactive arthritis. *British Medical Journal, 294,* 484.

Wofsy, C. B., Cohen, J. B., Hauer, L. P., Padian, N. S., Michaelis, B. A., Evans, L., et al. (1986). Isolation of AIDS-associated retrovirus from genital secretions of women with antibodies to the virus. *Lancet, 1,* 527–529.

World Health Organization. (2008). *HIV transmission through breastfeeding: A review of available evidence: 2007 update.* Geneva: World Health Organization.

World Health Organization. (2009). HIV and infant feeding. Retrieved March 20, 2009, from www.who.int/child_adolescent_health/topics/prevention_care/child/nutrition/hivif/en/index.html.

Working Group on Antiretroviral Therapy and Medical Management of HIV-Infected Children. (2009). Guidelines for use of antiretroviral agents in pediatric HIV infection. Retrieved March 20, 2009, from http://aidsinfo.nih.gov/contentfiles/PediatricGuidelines.pdf.

Worobey, M., Gemmel, M., Teuwen, D. E., Haselkorn, T., Kunstman, K., Bunce, M., et al. (2008). Direct evidence of extensive diversity of HIV-1 in Kinshasa by 1960. *Nature ,455,* 661–664.

Worobey, M., Santiago, M. L., Keele, B. F., Ndjango, J., Joy, J. B., Labama, B. L., et al. (2004). Origin of AIDS: Contaminated polio vaccine theory refuted. *Nature, 428,* 820.

Ziegler, J. V., Cooper, D. A., Johnson, R. O., & Gold, J. (1985). Postnatal transmission of AIDS-associated retrovirus from a mother to an infant. *Lancet, 1,* 896–897.

2 HIV Screening, Testing, and Counseling

DONNA M. GALLAGHER

BACKGROUND

The introduction and widespread use of HIV antibody testing began in 1985 with a primary goal of screening the blood supply and organs for donation to protect the public from exposure to HIV. Determining HIV serostatus was a critical piece of the differential diagnosis. Test results required confidentiality to safeguard patients from stigma and discrimination and, in some cases, physical and psychological harm. In addition, in those early years the lack of effective treatment for HIV and the associated opportunistic infections (OIs) diminished the desire for both patients and providers to aggressively pursue HIV testing as a routine practice. Pre- and posttest counseling was standard practice and considered an essential part of the testing process. In most U.S. states, separate, written informed consent was also required by law.

The original principles of HIV counseling and testing (HCT), also known as voluntary counseling and testing (VCT), were the widely accepted practice for over 20 years and were used primarily to guide counseling of persons seeking to know their HIV serostatus. Many people took advantage of the availability of testing but chose the anonymous option to avoid having their name associated with the fact that they were tested and/or linked to the results of the test. The availability of anonymous testing increased the number of tests performed but also created difficulties in identifying and referring for care those who were HIV positive. Tested persons moved from place to place and often were tested in several places, resulting in duplicate counting and incorrect state statistics. Many of those tested never returned to the test site to obtain their test results and, if tested anonymously, could not be located.

In 1993, the Centers for Disease Control and Prevention (CDC) recommended that HIV testing be used more frequently in acute care settings (Centers for Disease Control and Prevention [CDC], 1993). In addition, the practice of using names or unique identifiers to identify who was being tested was strongly recommended. These initial recommendations were written in response to data suggesting that approximately 25% of HIV-positive persons (an estimated 250,000 persons) were unaware of their status (Glynn & Rhodes, 2005) as well as the growing body of evidence demonstrating that late entry into care has long-term deleterious effects, often resulting in decreased survival (Flanigan & Beckwith, 2008). The responses to the CDC recommendations were generally unenthusiastic (CDC, 2001; Liebert, 2008; Obermeyer & Osborn, 2007). By 1996, the urgency to accomplish more widespread testing was amplified further as the availability and successful use of highly active antiretroviral therapies (HAART) demonstrated improved survival and became state-of-the-art HIV care (Palella et al., 1998).

In 2003, the CDC again revised the HIV testing recommendations and introduced the Advancing HIV Prevention Initiative (AHI) (CDC, 2003a, 2003b, 2005). This effort targeted emergency departments, urgent care centers, and walk-in clinics in demographic areas thought to have large numbers of persons known to be at high risk for HIV, particularly in areas with high numbers of injection drug users (IDUs) and minorities (Ehrenkranz et al., 2008; Hardwicke et al., 2008; Haukoos, Hopkins, & Byyny, 2008).

Prior to these revised recommendations, the predominant practice for HIV testing in clinical settings was based on clinical indications known to be associated with HIV, reported risk factors (e.g., injection drug use, unprotected sexual practice), or an individual's request for HIV testing. Because there are now medical as well as public health benefits associated with knowing one's HIV status, the CDC revised its 2003 recommendations in 2006, adding language urging providers to make HIV testing a routine practice (CDC, 2006). The practice of reporting the name of a person who tests positive for HIV is no longer optional for states receiving federal funding for HIV care. The formula used to determine the level of dollars that each state will receive to support care and medications is now tied to the number of individually named persons with HIV living in a state. Some states continue to offer anonymous testing, and many federal and state-funded counseling and testing programs are still in operation. Sites in these states spend significantly more time providing counseling, testing, and prevention information and urging persons who are HIV positive to gain access to health care.

The 2006 Revised Recommendations

The CDC's (2006) "Revised Recommendations for HIV Testing of Adults, Adolescents, and Pregnant Women in Health-Care Settings" urged "testing of all persons aged 13–64 irrespective of lifestyle, perceived risk, or local prevalence and be considered part of routine primary care" (p. 10). In these revised recommendations, the CDC recommended that HIV testing should also be used as a screening opportunity in acute care and other clinical settings and that HIV testing should be "opt out," meaning that unless a patient specifically declines to be tested, a test will be performed (Bartlett et al., 2008; Branson et al., 2006; CDC, 2006). The overall goal of these revised recommendations is to decrease the number of HIV-positive persons who are still unaware of their status and to promote earlier entry into HIV care. As with previous recommendations, adoption of these revised recommendations has been slow, as demonstrated by the fact that only an estimated 40 % of the U.S. population know their status or have ever been tested for HIV (Bartlett et al., 2008).

In 2008, the practice of HIV antibody testing is now well established and associated with both improved treatment outcomes and successful prevention strategies. HIV testing continues to be an essential component of a differential diagnosis. Advances in HIV testing technology now make it possible to receive test results in as little as 30 minutes or less and has led to the Substance Abuse and Mental Health Service Administration's (SAMHSA) Rapid HIV Testing Initiative and efforts of the CDC to reduce barriers to making HIV testing a routine part of health care (San Antonio-Gaddy et al., 2006; White et al., 2008).

TESTING FOR HIV-1 AND HIV-2

HIV testing is designed to be highly sensitive and specific. The method used for HIV testing is most often a measure of the presence of HIV antibodies in serum/plasma or oral mucosal exudates. EIA (enzyme immunoassay) and enzyme-linked immunosorbent assay (ELISA) have long been the standard for HIV screening. These tests have seen many transformations since they were first used in 1985. Improvements over time in both the sensitivity and specificity of the tests have made the tests more reliable and accurate tools. Through use of these tests, HIV antibodies can be detected in blood (most commonly used), saliva, or urine (less commonly used).

EIA and ELISA identify antibodies in a patient's serum/plasma but do not distinguish which specific antibodies are present. Most tests still require laboratory processing and have a moderately complex Clinical Laboratory Improvement Amendment (CLIA) status. Tests to detect HIV-1 (the retrovirus most commonly seen in North America, including the United States) and HIV-2 (also a retrovirus, seen most often in West Africa) have been available for some time, but not all patients were routinely tested for both. HIV-2 testing was used most often for patients from areas known to have HIV-2 prevalence and for patients whose clinical presentation differed from that of HIV-1. The U.S. blood supply and organ donations are screened for both HIV-1 and HIV-2. A nonreactive result from the initial ELISA screening test is considered to be HIV negative. Persons exposed after testing to an infected partner or partner of unknown HIV status should be retested. A reactive ELISA result is retested in duplicate and, if either duplicate test is reactive, the specimen undergoes confirmatory testing with a more specific test (e.g., Western blot or an immunofluorescence assay). An important principle for caregivers to know is that a nonreactive screening test does not necessarily mean that a tested person is uninfected with HIV. Because several months may pass before antibodies to HIV are at a detectable level (called the "window period"), some infected persons may test negative for infection on screening tests.

Rapid Testing

Rapid tests at the point of care now provide the results of an enzyme immunoassay in as little as 15 minutes (e.g., Clearview Complete HIV 1/2 and Clearview HIV 1/2 Stat-Pak). Rapid testing is a core component of the current concept that HIV testing should now be considered a screening strategy with the goal that "all patients should be tested at least once" (CDC, 2006). Key advantages of rapid testing are lower test cost and ease of use, test accuracy, posttest counseling on the day of testing, more rapid referral to medical treatment for those testing positive, and potential for those who test positive to change behaviors that might expose others to HIV (Shrestha et al., 2008). Because of reports of higher than expected false-positive results in some parts of the country, all positive tests are confirmed with a conventional ELISA and Western Blot. The CDC (2007) has issued quality-assurance guidelines for rapid

HIV testing. The Food and Drug Administration (FDA)–approved rapid tests (Table 2.1) to detect both HIV-1 and HIV-2 as one test are now available and are being used more routinely for the reasons cited above.

Prevention of Mother-to-Child Transmission (PMTCT)

The availability of rapid testing is critical when the results of the test will have an immediate impact on medical decisions, when the likelihood of a patient returning for the results is very low, and when the patient is in a labor and delivery setting (Franco-Paredes, Tellez, & del Rio, 2006). The urgency to know the HIV status of a pregnant woman in the labor and delivery setting is based on the success of interventions that reduce perinatal transmission. This test result is particularly important when a woman presents with unknown HIV status (Barbaci, Repke, & Chaisson, 1991; Chersich & Temmerman, 2008; Gross & Burr, 2003; Gruskin, Ahmed, & Ferguson, 2008). The opportunity to offer a medication intervention for an HIV-positive pregnant woman (required prior to, during, and after delivery) has proven to dramatically decrease the potential for transmission from mother to child. Studies have demonstrated that a significant number of vertical transmissions occur at the time of delivery, making the timing of treatment with antiretroviral medications critical (Institute of Medicine, 1999; Kriebs & Shannon, 2008). Current evidence demonstrates that the mother-to-child HIV transmission rate can be kept under 2% when women have received antiretroviral treatment prior to delivery and immediately after delivery. If a woman with a high viral load delivers a baby, the rate of transmission *without antiretroviral treatment* can be as high as 25% (Lindegren et al., 1999). (See Chapter 13 for a fuller discussion of prevention of mother-to-child transmission of HIV.)

Rapid test results are also used as part of the decision algorithm when determining the need for postexposure prophylaxis for health care workers and others potentially exposed to HIV in an occupational setting. Prior to the advent of rapid testing, a health care worker began postexposure prophylaxis (PEP) medication if the source patient didn't have an HIV test result in his or her medical record. Rapid testing can now eliminate the approximate two-week wait for results and potentially obviate the need for medication entirely.

The most recent technological advances in HIV testing such as the BED-HIV-1 Capture EIA Assay test (an in vitro quantitative enzyme assay) can clarify whether a new HIV-positive test represents new disease

Table 2.1

FDA-APPROVED RAPID HIV ANTIBODY SCREENING TESTS

TEST	SPECIMEN TYPE	CLIA CATEGORY	SENSITIVITY (95% C1*)	SPECIFICITY (95% C1)	MANUFACTURER	APPROVED FOR HIV-2 DETECTION
OraQuick ADVANCERapid HIV-1/2 Antibody Test	Whole blood (finger stick or venipuncture)	Waived	99.6% (98.5–99.9)	100% (99.7–100)	OraSure Technologies (www.orasure.com)	Yes
	Oral fluid	Waived	99.3% (98.4–99.7)	99.8% (98.6–99.9)		
	Plasma	Moderate complexity	99.6% (98.9–99.8)	99.9% (99.6–99.9)		
Uni-Gold Recombigen HIV	Whole blood (finger stick or venipuncture)	Waived	100% (99.5–100)	99.7% (99.0–100)	Trinity Biotech (www.unigoldhiv.com)	No
	Serum/plasma	Moderate complexity	100% (99.5–100)	99.8% (99.3–100)		
Reveal G3 Rapid HIV-1 Antibody Test	Serum	Moderate complexity	99.8% (99.2–100)	99.1% (98.8-99.4)	MedMira (www.medmira.com)	No
	Plasma		99.8% (99.0-100)	98.6% (98.4-98.8)		

Test	Specimen	Complexity	Sensitivity	Specificity	Manufacturer	Differentiates HIV-1/HIV-2
MultiSpot HIV-1/HIV-2	Serum/plasma	Moderate complexity	100% (99.9-100)	99.9% (99.8-100)	BioRad Laboratories (www.biorad.com)	Yes, differentiates HIV-1 from HIV-2
	HIV-2		100% (99.7-100)			
Clearview HIV-1/2 Stat-PAK	Whole blood	Waived	99.7%	99.9%	Inverness Medical Professional Diagnostics (www.inverness medical.com)	Yes
	Serum & Plasma	Non-waived	99.7%	99.9%		
Clearview COMPLETE HIV-1/2	Whole blood	Waived	99.7%	99.9%	Inverness Medical Professional Diagnostics (www.inverness medical.com)	Yes
	Serum & Plasma	Non-waived	99.7%	99.9%		

FDA-approved Rapid HIV Antibody Screening Tests. Health Research and Educational Trust. Prepared by K. Stanger and F. Margolin at HRET; M. Lampe, J. Clark & B. Branson at CDC. Retrieved July 2008 from http://www.hret.org/hret/programs/content/rpd1.pdf.

or late identification of old disease, thereby taking some of the guesswork out of the decision to treat early or wait. Advances in HIV testing technology will continue to expand the options for HIV testing. The CDC's 2006 revised recommendations for HIV testing and the availability of rapid testing technology have dramatically changed the HIV screening and testing landscape. Responsibility for testing is returning to the primary care setting and expanding to many other health care settings that may include nontraditional sites such as the local pharmacy, the neighborhood outreach van, and the dental office (Vernillo & Caplan, 2007). The HIV social context, however, still has elements of stigma and discrimination that continue to have a negative impact on the ability to make HIV testing normal (Wynia, 2006). However, scientific evidence shows that normalized testing and early diagnosis and treatment can result in improved quality of life and a relatively normal lifespan for people living with HIV (Campos-Outcalt et al., 2006).

Confirming HIV-Positive Tests

Currently, the standard procedure in the United States when an HIV test is positive (irrespective of the type of antibody test) is confirmation by a more specific test. A Western Blot (WB) is performed to identify specifically which of the individual proteins found on the HIV are present. If an EIA is positive and then confirmed with a WB, the tested person is confirmed to be HIV positive. However, in some low-resource countries where laboratory facilities may be limited, a WB may not be available; therefore, confirmation of a positive rapid test result is accomplished by administering another rapid test, preferably a different brand than that of the first rapid test. All FDA-approved rapid tests have been found to be highly sensitive and specific. The reported high specificity of rapid tests (Table 2.1) means that, if a rapid test is positive, the patient is most likely infected with HIV. The validity of rapid tests is dependent on the HIV prevalence of the population. It is mandatory to confirm an HIV-positive test with a more specific HIV test if the population tested has a low HIV prevalence, which makes the chances of false-positive tests more likely. The confirmatory test like the Western Blot will determine if the rapid test is a true positive.

RNA and DNA Testing

Polymerase chain reaction (PCR) assay is an extremely sensitive technique used to find specific HIV-1 nucleic acid sequences in a DNA form and RNA fragments that amplify in infected cells. PCR is used most frequently to evaluate newborns born to HIV-positive women to determine if a baby has antibodies from his or her infected mother or is in fact infected with HIV. PCR is not widely used in low-resource settings due to cost and lack of availability. Branched DNA (bDNA) assay measures HIV RNA in the plasma of infected patients and is also highly sensitive but expensive, which is a major determining factor when choosing which test will be used. The use of the p24 antigen test is a measure of the presence of HIV proteins but is less frequently used due to cost and the availability of other sensitive and more rapid tests, such as viral load.

Home Testing

An FDA-approved "home test" kit has been on the market since 1996 and initially was intended to provide confidentiality and remove the need for an individual to go to a test site. This test, which can be purchased on the Internet, is sold as "The Home Access HIV-1 Test System" or "The Home Access Express HIV-1 Test System." According to the U.S. FDA (2008):

> This approved system uses a simple finger prick process for home blood collection which results in dried blood spots on special paper. The dried blood spots are mailed to a laboratory with a confidential and anonymous personal identification number (PIN), and analyzed by trained clinicians in a laboratory using the same tests that are used for samples taken in a doctor's office or clinic. Test results are obtained through a toll free telephone number using the PIN, and post-test counseling is provided by telephone when results are obtained (¶9).

The cost of the test (approximately $75.00) slowed the expected popularity of the home test. The use of home testing has diminished further as rapid testing has become more widely available.

Window Period

The "window period" is the length of time after infection that it takes for a person to develop detectable antibodies using current testing methods. Most persons who are infected with HIV will seroconvert (i.e., react to HIV by creating antibodies to the virus) within the first three months following exposure, and many will serconvert within four weeks following infection. Only a few HIV-infected persons will take six months to seroconvert. During the window period, the standard tests for antibodies may not provide accurate results. Patients who have access only to antibody testing need to receive counseling that includes repeat testing at 3 and 6 months. If they have access to more specific tests, such as viral culture or viral load, they can receive clearance sooner. This is a particularly difficult waiting period for infants who have been born to HIV-positive mothers. Infants carry their mothers' immunity for approximately 18 months; thus they can test positive for HIV from birth until the period where they have developed their own immune system. If antibody testing is the only available test, it may be two years before it is known whether an infant is true positive or negative. The use of more specific tests such as PCR and bDNA can reduce this waiting time to a few months.

HIV Test Counseling

The CDC's revised recommendations (2006) suggest that testing should be a routine process that does not require special *pretest* counseling. Counseling is recommended only if an HIV test is positive (Beckwith et al., 2005; Bozzette, 2005; CDC, 2006; Hutchinson et al., 2006; Koo et al., 2006). This recommendation has not gained universal acceptance at this writing. Until the CDC's revised recommendations (2006) were promulgated, pre- and posttest counseling was a routine and widely accepted part of the HIV testing process. While the field is shifting to fully adopt the CDC's revised recommendations, several options are still available to persons seeking HIV testing. Several states continue to have anonymous test sites and walk-in sites that require a name but do not require identification. Some of these sites are able to offer free testing while others charge a small fee. A permanent record linking the test results to the name of the person being tested is not part of the process, so the results remain anonymous. Name-based reporting of HIV test results is a key element of the CDC's (2006) revised recommendations and is also tied to the formula funding provided through the Ryan White HIV Treatment Modernization Act.

Confidential Testing

Confidential testing is most often performed in a health care setting. When an HIV test is performed, the results are given to the patient and are placed in the medical record. Release of the test results is protected by the Health Insurance Portability and Accountability Act (HIPAA), and some state laws require patient consent to release the results. State laws change frequently and vary dramatically from state to state; thus providers need to know their state laws regarding testing (Goldschmidt & Neff, 2009; Hanssens, 2007; Wolf, Donoghoe, & Lane, 2007). The over-arching goal of testing is to provide tested individuals with test results and to facilitate access to the health care system as early as possible for those testing positive.

Anonymous Testing

For most of the past 25 years, federal and state funding has supported anonymous counseling and testing programs. Anonymous counseling and testing sites are generally located in settings that are outside the traditional health care system. Blood specimens and results are iden-tified only by codes. The movement away from anonymous testing is driven by the evidence that a higher percentage of people testing anon-ymously fail to return for their results, thereby delaying their entry into care and affecting overall survival (Anaya et al., 2008; Tesoriero et al., 2008). Currently, funding for HIV care is based on a formula that requires name-based reporting. Patients tested in anonymous or code-based programs are not counted when the formula is funded, leading to a reduction in funds awarded to a state. By 2008, all 50 states had converted to the name-based model, a shift that is likely to greatly reduce or even eliminate anonymous testing.

Pretest Counseling

Pretest counseling was the standard practice prior to the CDC's revised recommendations (2006). The pretest encounter is used to assess a person's readiness to test; to provide information, including a discussion of risk behaviors, the appropriateness of taking an HIV test, information about the process of testing including the time needed for test result (20 to 30 minutes for rapid test results, 2 to 14 days for standard ELISA); and to provide an overview of how the virus works and how transmission occurs as well as how to prevent transmission. Pretest counseling also includes a brief discussion of the impact of HIV on the immune system and demonstrates to those seeking testing the importance of knowing their status and what the results mean.

Standard pretest counseling is being replaced in many settings (e.g., emergency rooms, labor and delivery, outreach vans) that have adopted the CDC's revised recommendations (2006) with a variety of abbreviated approaches (Kurth et al., 2007; Shamos et al., 2008; Zetola et al., 2008). Many of these approaches include only a brief description of the HIV test, which will also serve as informed consent in states that have consent laws. Some approaches include interactive educational programs and/ or films, and some settings give the person written information while waiting to be tested. Most of these new models are designed to reduce the time burden on providers (Calderon et al., 2006; Sobo et al., 2008). Another alternative is the use of an "abbreviated pretest counseling tool" that can be accomplished in 5 minutes at the bedside or in a private area in a waiting room (see Table 2.2). As the practice of traditional 20 to 30 minute pretest counseling sessions is phased out in compliance with the CDC's revised recommendations (2006) on testing, there will surely be more tools available. Currently, several examples of these tools are available on the website (www.aidsetc.org) of the Health Resources and Services Administration (HRSA) AIDS Education and Training Centers (AETC).

Posttest Counseling

The primary goals when a person returns for an HIV test result are the immediate delivery of the information and support of the patient (see Table 2.3). After assessing the person's response to the HIV test results, the time can be used to reinforce information regarding the risk of transmission to his or her sexual partner(s) and providing a referral to a provider.

In the past, patients were advised to bring someone with them when they got their results to serve as a support. However, if the patient had a rapid test this preplanning may not be an option. Evaluation of a patient's response to his or her HIV results is critical and will guide the clinicians' referral decisions. A mental health referral may be more important than the primary care referral if a patient is mentally unstable after receiving the news of a positive test.

Posttest counseling is usually face-to-face and is conducted by a person who is knowledgeable about HIV resources and treatment. Historically, a posttest session was approximately one hour long and included a review of how the virus causes damage, how it is transmitted, the effect on the immune system, how to avoid transmission to sexual partners, safe handling for families, discussion of immediate treatment for pregnant women, and a plan for medical follow-up. Posttest counseling is part of the CDC's revised recommendation (2006). However,

Table 2.2

ABBREVIATED PRETEST COUNSELING

- Have you ever been tested for HIV before?
- If you have been exposed to HIV in the past month, today's test may not be accurate. The body needs 1 to 2 months to develop the antibodies that the test measures. You will need to test again in 3 to 6 months.
- HIV testing is routinely performed here along with many other tests.
- You will receive your results in 48 hours if a blood test is performed. If you have been told that you will have a rapid test, the results will be available in 30 to 60 minutes. If your test is positive, a confirmatory test will be performed.
- The results of the HIV test are given to you and the clinicians caring for you. The results will be kept confidential along with your medical records.
- HIV is a virus that is 100% preventable if exposure to the virus is avoided.
- HIV is passed to men and women during unprotected sexual intercourse, through exposure to blood, and by sharing needles to inject drugs.
- Pregnant women can pass the virus to their unborn child.
- If you suspect that you have been exposed to HIV, abstain from sexual intercourse or use barrier protection such as a condom is to avoid exposing your partner to HIV.
- HIV affects your immune system. The immune system helps to protect you when you have been exposed to viruses, including the common cold, the flu, and many other illnesses.
- Knowing your HIV test results will help you make future decisions about your care.
- There are medications to treat HIV infection that work best when taken early, before the virus damages your immune system.
- More information will be available when you receive your test results.

Local resources for more HIV information can be inserted here

in many settings today the session is time reduced, and patients may receive a significant amount of information in writing and a referral to a medical provider for follow-up. Part of the posttest counseling session is usually spent discussing ways to disclose the HIV-positive test result to a partner and to facilitate testing of the partner. Such counseling may also include strategies to inform other family members.

When counseling an HIV-positive injection drug user, information should include locations where clean needle exchange is available and reinforcement of information regarding risk of transmission via needle sharing.

Table 2.3

POSTTEST COUNSELING INFORMATION FOR PATIENTS

- Your HIV test result is positive, which means you have been exposed to HIV.
- A test will be performed to confirm this result.
- HIV is a virus that can be spread to others when having unprotected sexual intercourse with men and/or women, through exposure to the blood of an HIV-positive person, when sharing needles used to inject drugs, or from an HIV-positive pregnant woman to her unborn baby.
- Assistance is available if you would like help when telling your partner or any other family members about your HIV test.
- Use a condom (male/female) during sexual intercourse to reduce the risk of transmission to your sexual partner.
- Do not share needles or syringes. A list of needle exchange sites is below along with a list of drug treatment programs.
- Do not share razors, toothbrushes, tattoo needles, and/or body piercing needles.
- People with HIV are living long lives when they take care of their overall health. Powerful drugs have been successful at reducing the damage that HIV can do to the immune system if untreated. Early follow-up with a health care team will improve your chances of success with the HIV medications.
- Reducing your use of alcohol and cigarettes will improve your overall health while helping to keep your immune system healthy. Eating well, exercising, and sleeping will also improve your immune system health.
- It is helpful to avoid stress. Finding a friend or partner to support you is an important component of a successful care plan.

Referrals can be added here

In addition, information and referral (if possible) to a drug treatment program is a critical element of posttest counseling. A key goal is to have a patient leave a posttest counseling session with enough information to take the next step and enough support to avoid feelings of hopelessness.

IMPLICATIONS FOR NURSING PRACTICE

Nurses have played many key roles across the full spectrum of HIV care. However, some nurses have not been involved in testing and counseling and/or the actual process of testing due to the availability of dedicated HIV counseling and testing programs, HIV specialty clinics, and anonymous test sites. In addition, only patients identified to be "at risk" or those who requested testing were offered testing. These factors have limited the overall number of nurses who have counseling and testing experience.

The CDC's revised recommendations (2006) for HIV testing have significantly changed the HIV testing landscape from a risk-based model to a routine screening model. The goal of testing every person at least once in his or her lifetime can be accomplished only if nurses from every area of health care participate in the effort (Cohan et al., 2008; Mooney, 2008). Nurses will be expected to serve as patient advocates to insure that patients receive the information and referrals they will need when receiving HIV test results. Patients will rely on nurses to provide emotional support and guidance regarding treatment plans. Nurses in all areas of health care may find themselves involved in HIV testing, e.g., sharing results with a patient, providing a referral to care, administering HIV medications to a pregnant woman during labor to prevent transmission to her unborn child, counseling a teen about HIV prevention skills, teaching a patient about nutrition and exercise to maintain their immune system, and myriad other ways.

Some nurses have chosen to make HIV care their specialty area of practice. These nurses will serve as resources for other nurses who need support and guidance when one of their patients is found to be HIV positive; however, all nurses will need to have a basic understanding of HIV and a working knowledge of the implications of routine HIV testing in their work setting.

CONCLUSION

The identification of people infected with HIV is a critical step toward ending the spread of the HIV (Granich et al., 2008). Until routine HIV screening is fully implemented and the stigma associated with testing is no longer an issue, patients will need to have their rights safeguarded (Yeatman, 2007). The decision to test should be informed and voluntary. Nurses are in key positions as leaders, educators, and trusted providers to both facilitate HIV testing efforts and advocate for patients rights.

REFERENCES

Anaya, H. D., Hoang, T., Golden, J. F., Goetz, M. B., Gifford, A., Bowman, C., et al. (2008). Improving HIV screening and receipt of results by nurse-initiated streamlined counseling and rapid testing. *Journal of General Internal Medicine, 23*(6), 800–807.

Barbaci, M., Repke, J. T., & Chaisson, R. E. (1991). Routine prenatal screening for HIV infection. *Lancet, 337,* 709–711.

Bartlett, J. G., Branson, B. M., Fenton, K., Hauschild, B. C., Miller, V., & Mayer, K. H. (2008). Opt-out testing for human immunodeficiency virus in the United States. *Journal of the American Medical Association, 300*(8), 945–915.

Beckwith, C. G., Flanigan, T. P., del Rio, C., Simmons, E., Wing, E. J., Carpenter, C. C., et al. (2005). It is time to implement routine, not risk-based HIV testing. *Clinical Infectious Diseases, 40*(7), 1037–1040.

Bozzette, S. A. (2005). Routine screening for HIV infection--timely and cost-effective. *New England Journal of Medicine, 352*(6), 620–621.

Branson, B. M., Handsfield, H. H., Lampe, M. A., Janssen, R. S., Taylor, A. W., Lyss, S. B., et al. (2006). Revised recommendations for HIV testing of all adults, adolescents, and pregnant women in health-care settings. *Morbidity and Mortality Weekly Report Recommendations and Reports, 55*(RR-14), 1–17.

Calderon, Y., Haughey, M., Bijur, P. E., Leider, J., Moreno-Walton, L., Torres, S., et al. (2006). An educational HIV pretest counseling video program for off-hours testing in the emergency department. *Annals of Emergency Medicine, 48*(1), 21–27.

Campos-Outcalt, D., Mickey, T., Weisbuch, J., & Jones, R. (2006). Integrating routine HIV testing into a public health STD clinic. *Public Health Reports, 121*(2), 175–180.

Centers for Disease Control and Prevention. (1993). Recommendations for HIV testing services for inpatients and outpatients in acute-care hospital settings. *Morbidity and Mortality Weekly Report Recommendations Report, 42,* 1–6.

Centers for Disease Control and Prevention. (2001). *HIV counseling and testing in publicly funded sites: Annual report, 1997 and 1998.* Atlanta: Centers for Disease Control and Prevention, 2001. Available online at www.cdc.gov/hib/pubs/cts98.pdf.

Centers for Disease Control and Prevention. (2003a). Advancing HIV prevention: New strategies for a changing epidemic--United States. *Morbidity and Mortality Weekly Report, 52*(15), 329–332.

Centers for Disease Control and Prevention. (2003b). Incorporating HIV Prevention into the medical care of persons living with HIV. *Morbidity and Mortality Weekly Report, 52* (RR12), 1–24. Retrieved on March 20, 2009, from www.cdc.gov/mmwr/Preview/mmwrhtml/rr5212a1.htm.

Centers for Disease Control and Prevention. (2005). *Advancing HIV prevention: Progress summary, April 2003-September 2005.* Available online at www.cdc.gov/hiv/topics/prev_prog/AHP/resources/factsheets/progress_2005.htm.

Centers for Disease Control and Prevention. (2006). Revised recommendations for HIV testing of adults, adolescents, and pregnant women in health-care settings. *Morbidity and Mortality Weekly Report, 55*(RR-14). Available online at www.cdc.gov/mmwr/pdf/rr/rr5514.pdf.

Centers for Disease Control and Prevention. (2007). *Quality assurance guidelines for testing using rapid HIV antibody tests waived under the clinical laboratory improvement amendments of 1988.* Available online at http://www.cdc.gov/hiv/topics/testing/resources/guidelines/pdf/QA_Guidlines.pdf.

Chersich, M. F., & Temmerman, M. (2008). Increasing access to HIV testing for women by simplifying pre- and post-test counseling. *Current Women's Health Reviews, 4*(3), 172–179.

Cohan, D., Sarnquist, C., Gomez, E., Feakins, C., Maldonado, Y., & Zetola, N. (2008). Increased uptake of HIV testing with the integration of nurse-initiated HIV testing into routine prenatal care. *Journal of Acquired Immune Deficiency Syndromes, 49*(5), 571–571.

Ehrenkranz, P. D., Ahn, C. J., Metlay, J. P., Camargo, C. A. Jr., Holmes, W. C., & Rothman, R. (2008). Availability of rapid human immunodeficiency virus testing in academic emergency departments. *Academic Emergency Medicine, 15*(2), 144–150.

Health Research and Educational Trust. (2008). FDA-Approved Rapid HIV Antibody Screening Tests. Available online at http://www.hret.org/hret/programs/content/rpd1.pdf

Flanigan, T. P., & Beckwith, C. G. (2008). Routine HIV testing in jails is critical for the early diagnosis of HIV infection in men. *Clinical Infectious Disease, 47*(10), 1366.

Franco-Paredes, C., Tellez, I., & del Rio, C. (2006). Rapid HIV testing: A review of the literature and implications for the clinician. *Current HIV/AIDS Reports, 3*(4), 167–175.

Glynn, R., & Rhodes, P. (2005). Estimated HIV prevalence in the United States at the end of 2003 [abstract T1-B1101]. Programs and abstracts of the 2005 National HIV Prevention Conference, Atlanta. Available online at www.aegis.com/conferences/nhivpc/2005/t1-b1101.html.

Goldschmidt, R., & Neff, S. (2009). Compendium of State HIV testing laws—2009. Retrieved March 20, 2009, from www.nccc.ucsf.edu/StateLaws/Index.html.

Granich, R. M., Gilks, C. F., Dye, C., De Cock, K. M., & Williams, B. G. (2008). Universal voluntary HIV testing with immediate antiretroviral therapy as a strategy for elimination of HIV transmission: A mathematical model. *The Lancet, 373*(9657), 48–57.

Gross, E., & Burr, C. K. (2003). HIV counseling and testing in pregnancy. *New Jersey Medicine, 100*(Suppl. 9), 21–26.

Gruskin, S., Ahmed, S., & Ferguson, L. (2008). Provider-initiated HIV testing and counseling in health facilities--what does this mean for the health and human rights of pregnant women? *Developing World Bioethics, 8*(1), 23–32.

Hanssens, C. (2007). Legal and ethical implications of opt-out HIV testing. *Clinical Infectious Diseases, 45*(Suppl. 4), s232–239.

Hardwicke, R., Malecha, A., Lewis, S. T., & Grimes, R. M. (2008). HIV testing in emergency departments: A recommendation with missed opportunities. *Journal of the Association of Nurses in AIDS Care, 19*(3), 211–218.

Haukoos, J., Hopkins, E., & Byyny, R. (2008). Patient acceptance of rapid HIV testing practices in an urban emergency department: Assessment of the 2006 CDC recommendations for HIV screening in health care settings. *Annals of Emergency Medicine, 51*(3), 303–309.

Hutchinson, A. B., Branson, B. M., Kim, A., & Farnham, P. G. (2006). A meta-analysis of the effectiveness of alternative HIV counseling and testing methods to increase knowledge of HIV status. *AIDS, 20*(12), 1597–1604.

Institute of Medicine, National Research Council (1999). Reducing the odds: Preventing perinatal transmission of HIV in the United States. Washington, DC: National Academy Press.

Koo, D. J., Begier, E. M., Henn, M. H., Sepkowitz, K. A., & Kellerman, S. E. (2006). HIV counseling and testing: Less targeting, more testing. *American Journal of Public Health, 96*(6), 962–964.

Kriebs, J. M., & Shannon, M. (2008). HIV counseling and testing in pregnancy. *Journal of Midwifery & Women's Health, 53*(3), 256–257.

Kurth A., Spielberg F., Severynen A., & Holt, D. (2007, July 22–27). *A randomized controlled trial of computer counseling to administer rapid HIV test consent and counseling in a public emergency department: Final results.* Paper presented at a meeting of the International AIDS Society, Sydney, Australia.

Liebert, M. A. (2008). U.S. not achieving HIV testing goals. *AIDS Patient Care and STDs, 22*(12).

Lindegren, M. L., Byers, R. H., Thomas, P., Davis, S. F., Caldwell, B., Roges, M., et al. (1999). Trends in perinatal transmission of HIV/*AIDS in the United States. Journal of American Medical Association, 282*(6), 531–538.

Mooney H. (2008). Nurses told to radically expand HIV test levels. *Nursing Times, 104*(48), 1.

Obermeyer, C. M., & Osborn, M. (2007). The utilization of testing and counseling for HIV: A review of the social and behavioral evidence. *American Journal of Public Health, 97*(10), 1763–1774.

Palella, F., Delaney, K., Moorman, A., Loveless, M., Fuhrer, J., Satten, A., et al. (1998). Declining morbidity and mortality among patients with advanced human immunodeficiency virus infection. *New England Journal of Medicine, 338,* 853–860.

San Antonio-Gaddy, M., Richardson-Moore, A., Burstein, G. R., Newman, D. R., Branson, B. M., & Birkhead, G. S. (2006). Rapid HIV antibody testing in the New York state anonymous HIV counseling and testing program: Experience from the field. *Journal of Acquired Immune Deficiency Syndrome, 43*(4), 446–450.

Shamos, S. J., Mettenbrink, C. J., Subiadur, J. A., Mitchell, B. L., & Rietmeijer, C. A. (2008). Evaluation of a testing-only "express" visit option to enhance efficiency in a busy STI clinic. *Sexually Transmitted Diseases, 35*(4), 336–340.

Shrestha, R. K., Clark, H. A., Sansom, S. L., Song, B., Buckendahl, B., Calhourn, C. B., et al. (2008). Cost-effectiveness of finding new HIV diagnoses using rapid HIV testing in community-based organizations. *Public Health Reports, 123*(0), 94–100.

Sobo, E., Bowman, C., Halloran, J., Asch, S., Goetz, M. B., & Gifford, A. (2008). "A routine thing": Clinician strategies for implementing HIV testing for at-risk patients in a busy healthcare organization (and implications for implementation of other new practice recommendations). *Anthropology & Medicine, 15*(3), 213–225.

Tesoriero, J. M., Battles, H. B., Heavner, K., Leung, S. Y., Nemeth, C., Pulver, W., et al. (2008). The effect of name-based reporting and partner notification on HIV testing in New York state. *American Journal of Public Health, 98*(4), 728–735.

U.S. Food and Drug Administration. (2008). *Testing yourself for HIV-1, the virus that causes AIDS.* Retrieved January 29, 2009, from www.fda.gov/CbER/infosheets/hiv-home2.htm.

Vernillo, A. T., & Caplan, A. L. (2007). Routine HIV testing in dental practice: Can we cross the Rubicon? *Journal of Dental Education, 71*(12), 1534–1539.

White, D. A., Scribner, A. N., Schulden, J. D., Branson, B. M., & Heffelfinger, J. D. (2008). Results of a rapid HIV screening and diagnostic testing program in an urban emergency department. *Annals of Emergency Medicine,* [Epub ahead of print]. Abstract available online at http://www.annemergmed.com/article/S0196-0644(08)01844-1/abstract

Wolf, L. E., Donoghoe, A., & Lane T. (2007). Implementing routine HIV testing: The role of state law. *PLoS ONE, 2*(10).

Wynia, M. K. (2006). Routine screening: Informed consent, stigma and the waning of HIV exceptionalism. *American Journal of Bioethics, 6*(4), 5–8.

Yeatman, S. E. (2007). Ethical and public health considerations in HIV counseling and testing: Policy implications. *Studies in Family Planning, 38*(4), 271–278.

Zetola, N. M., Grijalva, C. G., Gertler, S., Hare, C. B., Kaplan, B., Dowling, T., et al. (2008). Simplifying consent for HIV testing is associated with an increase in HIV testing and case detection in highest risk groups, San Francisco January 2003–June 2007. *PLoS ONE, 3*(7).

3 The HIV Disease Trajectory

CARL A. KIRTON

INTRODUCTION

Infection with the human immunodeficiency virus (HIV) induces defects in the cell-mediated and humoral responses of the human host, thus rendering the host susceptible to opportunistic infections and neoplasms. The pathogenesis of HIV infection is highly complex but is essential knowledge for understanding the impact of this virus on the host's immune system and the development of treatments designed to impair viral replication and support immunologic recovery. Since the discovery of the disease in 1981, much has been learned about the natural history of HIV, the pathogenesis of HIV infection, and how therapy can impair the virus and restore host immunity. The purposes of this chapter are to summarize the current knowledge pertaining to the pathogenesis of HIV infection, to describe the natural history of HIV disease, and to provide an overview of HIV-related diseases and conditions.

CHARACTERISTICS OF HIV
Classification

HIV is a retrovirus. It is a member of the subfamily of retrovirus called lentivirus, one of the slow viruses of the *Retroviridae* family. (Other lentiviruses include the simian virus [SIV] and the feline immunodeficiency virus [FIV].) There are two known types of HIV viruses, HIV-1 and HIV-2. HIV-1 was first discovered in 1984, three years after the

71

first cases of AIDS were reported, followed in 1986 by the discovery of HIV-2 in West African AIDS patients. Both types are capable of causing disease in the human host, and the manifestations of disease caused by HIV-1 and HIV-2 are clinically indistinguishable. On a structural level, HIV-1 and HIV-2 have important genetic differences, primarily in the envelope gene (discussed below). HIV-1 is the predominate retrovirus seen worldwide, and HIV-2 is mainly seen in a few West African countries. Of the fewer than 68 cases of HIV-2 detected in the United States. from 1996 to 2006, all were in persons born in Africa or India (Kumar & Selik, 2007).

HIV-1

HIV-1 can be further subclassified into three groups: the "major" group M, the "outlier" group O, and the "new" group N. More than 90% of HIV-1 infections belong to HIV-1 group M (Spira et al., 2003). Group O appears to be restricted to west-central Africa; and group N, discovered in 1998 in Cameroon, is extremely rare. The viral envelope of group M is so diverse that there are at least nine genetically distinct subtypes (or clades) of HIV-1: subtypes A, B, C, D, F, G, H, J, and K. Occasionally, two viruses of different subtypes can meet in the cell of an infected person and mix together their genetic material to create a new hybrid virus. Many of these new strains do not survive for long, but those that infect more than one person are known as circulating recombinant forms (CRF). For example, the CRF A/B is a mixture of subtypes A and B. The HIV-1 subtypes and CRFs are distributed throughout the world, with the most widespread being subtypes A and C. Chapter 1 discusses the epidemiology of HIV in greater detail.

HIV-2

While HIV-1 is found around the world, the prevalence of HIV-2 is highest in West Africa. HIV-2 is believed to have first infected humans as early as the 1940s, jumping from sooty mangabeys to humans (zoonosis) as a result of bush meat hunting and slaughtering. Countries where HIV-2 is common include Cape Verde, Côte d'Ivoire (Ivory Coast), Gambia, Guinea-Bissau, Mali, Mauritania, Nigeria, Sierra Leone, Benin, Burkina Faso, Ghana, Guinea, Liberia, Niger, São Tomé, Senegal, and Togo. HIV-2 is also found in Angola and Mozambique. HIV-2 has a lower transmission rate and a less pathogenic course. When the genetic structures of

HIV-1 and HIV-2 are examined there is a 40% to 50% similarity. The differences between the two strains are discussed below (Levy, 2009).

VIRAL STRUCTURE AND GENETIC MATERIAL
HIV Structure

The HIV internal virus environment consist of two basic components: (1) a core of nucleic acid, called the genome, which contains two copies of single-stranded RNA, and (2) a protein component that surrounds the genome called a p24 capsid. The genome carries the genetic information of the virus, while the p24 capsid gives the virus its shape and offers protection to the genome. The outer shell of the virus is known as the viral envelope. The inner surface of the virus's envelope is coated by p17 protein. Embedded in the envelope is an outer protruding cap glycoprotein (gp) 120 and a stem gp41. The surface glycoprotein of enveloped virus plays a critical role in the initial events of viral infection, mediating virion attachment to cell and fusion of the viral and cellular membranes (Levy, 2007). Figure 3.1 depicts the organization of the HIV-1 virion.

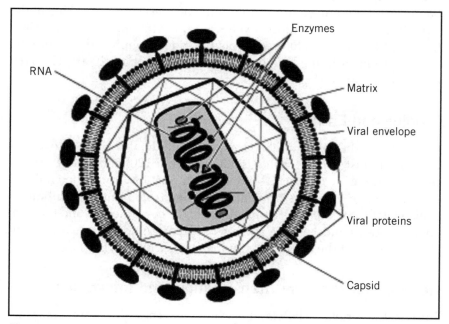

Figure 3.1 Structure of the human immunodeficiency virus.
Source: National Institutes of Health, National Human Genome Research Institute.

HIV Genetics

The HIV-1 genome is composed of nine genes (*gag, pol, vif, vpr, vpu, tat, rev, env nef*). The genes of HIV can be classified into three classes based on their function. There are structural proteins (Gag, Pol, and Env), regulatory proteins (Tat and Rev), and accessory proteins (Vpu, in HIV-1 only; Vpx, in HIV-2 only; Vpr, Vif, and Nef).

HIV LIFE CYCLE
HIV Attachment

HIV preferentially infects cells that express CD4 receptors and coreceptors (CCR5 and/or CXCR4); CD4 alone is insufficient to permit the entry of HIV-1. These target cells include dendritic cells, T-cells, and macrophages and are present in rectal, vaginal, penile, and oral mucosa, the most common sites for HIV infection (Turville et al., 2003). Dendritic cells (DC) play a major role in HIV transmission as they appear to be one of the first cell types infected after sexual transmission of HIV. Biologically, dendritic cell are antigen-presenting cells, which are important cells for initiating a primary immune response and trafficking of the virus to lymph nodes. Alternatively, HIV may be entered directly into the bloodstream and is filtered through regional lymph nodes where the virus reproduces in the lymph nodes (Grossman et al., 2006). The HIV life cycle is displayed in Figure 3.2.

Binding and Entry

On entry in the subepithelial compartment, HIV-1 entry into target cells is a multistep process that is initiated by gp120 binding to the CD4 receptor, usually CCR5 or CXCR4. This formation brings the viral and cell membrane into close proximity, allowing fusion of the membranes. Following fusion, the virus enters the cell, the core uncoats, and the core contents (two stands of RNA and reverse transcriptase) are released into the cytoplasm of the target cell (Sudharshan & Biswas, 2008).

Reverse Transcriptase, Translocation, and Integration

Reverse transcriptase (RT) is an enzyme that acts with a second enzyme, RNAse, to copy the viral RNA into DNA. The RT enzyme transcribes the two RNA strands into two stands of DNA, while the RNAse separates

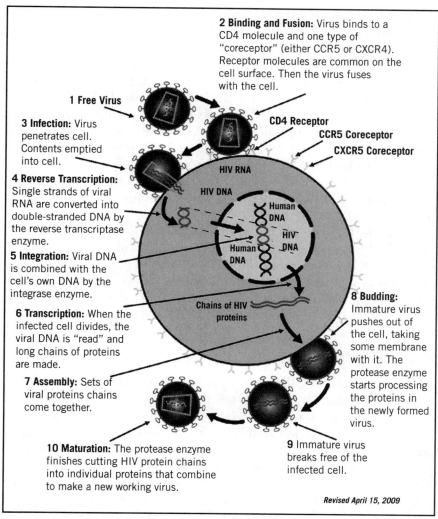

2 Binding and Fusion: Virus binds to a CD4 molecule and one type of "coreceptor" (either CCR5 or CXCR4). Receptor molecules are common on the cell surface. Then the virus fuses with the cell.

1 Free Virus

3 Infection: Virus penetrates cell. Contents emptied into cell.

CD4 Receptor

CCR5 Coreceptor

CXCR5 Coreceptor

4 Reverse Transcription: Single strands of viral RNA are converted into double-stranded DNA by the reverse transcriptase enzyme.

HIV RNA

HIV DNA

Human DNA

HIV DNA

Human DNA

5 Integration: Viral DNA is combined with the cell's own DNA by the integrase enzyme.

6 Transcription: When the infected cell divides, the viral DNA is "read" and long chains of proteins are made.

Chains of HIV proteins

8 Budding: Immature virus pushes out of the cell, taking some membrane with it. The protease enzyme starts processing the proteins in the newly formed virus.

7 Assembly: Sets of viral proteins chains come together.

10 Maturation: The protease enzyme finishes cutting HIV protein chains into individual proteins that combine to make a new working virus.

9 Immature virus breaks free of the infected cell.

Revised April 15, 2009

Figure 3.2 HIV life cycle. Source: AIDS InfoNet.

the DNA copies from the RNA. Reverse transcriptase sometimes makes mistakes reading the RNA sequence. The result is that not all viruses produced in a single infected cell are alike; but, rather, the process results in a variety of subtle molecular differences in the viruses' surface coat and enzymes. These molecular differences in surface coats create obstacles to vaccine production because vaccines are designed to produce antibodies that bind to very specific viral surfaces (Levy, 2007).

The double-stranded DNA, along with the gag proteins and integrase, is transported across the cell's nuclear pore and into the nucleus. This movement is mediated by the gag proteins. On entry into the nucleus, the integrase enzyme trims the viral DNA, cuts the host cell chromosomal DNA, and inserts the viral DNA into the host's chromosome. When HIV is integrated in the host DNA, the HIV is known as a provirus. The genes of the HIV are located in the central region of the proviral DNA, and these genes are flanked at both ends by long terminal repeats (LTRs). They are "sticky ends," which are used to insert the HIV genome into host DNA. They also act as promoter/enhancers. When integrated into the host genome, they influence the cell machinery that transcribes DNA, to alter the amount of transcription that occurs (Grigorov et al., 2005).

Once the HIV proviral DNA is integrated into the cell's chromosomal DNA, viral replication may enter a restricted, latent phase, depending on the state of activation of the infected cell. Activation stimuli, such as opportunistic pathogens or immunization induce the elaboration of cytokines that promote proviral transcription and subsequent viral replication (McMichael & Rowland-Jones, 2001).

Viral Transcription

On cellular activation, the provirus is transcribed into strands of RNA. Some of the strands are sliced by cellular enzymes to become messenger RNA (mRNA) that serves as the template for the synthesis of new virus particles. The strands left unspliced are the genomic RNA that will be packaged in the core of the new viral particles (Stine, 1997). Following proviral transcription, the Rev protein binds to the RNA transcripts and delivers them to ribosomes in the cytoplasm. At the ribosome, the mRNA is translated to polyproteins that will serve as the structural and regulatory protein of new virus particles. Under the influence of the Gag protein, the viral polyproteins are assembled in a long chain. Before these proteins become functional, they must be cut from the longer polypeptide chain. Viral protease cuts the long chain into its individual proteins (Stine, 1997).

Viral Synthesis and Budding

The viral proteins accumulate at the plasma membrane, and the two genomic RNA copies become encapsidated by the gag proteins. The viral particles begin to bud from the host cell and acquire their lipid envelopes from the plasma membrane. The HIV particles break out of the host cells, collecting a membrane with gp120 receptors in it as they leave (Stine, 1997)

EARLY VIROLOGIC EVENTS

Following acute infection, HIV-1 RNA can be measured in the plasma in virtually all infected people. Soon after infection, rapid virus production, unopposed by an effective host immune response, results in plasma viremia of 10^6 to 10^7 HIV-1 RNA copies per milliliter. Each day as many as 10 billion virus particles are produced by HIV-infected cells (Ho, Neumann, & Perelson, 1995). During acute infection, HIV is rapidly disseminated to the lymph node by infected macrophages, resting CD4 cells, activated CD4 cells, and dendretic cells. The function of the lymphoid organs is to filter and trap invading pathogens and present them to immune competent cells. In early-stage HIV disease, the virus is trapped on the follicular dendritic cell (FDC) network of the germinal centers of lymphoid tissue. CD4 cells that migrate into the area to provide help in the germinal center are susceptible to infection by these virions. In the early stage of disease, the FDC network is relatively intact. Over time, the lymphoid tissue begins to involute, and early degeneration of FDCs is observed. The trapping ability of these FDCs is compromised. In advanced-stage disease, there is dissolution of the FDC network; virus can no longer be effectively trapped and spills over readily into the circulation. At this stage, there is loss of HIV-specific immune responses as well as loss of the ability to respond to other pathogens, and profound immunosuppression ensues (Levy, 2007).

EARLY IMMUNLOGIC EVENTS
CD4 Cells: Lymphocyte Dynamics

T lymphocytes fall into two categories: antigen-naïve ("naïve") and antigen-experienced ("memory") cells. Memory cells can further be classified as "central" memory cells and "effector" memory cells. The former are recirculated through blood and lymphatic fluids to secondary lymphatic tissue and the latter, once they leave the lymphatic tissues, do not have the ability to recirculate. The first phase of HIV infection (the first few weeks after HIV transmission) is characterized by rapid and massive directly HIV-mediated loss of "effector" memory CD4 T helper cells, which express CD4 and CCR5 coreceptors. Acute infection does not efficiently target resting central and memory-naïve T-cells, which do not significantly express the CCR5 coreceptor. It is not yet known whether this rapid effector cell depletion or a direct influence of HIV virons and viral gene protein next trigger both a humoral and a cellular immune response against HIV infection (McMichael & Rowland-Jones, 2001).

Cellular Immune Response

During primary infection and normally prior to seroconversion, activation of HIV-1–specific cytotoxic CD8+ T lymphocytes (CTL) occurs to control viral replication. The CTL response is the most important and the most effective immune system response in controlling viral replication. There are various mechanisms by which CTL-mediated virus inhibition occurs. The first mechanism is to directly lyse infected cells before any new virus are produced. The second mechanism is the interaction of Fas ligand (FasL) on the CTL surface with Fas molecules on target cells resulting in apoptotic lysis of infected cells. The third mechanism occurs through the ability of CTL to bind to HIV-1 infected cells and to release noncytotoxic antiviral acting compounds (also called soluble factors) such as interferon-alpha and chemokines. Soluble factors compete with HIV-1 for the CCR5 coreceptor and have shown to be capable of inhibiting infection of CD4 T lymphocytes (Wagner, 1998; Yang et al., 1997). The pivotal role of specific CTL for the control of viral replication is supported by the observation that individuals infected with HIV and without any significant disease progression (see following discussion) frequently show extraordinary strong qualitative and quantitative HIV-1–specific CTL response.

Despite the presence of a robust cellular immune response in most HIV-infected individuals, disease progression typically occurs. Several mechanisms have been suggested to explain the inability of HIV-1–specific CTL to suppress and eradicate HIV over the long term: downregulation of HLA class I molecules (Collins et al., 1998); HIV's ability to mutate to variants that escape CTL detection; sequestration of the virus to protected compartments (e.g., brain); switch of the virus to CXCR4 receptor; upregulation of the fas ligand, causing apoptoptosis of the CTL (McMichael & Phillips, 1997). Additionally, the cellular immune response is dependent on the presence of HIV-1–specific helper CD4 cells, which in HIV-1 infection may be infected and depleted in early infection, resulting in the progressive loss of an effective CTL response.

Humoral Immune Response

The contribution of specific humoral immune response appears to play a minor role in controlling HIV-1 infection. Neutralizing antibodies are generally not detected during acute infection and appear only after the drop of initial viremia. Early neutralizing antibodies tend to be of low titers, are not present in all patients, and are only able to neutralize a limited range of HIV isolates. Therefore the contribution of HIV-1–specific humoral response in limiting disease during the acute phase of infection is still a matter of debate. HIV-1–specific antibodies, however, play a key role in the removal of virus from circulation, by sequestering viruses as immune complexes in the follicular dendritic cells network of the lymph node (Cao & Walker, 2000).

CHRONIC IMMUNE SYSTEM ACTIVATION

Chronic immune system activation is characterized by an excessive/aberrant immune activation and is the known to be the driving force behind for HIV-associated immune dysfunction (Sodora & Silvestri, 2008). The period of chronic immune system activation is marked by a reduction of viral replication from a peak to a set level; this stage is often thought of as the chronic phase of HIV infection. The exact mechanism behind this generalized immune activation and transition from acute to chronic phase transition has yet to been determined, and it is now widely accepted that persistent immune activation has a central role in driving progression from HIV to AIDS. Historically, some scientists thought that CD4 cell loss leading to AIDS was a result of the immune system's homestatic responses to keep up with the rate of loss of CD4 cells. This model, however, was overly simplistic and was challenged by the recognition that chronic immune system activation and dysfunction is present to chronic illness (Levy, 2009).

The chronic immune activation state is characterized by (1) increased frequency of CD4 cells expressing activation markers; (2) increased production of proinflammatory cytokines; and (3) increased turnover of T and B lymphocytes, NK cells, and accessory cells. Why HIV infected individuals are unable to effectively control the level of immune activation and why it does not resolve are unknown and continue to be investigated (Appay & Sauce, 2008).

Why is the HIV-induced immune activation so disruptive to the immune system? Because HIV is known to replicate more efficiently in activated CD4 T lymphocytes, chronic immune activation is probably instrumental in sustaining viral replication by providing available targets for HIV replication. In this context, the preferential activation, infection, and killing of HIV-specific CD4 T cells are probably detrimental because these processes result in the loss of CD4 T cell help, potentially contributing to the exhaustion/failure of CD8-mediated cytotoxic T lymphocytes' responses to the virus. Another consequence of HIV-associated chronic immune activation that may have negative consequences in the long term is the expansion of activated "effector" T (TE) cells of both CD4 and CD8 lineages. The expansion of a pool of fast-replicating but short-lived CD4 TE cells may indirectly facilitate CD4 T cell depletion. First, the expansion of CD4 TE cells may come at the expense of the naïve and memory T cell pools. A continuous drain from these pools could, in turn, result in a reduced capacity of the immune system to generate primary and memory responses to antigens. Chronic immune activation may also result in the proliferative senescence of the T cell pool, particularly at the level of CD4 central memory T cells. Second, expansion of activated TE cells may be accompanied by the production of proinflammatory and proapoptotic cytokines that complete the vicious cycle sustaining the generalized immune activation associated with pathogenic HIV infections. Third, the chronic proinflammatory environment also has multiple suppressive effects at different levels. HIV interferes with the function of several immune cell types, such as B cells, NK, dendritic cells, and monocytes, and may impair the regenerative capacity of the immune system at the levels of bone marrow, thymus, and lymph nodes (Grossman et al., 2006). Expansion of our understanding of the mechanism and causes immune system activation is important and could represent an important therapeutic strategy against control of immune dysfunction that accompanies HIV infection.

THE STAGES OF HIV DISEASE

Primary Infection (or Acute Infection)

Primary (or "acute") HIV infection is the first stage of HIV disease, typically lasting only a week or two, when the virus first establishes itself in the body. Symptoms, typically of a flulike nature, occur in 50 to 90% of patients during this period. These symptoms, which usually last no more than several days, might include fevers, chills, night sweats, myalgias and arthralgias, pharyngitis, and rashes (Kahn & Walker, 1998; Perlmutter, Glaser, & Oyugi, 1999). Because primary HIV infection may resemble infectious mononucleosis, influenza, severe streptococcal pharyngitis, viral hepatitis, toxoplasmosis, or even secondary syphilis, a diagnosis of HIV infection may be missed.

Blood taken during the acute phase of HIV infection may show lymphopenia and thrombocytopenia. The CD4 count usually remains normal during this period. The HIV-1 antibody tests will often be negative, as they do not become positive until antibodies are produced in response to the infection. (Also see Chapter 2). HIV-1 RNA level (viral load) may be measured by polymerase chain reaction (PCR), which is 95 to 98% sensitive for HIV. This test become positive within two weeks of infection (depending on the testing method used) and is often used to diagnosis acute infection. During the symptomatic phase of acute HIV infection, the viral RNA shows in excess of 50,000 copies per mL. If viral RNA quantification is not available, a serum or plasma p24 antigen test may be used to detect viral infection before the appearance of HIV antibodies.

Seroconversion

The term *seroconversion* refers to the period of time when an HIV-infected person's immune system responds to the infection by producing antibodies to the virus. Most people develop antibodies within three months after infection, and in rare cases it may take up to six months for antibodies to appear. If the HIV-1 antibody test (ELISA) is done before seroconversion is complete, it may give a false-negative result because sufficient antibodies have not yet been developed. A three-month window period between infection and production of antibodies is normal for most of the population. Blood taken during the seroconversion phase of HIV infection may show various CD4 cell counts levels. The typical pattern is for the CD4 cell count to remain within normal levels, and in some cases the CD4 cell count can decrease to levels where the patient is severely immunocompromised. The HIV-1 antibody tests (ELISA and Western blot test) will be positive. The quantitative plasma HIV-1 RNA level (viral load) now declines after surging to extreme highs during the period of acute infection.

The Asymptomatic Stage (or Chronic HIV Infection)

After seroconversion, most people infected with HIV continue to look and feel completely well for long periods, usually for many years. Although this period is characterized by relative wellness and few symptoms, HIV is still very active (see preceding discussion of chronic immune system activation) and is continuing to weaken the immune system during this stage. In the absence of treatment the viral load is maintained at a relatively stable level (called the set point), generally below 20,000 copies per mL, and the CD4 cell count will slowly decline each year in most infected persons. The set point is commonly used to determine the risk for disease progression; individuals with higher set points are at higher risk for faster disease progression (Kelley, Barbour & Hecht, 2007). In the absence of treatment, this stage can last ten years or longer.

HIV Symptomatic Disease

When the immune system is compromised by HIV infection, many people begin to experience HIV disease symptoms, often mild or subtle in nature. Typical problems include oral or vaginal thrush, recurrent herpetic eruptions on the mouth or genital areas, fevers, diarrhea, and weight loss. These problems often lead to an initial HIV diagnosis. In the absence of treatment during this period, the viral load may remain stable; but typically the viral load will increase, and the CD4 cell count may decline from the value seen during the asymptomatic period. While there is still some disagreement among practitioners and researchers, increasing evidence suggests that individuals with symptomatic disease should be offered antiretroviral therapy at any CD4 cell count (Kitahata et al, 2009; Sax & Baden, 2009).

AIDS

According to the Centers for Disease Control and Prevention (CDC, 2008), laboratory-confirmed HIV infection must be present before a diagnosis of AIDS can be given:

> For adults and adolescents (aged ≥13 years), the case definitions for HIV infection and AIDS have been revised into a single case definition for HIV infection that includes AIDS and incorporates the HIV infection classification system. Laboratory-confirmed evidence of HIV infection is now required to meet the surveillance case definition for HIV infection, including stage 3 HIV infection (AIDS). Diagnostic confirmation of an AIDS-defining condition alone [See Table 3.1] without laboratory-confirmed evidence of HIV infection, is no longer sufficient to classify an adult or adolescent as HIV infected for surveillance purposes. The 2007 World Health Organization (WHO) revised surveillance case definition for HIV infection also requires laboratory confirmation of HIV infection.

Table 3.1

AIDS-DEFINING CONDITIONS

- Bacterial infections, multiple or recurrent*
- Candidiasis of bronchi, trachea, or lungs
- Candidiasis of esophagus†
- Cervical cancer, invasive§
- Coccidioidomycosis, disseminated or extrapulmonary
- Cryptococcosis, extrapulmonary
- Cryptosporidiosis, chronic intestinal (>1 month's duration)
- Cytomegalovirus disease (other than liver, spleen, or nodes), onset at age >1 month
- Cytomegalovirus retinitis (with loss of vision)†
- Encephalopathy, HIV related
- Herpes simplex: chronic ulcers (>1 month's duration) or bronchitis, pneumonitis, or esophagitis (onset at age >1 month)
- Histoplasmosis, disseminated or extrapulmonary
- Isosporiasis, chronic intestinal (>1 month's duration)
- Kaposi sarcoma†
- Lymphoid interstitial pneumonia or pulmonary lymphoid hyperplasia complex*†
- Lymphoma, Burkitt (or equivalent term)
- Lymphoma, immunoblastic (or equivalent term)
- Lymphoma, primary, of brain
- *Mycobacterium avium* complex or *Mycobacterium kansasii*, disseminated or extrapulmonary†
- *Mycobacterium tuberculosis* of any site, pulmonary,†§ disseminated,† or extrapulmonary†
- *Mycobacterium*, other species or unidentified species, disseminated† or extrapulmonary†
- *Pneumocystis jirovecii* pneumonia†
- Pneumonia, recurrent†§
- Progressive multifocal leukoencephalopathy
- *Salmonella* septicemia, recurrent
- Toxoplasmosis of brain, onset at age >1 month†
- Wasting syndrome attributed to HIV

* Only among children aged <13 years. (CDC. 1994 Revised classification system for human immunodeficiency virus infection in children less than 13 years of age. MMWR 1994;43[No. RR-12].)
† Condition that might be diagnosed presumptively.
§ Only among adults and adolescents aged >13 years. (CDC. 1993 Revised classification system for HIV infection and expanded surveillance case definition for AIDS among adolescents and adults. MMWR 1992;41[No. RR-17].)

Source: Centers for Disease Control and Prevention. (2008). Appendix A: AIDS—Defining Conditions, 57(RR10), 9.

For children younger than 18 months of age, the CDC (2008) has concluded that " . . . children in this age group whose illness meets clinical criteria for the AIDS case definition but does not meet laboratory criteria for definitive or presumptive HIV infection are still categorized as HIV infected when the mother has laboratory-confirmed HIV infection".

Persons with laboratory-confirmed HIV infection frequently experience one or more "AIDS-defining conditions" (Table 3.1) (CDC, 2008).

During this phase the lymphoid tissue has mostly been replaced by fibroid tissue, and virus trapping by the lymphatic tissue is minimal or absent, resulting in an increased level of virus in the peripheral blood. The viral load is found to be markedly elevated, and there is marked deterioration of the immune system, resulting in a CD4 cell count that is often $< 200/mm^3$. Immune-compromised HIV-positive individuals may experience opportunistic infections (called "opportunistic" because they are caused by organisms that do not ordinarily induce illness in people with normal immune systems but take the "opportunity" to flourish in people with compromised immune systems). Some of the most common opportunistic infections include Pneumocystis jirovecii pneumonia (formerly known as pneumocystis carinii pneumonia [PCP]), Mycobacterium avium complex (MAC) disease, cytomegalovirus (CMV), toxoplasmosis, and candidiasis (see Table 3.2). In addition to the infectious diseases listed in Tables 3.1 and 3.2, persons with AIDS are at greater risk of developing a number of neoplasms, including Kaposi sarcoma, non-Hodgkin lymphoma, and invasive cervical cancer in women. Clinicians have also observed an increased risk other neoplasms (e.g., lung, liver, colorectal, and skin cancers) in persons with HIV/AIDS. The treatment of persons with AIDS having an opportunistic disease may be complicated; the outcome of such treatment is not readily predictable because some interventions are experimental in nature, and response to treatment varies widely. Over the years of the pandemic, a number of treatments have been developed to prevent and treat opportunistic infections in HIV-infected adults, adolescents, and children (CDC, National Institutes of Health, and the HIV Medicine Association of the Infectious Diseases Society, 2008a, 2009a). The CDC has also developed recommendations to help patients avoid exposure to or infection from opportunistic pathogens (CDC, 2009). In addition to these opportunistic conditions, HIV-related treatment with antiretroviral agents may predispose persons living with HIV/AIDS to other conditions (e.g., diseases stemming from HAART-associated hyperlipidemia and hyperglycemia). Without treatment, death usually occurs between two and five years after an AIDS diagnosis.

Table 3.2

OPPORTUNISTIC INFECTIONS IN THE IMMUNOCOMPROMISED HOST*

ORGANISM	PROBABLE INFECTION SITE	SIGNS AND SYMPTOMS	TREATMENT
Bacteria			
Neisseria meningitidis	Meningitis, pneumonia, purulent conjunctivitis, sinusitis, endocarditis, genital infections	Arthralgias and myalgias, hypotension, petichial rash, thrombosis, and hemorrhage	Penicillin or third- or fourth-generation cephalosporins
Corynebacterium diphtheriae	Upper respiratory, wounds, skin, occasional GI tract in immunocompromised host	Skin disorders, membranous covering on tissues	Vancomycin, penicillin, or erythromycin
Actinobacteria	Abscesses head and neck, thorax, or abdomen	Painful indurated swelling in mouth or neck, fistulas, bowel obstruction	Doxycycline, ceftriaxone, ampicillin, or erythromycin
Nocardia	Pulmonary infection, arthritis, cardiac, abdominal	Mucopurulent sputum, night sweats, fistulae	Cotrimoxazole for 12–18 months or high-dose sulfonamides, amikacin, ceftriaxone
Enterobacteriae	Diarrhea, colitis, bacteria	Watery diarrhea with blood or pus and abdominal cramping, blood infections, peritonitis of GI tract connection with abdomen, urinary tract infection with GI contamination	Ampicillin, third- or fourth-generation cepahlosporins, carbapenams, fluoroquinolone, azithromycin, cotrimoxazole
Mycobacterium tuberculosis	Cavitating lung lesions with apical localization most common; skin, liver, or renal tuberculosis	Persistent cough, lymphadenopathy, pleural effusions, intermittent fevers, night sweats, increased liver enzymes	Isoniazid with Pyridoxine or rifamycin or rifabutin
Mycobacterium avium-intracellulare	Milder pneumonitis than muscular tuberculo-sis, lymphadenitis	Gradual-onset fever, night sweats, anorexia, weight loss, diarrhea, weakness	None, oral 5-fluorocytosine, or possibly amphotericin B or liposomal amphotericin B

The reader should consult the latest treatment regimen for prescribing guideline.

(continued)

Table 3.2

OPPORTUNISTIC INFECTIONS IN THE IMMUNOCOMPROMISED HOST *continued*

ORGANISM	PROBABLE INFECTION SITE	SIGNS AND SYMPTOMS	TREATMENT
Fungi			
Candida albicans, tropicalis, and kruzei	Nails, skin, mucous membranes (oral, esophageal, vaginal, GU), bacteremia	Scaly, erythematous rash of skin, cream/yellow lacelike irregular lesion, white discharge	Topical antifungals, such as nystatin, azole antifungals, amphotericin B, amphotericin with or without 5- fluoro-cytosine, liposomal amphotericin, caspofungin
Aspergillus	Corrosive fungal ball in lungs, ear, cornea, sinuses, brain, or liver abscess	Cough, blood tinged sputum, red and swollen eyes	Amphotericin with or without 5-fluoro-cytosine, liposomal amphotericin, voriconazole, caspofungin
Cryptococcus neoformans	Pulmonary, meningitis	Rare pulmonary symptoms, frontal head ache and progressive neurological decline in meningitis	None, oral 5-fluoro-cytosine, or possibly amphotericin B or liposomal ampho-tericin B
Blastomyces	Bronchopneumonia, bacteremia	Viral pulmonary symp-toms, painless skin macules, abscesses	Amphotericin B or liposomal ampho-tericin B
Histoplasma capsulatum	Pneumonitis with other inflammatory reactions, pleural effusions, pericardi-tis, sinusitis	Fever, headache, chills, cough, chest pain, sore throat, GI distress	Itraconazaole or Amphotericin B or liposomal ampho-tericin B

Table 3.2

OPPORTUNISTIC INFECTIONS IN THE IMMUNOCOMPROMISED HOST *continued*

ORGANISM	PROBABLE INFECTION SITE	SIGNS AND SYMPTOMS	TREATMENT
Viruses			
Herpes simplex	Type I—gingivo-stomatitis, extra-oral lesions Type II—genital, extragenital. Either may disseminate; and, in patients who are immunocompromised, both types are found in any body location. Herpes simplex virus, pneumonia, and meningitis are not uncommon in the immunocompromised	Oral or extra-oral ulcers with raised outer border, extra-oral or genital vesicles with crusting and clear drainage. Occasional erythema. Paresthesias and pain in the area.	Valacyclovir, famciclovir, or acyclovir
Varicella-zoster virus	Unilateral skin eruptions around the thorax or vertically on legs or arms	Fever, malaise, severe deep pain, pruritis, paresthesias in the area involved even before the small red nodular lesions filled with fluid or pus are present. Lesions occur in a vertical fashion	Valacyclovir, famciclovir, or acyclovir
Cytomegalovirus	Lungs, liver, GI tract, retina, central nervous system. May occur less commonly as a septicemia	Mild, nonspecific flulike symptoms are typical of primary infection, although immunocompromised hosts exhibit localized infections present as respiratory dis-tress with diffuse chest X-ray infiltrates, diarrhea, elevated transaminases, organ specific dysfunction	Ganciclovir, acyclovir, cytomegolovirus immunoglobulin,
Respiratory synctival	Usually infects lower respiratory tract, but mild to moderate upper respiratory infection may occur	Low-grade fever, rhinitis, nonproductive cough, fatigue, myalgias, arthralgias are symptoms of primary infection.	Ribavirin with or without immunoglobulin

(continued)

Table 3.2

OPPORTUNISTIC INFECTIONS IN THE IMMUNOCOMPROMISED HOST *continued*

ORGANISM	PROBABLE INFECTION SITE	SIGNS AND SYMPTOMS	TREATMENT
Parasites			
Pneumocystis jirovecii	Primarily alveolar or parenchymal lung infection	Low-grade fever, cough, mild hypoxemia, dyspnea, minimal sputum, progressive infiltrates and respiratory symptoms	Trimethoprim-sulfamethoxazole, or alternatively pentamadine, pyrimethamine sulfa, or dapsone.
Legionellosis *(Legionella)*	Primarily diffuse interstitial pneumonia, possibly GI tract	High-spiking fevers, dyspnea, hypoxemia, large amounts of white sputum, wide-spread infiltrates on chest X-rays	Fluoroquinolones, azithromycin, erythromycin with or without rifampin, clarithromycin
Mycoplasma	Primarily cavitating pneumonia, although liver infections or bacteremia have been noted	High fever, cough with large amount of sputum, lobular pneumonia	Erythromycin, azithromycin, clarithromycin fluoroquinolone, doxycycline,
Toxoplasma gondii	Generalized infection, encephalitis, myocarditis, hepatitis, and pneumonitis	Fever and monolike syndrome, delirium, maculopapular rash (especially palms and soles of feet)	Trimethoprim-sulfamethoxazole Pyrimethamine with folinic acid and sulfadiazine, with clindamycin added in refractory patients
Cryptosporidium	GI tract, cholecystitis	Watery diarrhea, cramping abdominal pain, weight loss, anorexia, nausea, vomiting, malaise	No specific antimicrobials are known to be effective; antidiarrheal agents

Source: Centers for Disease Control and Prevention, National Institutes of Health & the HIV Medicine Association of the Infectious Diseases Society. (2009). Guidelines for prevention and treatment of opportunistic infections in HIV-infected adults and adolescents. Retrieved April 12, 2009, from www.cdc.gov/mmwr/pdf/rr/rr58e324.

Variations to HIV trajectory: Long-Term Nonprogressors

Crucial to our understanding of HIV pathogenesis is the study of individuals who remain healthy in the absence of antiretroviral therapy. Individuals who maintain normal CD4 T-cell counts in the absence of therapy have been described as "long-term nonprogressors" (LTNP) and represent less than 5% of infected individual (Madec et al., 2009). Because many factors may contribute to limiting disease progression, investigators have increasingly defined HIV controllers based on plasma HIV RNA levels rather than on CD4 counts or survival time alone. Two distinct groups of HIV controllers have been described based on plasma viral load measurements: those who maintain HIV RNA below detectable limits (i.e., <50 copies/mL), designated as "elite controllers," and those with persistently detectable yet low plasma HIV RNA (i.e., 50 to 2000 copies/mL), designated as "viremic controllers." Elite controllers are believed to represent <1% of the HIV-infected population (Levy, 2009).

LTNP represent an ideal population to study from genetic, immunologic, and viral perspectives in attempts to understand how to control or treat HIV infection. Factors that have been identified as contributing to long-term survival are (Levy, 2009):

- Infection with a low replicating virus or an attenuated HIV strain (nef-mutated) with a reduced replicative ability
- Strong cell-meditated anti-HIV immune response, particularly CD8+ cell cytotoxic and noncytotoxic antiviral activity
- Genetic background (e.g., receptor polymorphism—*HLA-B57; B27* and immune response)
- Lack of one CCR5 allele

CONCLUSION

Since the early years of the HIV epidemic, tremendous progress has been made in understanding host defense mechanisms, the behavior of the virus in the human host, and the mechanisms behind immune system dysfunction.. This information, taken together with current insights into the tremendous variability of the disease course, as well as host and viral factors that may influence clinical outcomes, offers promise for the development of new therapeutic strategies, including the discovery and use of vaccines.

REFERENCES

Appay, V., & Sauce, D. (2008). Immune activation and inflammation in HIV-1 infection: Causes and consequences. *Journal of Pathology, 214,* 231–241.

Cao, H., & Walker, B. (2000). Immunopathogenesis of HIV-1 infection. *Clinics in Dermatology, 18,* 401–410.

Centers for Disease Control and Prevention. (2008). Revised surveillance case definitions for HIV infection among adults, adolescents, and children aged <18 months and for HIV infection and AIDS among children aged 18 months to <13 years—United States, 2008. *Morbidity and Mortality Weekly Report, 57*(RR10), 1–8.

Centers for Disease Control and Prevention. (2009). Recommendations to help patients avoid exposure to or infection from opportunistic pathogens. *Morbidity and Mortality Weekly Report, 58,* 199–207. Retrieved April 6, 2009, from www.cdc.gov/mmwr/preview/mmwrhtml/rr58e324a2.htm.

Centers for Disease Control and Prevention, National Institutes of Health & the HIV Medicine Association of the Infectious Diseases Society. (2008). Guidelines for prevention and treatment of opportunistic infections among HIV-exposed and HIV-infected children. Retrieved April 3, 2009, from http://aidsinfo.nih.gov/contentfiles/Pediatric_OI.pdf.

Centers for Disease Control and Prevention, National Institutes of Health & the HIV Medicine Association of the Infectious Diseases Society. (2009). Guidelines for prevention and treatment of opportunistic infections in HIV-infected adults and adolescents. Retrieved April 3, 2009, from www.cdc.gov/mmwr/pdf/rr/rr58e324.pdf.

Collins, K., Chen, B., Kalams, S., Walker, B., & Baltimore, D. (1998). HIV-1 Nef protein protects infected primary cells against killing by cytotoxic T lymphocytes. *Nature, 391*(6665), 397–401.

Grigorov, B., Muriaux, D., Argirova, R. Darlix, J. (2005). New insights into human immunodeficiency virus - type 1 replication. *Biotechnolology & Biotechnology Equipment, 19,* 3–15.

Grossman, Z., Meier-Schellersheim, M., Paul, W. & Picker, L. (2006). Pathogenesis of HIV infection; what the virus spares is as important as what is destroys. *Nature Medicine, 12,* 289-295.

Ho, D., Neumann, A., & Perelson, A. (1995) Rapid turnover of plasma virions and CD4 lymphocytes in HIV-1 infection. *Nature, 373,* 123–126.

Kahn, J. O., & Walker, B. D. (1998). Acute human immunodeficiency virus type 1 infection. *New England Journal of Medicine, 339,* 33–39.

Kitahata, M. M., Gange, S. J., Abraham, A. G., Merriman, B., Saag, M. S., Justice, A. C., et al. (2009). Effect of early versus deferred antiretroviral therapy for HIV on survival. *New England Journal of Medicine, 360,* DOI: 10.1056/NEJMoa0807252.

Kelley, C., Barbour, J., & Hecht, F. (2007). The relation between symptoms, viral load, and viral load set point in primary HIV infection. *Journal of Acquired Immune Deficiency Syndromes, 45,* 445–448.

Kumar, L., & Selik, R. (2007, December 5–7). Epidemiology of HIV-2 infection in the U.S., 1996–2006. Paper presented at 2007 HIV Diagnostics Conference, Atlanta, GA. Retrieved April 15, 2009 from www.hivtestingconference.org/powerpoint/1_Kumar.pps#257,2, Outline.

Levy, J. (2007). *HIV and the pathogenesis of AIDS* (3rd ed.). Washington, DC: American Society of Microbiology.

Levy, J. (2009). HIV pathogenesis: 25 years of progress and persistent challenges. *AIDS, 23,* 147–160.

Madec, Y., Boufassa, F., Avettand-Fenoel, V., Hendou, S., Melard, A., Bouchert, S., et al. (2009). Early control of HIV-1 infection in long-term nonprogressors followed since diagnosis in the ANRS SEROCO/HEMOCO cohort. *Journal of Acquired Immune Deficiency Syndromes, 50,* 19–26.

McMichael, A., & Phillips, R. (1997) Escape of human immunodeficiency virus from immune control. *Annual Review of Immunology, 15,* 271–296.

McMichael, A., & Rowland-Jones, S (2001). Cellular immune response to HIV. *Nature, 410,* 980–987.

Perlmutter, B. L., Glaser, J. B., & Oyugi, S. O. (1999). How to recognize and treat acute HIV syndrome. *American Family Physician, 60,* 535–542, 545–546.

Sodora, D., & Silvestri, G (2008). Immune activation an AIDS pathogenesis. *AIDS, 22,* 439–446.

Sax, P., & Baden, L. (2009, April 1). When to start antiretroviral therapy—Ready when you are? *New England Journal of Medicine.* Retrieved April 15, 2009, from http://content.nejm.org/cgi/content/full/NEJMe0902713.

Spira, S., Wainberg, M., Loemba, H., Turner, D., & Brenner, B. (2003). Impact of clade diversity on HIV-1 virulence, antiretroviral drug sensitivity and drug resistance. *Journal of Antimicrobial Chemotherapy, 51,* 229–240.

Stine, G. J. (1997). *AIDS Update 1997.* Saddle River, NJ: Prentice Hall.

Sudharshan, S., & Biswas, J. (2008) Introduction and immunopathognesis of acquired immune deficiency syndrome. *Indian Journal of Ophthalmology, 56,* 357–362.

Turville, S., Wilkinon, J., Cameron, P., Dable, J., & Cunninghham, A. (2003). The role of dendritic cell C-type lectin receptors in HIV pathogenesis. *Journal of Leukocyte Biology, 74,* 710–718.

Wagner, L., Yang, O., Garcia-Zepeda, E., Ge, Y., Kalams, S., Walker, B., et al. (1998). Beta-chemokines are released from HIV-1-specific cytolytic T-cell granules complexed to proteoglycans. *Nature, 391*(6670), 908–911.

Yang O., Kalams, S., Trocha, A., Cao, H., Luster, A., Johnson, R., et al. (1997). Suppression of human immunodeficiency virus type 1 replication by CD8+ cells: Evidence for HLA class I-restricted triggering of cytolytic and noncytolytic mechanisms. *Journal of Virology, 71,* 3120–3128.

4

Ethical and Legal Dimensions of the HIV/AIDS Pandemic

JERRY D. DURHAM

The HIV/AIDS epidemic has created ethical dilemmas for infected persons, caregivers, and society as a whole. Early in the epidemic, Mills and associates (1986) summarized these dilemmas:

> For the individual, measures to control the spread of AIDS may invade privacy, constrain sexual conduct and procreation, and limit liberty. For the public, AIDS retrovirus infection continues to spread, especially among high-risk groups, and is often fatal . . . We therefore believe that AIDS poses the most profound issues of constitutional law and public health since the Supreme Court approved compulsory immunization in 1905 (Mills, Wofsy, & Mills, 1986, p. 931).

Over the course of the pandemic, policy makers in the United States and around the globe have addressed many of these ethical dilemmas by developing and implementing policies and laws that attempt to balance the rights of individuals affected by the epidemic with the interests of the broader community and the practice of public health. Many of these responses, in the words of Brandt (1986, 1988), have revealed this nation's deepest cultural, social, and moral values, serving as a kind of litmus test of America's humanity. A central ethical issue of the HIV/

93

AIDS pandemic is need to protect the individual rights of those with HIV infection while at the same time attending to the rights of those who not infected. Former U.S. Surgeon General Everett Koop (1988) noted presciently early in the pandemic that if America's leaders could balance individual freedom and public interest with fairness and understanding, ". . . we may give the world something as precious as the scientific breakthrough we all seek in prevention and treatment" (p. 311).

Early in the pandemic, the reactions of some segments of American society to HIV/AIDS were a source of concern to civil libertarians who feared that such reactions would lead to undue restrictions of infected individuals' liberties. In their book exploring ethics and public policy concerns generated by AIDS, Pierce and VanDeVeer (1988) pose two critical questions:

1 "When is it all right, if ever, to interfere with the capacity of competent people to direct their own lives?" and
2 "When is it permissible to infringe upon the liberties of others in order to protect them, presumably from themselves, and to protect society from them or their actions?"

Proposals such as mandatory HIV screening/testing and barring HIV-positive individuals from certain jobs, occupations, and activities interfere with the choices or acts of others and are thus ethically problematic. While many of these concerns have lessened over the course of the pandemic as HIV/AIDS has affected large numbers of persons around the world, thus becoming somewhat more "normalized" as a chronic health condition, nonetheless infringements on human liberty and human rights remain important ethical concerns.

Because HIV transmission arises mainly as a result of behaviors, beliefs about what constitutes permissible constraints on such behaviors have inevitably influenced decisions about permissible strategies and public policies to address HIV-related questions (Pierce & VanDeVeer, 1988). These decisions raise additional questions about beneficence, respect for persons, autonomy, intimacy, and privacy, to list only the most obvious ethical concerns. But the understanding and rational use of principles that help determine when it is ethically defensible to restrict the liberties of others are insufficient in the HIV pandemic. In the emotional climate attendant to the HIV epidemic, rational thought does not always prevail. As Rowland (1986, p. 44) has noted, "[the] power of prejudice can be chillingly greater than the power of logic."

BALANCING INDIVIDUAL RIGHTS WITH THE PUBLIC GOOD

Balancing individual rights with societal benefits has received considerable attention in America's legal system (Fairchild et al., 2007). For over 100 years jurists have sought to balance society's interest in controlling communicable disease against society's claim of liberty. Until the passage of the Fourteenth Amendment to the Constitution, however, Americans had little protection against the abuse of individual civil liberty (Merritt, 1986). However, since 1940 the courts have recognized that individuals have certain fixed rights—even when these endanger others (Merritt, 1986). Moreover, the courts have grown increasingly wary of medical experts' claim that certain persons are dangerous (e.g., the mentally ill) or that certain procedures are essential to the promotion of public health.

This key role of the courts was demonstrated in March 1998 when the U.S. Supreme Court held in *Bragdon v. Abbott* that HIV is impairment and, therefore, HIV-infected persons are covered by the Americans with Disabilities Act, which prohibits discrimination against persons with perceived or actual disabilities. In an earlier decision, *The School Board of Nassau County, Florida v. Arline*, the U.S. Supreme Court held that discrimination against a handicapped person, in this case a teacher with tuberculosis, on the basis of fears deriving from the handicap's contagious nature, violated the Federal Rehabilitation Act of 1973 (Banta, 1987). This decision was widely construed to apply to people with AIDS. The Supreme Court held in the Arline case that persons with a contagious disease may be covered by the Rehabilitation Act and that each such person needed to have an "individualized inquiry" to determine the workplace risk to others and whether reasonable accommodation was possible (Webber, 2007). Subsequent federal court decisions have supported this important case and have gone even further, generally holding that HIV infection also can be construed as a handicap, and thus these decisions afford greater protection for some individuals from discrimination (National Gay Rights Advocates & National Lawyers Guild AIDS Network, 1988).

According to Jayasuriya (1988), AIDS-related laws can be placed in three broad categories: product-related laws, behavior- and attitude-oriented laws, and institution-oriented laws. In the first category, product-related laws seek to protect supplies of products (e.g., semen, tissue, blood, condoms). In the second category, behavior- and attitude-oriented laws are aimed at reducing high-risk behaviors, making it an offense to engage in sex while infected; requiring compulsory screening, quarantine, and contact tracing; and providing for deportation and for the refusal of visas. Laws in this category generate the greatest controversy and are most likely to be challenged in court by individuals. In the third category, institution-oriented laws seek to promote research, education, counseling, and care of people with AIDS. Laws that prevent discrimination against HIV/AIDS may also be included in this category. Hamblin (1991) has articulated three models by which laws can be incorporated into HIV/AIDS policies:

- The traditional proscriptive model that penalizes certain forms of conduct;
- The protective model that upholds the rights and interests of those infected with HIV or at risk of infection; and
- The instrumental model that uses the law to effect changes in values and patterns of social interaction that lead to susceptibility to HIV infection.

Most of the laws, at least those in the United States, can be broadly classified into one or more of the categories proposed by Jayasuriya (1988) or Hamblin (1991).

The AIDS litigation Project's review of 600 cases of persons with HIV/AIDS in federal and state courts found that subsets of litigation involved HIV/AIDS in the public health and health care systems (Gostin & Webber, 1998). These cases related to testing and reporting; privacy and control of information about a person's HIV status, including the duty to warn and the right to know; physician standards of care in prevention and treatment; discrimination and access to health care; exclusion and isolation of HIV positive persons; the rights of persons living with HIV/AIDS (PLWH) in the areas of employment, disability benefits, housing, public accommodations, commercial establishments, and the military; and efforts by infected individuals to obtain needed public benefits. Federal and state laws address various areas of law and public policy including the following:

- Public health issues, e.g., state quarantine powers, restriction of sexually oriented commercial activities, legal restrictions to prevent transmission (such as mandatory testing);
- Criminal behaviors, e.g., intentional infection of another with HIV, criminal assault by PLWH, sodomy;

- Immigration;
- Prisons/jails, e.g., HIV testing of inmates, segregation of HIV-positive inmates, privacy rights, access to health care, and early release; and
- Schools and educational programs, e.g., curriculum content, condom distribution, and abstinence-only sex education programs, rights of HIV-positive students) (Webber, 2007).

Several law practices and centers specialize in providing legal services for PLWH. The Center for HIV Law and Policy in New York City, for example, lists a range of legal issues and concerns of PLWH for whom they provide services that address such area as advance directives and wills; insurance issues (e.g., HIPAA issues, insurance availability, policy rescission, discrimination in coverage, denial of claims, confidentiality of insurance-related information, and viatical settlements); blood, organ, and semen donation; confidentiality; family law (e.g., guardianship issues, powers of attorney, adoption issues, and HIV-positive parent's visitation rights); and racial justice. At least one U.S. HIV-related legal center, the HIV Law Project, also located in New York City, focuses on the legal needs of low-income PLWH, especially women, children, and the homeless. Because of court challenges to many laws, Jayasuriya (1988) believes that future laws will be carefully evaluated in terms of medical, scientific, and technological readiness and validity; constitutional, ethical, cultural, and social acceptability; political expediency; and economic feasibility.

In more recent years, much of the discussion around HIV-related law and public policy has focused on the human rights of PLWH (Gruskin & Tarantola, 2002; Patterson & London, 2002; Stone & Gostin, 2004; Tarantola, 2008 UNAIDS, 2007). According to Stone and Gostin (2004, p. 2):

> As the pandemic has progressed, it has become apparent that human rights law is relevant not only to the treatment of infected individuals but also to wider polices that influence vulnerability to HIV/AIDS, as populations that are discriminated against, marginalized, and stigmatized are at a greater risk of contracting the disease. A central tool in fighting the pandemic therefore must be to strengthen the recognition of the human rights of all people.

Patterson and London (2002) assert that human rights law can help shape responses to the HIV/AIDS pandemic by (1) providing a framework on which governments can formulate laws and policies integrating public health objectives and human rights; (2) providing a basis for nongovernment organizations to monitor governments' performance in their policies and programs to ensure that public health programs do not violate human rights; and (3) by speaking to the obligations of public health practitioners for protecting and promoting health at a population level.

Human rights flow from principles and standards derived from moral philosophy, which guided the Universal Declaration of Human Rights (UDHR) in 1948 in response to the atrocities of World War II (Tarantola, 2008). Other important treaties and conventions followed the UDHR and have further contributed to consensus on global justice and human rights, including:

- The Convention on the Elimination of All Forms of Racial Discrimination (United Nations, adopted in 1965)
- The International Covenant on Economic, Social and Cultural Rights (United Nations, adopted in 1966)
- The International Covenant on Civil and Political Rights (United Nations, created in 1966 and entered into force in 1976)
- The Covenant on Economic, Social and Cultural Rights (United Nations, Adopted in 1966 and entered into force in 1976)
- Declaration of Alma-Ata (International Conference on Primary Health Care, adopted in 1978)
- The Convention on the Elimination of All Forms of Discrimination against Women (United Nations, adopted in 1979)
- The Convention on the Rights of the Child (United Nations, adopted in 1989)
- The Commission on Human Rights (UNAIDS), *Protection of human rights in the context of human immunodeficiency syndrome (HIV) and acquired immunodeficiency syndrome (AIDS)* (United Nations Resolution, adopted in 1999)
- United Nations Declaration of Commitment on HIV/AIDS (United Nations, adopted in 2001)

A growing interest in international human rights has also been fostered by various movements of the 1960s, including the involvement of civil society in humanitarian health emergencies, which resulted in the creation of several nongovernment organizations (Tarantola, 2008). Other movements that promoted a growing interest in human rights included the U.S. civil rights movement, the feminist movement, and the gay rights movement. The crumbling of certain world ideologies in the late 1980s, which allowed for the rise of new paradigms to guide public policy and international relations, and the emergence of HIV/AIDS as a pandemic also played a role in the linkage of health and human rights at the end of the twentieth century (Tarantola, 2008).

Human rights "are broadly concerned with defining the relationship between individuals and the state" (Gruskin & Tarantola, 2002, p. 2). The first article of the UDHR provides the foundation for the articles that follow: "All human beings are born free and equal in dignity and rights. They are endowed with reason and conscience and should act towards one another in a spirit of brotherhood." With a focus on the rights and freedoms of all human beings, human rights include civil and political rights (e.g., freedom of expression) and social, cultural, and economic rights (e.g., right to health care and education). As international norms, human rights serve to protect people throughout the world from severe political, legal, and social abuses. Provisions for enforcement of international human rights treaties are generally weak, although some treaties do provide for complaints about a state's alleged violation of a treaty (Patterson & London, 2002). While many nations are unable to fulfill all rights immediately because of limited resources and other constraints, governments are publicly accountable for their actions vis-à-vis HIV/AIDS and have responsibilities at three levels:

- They must respect human rights;
- They must protect human rights;
- They must fulfill human rights (Gruskin & Tarantola, 2002; Tarantola, 2008).

International organizations such as Human Rights Watch and Amnesty International (founded in 1978 and 1961, respectively) have sought to defend and protect human rights around the world through such activities as research, advocacy, lobbying, and mass demonstrations. Still another human rights organization, Physicians for Human Rights (PHR), was founded in 1986 on the belief that "health professionals . . . are uniquely positioned to investigate the health consequences of human rights violations and work to stop them." In keeping with this belief, PHR "mobilizes health professionals to advance health, dignity, and justice and promotes the right to health for all."

According to UNAIDS (n.d., ¶.7,9,10), PLWH around the world should entitled to a number of human rights, including those in marginalized populations (e.g., sex workers, people who use drugs, prisoners). These human rights include the following:

- Right to nondiscrimination and equality before the law;
- Right to liberty, security of person and freedom from cruel, inhuman, and degrading treatment, including right not to be arrested and imprisoned on the basis of HIV status;
- Right to health, including right not to be denied health care or treatment on the basis of HIV status;
- Right to participate in public life, including participation in HIV policy formulation and implementation;
- Right to marry and found a family, regardless of HIV status;
- Right to education, i.e., right not to be thrown out of school on the basis of HIV status;
- Right to work, i.e., right not to be fired on the basis of HIV status;
- Right to social security, assistance, and welfare, i.e., right not to be denied these benefits on the basis of HIV status;
- Right to freedom of movement, regardless of HIV status; and
- Right to seek and enjoy asylum, regardless of HIV status.

In the course of implementing measures to ensure the health of the public, certain measures (e.g., those that seek to curb the spread of disease) may place restrictions on human rights. In limiting human rights to achieve a greater public good, the government is expected to meet the following "Siracusa Principles," promulgated by the U.N. Economic and Social Council, before implementing the restriction(s):

1   The restriction is provided for and carried out in accordance with the law;
2   The restriction is in the interest of a legitimate objective of general interest;
3   The restriction is strictly necessary in a democratic society to achieve the objective;
4   There are no less intrusive and restrictive means available to reach the same goal; and
5   The restriction is not imposed arbitrarily, i.e., in an unreasonable or otherwise discriminatory manner (Gruskin & Tarantola, 2002, p. 5).

In the early years of the pandemic, the HIV-related human rights concerns were focused on the rights of individuals, e.g., discrimination of PLWH. Over time, however, as HIV was linked to neglect and violation of human rights, which were seen as root causes of the epidemic, a greater emphasis was placed on the full range of social, political, and cultural factors that affect HIV/AIDS (Patterson & London, 2002). The three-day Millennium Summit of 150 world leaders, held in New York City in September 2000, signaled a new emphasis on economic and social rights as basic human rights.

In 2008, world leaders came together again to articulate the Millennium Development goals that aim by 2015 to implement an action plan that seeks to promote poverty reduction, education, maternal health, and gender equality and to combat child mortality, AIDS, and other diseases. These foci would seem to seek placing greater emphasis on economic security as a fundamental basis for human dignity while still maintaining the importance of geopolitical human rights. As a result of this shift, public health policies and organizations have begun to place greater emphasis on social and health care justice relative to the HIV/AIDS pandemic. For example, in recognition of the socioeconomic disparities that exist between resource-limited and resource-rich nations, several international efforts have been mounted to increase access to HIV-related medications and care (e.g., the Global Fund to Fight AIDS, Tuberculosis, and Malaria; the President's Emergency Plan for AIDS Relief [PEPFAR]; the Treatment Action Campaign [TAC]; and changes in drug pricing policies to allow for great access to antiretroviral therapy).

STIGMATIZATION AND BLAME

In the early years of the HIV/AIDS epidemic, the public's initial reaction to AIDS outweighed the real dangers to the general public. According to Herek (2005), "Early surveys of public opinion revealed widespread fear of the disease, lack of accurate information about its transmission, and willingness to support draconian public policies that would restrict civil liberties in the name of fighting AIDS" (pp. 121–122). HIV/AIDS-related stigma has been correlated with age (younger = less stigma), education level (less education = more stigma), personal contact with a PLWH (personally knowing someone with HIV/AIDS = less stigma), knowledge about HIV transmission (more knowledge = less stigma), and attitudes toward homosexuality (more favorable attitudes toward gays = less stigma) (Herek, 2005). While AIDS-related stigma has decreased since the pandemic first started, such stigma remains an important concern (Darrow et al., 2008; Parker & Aggleton, 2003). That HIV/AIDS-related stigma is a worldwide problem is documented by the dozens of presentations on this topic at the XVII International AIDS Conference held in Mexico City in 2008.

Because AIDS first appeared in this country among a group of persons that sociologists labeled as "pariahs," many came to believe that AIDS mirrored the moral defilement of its "victims." This stigmatized pariah status evolved because HIV/AIDS was viewed as a disease that was caused by a behavior or behaviors that were both avoidable and immoral; it was unalterable or degenerative, resulting in death; it was seen as contagious or placing others in harm's way (a result of an overestimation of HIV risk); and some PLWH had conditions that were repellant or upsetting with biomedical manifestations of disease, especially near the end of their lives. This social history of the disease led many persons having contact with individuals known to have AIDS to consciously or unconsciously engage in distancing behaviors, both verbal and nonverbal (e.g., avoidance), further reinforcing the stigmatized status and isolation of persons with AIDS. (Also see Chapter 11.)

While few caregivers, at least in the United States, now refuse to provide care for PLWH, many persons, especially early in the history of the pandemic, stigmatized PLWH as a result of homophobia, unrealistic fears of contagion, death anxiety, moral outrage, religious beliefs, and cultural and/or racial prejudice (Barrick, 1988; Brock, 1986; Clavreul, 1983; Douglas, Kalman, & Kalman, 1985; Pomerance & Shields, 1989). These negative attitudes and misconceptions, which stem from fears, perceptions about mode of infection, a lack of knowledge, and/or prejudicial beliefs, may also held by some caregivers and can present a formidable barrier to compassionate care of people with AIDS (D'Augelli, 1989; Douglas et al., 1985; Earl & Penney, 2003; Gerbert et al., 1989; Kalman, 1988; Li, Scott, & Li, 2008; Pomerance & Shields, 1989; Rondahl, Innala, & Carlson, 2003; Tyer-Viola, 2007; Watkins & Gray, 2006). Fear of AIDS stigma may affect HIV diagnosis and treatment. Some at-risk persons, out of concern for this stigma, may choose to avoid HIV testing and participation in risk-reduction education. Fear of AIDS stigma may also result in some HIV-positive persons entering treatment late or not adhering to prescribed treatment regimens (Fikremariam, 2004). These individuals may choose to keep their at-risk status or their HIV-positive status secret rather than endure blame, ridicule, shame, and ostracism, thereby placing others, including their sexual or drug-sharing partners, at risk of infection as well (Valdiserri, 2002; Vanable et al., 2006).

For the welfare of their patients and for their own mental well-being, health care workers should participate in programs to increase their knowledge of HIV/AIDS, reduce their AIDS anxiety and stigma, and deal with prejudicial feelings and beliefs (Beanet al., 1989). Multiple approaches have been implemented to reduce HIV/AIDS-related stigma (Klein, Karchner, & O'Connell, 2002). In their review of interventions to reduce HIV/AIDS-related stigma, Brown, Trujillo, and Macintyre (2001) concluded that, while stigma can't be completely eliminated, some interventions do reduce stigma. Adding at least one intervention, such as coping skills or counseling, to a knowledge-enhancement intervention can synergistically change attitudes and behaviors. The following stigma-reduction interventions have been implemented: information-based approaches (e.g., peer education, guided group discussions, and media advertisements); coping skill acquisition (e.g., role play, scripting, master imagery, and reframing/relaxing techniques); counseling approaches (e.g., one-on-one and support groups); and contact with affected groups (e.g., live testimonials, live interaction with PLWH, and visualization of being a PLWH) (Brown et al., 2001). Brown, Trujillo, and Macintyre (2001) also concluded that:

- Interventions in developing countries have tended to be community based, unlike those in the United States that are more individual oriented;
- Many intervention studies in developing countries were not rigorously evaluated, and few studies assessed sustained changes and attitudes over time; and
- Stigma-reduction interventions or combinations of such interventions have been shown to reduce stigma.

Although the general public has become increasingly informed about HIV/AIDS, a significant percentage of Americans still hold misconceptions about HIV transmission, prevention, and treatment (The public's knowledge and perceptions, 2006). Fear of contagion neither adequately explains nor justifies stigmatization of people with HIV/AIDS. Because Americans are increasingly knowledgeable about AIDS, what explains the hateful behaviors of some toward people with AIDS? Do they simply not trust the reassurances of scientists, government officials, and health experts about their own risk of becoming infected through casual contact? It is more likely that these individuals hold deeply prejudicial views about those groups of people who have been disproportionately affected by HIV (Pryor, 1988). Unfortunately, these prejudicial beliefs may impede conventional educational efforts to deal successfully with fear of AIDS. To the extent that these negative reactions are a function of symbolic factors, they are likely to persist even in the absence of fears about contagion.

Another factor influencing ethical decisions making is the Judeo-Christian heritage of most Americans, a tradition brimming with lessons of sin and punishment. In this tradition, blame may be heaped on those who, because they did bad things, became ill, and sometimes even on those having a special relationship with the ill (Sabatier, 1988). In this view, God punishes as a warning to others about the wages of sin. Those not accepting responsibility for or not in control of their behaviors are held accountable for the consequences. While some religions have moved away from this conservative perspective to a more postmodern worldview over the course of the HIV pandemic, still others continue to shun and even condemn the PLWH for their illness.

Gay people, who have been linked in the public's mind to the HIV pandemic from its onset, are often blamed for their orientation, as well as for their behaviors, and made to feel that this orientation is unnatural or, if seminormal, at least should not be acted on. Such thinking denies gay people the right to enjoy the same human potential as straight people, that is, the freedom to live sexual lives that reflect their natural orientation. This attitude of blame is also reflected in the dogma of some organized religions that follow the dictum of "hate the sin, love the sinner." This posture can be thought of as being tantamount to telling a person of color, "we hate the color of your skin, but we love you as a person." Those holding the "hate the sin, love the sinner" position believe they are being kind and following the teachings of their religion, but this thinking is all too telling of why so many gay people are estranged from organized religion in America. To be told that one's sexual orientation is unacceptable is, in the view of many gay people, to be told that they themselves are unacceptable. The price of acceptance, i.e., the denial of self, is a price too high for many to pay.

DISCRIMINATION AGAINST PEOPLE WITH HIV/AIDS

Former UNAIDS executive director Peter Piot and colleagues (2009) have recently noted that the international community underestimated "the extent to which stigma and discrimination—against people living with HIV/AIDS and those most vulnerable to it—would remain formidable obstacles to tackling AIDS" (p. 1). This discrimination, the authors say, has resulted in ostracism, violence, eviction, loss of employment, and restrictions on travel. HIV-related discrimination has been defined by UNAIDS (2007) as "the unfair and unjust treatment of an individual based on his or her real or perceived HIV status" (p. 9). Discrimination against persons living with HIV/AIDS results from the stigma associated with HIV/AIDS. As recently as 2003, UNAIDS (2003) reported that 40% of countries (including half of the countries in sub-Saharan Africa) had not adopted antidiscrimination laws to protect persons living with HIV/AIDS. Such discrimination serves as "roadblocks" to prevention, treatment, care, and support of PLWH (UNAIDS, 2007). Discrimination can take many forms, including travel restrictions (several dozen countries have travel restrictions in place for HIV-positive people [U.N. Secretary, 2008]), employment discrimination, refusal to provide care, housing discrimination, discrimination in public accommodations, and bullying (UNAIDS, 2000b). HIV-related stigma and its resulting discrimination disproportionately affect socially vulnerable groups (e.g., sex workers and men who have sex with men), including women and girls who may have fewer coping resources and may be more susceptible to violence (UNAIDS, 2007).

Some of the key causes of the discrimination resulting from stigma include a lack of awareness and knowledge of the harmful effects of stigma/discrimination, fear of acquiring HIV infection from everyday contact with infected persons, and linking HIV-infected persons to behaviors considered immoral or improper (UNAIDS, 2007). UNAIDS (2007) has endorsed several promising approaches to reduce stigma/discrimination: empowerment of people living with HIV; provision of updated education about HIV; and fostering activities that bring direct or indirect interaction between PLWH and key audiences. At the national and international levels, UNAIDS (2007) has advocated for a range of actions that could potentially reduce stigma/discrimination.

Important legal decisions have established that persons with HIV/AIDS are legally disabled and are protected by both state and federal laws prohibiting discrimination on the basis of handicap (e.g., the Americans with Disabilities Act; the Rehabilitation Act of 1973; the Federal Civil Rights Acts of 1964 and 1991). The U.S. Equal Employment Opportunity Commission (EEOC) is responsible for enforcing all employment-

Table 4.1

AIDS/HIV ANTI-DISCRIMINATION RESOURCES

- AIDS Legal Referral Panel (ALRP): www.alrp.org/article.php?list=type&type=4
- American Civil Liberties Union: www.aclu.org/
- Department of Justice (ADA Enforcement): www.ada.gov/enforce.htm
- Gay and Lesbian Advocates & Defenders:
  www.glad.org/work/initiatives/c/civil-rights-project/
- International Gay and Lesbian Human Rights Commission (IGLHRC):
  www.iglhrc.org/cgi-bin/iowa/content/about/index.html
- Lambda Legal: www.lambdalegal.org/
- National Health Law Program: www.healthlaw.org/
- Office of Civil Rights: www.ed.gov/about/offices/list/ocr/index.html
- National Lawyers Guild, National Office: www.nlg.org/
- U.S. Equal Employment opportunity commission: www.eeoc.gov/
- U.S. Department of Housing and Urban Development:
  www.hud.gov/complaints/index.cfm

---

related discrimination laws. In addition, most states have laws prohibiting discrimination on the basis of handicap and/or disability. The passage of laws at the local, state, and federal levels that affect the lives of persons with HIV/AIDS has led to the need to be informed about organizations that assist persons experiencing discrimination and other legal problems because of their status. A partial list of federal and nongovernmental organizations that assist in preventing discrimination against PLWH is displayed Table 4.1.

JUSTICE AND HIV/AIDS

Justice in health care generally focuses on questions of a right to health care, fairness in access to care, and distribution of resources (Gostin, 2007; Powers & Faden, 2006). Philosophers and bioethicists in various camps--conservative, liberal, libertarian, and utilitarian--have shaped debate about health care justice. A fuller understanding of personal and societal vulnerability to HIV/AID—Soften connected to risk behaviors resulting from social oppression and discrimination—raises compelling questions of a fundamental nature about health care justice. Because in the United States PLWH are likely to come from the ranks of marginalized populations—racial minorities, gay men, injection drug users, the impoverished, the homeless and mentally ill, and poor women—it is not difficult to see that concerns for health care justice will remain paramount in ethical debates relative to the pandemic.

The ways in which health care justice is achieved, or not achieved, can mean the difference between living and dying for PLWH. If nothing else, the HIV/AIDS pandemic has caused the world's leaders and policy-makers to reflect on and to deal more constructively with issues of health care justice. The HIV/AIDS epidemic

- Illustrates the limits of health resources;
- Reminds us that we may not have an infinite capacity to provide needed care for every sick person;
- Reminds us that we may have to make uncomfortable decisions about the distribution of our health care resources; and
- Reminds us that we live in a sometimes unjust society, which struggles to make good on its promises of justice for all.

The daily challenges of PLWH underscore the difficulties millions face in achieving health care justice in the U.S. and around the globe. For example, in the United States, those with insurance can generally obtain the resources they need for adequate health care, while an estimated 46 million Americans (18% of the U.S. population of adults under the age of 65) lacking insurance must settle for no health care or less than adequate health care (DeNavas-Walt, Proctor, & Smith, 2008). Justice rings hollow for millions of American denied access to adequate health care because they lack insurance, because they are unemployed or unemployable, because their employer does not offer insurance coverage, or because they cannot afford to pay their share of the insurance premium of their employer's insurance. In resource-limited nations, millions of persons do not have access to HIV testing, and many millions more lack adequate access to antiretroviral drug treatment and to health care providers with the expertise to treat their condition (Boulle & Ford, 2008; Harries, Schouten, & Libamba, 2006).

Before one can fully consider how to achieve health care justice for PLWH, one must attempt to respond to a more basic question: Is health care special? Daniels (1985) has suggested that one way to understand this question is to ask whether health care services should be viewed as we view other commodities—items bought or sold in the marketplace. Should society allow inequalities in access to health care services to vary with whatever economic inequalities are permissible according to principles of distributive justice? Or is health care in some way special and not to be treated like other commodities (e.g., cars or personal computers) whose exchange is affected by market conditions? The fact that tens of millions of Americans are uninsured or underinsured would seem to argue that, while as a nation we may believe that everyone should have adequate health care, in the United States, health care is a barterable commodity.

Daniels (1985) has raised some of the following questions related to health care justice:

1 Is health care a right to which everyone is entitled?
2 What kinds of health care services will/should exist in a society?
3 Who will get these services and on what basis?
4 Who should deliver these services?
5 How will the burdens of financing these services be distributed?

If one claims that PLWH have a right to health care, hard questions must still be answered. For example:

1 What share of America's total health resources should be allocated to AIDS?
2 To which areas should this allocation of resources be made—prevention, direct care, research? Which one is a priority, given that health care resources are not infinite?
3 Who should be entitled to make decisions about resource allocation—the federal government, states, local government? Should the federal government set aside a special fund for HIV/AIDS care and distribute these funds to states according to the number of needy persons in those states?
4 What constitutes a fair share of the health budget for HIV/AIDS? Is it fair to divert resources from other health areas to AIDS?
5 What level of care, if any, is the government morally obligated to provide for PLWH? If health care is special and if some level of care should be guaranteed for all, how does one ensure that health care providers will embrace concepts of justice?

The tension generated in efforts to balance provider autonomy, power, and special interests with efforts to establish health care justice is not easily resolved. If PLWH are to have access to adequate health care, it would seem that several concerns related to human resources also need to be addressed (Daniels, 1985):

1   What are the ethical duties of providers to deliver care to people with AIDS?

2   In what ways does a duty (or perhaps even a legal requirement) to provide care infringe on the liberties of providers?

3   Do the requirements of health care justice improperly infringe upon the economic interests of certain provides?

4   Do some types of health care providers have a greater obligation than others in helping to achieve health care justice? Do all equally have a social contract to provide care?

5   Do providers have an obligation to treat people with AIDS regardless of their ability to pay? Or do only some providers have this obligation?

6   Do practitioners have a moral or legal obligation to work in a specialty of need because there is an inadequate number of specialists in that area?

Whether this nation will have the requisite human resources to care for PLWH in future years is unclear. Should Congress pass legislation that ensures at least a minimum level of health care for all Americans, who will provide care to the millions of health care consumers who are now uninsured but who would certainly have an expectation of access to health care? A burgeoning shortage of nurses and physicians raises compelling questions about the delivery of adequate care for persons with AIDS. These concerns, among others, are of considerable interest several organizations that seek to advance social justice within health care, including the Institute for Health and Social Justice (http://pih.org/what/advocacy.html), the Health Equity and Social Justice Strategic Direction Team of the National Association of County and City Health Officials (www.naccho.org/topics/justice/mission.cfm), the National Center on Minority Health and Health Disparities (http://ncmhd.nih.gov/), and FACE AIDS (www.faceaids.org/whatwedo).

PRIVACY AND CONFIDENTIALITY

Since the beginning of the HIV epidemic in the United States, ethicists and advocates of PLWH have expressed concerns about privacy and confidentiality as these concepts relate to the epidemic. Concerns related to privacy and confidentiality stem from the conflict between individual rights and public good. According to the U.S. Department of Health and Human Services, the Office for Civil Rights (OCR) has responsibility for enforcing the Privacy Rule under the Health Insurance Portability and Accountability Act of 1996 (HIPAA), which protects the privacy of individually identifiable health information, and the confidentiality provisions of the Patient Safety Act, which protects identifiable information being used to analyze patient safety events and improve patient safety (See ftp.hrsa.gov/hab/hipaa04.pdf and www.hhs.gov/ocr/privacy/index.html for more information). Privacy and confidentiality, as these relate to HIV, are also a core concern of the American Civil Liberty Union's AIDS Project (www.aclu.org/hiv/privacy/index.html). The Electronic Privacy Information Center (EPIC) online guide to privacy resources provides a comprehensive listing of privacy-related resources (http://epic.org/privacy/privacy_resources_faq.html).

Privacy may be thought of as the freedom of the individual to pick and choose for him- or herself the time and circumstances under which, and the extent to which, his or her attitudes, beliefs, behaviors, and opinions are shared or withheld from others (Kelman, 1977). Some ethicists maintain that privacy is a conditional right, while others believe that privacy is a basic human need and as such is on par with rights rooted in other basic human needs. While privacy is not mentioned in either the Constitution or Bill of Rights, it has been recognized, primarily since the mid-1960s, by the Supreme Court as a right (Grad, 2005). In law, as articulated by Justice Louis Brandeis in the 1890s, privacy is conceptually linked to "the right to be left alone" (Laurant, 2003). In addition, privacy is protected in the Universal Declaration of Human Rights, the International Covenant on Civil and Political Rights, and in other human rights treaties.

Privacy may be thought of as "decisional privacy," that is, the right to make decisions about one's body and health care treatment, and "informational privacy," or the right to limit and control others' knowledge of intimate facts about our lives, including state of health (Grad, 2005). Informational privacy is closely linked to the concept of confidentiality. Ordinarily intrusions into privacy, in either research or clinical care, require informed consent. Although most social injuries result from breaches in confidentiality, invasions of privacy also carry considerable risk. This risk includes the following concerns of research subjects:

That public exposure of their views and actions may have damaging consequences for them; that the procedures used to elicit information may
deprive them of control over their self-preservation; and that research
may probe into areas that constitute their private space, overstepping the
boundary between self and environment (Kelman, 1977, p. 169).

Researchers and caregivers often inquire into the most private
and intimate aspects of their subjects'/patients' lives. Rawnsley (1980)
has noted that the hospital provides a laboratory of sorts in which the
invasion of privacy may be epidemic. Early in their education, health
providers learn that they do not ordinarily intrude into an individual's
privacy without obtaining informed consent. But outside the hospital
in daily life, persons are often asked to provide information about their
lives that may eventually lead to the denial of health or life insurance on
the basis of suspected HIV infection. Ought insurance companies, for
example, have the right to obtain this personal information, the right to
test blood samples with or without the individual's knowledge, the right
to examine the medical and social histories in search of factors that tip
them off to the true nature of an AIDS-related illness? The answers
to such questions may rest partially on society's willingness to sanction
intrusions into privacy. Concerns about both privacy and confidentiality,
as well as autonomy, are at the center of debate about the Centers for
Disease Control and Prevention's revised recommendations (CDC,
2006a) for "routine" HIV testing of adults, adolescents, and pregnant
women in health care settings (Bayer & Fairchild, 2006; Gostin, 2006,
2007; Rennie & Behets, 2006).

Confidentiality, although sometimes used interchangeably with
privacy, may be thought of as the mode of management of private
information. To contrast the two concepts, an individual may share
private information with a caregiver, but that caregiver is expected
to keep this information *confidential*, that is, to refrain from sharing
this information without the individual's written authorization or
some other compelling justification. Throughout the history of the
HIV pandemic, there have been many reported instances of private
information about persons with HIV/AIDS being shared inappropriately or inadvertently with others. It follows, therefore, that the
greater the number of persons who have knowledge of private information, the greater the risk that confidentiality will be breached.
With the advent of computer-based patient records, employees
of hospitals—including those without a "need to know"—can gain

access to private information about patients and share that information with unauthorized persons. In addition, hackers have gained access to patient records at hospitals and other health care settings because of vulnerabilities in the facilities' information technology system. President Obama's economic recovery plan includes a proposal to spend billions of dollars to accelerate the use of computerized medical records in hospitals, physicians' offices, and other health care settings, with the aim of reducing costs and improving quality of care; however, as greater numbers of persons are able to gain access to patient records, efforts to protect private patient information, including reliable technological measures, appropriate institutional policies, and governmental regulations—as well as adequate penalties to serve as deterrents—will need to be in place.

The Presidential Commission on the Human Immunodeficiency Virus Epidemic (1988) issued the following statement regarding the need to maintain confidentiality on matters related to HIV/AIDS:

> The rigorous maintenance of confidentiality is considered critical to the success of the public health endeavor to prevent the transmission and spread of HIV infection. . . . An effective guarantee of confidentiality is the major bulwark against that fear [of discrimination]. A federal statute that carefully balances the need for confidentiality of HIV information against the protection of public health is a necessary and appropriate response to confidentiality concerns (p. 126).

The Health Insurance Portability and Accountability Act of 1996 provides the greatest protection for the confidentiality of private health information. In addition, numerous state laws speak to the confidentiality of HIV-related information (Gostin, Lazzarini & Flaherty, 1997). Many states have (1) strengthened confidentiality standards to protect HIV-infected persons from discrimination, (2) supported anonymous HIV testing, (3) included AIDS under laws protecting the handicapped, and (4) limited health officials' power to quarantine and isolate those with communicable disease while strengthening due process for those who are infected (Eubanks, 1988).

SCREENING AND TESTING FOR HIV

According to Bayer and Fairchild (2006), the CDC's 2006 recommendations for "routine" HIV testing have heralded the end of the "exceptionalism" that has distinguished AIDS from other communicable diseases relative to public health policy. Although the CDC's recommendations for more routine testing might appear to some to be an action aimed at treating HIV like other communicable diseases, HIV testing continues to raise significant ethical issues, including concerns about intrusions into privacy and about confidentiality of results. State laws regarding HIV testing, including the issues of consent, confidentiality, and noti-fication decisions, vary widely (Brown, 2008). Some states cannot fully implement the CDC's 2006 recommendations regarding "routine" HIV testing without changes or additions to current laws (Brown, 2008).

Provision of confidentiality is critical to the success of name-based reporting of persons who are HIV infected. As of April 2008, all 50 states, the District of Columbia, and 5 dependent areas use the same confidential name-based reporting system to collect HIV and AIDS data (CDC, 2008). The CDC (2006b) has issued detailed guidelines to ensure the security and confidentiality of HIV/AIDS surveillance data. The National HIV/AIDS Clinicians' Consultation Center (Goldschmidt & Neff, 2009) has published a compendium, updated every two months, of state HIV testing laws that includes information about confidentiality, anonymous testing, and consent.

Since testing became available in 1985, the World Health Organization has maintained that such testing must be confidential, accompanied by counseling, and conducted only with informed consent. UNAIDS's (2009) current position regarding HIV testing is captured in the following statement:

> UNAIDS does not support mandatory testing of individuals. All testing, whether client or provider-initiated, should be conducted under the condi-tions of the "Three Cs": involve informed consent, be confidential, and include counselling. Recognizing the urgency of connecting HIV positive people to prevention, treatment, care and support, UNAIDS and the World Health Organization released in May 2007 operational guidance on provider-initi-ated HIV testing and counseling in health facilities. The guidance is in line with the 2004 UNAIDS/WHO Policy Statement on HIV testing and recom-mends that traditional voluntary testing and counselling be supplemented by provider-initiated testing in all health settings in generalized HIV epidemics, and in selected health facilities (such as tuberculosis, sexual health or ante-natal health clinics) in areas with low or concentrated HIV epidemics (¶ 3).

Granich and colleagues (2009) have proposed a model of annual voluntary testing and immediate antiretroviral therapy that, according to the proposed model, could effectively control disease transmission and eventually eliminate HIV infection. By 2016 this approach, according to the proposed model, would reduce the incidence of HIV and mortality to less than one case per thousand people per year and would reduce the prevalence of HIV to less than 1% within 50 years. Implementation of the model would require testing with a limited population first and, if successful, would require significant funding. De Cock and colleagues (2003) have made a similar proposal to expanded voluntary testing in Africa to stem the pandemic on that continent.

Mandatory testing of some segments of the population (e.g., athletes, prisoners, health care providers, and pregnant women) is controversial. In cases where such testing has been proposed or has been implemented, the core argument in favor of such testing rests on the protection of other parties (e.g. other athletes, prison guards and other prisoners, patients, and fetuses) who might be exposed unavoidably to infection from another infected person. Early arguments against mandatory HIV testing focused on problems of false-negative and false-positive test results as a reason for not requiring widespread testing. Early in the epidemic, those ethicists arguing against mandatory screening usually alluded to technical difficulties in the testing process. As diagnostic tests have seen improvements in sensitivity and specificity, become less costly, and produced results more quickly (see Chapter 2), these earlier concerns have faded away. Today legal arguments relative to mandatory testing focus on such constitutional issues as due process, equal treatment, informed consent, reasonable search and seizure, reproductive rights, and privacy rights (Nicholson, 2002). In recent years, partially in response to the advent of effective perinatal antiretroviral treatment, several states have considered or passed laws mandating HIV testing of pregnant women (or newborn infants of their untested mothers) in efforts to prevent mother-to-child transmission. Research suggests that many pregnant women tested were unaware that they were HIV positive (Simpson & Forsyth, 2007). Nicholson (2002) has captured the most salient ethical concerns of mandatory testing of pregnant women:

> The ethical considerations of mandatory testing often go hand-in-hand with many of the legal issues. Is it right to compel a pregnant woman to have an HIV test? Is it right to allow a fetus to go untreated for a fatal disease if the treatment is proven and readily available? Would testing discriminate unjustly against particular racial or socioeconomic groups? Is it ethical compel a pregnant woman to get an HIV test, and then allow

her to decline treatment for herself and her baby if she tested positive for the virus? (p. 175)

In spite of the likelihood that mandatory HIV testing would undoubtedly identify many women who were previously unaware of their HIV positive status, Durojaye (2008) has raised questions about human concerns rights (e.g., health and reproductive care and nondiscrimination) that such testing may infringe on, rights that are guaranteed in the Protocol to the African Charter on the Rights of Women, among other human rights instruments.

Testing of persons for a communicable disease generally rests on the belief that infected individuals need to be identified so that these individuals can be counseled to reduce the health risk to themselves and others. Testing for HIV is often encouraged so that carriers can be identified and educated to change behaviors that might pose a risk to others. But others' knowledge of HIV status is not a prerequisite to the provision of education that potentially leads to changing high-risk behaviors. Nor is knowing one's own HIV status a prerequisite to the adoption of behaviors that reduce or eliminate the risk of acquiring an HIV infection. One can argue that information about HIV and AIDS, and particularly information on the prevention of infection, should be widely available for all persons, particularly for populations identified at highest risk, regardless of HIV status.

Having information about one's own or another's HIV status generates hard questions:

1   Who has or should have access to this information?
2   Who should be informed when an individual is found to be HIV seropositive? An employer, fellow prisoners and guards, school personnel, a sexual partner, parents, insurance companies, patients of an infected health care worker? Should health care workers, police officers and fire fighters, morticians, or teachers be informed so that they can take precautions in the event they are exposed to body fluids? Or put another way, are HIV test results private information, or do certain others have the right to this information?
3   Should one be required to identify individuals who have been placed at risk of infection through sexual contact, intravenous drug sharing, or other exposure? (Health care providers, particularly physicians and public health workers, are concerned

about a duty to warn sexual partners of infected persons and often cite the 1976 legal decision in *Tarasoff v. The University of California,* which imposed a duty on psychotherapists to warn third parties from the potentially dangerous acts of their clients [Perry, 1989; Zonana, 1989]).

4 When and how should an HIV-positive parent inform her or his child of the parent's HIV status or inform an infected child of his or her HIV-positive status?

On the one hand, infected individuals may risk negative reactions by others and the loss of social status, insurance, or employment if their infected status becomes known. On the other hand, not knowing that one is infected can potentially mean that lifesaving or life-prolonging therapy is not implemented until late in the course of infection. Under such circumstances an individual may have missed the opportunity to prolong his or her life or that of another at risk of infection because early treatment was not begun. Despite many challenges related to an HIV diagnosis, increasingly individuals who are at some level of risk for HIV infection are being urged to seek HIV testing so as to avail themselves of counseling and early treatment; however, even when the risk for infection is high, some persons decide not to be tested because of greater concerns about losses that might occur were this information to be shared with others. The implementation of "opt-out" testing (CDC, 2006a) (see Chapter 2) is likely to increase the administration of HIV tests in acute and other health care settings, leading to the identification of HIV-positive persons who were previously unaware of their infection.

Contact tracing is the identification of persons who may have come into contact with a person harboring an infectious disease. Contact tracing of sexual or needle-sharing partners of HIV-positive persons is controversial. According to Furner and Gold (2004), "Contact tracing raises many issues for clinicians, and for patients . . . includ[ing] confidentiality, identification of asymptomatic HIV infected individuals, giving positive results, access to counselling, impact of local legislation, impact of cultural factors and the establishment of appropriate clinic processes for contact tracing" (¶ 1). Most states provide no clear statutory authority for public health authorities to trace contacts of HIV-infected persons. Contact tracing of potentially infected individuals is difficult because some infected persons have had numerous anonymous contacts. Moreover, because of the long incubation associated with AIDS, it is sometimes difficult for persons to remember all of their contacts within the past five years and for public health officials to locate these contacts. It has also been pointed out that each contact traced is costly to taxpayers. Somecritics of HIV contact tracing have argued that contact tracing cannot be implemented because there simply are not adequate numbers of trained personnel to carry out such tracing programs. In an effort to assist local and state health departments, the CDC (1998) has provided guidance for partner notification and referral services. According to principles of this guidance, partner notification must be voluntary, confidential, scientifically based, and culturally appropriate.

In those areas of the United States where partner notification is being implemented, HIV-positive persons are encouraged to provide voluntarily the names of sexual partners or needle-sharing partners who may have been placed at risk of HIV infection. Exposed persons are notified of the exposure but are not provided the name(s) of the HIV-positive person or persons. While privacy rights continue to be a concern, partner notification has increased since 2003 when the CDC issued an HIV-prevention strategy highlighting partner notification. Mandatory partner notification, as required, for example, in New York State (Office of Program Evaluation and Research, 2006), continues to be debated around such issues as duty to warn, the right to know, the mandate to protect public health, and rights to privacy and confidentiality (Ellison, 2004).

THE DUTY TO CARE

Still another ethical issue related to the care and treatment of PLWH is concerned with whether health care workers have the right to refuse to provide services to these individuals. Ethical debates related to health care professionals' duty to treat during an epidemic generally revolves around how risks should be distributed among health care professionals, conflicts that arise between professional duties and family duties, and the forms of support that societies owe health care workers during epidemics (Dwyer, 2008). More recently, some scholars have argued that the usual compelling arguments for a duty to treat (e.g., expressed consent, implied consent, special training, reciprocity [or social contract view], and professional oaths and codes) need to be carefully considered for their application during an epidemic (Malm et al., 2008). Early in the pandemic some nurses, physicians, dentists, and other health care providers refused to provide care to AIDS patients because of fear of contracting HIV or other reasons. Some health care workers were reported to have resigned rather than render such care. These health care providers were apparently concerned for their safety and possibly that of their families. Such concerns have now decreased considerably in the face of more accurate knowledge about AIDS and its transmissibility, established infection control guidelines, better treatments for HIV/AIDS, and the extremely low risk to health care workers providing care for PLWH.

Nurses' ethical duty to care for PLWH is supported by the American Nurses Association's (ANA) *Code of Ethics for Nurses* (2001) and the International Council of Nurses' *Code of Nurses* (2006). These codes underscore nurses' historical service to all persons, regardless of nationality, creed, race, color, age, sex, social/economic status, and illness. The ANA Committee on Ethics (1986) prepared a "Statement Regarding Risk Versus Responsibility in Providing Nursing Care," which states in part that "accepting personal risk which exceeds the limits of duty is not morally obligatory; it is a moral option." This statement notes that the differentiation between benefiting another as a moral duty and benefiting another as a moral option is found in four fundamental criteria:

1   The patient is at significant risk of harm, loss, or damage if the nurse does not assist.
2   The nurse's intervention or care is directly relevant to preventing harm.
3   The nurse's care will probably prevent harm, loss, or damage to the patient.
4   The benefit the patient will gain outweighs any harm the nurse might incur and does not present more than minimal risk to the health care provider.

On the basis of this statement, nurses presumably must determine whether patient benefit outweighs harm to the nurse. On the basis of present scientific data, the risk of harm to the nurse caring for a person with HIV/AIDS is negligible if well-established infection control measures are followed. Freedman (1988) points out that the committee's statement does not define minimal risk; thus the level or quantity of risk a nurse is obligated to accept remains vague.

Plumeri (1984) has noted that physicians may legally and ethically decline to treat persons with AIDS because a physician has neither a legal duty to treat a patient nor an obligation to accept as a patient all those who seek his or her services. The physician's legal duty to treat arises only on the creation of a physician–patient relationship. This legal tenet is supported by the American Medical Association's Principles of Medical Ethics (2001), Principle VI, which states, "A physician shall, in the provision of appropriate patient care, except in emergencies, be free to choose whom to serve, with whom to associate, and the environment in which to provide medical care." Moreover, according to Plumeri (1984), the physician may sever his or her professional relationship with persons with AIDS without risking charges of abandonment if the physician's services are no longer needed, if the termination occurs by mutual consent, if the termination is by unilateral action of the patient, or if it is by withdrawal by the physician after proper notification. Other reasons that may contribute to a physician's decision not to treat a patient include the physician's lack of expertise relative to the patient's condition, a religious or moral objection to the care being sought by the patient, lack of cooperation or unruliness on the part of the patient, and nonpayment by the patient, the latter only in nonemergency situations (Katz & Paul, 2002). In actuality, however, few physicians and other health care providers now refuse to treat PLWH, although some may still experience discomfort in doing so. The physician's duty to treat has been summarized by Sokol (2008) who concluded that " . . . the duty should be discharged unless it conflicts with one or more duties with great moral force" (p. 28).

END-OF-LIFE CARE

Since the advent of antiretroviral treatment for HIV infection, HIV disease has become increasingly a chronic condition with exacerbations, remissions, and eventual death. Many PLWH may succumb to other conditions linked to HIV disease (e.g., opportunistic infections and/or to an age-related conditions). End-of-life care poses a number of ethical dilemmas for PLWH and their caregivers (Harding et al., 2003). Ethical concerns related to progression of HIV disease and end-of-life care are prominent because (1) the care provider and patient (and the patient's family or proxy) may not always agree on the treatment course to follow; (2) persons with AIDS may become mentally incapable of making decisions; and (3) decision-making guidelines are difficult to follow in view of the high stress related to the care of persons with AIDS (Steinbrook et al., 1986). As HIV disease progresses, care providers and patients (and their families) may not agree on the goals of care, especially as these relate to the dichotomy between palliative versus curative treatment

(Selwyn & Rivard, 2003). Other end-of-life ethical concerns include the patient's right to life-sustaining therapy, the patient's right to refuse medical treatment, the futility of medical treatment, and assisted suicide (sometimes called "dignity death") (Walker, 1999).

Ideally, medical treatment of PLWH should be jointly determined by the patient and his or her care provider because preferences for care cannot be accurately predicted without discussion; however, many PLWH are ambivalent about discussing end-of-life care (Steinbrook et al., 1986). Some PLWH have drawn up living wills to ensure that their desires are carried out, although the nature of these instruments varies greatly from state to state (most states have enacted "death with dignity" or "living will" acts), and these wills raise additional ethical concerns (Ney, 1989). The Patient Self-Determination Act, which allows patients to specify their end-of-life wishes via advance directives, requires hospitals and other health care organizations that receive federal funds to tell patients of their rights under the applicable state law to make end-of-life medical decisions. Some terminally ill persons, including PLWH, would like a "dignity death," but at this time only three states--Washington, Oregon, and Montana--allow for assisted suicide, and many care providers decline to participate in such end-of-life treatment.

In some cases, staff and/or significant others must make treatment choices that affect the outcome of the patient's life. One study involving more than 1,400 PLWH found that more than half were at risk of needing to make end-of-life decisions without having discussed their preferences with their care providers (Wenger et al., 2001). When decisions are made by other persons without the patient's wishes being known, value judgments may inappropriately affect decision making. PLWH should consider appointing a trusted person as their durable power of attorney so that if they are unable to make decisions about their health care and other matters, this appointee can carry out their wishes. Many persons with AIDS prefer to appoint their friends or partners, rather than relatives, as substitute decision makers (Steinbrook et al., 1986).

HIV/AIDS RESEARCH: KEY ETHICAL CONCERNS

Numerous ethical concerns have been raised regarding research and experimental treatment of individuals with AIDS. In the conduct of research involving human subjects, the researcher is always concerned

by respect for persons, beneficence, and justice, among other principles (Macklin & Friedland, 1986). Because HIV research often involves
vulnerable and marginalized populations, researchers must confront a
range of challenges in enrolling subjects in research while at the same
time ensuring that these subjects' rights are scrupulously protected. In
recent years, much of the attention related to the ethics of HIV/AIDS
research has focused on biomedical research sponsored by pharmaceutical companies and academic institutions located in resource-rich
countries and carried out in resource-poor countries. Such research has
raised a number of ethical concerns, including equitable distribution of
benefits, confidentiality, obligations of sponsors (e.g., compensation of
subjects), exploitation of vulnerable subjects, voluntariness, coercion,
deception, undue inducement, inadequate disclosure, and subjects'
poor understanding of the research and its risks, among a host of other
concerns (Council for International Organizations of Medical Sciences,
2002; Emanuel, Currie & Herman, 2005; Emanuel et al., 2004; Macklin,
2004; MacQueen & Karim, 2007; Nuffield Council on Bioethics, 2005;
Pacea & Emanuelb, 2005; Shapiro & Meslin, 2001; Shah, 2006; Varmus
& Satcher, 1997). Commenting on such biomedical research, Varmus
and Satcher (1997) hold that "Trials that make use of impoverished
populations to test drugs for use solely in developed countries violate
our most basis understanding of ethical behavior" (p. 1003). In her 2004
book on double standards of such research, Macklin (2004) posed the
following key questions:

1   How can biomedical research be designed and conducted so as
    to contribute to the health needs of developing countries and at
    the same time contain adequate protections for the rights and
    welfare of the human subjects recruited for these studies?
2   If a particular study may not be conducted in the sponsoring
    country for ethical reasons, is it acceptable to carry out an
    identical study in a developing country and, if so, with what
    justification?
3   When completed research yields successful products, what
    obligations, if any, do the sponsors have to the community or
    country where the research was conducted?
4   Should the provisions of the international ethical guidelines for
    research, such as the Declaration of Helsinki, be interpreted
    and applied in the same way in resource-poor countries as they
    are in wealthier countries?

As a result of these concerns and after long debate, the Declaration of Helsinki was revised by the World Medical Association, although ethicists continue to debate the interpretation of this document as it applies to research in resource-poor countries. The Council for International Organizations of Medical Sciences (CIOMS) has published *International Ethical Guidelines for Biomedical Research Involving Human Subjects* (2002), which seeks to provide ethical principles of research with human subjects that are universal and culturally relevant. In addition, UNAIDS (2000a) has published guidelines for researchers conducting research on vaccines for HIV/AIDS. The International Conference on Harmonisation (1997) has produced a guideline that assists the pharmaceutical industry in conducting ethically sound research. As another level of protection of human subjects in clinical trials in resource-poor countries, HIV/AIDS research may be reviewed by Community Advisory Boards (CAB). The Fogarty/CFAR Research Ethics Website (http://bms.brown.edu/fogarty/codes.htm#reports) provides links to the many of the salient U.S. and international ethics codes and regulations that are of interest to researchers conducting HIV-related research.

Over the years, the HIV/AIDS research literature has focused on several areas of ethical and legal concern to researchers, including:

- Collecting, storing, and protecting confidential data;
- Minimizing the intrusiveness of research;
- Obtaining informed consent from subjects who may have diminished capacity or are unable to give consent;
- Knowing when a need exists to warn third parties of a subject's behavior that may harm these third parties;
- Reporting illegal behavior observed in the course of research (e.g., drug use, sex work);
- Considering how to promote access to clinical trials;
- Designing research that is both scientifically rigorous and ethically principled;
- Conducting research in resource-limited countries where ethical principles of research may differ from those of the researchers;
- Designing and conducting research involving hard-to-reach populations (e.g., the homeless and injection drug users).

Beneficence may be thought of as treating people in an ethical manner not only by respecting their decisions and protecting them from harm but also by making efforts to secure their well-being (National Commission for the Protection of Human Subjects, 1979). Beneficence is expressed by efforts to do no harm, to maximize possible benefits, and to minimize possible harms. In achieving these goals, one often does a risk-benefit analysis. However, learning what will benefit may require exposing individuals to risk. In clinical trials of drugs to treat HIV, for example, the subject may be exposed to considerable risk of harm. Macklin and Friedland (1986) hold that the obligations imposed on researchers by the principle of beneficence are not entirely patient centered. They point out that divided loyalties constitute a potential hazard of all clinical research. Allowing patients to take second place, they believe, can be ethically justified by the *respect-for-persons* principle. Other critics believe that there are no ethical grounds for conducting randomized, controlled trials with persons with AIDS in the effort to find efficacious drug therapies.

The ethical principle of *justice* asks, among other research-related questions, "Who ought to receive the benefits of research and bear its burdens?" Fair selection of subjects for study is one issue related to this principle. Taking steps to ensure that both risks and benefits are equally distributed among the at-risk population is another. Given the possibility that experimental drug therapy might prolong or save the lives of PLWH, should the FDA more quickly approve those experimental drugs that have not been proven to be both safe and effective prior to being used in clinical trials with AIDS patients? What criteria should be used in determining when a drug is both safe and effective against HIV or AIDS? It remains to be seen, in the case of HIV, what harms or benefits will accrue from efforts of the Food and Drug Administration (1997) to expedite the review of new antiretroviral drugs (or generic versions of these drugs).

Many experts believe that the most probable way of eliminating AIDS, or at least limiting its future spread, is the creation of a vaccine; however, testing such vaccines raises important logistical and ethical issues (Loue & Pike, 2007; Simon, Maghboeba, & van Stade, 2007). The lack of an animal model and the high mutability of the virus present formidable obstacles to such research. In addition, for an HIV vaccine to reach a phase III clinical trial, thousands of volunteers from marginalized populations will need to be recruited to participate in the research (Kegeles et al., 2006). Multiple obstacles stand in the way of a safe and effective HIV vaccine, including those elucidated by Johnston and Fauci (2008, p. 890):

■ The window for the immune system to clear the initial vaccine is narrow because HIV integrates and establishes latent infection within days or weeks.

- Destruction of CD4+ cells begins early after infection.
- Enormous genetic diversity and mutations that occur with replication enable HIV to avoid immune surveillance.
- Conserved antibody targets on the outer envelope protein are "hidden" from immune recognition.

Since the beginning of the HIV pandemic, several dozen possible vaccines have entered phase I or phase II of clinical trials in the United States. In 2007, at least 13 candidate vaccines that induce primarily T-cell responses were in phase I or phase II clinical trials (Johnston & Fauci, 2007). In 2005, the global investment in HIV vaccine research and development was estimated to be $759 million. By March 2007, the National Institutes of Health, which spend about $600 million annually on such vaccines, had supported 99 HIV vaccine trials involving more than 26,000 subjects (Steinbrook, 2007).

Testing of vaccines faces a number of important ethical and legal challenges (Berkley, 2003; Maddren, 2003; Osborn, 1986; Shapiro & Stein, 2004; Waldholz & Bishop, 1986). For example, in the early stages of such research researchers enroll uninfected subjects, some of whom will become infected with HIV during the trial. Researchers must grapple with care-related issues (including the level of care to be provided, by whom, and for how long) for these infected research subjects (Berkley, 2003). The AIDS Vaccine Clearinghouse (n.d.), in writing about ethical challenges of conducting HIV vaccine research, has summarized a key challenge in conducting such research with vulnerable populations who potentially might benefit from such research:

> For large-scale clinical trials in particular, it's important that the study population . . . reflect the diversity of people who will use a vaccine in the future. Researchers must determine if there will be any differences in how the vaccine works in different populations. If too few individuals of a particular group (like women or adolescents) are included in a trial, it is not possible to determine the nature of any differences, should any occur, among that group. (¶ 3)

In working with these vulnerable and marginalized populations, HIV vaccine researchers have to deal with such issues as complete and thorough disclosure of risks and benefits, the health literacy of subjects, trust, confidentiality, side effects and safety, contracting HIV from the vaccine, possible vaccine-induced progression of HIV, family concerns, and insurability (Kegeles et al., 2006). As noted earlier, one major problem lies in the recruitment of thousands of volunteers and monitoring them for years to ascertain that the vaccine is both effective and harmless. Another concern centers on the possible exploitation of subjects in developing countries or among other populations where AIDS is endemic. Trials in pediatric populations raise an additional set of ethical concerns. Among the many problems to overcome is testing vaccines for AIDS are the following (Mariner & Gallo, 1987):

1   Volunteers will produce antibodies to AIDS and thus may be at higher risk for discrimination, even though they may not have the disease.
2   Those at highest risk for the disease and most likely to volunteer for vaccine trials may already have antibodies—thus obtaining healthy volunteers who are at risk may be difficult.
3   Scientists are ethically bound to educate volunteers to avoid practices that increase their risk of AIDS. Scientists worry about how to identify at an early age those persons who would benefit from vaccination before they engage in high-risk behaviors. Persuading the vaccinated and unvaccinated volunteers in the trial to avoid exposure to the virus would thus require a much longer period of time to determine any statistical significance between the two groups.
4   Some scientists fear the AIDS vaccines under study might cause cancer or other undesired side effects in volunteers. Because of liability concerns, finding a manufacturer for such a high-risk vaccine may be difficult. Providing liability protection for health care workers who administer experimental vaccines may also be problematic.

Over time, researchers conducting HIV-related studies have increasingly come to understand that such research must address both needs of the communities participating in the research and the relevance of such research to these communities (Auerbach & Coates, 2000; MacQueen et al., 2004). Because of the public interest in solving this health problem, research participants may have mixed interests. On the one hand they often wish to preserve their anonymity, while on the other hand they want to increase knowledge about the causes and treatment of the disease. Research involving vulnerable and marginalized populations brings into sharp focus the issues and dilemmas regarding privacy. These dilemmas highlight the conflicts between the individual's right to privacy and some social good.

Researchers' efforts require the consent and cooperation of those having or at risk of acquiring HIV infection. While some individuals participate in research for altruistic reasons, they often fear that their participation in research or experimental treatment could pose the risk of identification, disenfranchisement, and even arrest for criminal activities. These fears are particularly strong for those whose sexual preferences or drug use has not been publicly acknowledged. Years of discrimination, rejection, and stigmatization, plus mistrust of the medical and government establishments, lead some potential subjects to question researchers' ability to guarantee their anonymity and confidentiality.

Research involving PLWH may produce uncontrolled consequences. Makarushka (1976), in writing about the uncontrolled consequences of research, maintains that "the mere fact that research is being conducted may be interpreted as indicating that the known subjects or members of the groups they are assumed to represent should be assigned a sick role by others" (p. 65). Once such groups have been identified in the public arena, "sanctions by the general public and policy-makers may be levied against subjects and the groups they are believed to represent" (p. 65). The popular press has provided numerous examples of discrimination against gay persons and others perceived as being at risk of contracting AIDS. The wide dissemination of research findings of subjects from groups perceived to be at risk of HIV infection will undoubtedly produce additional "unintended" harm to members of those groups.

Researchers and clinicians who are insensitive to the concerns of PLWH can potentially do great harm. Because PLWH are well aware of the serious nature of their disease, they may be highly vulnerable to the requests of clinicians and researchers seeking to conduct research with them. Awareness of this increased vulnerability should compel researchers and caregivers to seek means to assure the confidentiality of collected data, to minimize intrusions into the most private areas of these persons' lives, to consider how these findings may influence the lives of PLWH and the course of public policy, and to follow published guidelines for research involving persons with AIDS (Bayer, Levine, & Murray, 1984).

Because the social and personal risks for PLWH may be high, these individuals should be fully informed about all aspects of the study and any known risk to them, including how collected data may be used and who will have access to these data. If researchers and clinicians are unwilling or unable to provide potential subjects with detailed information that they can understand, subjects should carefully weigh the benefits of their participation versus the possible risks. They should not be easily swayed by the argument that public good supersedes the freedom and privacy of individual citizens whose rights in this society are not barterable.

CONCLUSION

The present HIV/AIDS pandemic has created ethical dilemmas and raised legal issues that profoundly affect the lives of all of the world's citizens. A major concern of ethicists relative to the pandemic is the balance between rights and duties of infected individuals and those of the greater society. The tension generated by efforts to balance these rights has led to policy formation and passage of laws influencing many aspects of people's lives. Protecting the human rights of PLWH around the globe, many of whom come from marginalized populations, is increasingly important if the pandemic is to be controlled. Conducting research with PLWH creates special challenges for researchers who are obligated to observe well-established ethical guidelines. Because of their historical roles as patient advocates and direct care providers, nurses, and particularly those in leadership positions, should join dialogues with their colleagues in medicine, government, philosophy, and law that concern HIV-related ethical and legal issues affecting their lives, the lives of PLWH, and ultimately the lives of all citizens of the world.

REFERENCES

The AIDS Vaccine Clearinghouse. (n.d.). Overview. Retrieved on March 25, 2009, from www.aidsvaccineclearinghouse.org/communities.htm.

American Medical Association. (2001). Principles of medical ethics. Chicago: Author.

American Nurses Association. (2001). *Code of ethics for nurses with interpretative statements.* Silver Spring, MD: Author.

American Nurses Association Committee on Ethics. (1986). Statement regarding risk versus responsibility in providing nursing care. Kansas City: Author.

Auerbach, J. D., & Coates, T. J. (2000). HIV prevention research: Accomplishments and challenges for the third decade of AIDS. *American Journal of Public Health, 90,* 1029–1032.

Banta, W. (1987). *AIDS in the workplace.* Lexington, MA: Lexington Books.

Barrick, B. (1988). The willingness of nursing personnel to care for persons with AIDS syndrome. *Journal of Professional Nursing, 4*(5), 366–371.

Bayer, R., & Fairchild, A. (2006). Changing the paradigm for HIV testing: The end of exceptionalism. *New England Journal of Medicine, 355,* 647–651.

Bayer, R., Levine, C., & Murray, T. (1984). Guidelines for confidentiality in research in *AIDS. IRB, 6,* 1–7.

Bean, J., Keller, L., Newberg, C., & Brown, M. (1989). Methods for the reduction of AIDS social anxiety and social stigma. *AIDS Education and Prevention, 1*(3), 194–221.

Berkley, S. (2003). Thorny issues in the ethics of AIDS vaccine trials. *The Lancet 362,* 992.

Boulle, A., & Ford, N. (2008). Scaling up antiretroviral therapy in developing countries: What are the benefits and challenges? *Postgraduate Medical Journal, 84*(991), 225–227.

Brock, R. (1986). On a nursing AIDS task force: The battle for confident care. *Nursing Management, 17*(3), 67–68.

Brandt, A. (1988). AIDS: From social history to social policy. *Law, Medicine, and Health Care, 14*(5–6), 231–242.

Brandt, A. (1986). AIDS: From social history to social policy. *Law, Medicine, and Health Care, 14* (5-6), 231-242.

Brown, J. (2008). The changing landscape of state legislation and expanded HIV testing. *Public Health Reports, 123* (Suppl. 3), 16–20.

Brown, L., Trujillo, L., & Macintyre, K. (2001). *Interventions to reduce HIV/AIDS Stigma: What have we learned?* New York: Population Council. Retrieved on March 10, 2009, from www.popcouncil.org/pdfs/horizons/litrvwstigdisc.pdf.

Centers for Disease Control and Prevention. (1998). HIV Partner Counseling and Referral Services—Guidance. Retrieved on March 30, 2009, from www.cdc.gov/hiv/resources/guidelines/pcrs/index.htm.

Centers for Disease Control and Prevention. (2006a). Revised recommendations for HIV testing of adults, adolescents, and pregnant women in health-care settings. *Morbidity and Mortality Weekly Report, 55*(RR-14). Available online at www.cdc.gov/mmwr/pdf/rr/rr5514.pdf.

Centers for Disease Control and Prevention. (2006b). Technical Guidance for HIV/AIDS Surveillance Programs, Volume III: Security and Confidentiality Guidelines. Retrieved March 25, 2009, from www.cdc.gov/hiv/topics/surveillance/resources/guidelines/guidance/index.htm.

Centers for Disease Control and Prevention. (2008). HIV infection reporting. Retrieved on March 30, 2009, from www.cdc.gov/hiv/topics/surveillance/reporting.htm.

Clavreul, G. (1983, October). *An evaluation of AIDS apprehension among nursing personnel and its observed effects upon the levels of patient care quality.* Unpublished study presented at the National Conference on the Acquired Immune Deficiency Syndrome, National Institutes of Health, Washington, DC.

Council for International Organizations of Medical Sciences. (2002). *International Ethical Guidelines for Biomedical Research Involving Human Subjects.* Geneva: World Health Organization.

Daniels, N. (1985). *Just health care.* Cambridge, U.K.: Cambridge University Press.

Darrow, W., Montanea, J., Uribe, C., Sanchez-Brana, E., Obiaja, K., Gladwin, H., et al. (2008, August 3–4). *The persistence of AIDS-related stigma.* Paper presented at the XVII International AIDS Conference, Mexico City.

D'Augelli, A. (1989). AIDS fears and homophobia among rural nursing personnel. *AIDS Education and Prevention, 1*(4), 277–284.

De Cock, K., Marum, E., & Mbori-Mgacha, D. (2003). A serostatus-based approach to HIV/AIDS prevention and care in Africa. *The Lancet, 362*(9398), 1847–1849.

DeNavas-Walt, C., Proctor, B., & Smith, J. (2008). Income, poverty, and health insurance coverage in the United States: 2007. Washington, DC: U.S. Government Printing Office. Retrieved on March 20, 2009, from www.census.gov/prod/2008pubs/p60-235.pdf.

Douglas, C., Kalman, C., & Kalman, T. (1985). Homophobia among physicians and nurses: An empirical study. *Hospital and Community Psychiatry, 36*(12), 1309–1310.

Durojaye, E. (2008). Addressing human rights concerns raised by mandatory HIV testing of pregnant women through the Protocol to the African Charter on the Rights of Women. *Journal of African Law, 52,* 43–65.

Dwyer, J. (2008). Developing the duty to treat: HIV, SARS, and the next epidemic. *Journal of Medical Ethics, 34,* 7–10.

Earl, C. E., & Penney, P. J. (2003). Rural nursing students' knowledge, attitudes, and beliefs about HIV/AIDS: A research brief. *Journal of the Association of Nurses in AIDS Care, 14*(54), 70–73.

Ellison, B. (2004). Reexamining mandatory HIV partner notification in Florida. *Florida Public Health Review, 1,* 56–58.

Emanuel, E., Currie, X., & Herman, A. (2005). Undue inducement in clinical research in developing countries: Is it a worry? *The Lancet, 366,* 336–340.

Emanuel, E. J., Wendler, D. Killen, J., & Grady, C. (2004). What makes clinical research in developing countries ethical? The benchmarks of ethical research. *Journal of Infectious Diseases, 189,* 930–937.

Eubanks, P. (1988, October 20). States have one goal, many paths, to fight AIDS. *Hospitals, 62,* 68.

Fairchild, A., Gable, L., Gostin, L., Bayer, R., Sweeney, P., & Janssen, R. (2007). Public goods, private data: HIV and the history, ethics, and uses of identifiable public health information. *Public Health Reports, 122,* 7–15.

Fikremariam, G. F. (2004, July 11–16). *Stigma and discrimination as barrier to HIV/AIDS treatment and care.* Paper presented at the XV International AIDS Conference, Bangkok, Thailand.

Food and Drug Administration. (1997). Expanded Access and Expedited Approval of New Therapies Related to HIV/AIDS. Retrieved on March 30, 2009, from www.fda.gov/oashi/aids/expanded.html.

Freedman, B. (1988). Health professions, codes, and the right to refuse to treat HIV-infectious patients. *Hastings Center Report, 18*(2), 20–25.

Furner, V., & Gold, J. (2004, July 11–16). *Contact tracing: A useful strategy for HIV prevention?* Paper presented at the XV International Conference on AIDS. Bangkok, Thailand, abstract no. E11866.

Gerbert, B., Maguire, B., Badner, V., Altman, D., & Stone, G. (1989). Fear of AIDS: Issues for health professional education. *AIDS: Education and Prevention, 1*(1), 39–53.

Goldschmidt, R., & Neff, S. (2009). Compendium of state HIV testing laws—200. Retrieved on March 25, 2009, from www.nccc.ucsf.edu/StateLaws/Index.html.

Gostin, L. (2006). HIV screening in health care settings: Public health and civil liberties in conflict? *Journal of the American Medical Association, 296,* 2023–2025.

Gostin, L. (2007). Why should we care about social justice? *Hastings Center Report, 37*(4), 3.

Gostin, L., Lazzarini, Z., & Flaherty, K. (1997). Legislative survey of state confidentiality laws, with specific emphasis on HIV and immunization. Retrieved on March 20, 2009, from http://epic.org/privacy/medical/cdc_survey.html.

Gostin, L., & Webber, D. (1998). HIV infection and AIDS in the public health and health care systems: The role of law and litigation. *Journal of the American Medical Association, 279,* 1108–1113.

Grad, F. P. (Ed.). (2005). *The Public Health Law Manual.* Washington, DC:American Public Health Association.

Granich, R. M., Gilks, C. F., Dye, C., De Cock, K. M., & Williams, B. G. (2009). Universal voluntary HIV testing with immediate antiretroviral therapy as a strategy for elimination of HIV transmission: A mathematical model. *The Lancet, 373*(9657), 48–57.

Gruskin, S., & Tarantola, D. (2002). Human rights and HIV/AIDS. HIV *InSite Knowledge Base.* Retrieved on March 7, 2009, from http://hivinsite.ucsf.edu/InSite?page=kb-08-01-07.

Hamblin, J. (1991). The role of the law in HIV/AIDS Policy, *AIDS, 5,* (Suppl. 2), 239–243.

Harding, R., Stewart, K., Marconi, K., O'Neill, J. F., & Higginson, I. J. (2003). Current HIV/AIDS end-of-life care in sub-Saharan Africa: A survey of models, services, challenges and priorities. *BMC Public Health, 3*(33). Published online October 23, 2003: doi:10.1186/1471-2458-3-33.

Harries, A.D., Schouten, E.J., & Libamba, E. (2006). Scaling up anti-retroviral treatment in resource-poor settings. *The Lancet, 367*(9525), 870–1872.

Herek, G. M. (2005). AIDS and stigma. In P. Conrad (Ed.), *The sociology of health & illness: Critical perspectives* (122–129). New York: Macmillan.

International Conference on Harmonisation. (1997). Retrieved on March 30, 2009, from www.ich.org/cache/compo/276-254-1.html.

International Council of Nurses. (2006). *The ICN code of ethics for nurses.* Geneva: Author.

Jayasuriya, D. (1988). AIDS-related health legislation. In A. Fleming, M. Carballo, D. FitzSimons, M. Bailey, & J. Mann (Eds.), *The Global Impact of AIDS* (pp. 313–316). New York: Alan R. Liss.

Johnston, P., & Fauci, A. (2007). An HIV vaccine—evolving concepts. *New England Journal of Medicine, 356,* 2073–2081.

Johnston, P., & Fauci, A. (2008). An HIV vaccine—challenges and prospects. *New England Journal of Medicine, 359,* 888–890.

Kalman, T. (1988). Homophobia among physicians and nurses. *American Journal of Psychiatry, 144*(1), 1514–1515.

Katz, L., & Paul, M. B. (2002, February). When a physician may refuse to treat a patient? *Physician's New Digest.* Retrieved on March 25, 2009, from www.physiciansnews.com/law/202.html.

Kegeles, S. M., Johnson, M. O., Strauss, R. P., Ralston, B., Hays, R. B., & Metzger, D. D. (2006). How should HIV vaccine efficacy trials be conducted? Diverse U.S. communities speak out. *AIDS Education and Prevention, 18,* 560–572.

Kelman, H. (1977). Privacy and research with human beings. *Journal of Social Issues, 33*(3), 169–195.

Klein, S. J., Karchner, W. D., & O'Connell, D. A. (2002). Interventions to prevent HIV-related stigma and discrimination: Findings and recommendations for public health. *The Journal of Public Health Management and Practice, 8*(6), 44–53.

Koop, C. E. (1988). Individual freedom and the public interest. In A. Fleming, M. Carballo, D. FitzSimons, M. Bailey, & J. Mann (Eds.). *The global impact of AIDS* (pp. 307–312). New York: Alan R. Liss.

Laurant, C. (2003). Privacy and human rights 2003: Overview. Retrieved March 20, 2009, from www.privacyinternational.org/survey/phr2003/overview.htm.

Li, Y., Scott, C. S., & Li, L. (2008). Chinese nursing students' HIV/AIDS knowledge, attitudes and practice intentions. *Applied Nursing Research, 21,* 147–152.

Loue, S., & Pike, E. C. (2007). *Case studies in ethics and HIV research.* New York: Springer.

Macklin, R. (2004). *Double standards in medical research in developing countries.* Cambridge, U.K.: Cambridge University Press.

Macklin, R., & Friedland, G. (1986), AIDS research: The ethics of clinical trials. *Law, Medicine and Health Care, 14*(5–6), 273–280.

MacQueen, K. & Karim, Q. (2007). Practice brief: Adolescents and HIV clinical trials: Ethics, culture, and context. *Journal of the Association of Nurses in AIDS Care, 18*(2), 78–82.

MacQueen, K., Shapiro, K., Karim, Q., & Sugarman, J. (2004). Ethical Challenges in International HIV Prevention Research. *Accountability in Research, 11*(1), 49–61.

Maddren, C. A. (2003). AIDS vaccines: Balancing human rights with public health. *Temple International Comparative Law Journal, 17*(1), 277–302.

Makarushka, J. (1976). The requirement of informed consent in research on human subjects: The problem of the uncontrolled consequences of health-related research. *Clinical Research, 24,* 64–66.

Malm, H., May, T., Francis, L. P., Omer, S. B., Salmon, D. A., & Hood, R. (2008). Ethics, pandemics, and the duty to treat. *American Journal of Bioethics, 8*(8), 4–19.

Mariner, W., & Gallo, R. (1987). Getting to market: The scientific and legal climate for developing an AIDS vaccine. *Law, Medicine, & Health Care, 15*(1–2), 17–26.

Merritt, D. (1986). The constitutional balance between health and liberty. *Hastings Center Report, 16*(6), 2–10 (Suppl.).

Mills, M., Wofsy, C., & Mills, J. (1986). The acquired immunodeficiency syndrome: Infection control and public health law. *New England Journal of Medicine, 314*(14), 931–936.

National Commission for the Protection of Human Subjects. (1979). *Belmont report.* Washington, DC: Department of Health and Human Services.

Nation Gay Rights Advocates & National Lawyers Guild AIDS Network. (1988). *AIDS practice manual: A legal and educational guide,* 2nd ed. San Francisco: Authors.

Ney, C. (1989). Living wills: The ethical dilemmas. *Critical Care Nurse, 9*(8), 20–41.

Nicholson, E. (2002). Mandatory HIV testing of pregnant women: Public health policy considerations and alternatives. *Duke Journal of Gender Law & Policy, 9,* 175–191.

Nuffield Council on Bioethics. (2005). *The ethics of research related to healthcare in developing countries: A follow-up discussion paper.* London: Author.

Office of Program Evaluation and Research. (2006). Impact of New York's HIV reporting and partner notification law: General findings report. Retrieved March 25, 2009, from www.health.state.ny.us/diseases/aids/regulations/notification/hivpartner/docs/impactreport.pdf.

Osborn, J. (1986). The AIDS epidemic: Multidisciplinary trouble. *New England Journal of Medicine, 314*(12), 779–782.

Pacea, C., & Emanuelb, E. (2005). The ethics of research in developing countries: Assessing voluntariness. *The Lancet, 365*(9453), 11–12.

Parker, R., & Aggleton, P. (2003). HIV and AIDS-related stigma and discrimination: A conceptual framework and implications for action. *Social Science & Medicine, 57,* 13–24.

Patterson, D., & London, L. (2002). International law, human rights, and HIV/AIDS. *Bulletin of the World Health Organization, 80,* 964–969.

Perry, S. (1989). Warning third parties at risk of AIDS: APA's policy is a barrier to treatment. *Hospital and Community Psychiatry, 40*(2), 158–161.

Pierce, C., & VanDeVeer, D. (1988). *AIDS: Ethics and public policy.* Belmont, CA: Wadsworth.

Piot, P., Kazatchkine, M., Dybul, M., & Lob-Levyt, J. (2009). AIDS: Lessons learnt and myths dispelled. *The Lancet,* published online March 20, 2009: doi:10.1016/S0140-6736(08)61345-8.

Plumeri, P. (1984). The refusal to treat: Abandonment and AIDS. *Journal of Clinical Gastroenterology, 6,* 281–284.

Pomerance, L., & Shields, J. (1989). Factors associated with hospital workers' reactions to the treatment of persons with AIDS. *AIDS Education and Prevention, 1*(3), 184–193.

Powers, M., & Faden, R. (2006). *Social justice: The moral foundations of public health.* New York: Oxford University Press.

Presidential Commission on the Human Immunodeficiency Virus Epidemic. (1988). *Report of the Presidential Commission on the human immunodeficiency virus epidemic.* Washington, DC: Author.

Pryor, J. (1988, October). Attitudes toward persons with AIDS: A mixture of fear and loathing. Paper presented at the Midwest Conference on the Social Implications of AIDS, Normal, IL.

The public's knowledge and perceptions about HIV/AIDS. (2006). *Kaiser Public Opinion spotlight.* Retrieved on March 11, 2009, from www.kff.org/spotlight/hiv/upload/Spotlight_Aug06_Knowledge-2.pdf.

Rawnsley, M. (1980). The concept of privacy. *Advances in Nursing Science, 2*(2), 25–31.

Rennie, S., & Behets, F. (2006). Desperately seeking targets: The ethics of routine HIV testing in low-income countries. *Bulletin of the World Health Association, 84*(1), 52–57.

Rondahl, G., Innala, S., & Carlson, M. (2003). Nursing staff and nursing students' attitudes toward HIV-infected and homosexual HIV-infected patients in Sweden and the wish to refrain from nursing. *Journal of Advanced Nursing, 41,* 454–461.

Rowland, C. (1986, April 1). The call of quarantine. *The Advocate, 443,* 42–46.

Sabatier, R. (1988). *Blaming others.* London: Panos Institute.

Selwyn, P. A., & Rivard, M. (2003). Palliative care for AIDS: Challenges and opportunities in the era of highly active anti-retroviral therapy. *Innovations in End-of-Life Care, 4*(3). Available online at www2.edc.org/lastacts/archives/archivesMay02/innovbios.asp.

Shapiro, H. T., & Meslin, E. M., (2001). Ethical issues in the design and conduct of clinical trials in developing countries. *New England Journal of Medicine, 345,* 139–142.

Shapiro, R. S., & Stein, R. E. (2004). Ethical and legal issues in AIDS vaccine trials. *Human Rights, 31*(4), 20–22.

Shah, S. (2006). *The body hunters.* New York: The New Press.

Simon, C., Maghboeba, M., & van Stade, D. (2007). Ethical challenges in the design and conduct of locally relevant international health research. *Social Science & Medicine, 64,* 1960–1969.

Simpson, J., & Forsyth, B. (2007). State-mandated HIV testing in Connecticut: Personal perspectives of women found to be infected during pregnancy. *Journal of the Association of Nurses in AIDS Care, 18*(5), 34–46.

Sokol, D. (2008). Ethics and epidemics. *American Journal of Bioethics, 8*(8), 28–29.

Steinbrook, R. (2007). One step forward, two steps backward—Will there ever be an AIDS vaccine? *New England Journal of Medicine, 357,* 2653–2655.

Steinbrook, R., Lo, B., Moulton, J., Saika, G., Hollander, H., & Volberding, P. (1986). Preferences of homosexual men with AIDS for life-sustaining treatment. *New England Journal of Medicine, 314*(7), 457–460.

Stone, L., & Gostin, L. (2004). Using human rights to combat the HIV/AIDS pandemic. *Human Rights Magazine, 31*(4), 2–3, 22.

Tarantola, D. (2008). Global justice and human rights: Health and human rights in practice. *Global Justice: Theory Practice Rhetoric, 1,* 11–26.

Tyer-Viola, L. A. (2007). Obstetric nurses' attitudes and nursing care intentions regarding HIV-positive pregnant women. *Journal of Obstetrical, Gynecological and Neonatal Nursing, 36,* 398–409.

UNAIDS (n.d.) *Human rights and HIV.* Retrieved on March 7, 2009, from www.unaids.org/en/PolicyAndPractice/HumanRights/20070601_reference_group_HIV_human_rights.asp.

UNAIDS. (2000a). *Ethical considerations in HIV preventive vaccine research.* Geneva: Author.

UNAIDS. (2000b). Protocol for identification of discrimination against people living with HIV. Retrieved March 27, 2009, from http://data.unaids.org/Publications/IRC-pub01/jc295-protocol_en.pdf.

UNAIDS. (2003). Combating stigma and discrimination is vital to improving access to HIV/AIDS care, says UNAIDS and WHO. Retrieved March 25, 2009, from http://data.unaids.org/Media/Press-Releases01/kampala_pr_26oct03_en.pdf.

UNAIDS/WHO. (2004). UNAIDS/WHO policy statement on HIV testing. Retrieved on March 20, 2009, from www.who.int/hiv/pub/vct/en/hivtestingpolicy04.pdf.

UNAIDS. (2007). Reducing HIV stigma and discrimination: A critical part of national AIDS programmes. Retrieved March 25, 2009, from http://data.unaids.org/pub/Report/2008/jc1420_stigma_discr_en.pdf.

UNAIDS. (2009). HIV testing and counseling. Retrieved March 20, 2009, from www.unaids.org/en/PolicyAndPractice/CounsellingAnd Testing/default.asp.

U.N. Secretary-General calls for end of discrimination against, travel restrictions on people living with HIV/AIDS. (2008). Retrieved March 29, 2009, from www.thebody.com/content/legal/art47069.html.

Valdiserri, R. O. (2002). HIV/AIDS stigma: An impediment to public health. *American Journal of Public Health, 92,* 341–342.

Vanable, P. A., Carey, M. P., Blair, D. C., & Littlewood, R. A. (2006). Impact of HIV-related stigma on health behaviors and psychological adjustment among HIV-Positive Men and Women. *AIDS and Behavior, 10,* 473–482.

Varmus, H., & Satcher, D. (1997). Ethical complexities of conducting research in developing countries. *New England Journal of Medicine, 337,* 1003–1005.

Waldholz, M., & Bishop, M. (1986, April 14). Testing as AIDS vaccine in people may be tougher than creating it. *Wall Street Journal,* p. 25.

Walker, R. M. (1999). Ethical issues in end-of-life care. *Cancer Control, 6*(2), 162–167.

Watkins, S., & Gray, J. (2006). Human immunodeficiency virus/acquired immune deficiency syndrome: A survey of knowledge, attitudes, and beliefs of Texas registered nurses in the 21st century. *Journal for Nurses in Staff Development, 22,* 232–238.

Webber, D. (2007). *AIDS and the law.* New York: Aspen Publishers.

Wenger, N. S., Kanouse, D. E., Collins, R. L., Liu, H., Schuster, M. A., & Gifford, A. L., et al. (2001). End-of-life discussions and preferences among persons with HIV. *Journal of the American Medical Association, 285,* 2880–2887.

Zonana, H. (1989). Warning third parties at risk of AIDS: APA's policy is a reasonable approach. *Hospital and Community Psychiatry, 40*(2), 162–164.

Preventing, Diagnosing, and Managing HIV Disease

5
Prevention of HIV Infection in the 21st Century

SANDE GRACIA JONES
CAROL A. "PAT" PATSDAUGHTER

In June 1982, Dr. William Darrow, a behavioral scientist at the Centers for Disease Control and Prevention's (CDC) sexually transmitted disease (STD) unit, was able to "connect the dots" from Patient Zero and demonstrate that HIV in homosexual men was sexually transmitted (Jones & Messmer, 2001, p. 219). Darrow, now a professor at Florida International University in Miami, FL, reflected on the issue of HIV prevention during a 1996 interview: "The riddle is, why is it that 15 years later we haven't seemed to progress? What can we do to stop the spread of AIDS? And, more importantly, why don't people change their behaviors?" (Ojito, 1996, p. 10).

More than a decade later, Darrow's concerns remain relevant. Although scientists know how HIV is transmitted, new cases of HIV infection occur globally every year. Knowing the "how" of HIV transmission has not been enough to stop the epidemic. In fact, the CDC (2008d) announced that their original estimate of 40,000 new cases of HIV infection in the United States per year was an underestimate. The new HIV incidence surveillance system has revealed that the epidemic is much worse (56,300 new infections in 2006), particularly among African Americans, Hispanics, and gay and bisexual men of all races/ethnicities.

In the 21st century, researchers and health care providers are now looking at combinations of biomedical, behavioral, and structural interventions to end the epidemic. However, there are major global challenges for HIV prevention. For example, over two-thirds of young men and women around the world do not have adequate knowledge about HIV; only one-third of HIV-infected pregnant women receive antiretroviral therapy;

139

and injecting drug users (IDUs) and men who have sex with men (MSM) still have poor access to HIV-preventive services (Horton & Das, 2008). Early prevention successes evolved from collective responses generated by people living with HIV/AIDS. Along with community groups, they confronted the stigma, discrimination, and denial associated with the disease (Merson et al., 2008). Moving forward, a global response to HIV prevention involving social factors such as sexual behavior, injecting drug use, and gender inequalities will be needed to fully address the HIV/AIDS pandemic (Merson et al., 2008).

Twelve years after Darrow's 1996 remarks, the Joint United Nations Programme on HIV/AIDS (UNAIDS) focused on the same questions for HIV prevention. Although a large body of knowledge has been developed over the past 25 years regarding HIV transmission and how to prevent infection, the problem remains that nearly 7,000 people around the world become infected with the virus every day (Piot et al., 2008). The international response to HIV prevention has gained some momentum due to three factors: (1) the availability of treatment with antiretroviral drugs, (2) the recognition that the pandemic has both development and security implications, and (3) a substantial increase in financial resources brought about by new funders and funding mechanisms (Merson et al., 2008, p. 475). The challenge is to develop and implement an effective HIV prevention global movement that supports not only biomedical strategies but also a combination of behavioral and structural approaches based on both scientifically derived evidence and the wisdom and ownership of communities (Merson et al., 2008).

This chapter will explore HIV prevention in the 21st century. It will begin with a brief review of routes of HIV transmission and subsequently discuss HIV prevention from biomedical, behavioral, and structural perspectives. Finally, this chapter will review some of the evidence-based interventions that have been recommended by the CDC as models for specific populations.

Readers may wish to review the *2008 Compendium of Evidence-Based HIV Prevention Interventions* developed through efficacy reviews by the Centers for Disease Control and Prevention (2008a) as a companion document to this chapter.

HIV TRANSMISSION

Routes of HIV transmission are usually classified into three modes: sexual transmission, transmission through blood and body fluids, and maternal-child transmission. HIV is primarily found in the blood, semen, or vaginal fluid of an infected person and is transmitted through exposure to HIV-infected blood or body products. HIV is spread by sexual contact with an infected person, by sharing needles and/or syringes (primarily used for drug injection) with someone who is infected, or through transfusions of infected blood or blood clotting factors (which are now extremely rare in countries where blood is screened for HIV antibodies). Babies born to HIV-infected women may become infected before or during birth or through breast-feeding after birth. A person may be at risk for HIV because of any of the following behaviors or conditions: (1) injected drugs or steroids during which equipment (e.g., needles, syringes, cotton, water) and blood were shared with others; (2) unprotected vaginal, anal, or oral sex (i.e., sex without using condoms) with men who have sex with men, multiple partners, or anonymous partners; (3) exchange of sex for drugs or money; (4) receipt of a diagnosis of, or treatment for, hepatitis, tuberculosis (TB), or a sexually transmitted disease such as syphilis; (5) blood transfusion or receipt of clotting factor between 1978 and 1985; (f) and/or unprotected sex with someone who has any of the risk factors listed above (CDC, 2008b, ¶ 3).

In the health care setting, workers have been infected with HIV after being stuck with needles containing HIV-infected blood or, less frequently, after infected blood gets into a worker's open cut or a mucous membrane (i.e., the eyes or inside of the nose). However, there has been only one instance of a patient being infected by a U.S. health care worker who had HIV (CDC, 2007a).

Behavioral variables are often examined in HIV prevention studies. However, to be truly effective, HIV prevention must move beyond simply looking at these behavioral variables. Effective HIV prevention planning must also demonstrate insight regarding the influence of the pervasive cultural, sociodemographic, socioeconomic, gender-specific, and relational factors that mediate risky sexual and drug-related behaviors (Exner et al., 2003; O'Leary & Wingood, 2000). Additionally, HIV prevention strategies must be grounded and implemented in the language of the target population. For example, Alberto Santana, Director of the National Alliance of State and Territorial AIDS Directors (NASTAD), has emphasized that specific strategies are needed to teach prevention and reach the diverse Hispanic communities in states such as Florida, New York, and California. Santana noted "the way you develop prevention methods for Cuban-Americans in Miami-Dade County would be different from how you develop prevention messages to Columbians and Venezuelans just in terms of the language that you use" (Hernandez, 2003, ¶ 1).

Sexual Transmission

All sexually active people are at risk for HIV, although denial of risk is common among many groups. Sexual transmission of HIV is a risk not only for adolescents and young adults but also for older adults and senior citizens due to the availability of drugs to treat erectile dysfunction (ED) (Jones et al., 2007). Both heterosexuals and homosexuals (i.e., MSM, women who have sex with women [WSW]) are at risk for HIV and other STDs. High-risk sexual practices include unprotected vaginal, anal, or oral sex (i.e., sex without using condoms or protective barriers), especially with multiple partners or anonymous partners. The existence of STDs also increases the risk of HIV transmission (CDC, 2007e). Persons who exchange sex for money, drugs, or essential commodities, particularly those who have been forced into this position, are at risk for HIV/STD transmission due to inability to negotiate or enforce condom use. Other socioeconomic or situational factors include the use of mood-altering substances, which may cause impairment of judgment in sexual encounters. A particularly high-risk situation that has occurred with MSMs is sexual encounters while simultaneously using recreational drugs, such as crystal methamphetamine, with sex-enhancing drugs, such as sildenafil (Viagra) (Elford, 2006).

Prevention measures include the use of physical barriers (e.g., male and female condoms, dental dams) and chemical barriers (e.g., experimental vaginal and rectal microbicides). Safer-sex behavioral practices include abstinence, monogamy/being faithful, consistent and correct use of barrier devices, and avoidance of mood-altering drugs. Effective prevention methods must also include education about risk factors and situational contexts that can lead to sexually transmitted HIV.

Barrier Devices

The CDC (2007a) has reported that male latex condoms are highly effective against HIV transmission when used consistently (i.e., every time) and correctly. The proper and consistent use of latex or polyurethane condoms when engaging in oral, vaginal, or anal sexual intercourse can greatly reduce a person's risk of acquiring or transmitting STDs, including HIV. While natural membrane (e.g., "skin" or lambskin) condoms are effective for contraception, they are not effective against HIV. These condoms contain natural pores, and laboratory studies have demonstrated that the HIV virus can pass through the pores.

Condoms, which are classified as medical devices, are regulated by the Food and Drug Administration (FDA) (CDC, 2007a). The FDA regulations include provisions for U.S. condom manufacturers to test latex condoms for defects, including holes, before they are packaged. Several studies of correct and consistent condom use in the United States have shown that latex condom breakage rates are less than 2%. Even when condoms do break, one study showed that more than half of such breaks occurred prior to ejaculation (CDC, 2007a).

An important step in effective male condom use is knowing how to properly apply a condom. With abstinence-only education taught in many U.S. school systems, young people—both young men and women—may not have learned condom use skills (Jones et al., 2008a). A study of 158 undergraduate college students revealed that condom breakage/slippage was associated with never having received instruction on correct condom use, more than one sex partner, and more frequent use of condoms as well as partner(s) being less than highly motivated to use condoms. Students using condoms without proper lubrication and those experiencing loss of erection during sex were more likely to report slippage (Yarbel et al., 2004). A study of heterosexual college men found that:

- 60% did not discuss condom use with their partner before sex;
- 42% reported they wanted to use condoms but did not have any available;
- 43% put condoms on after starting sex;
- 15% removed condoms before ending sex;
- 40% did not leave space at the tip;
- 30% placed the condom upside down on the penis and had to flip it over; and
- 32% reported losing erections with condom use (Crosby et al., 2002).

Besides loss of erection, other barriers to condom use include embarrassment when purchasing condoms and lack of income to purchase condoms (Crosby et al., 2008; Essien et al., 2005; Graham et al., 2006; Moore et al., 2008).

Women may wish to consider using the female condom (called "FC1") when a male condom cannot be used or if there is a latex allergy.

The FC1, approved by the Food and Drug Administration (FDA) in 1993, is available worldwide, although sometimes in limited quantities. About 35 million (or 90% of all FC1s) were distributed in resource-poor countries in 2008 (Graham, 2008). In the United States, the female condom has a retail cost of $1.15 to $2.75 (depending on distribution source), compared to a cost of 80 cents in resource-poor countries (Graham, 2008). Depending on the country, the female condom has various brand names, including Reality, Femidom, Dominique, Femy, Myfemy, Protectiv', and Care. The polyurethane 6.5-inch-long FC1 is lubricated but has no spermicide. A new 30% less expensive version of the current female condom, called the FC2, gained approval of an FDA advisory panel in December 2008, potentially leading to a broader distribution and use of this newer version of the FC. The FC2 is made of nitrile rubber, commonly used for making medical examination gloves.

The female condom has been distributed and extensively studied in Brazil and Africa. Although an FC may not be the preferred method of protection for the majority of women, the female condom may be a valuable option for some women if provided with access, proper education, and promotion (Barbosa et al., 2007; Napierala et al., 2008). Although the female condom has been promoted as a "female-controlled" method of protection, a U.S. study on the female condom with young urban men and women aged 15 to 20 found that the women were concerned about contraceptive effectiveness, side effects, and availability (i.e., over the counter vs. provider controlled) of the female condom and classified the female condom and the male condom as the same in terms of being "male-controlled" versus "female-controlled" (Latka, Kapadia, & Fortin, 2008). Other concerns that have been expressed with the female condom included lack of knowledge, difficulty in insertion, slippage during intercourse, and price (i.e., in U.S. retail drug stores, the FC costs more than three to four times more than a male condom).

The use of hormonal contraceptives (i.e., birth control pills) may be a factor for decreased or inconsistent condom use in women. A study of women who started using either the pill or depot medroxyprogesterone acetate (DMPA) found that of the women who had used condoms consistently before starting on DMPA or the pill, 54% discontinued consistent use after taking these contraceptives. Seventy-five percent of women in nonmonogamous relationships were inconsistent condom users, although nearly a third had been consistent condom users prior to beginning a hormonal contraceptive method (Sangi-Haghpeykar, Posner, & Pointdexter, 2005). Therefore, a priority for prevention education for women of childbearing age is the need for dual-method protection, emphasizing the use of the birth control pill to prevent contraception combined with the use of a condom to prevent infection with HIV or other STDs. Furthermore, education for postmenopausal women and their partners must also focus on the need to use condoms to prevent infection, even though contraception is no longer a concern.

HIV prevention education should also include information warning against the use of vaginal contraceptives/spermicides containing nonoxynol 9 (N9). In 2007, the FDA published warning statements and other labeling information for all over-the-counter (OTC) vaginal contraceptive drug products (also known as vaginal contraceptives/spermicides) containing N9. These warning statements advised consumers that vaginal contraceptives/spermicides containing N9 do not protect against HIV or STDs. The warnings and labeling information also advised consumers that use of vaginal contraceptives and spermicides containing N9 could irritate the vagina and rectum and may increase the risk of getting HIV from an infected partner (FDA, 2007).

Other types of barrier devices include the use of dental dams or natural latex rubber sheets for oral sex. Some inventive persons have used saran or plastic wrap as a barrier device or cut open a condom and laid it out flat. However, it is important to note that the efficacy of dental dams and other barrier devices has not been evaluated by the FDA.

STDs

Studies have shown that individuals who are infected with STDs are at least two to five times more likely than uninfected individuals to acquire HIV infection if they are exposed to the virus through sexual contact (CDC, 2008f). The CDC/Health Services Resources Administration (HRSA) Advisory Committee on HIV/AIDS and STD Prevention (CHAC) has recommended that early detection and treatment of STDs should be only one component of a comprehensive HIV prevention program, which also must include a range of biomedical, behavioral, and social interventions. CHAC has also recommended that:

- Early detection and treatment of curable STDs should become a major, explicit component of comprehensive HIV prevention programs at national, state, and local levels;
- In areas where STDs that facilitate HIV transmission are prevalent, screening and treatment programs should be expanded;

- HIV testing should always be recommended for individuals who are diagnosed with or suspected to have an STD; and
- HIV and STD prevention programs in the United States, together with private and public sector partners, should take joint responsibility for implementing these strategies. (CDC, 2008f, ¶ 2–3)

Heterosexual Transmission in Adolescents and Young Adults

A variety of factors are associated with risk for HIV in heterosexual young people. These include denial of risk coupled with desire for intimacy and an inability to integrate general knowledge of HIV risk into their personal interactions (O'Sullivan, Udell, & Patel, 2006). Results from the 2007 Youth Risk Behavior Surveillance System (YRBSS) survey indicated that 47.8% of high school students have had sexual intercourse in their lifetime. Additionally, 35.0% of high school students were currently sexually active, and 38.5% of these students had not used a condom during their last sexual intercourse (Eaton et al., 2008).

College-aged heterosexuals are also at risk for HIV due to high levels of sexual activity, decreased use of condoms, serial monogamy, and developmental issues such as feelings of invincibility and low perceived risk (Lewis, Malow, & Ireland, 1997; Opt et al., 2007; Roberts & Kennedy, 2006). HIV risk for ethnic minorities, such as Hispanic students, may be compounded by normative behaviors, gender roles, and cultural beliefs that affect their sexual practices (Gurman & Borzekowski, 2004; Jones et al., 2008a; Marin, 2003; Peragallo et al., 2005; Schiffner & Buki, 2006; Villarruel, Jemmott, & Jemmott, 2005).

The concept of romantic love may hinder risk assessment and safer-sex negotiation, particularly in young women (East et al., 2007). A study of first-semester nursing college students at a historically black college and university (HBCU) revealed that the students knew that HIV was a serious disease that could result in death (Adepoju, Watkins, & Richardson, 2007). However, the students also self-reported that they were willing to submit to the sexual demands of their partners, even when they refused to wear condoms. Over half of the females also stated that using a condom might diminish their feelings during the sexual experience, and they thought that it was important that this did not happen. In terms of prevention, the study findings demonstrated the need to incorporate intensive HIV/AIDS education into college curricula, including strategies that motivate students to use condoms in all sexual encounters and ways to negotiate safer sex.

Mood-altering substances may also influence unsafe sexual practices. Gullette and Lyons (2006) found that college students with low self-esteem consumed more alcohol, had more sexual partners, and had more HIV risk-taking behaviors than other students. A study that explored high-risk sexual behavior among 1,130 students at a South Florida minority-serving university showed that past-month alcohol use and illicit drug use were significantly associated with both risky and consistently risky sexual behavior (Trepka et al., 2008). These study findings demonstrated the need to address the use of alcohol and other drugs on campuses when planning interventions to promote safer sexual behavior.

The consumption of energy drinks has become popular on college campuses in the United States (Malinauskas et al., 2007).

A new phenomena that has emerged on campus is the consumption of alcohol mixed with energy drinks. College students perceive that energy drink consumption lessens subjective intoxication when consumed with alcohol. However, a study found that students who reported consuming alcohol mixed with energy drinks had significantly higher prevalence of alcohol-related consequences, including being taken advantage of sexually and taking advantage of another person sexually (O'Brien et al., 2008).

From an international perspective, socioeconomic factors may influence safer sex practices. A study of 4,800 young people aged 14 to 22 in Cape Town, South Africa, showed that social resources in households and communities mediated HIV risk behaviors (Camlin & Snow, 2008). Mothers' financial support for clothing, school fees and uniforms, and pocket money was associated with condom use, particularly among young women, suggesting that material need increased vulnerability to higher-risk behaviors.

Heterosexual Transmission in Older Adults

Many persons mistakenly believe that heterosexual older adults are not at risk for HIV/AIDS, and many older people do not perceive themselves to be at risk for HIV infection (Linsk, 2000; Longo et al., 2008; Williams & Donnelly, 2002). Gott (2001) studied men over age 50 and found that many participants reported that they had not received very much information on HIV and sexually transmitted diseases, and 7% engaged in behaviors that placed them at risk for a sexually transmitted disease. Older adults may reenter the dating scene after divorce or the death of a spouse, may not consider the need to use condoms, and may have misperceptions about their vulnerability to HIV (Falvo & Norman, 2004). In a study of older adults, Maes and Louis (2003) found that although respondents recognized the seriousness of AIDS, they did not believe that they were susceptible to the disease, even though 10% reported sexual activity outside of a long-term relationship.

To learn more about older adults' sexual beliefs, focus groups were conducted with older adults to discuss sexuality and sexual practices of older adults (Klein et al., 2001). The older adults' perceptions about sexuality and aging included:

1   Persons age 50 year of age and older, especially those expe-
    riencing life transitions, expose themselves to HIV infection
    through unprotected sexual behaviors.
2   Persons age 50 years of age and older may have sexual relations
    with people younger or older than themselves, but tend to have
    sexual relations with people of the same race.
3   Older adults may be more reluctant to discuss their sexual prac-
    tices than younger people.

The advent of effective erectile dysfunction (ED) pharmacotherapy has placed older adults at risk for HIV and other STDs (Karlovsky, Lebed, & Mydlo, 2004). Older heterosexual males using sildenafil or other ED drugs may be at risk for sexually acquired HIV because they lack factual knowledge of HIV transmission and may not perceive themselves as at risk for or susceptible to HIV (Palmer, 2000; Paniagua, 1999). Additionally, older men may use ED drugs with sexual partners who are not their primary partners (i.e., extramarital affairs, one-night casual encounters, paid encounters with sex workers). A study of heterosexual men aged 50 years of age and older using prescribed ED drugs found that men had misperceptions about HIV transmission, and some men in stable marital relationships used sildenafil during extramarital affairs (Jones et al., 2008b).

Older women are also at risk for HIV and STDs, although they may not perceive themselves to be at risk. Although older women need safer-sex messages, they may not listen to them (Palmer, 2000). Older women outnumber men, making women less likely to put a relationship at risk by insisting on use of a condom. Additionally, recently widowed or divorced older women who were married for decades may have never practiced safer sex in their lifetime and are unaccustomed to thinking about noncontraceptive protection. Women may also be oblivious to the risky behavior patterns of their male partners, who may go outside the relationship for sex (Palmer, 2000). Cultural and gender roles may also affect older women's safer-sex practices. For example, a study of older adult inner-city Latinos and Latinas revealed that women were significantly less likely to have experience with condoms than men; additionally, machismo, lack of perceived risk, and perceived ineffectiveness were identified as potential barriers to condom use (Hillman, 2008).

Substance use and abuse are cofactors for unsafe sex, and HIV risk in older persons may be related to drug and alcohol use (Williams & Donnelly, 2002). In the years 2000 to 2001, approximately one-third of the U.S. elderly population—about 11 million persons—consumed alcohol (Breslow, Faden, & Smothers, 2003). Specific later-life social contexts and coping dificulties are risk factors for late-life drinking problems among both women and men (Moos et al., 2004). A study of prescription drug use in the United States found that risk factors associated with problem use of prescription drugs included older age, persons in poor to fair health, and daily alcohol drinkers (Simoni-Wastila & Strickler, 2004).

Heterosexual Transmission in Women

Women are at risk for HIV acquisition due to both physiological and psychosocial factors. From a physiological perspective, women are more likely to acquire HIV for several biological reasons:

1   There is a more exposed surface area in the female genitals (i.e., sex organs) than in the male genitals.
2   There are higher levels of HIV in semen than in vaginal fluids.
3   More semen is exchanged during sex than vaginal fluids (Office on Women's Health, 2008).

Additionally, societal and economic factors influence women's risk for HIV. A study of women in India found that HIV-positive women were significantly more likely to report marital dissatisfaction, a history of forced sex, domestic violence, depressive symptoms, and husband's extramarital sex when compared to HIV-negative women (Gupta et al., 2008). Findings also indicated that specific factors related to the quality of the marital relationship may be related to HIV-related risks for women.

Gender roles also affect women's risk for HIV. Bertens and colleagues (2008) conducted a qualitative study to describe and understand gender roles and the relational context of sexual decision making and safer sex negotiation among Afro-Surinamese and Dutch Antillean women in the Netherlands. In negotiating safer sex with a partner, women reported encountering ambiguity between being respectable and being responsible. The need to be respectable inhibited negotiation practices because there was no perceived need for respectable, virtuous women to use condoms. Respectable women would participate only in serious monogamous relationships, which they considered to be inherently safe. Safer sex negotiation was limited by women's desire to feel like a woman, "to tame the macho-man" and constrain him into a steady relationship (p. 547). Respectability appeared to enforce silence about men's sexual infidelity. The researchers concluded that this ambiguity due to cultural values and gender roles should be considered when developing HIV/STD prevention programs. Additionally, raising awareness of power imbalances and conflicting roles and values may support women in safer sex decision making.

Consistent with the Netherlands study findings, safer sex practices of Hispanic women may be affected by gender differences, ethnicity roles, and normative beliefs (Jemmott, Jemmott, & Villarruel, 2002; Marin, 2003). Jones and colleagues (2008a) conducted focus groups with Latina nursing students to discover their perceptions regarding contemporary barriers to safer sex practices for Latina students in South Florida. A major theme that emerged from the focus groups was "With Latinas, it's all about being La Senorita" (p. 315). This phrase referred to the gender-specific Hispanic concept of a woman's role post-nina (i.e., little girl), which commenced on the Latina's 15th birthday (i.e., quince anos) and ended with becoming "La Senora" (i.e., a married woman). "La Senorita" was expected to remain a virgin until marriage, while a male in this same age group was expected to become sexually experienced (i.e., machismo). While the young women did not condone male sexual activity, it was often quietly accepted and even expected. The dual expectations of "La Senorita" were to remain a virgin while attracting and keeping a sexually active male who would become her husband. These potentially competing expectations could lead to unsafe sexual practices. This concept varied among Hispanic ethnic groups and was influenced by the females' socioeconomic status, educational status, and level of acculturation. The concept was also greatly influenced by parental expectations. Other traditional beliefs related to sex and gender roles (e.g., men being unable to control their sexual desires; women pleasing men rather than considering their own desires) may contribute to high-risk sexual activity. Thus, men may be encouraged to have multiple sex partners, while women face emotional consequences when they request use of a condom, which becomes a signal of their promiscuous sexual behavior.

The influence of gender roles on safer-sex practices has also been noted with Caribbean women. In a study of HIV/AIDS prevention practices among recent-immigrant, single Jamaican women, Gillespie-Johnson (2008) found that the women did not perceive themselves as susceptible to HIV. Although participants were not sure of a mutually monogamous relationship, they did not use condoms, and talking about sexual issues was viewed as taboo. Barriers to condom use included lack of condom negotiation skills, fear of losing their relationship, and fear of physical or mental abuse from their significant other.

Nonvolitional sex is sexual behavior that violates a person's right to choose when and with whom to have sex and in which sexual behaviors to engage. Extreme examples of nonvolitional sex include rape, forced sex, childhood sexual abuse, and sex trafficking (Kalmuss, 2004). Gender and power inequities can lead to nonvolitional sex, placing women around the world at risk for HIV (González-Guarda, Peragallo, & Vasquez, 2008; Weidel, Provencio-Vasquez, & González-Guarda, 2008). For example, a study of female African American adolescents revealed that the girls who reported a history of sexual abuse or molestation were more likely to think that condoms interfered with sexual pleasure and were less likely to think that condoms were important to partners than girls with no history of sexual abuse (Hall et al., 2008). Additionally, the girls with a history of sexual abuse reported more instances of unprotected vaginal sex and more lifetime sex partners.

The trafficking (i.e., selling or trading) of young women and children for prostitution and other forms of sexual exploitation is one of the most significant human rights abuses in contemporary society (Hodge, 2008) and is a global concern (also see chapter 16). A study of 580 brothel-based sex workers in eastern India found that one in every four sex workers (24%) had joined the profession by being trafficked (Sarkar et al., 2008). Violence early in the profession was more prevalent among the trafficked victims, including women sold by their family members, compared to women who voluntarily joined the profession. Furthermore, HIV infection was significantly associated with sexual violence.

Female-initiated HIV prevention methods are needed, particularly in developing countries where gender and power inequities place women at risk for HIV. However, there are few female-initiated HIV prevention devices beyond the previously mentioned female condom. Although research over the past decade has focused on vaginal microbicides, none have been found to be effective to date (Cutler & Justman, 2008; Poynten et al., 2008). For example, a completed Phase III study found that carrageenan (Carraguard) alone was safe to use vaginally but was not effective at preventing HIV infection when compared with a placebo gel. Carrageenan is now being studied in combination with other investigational microbicides to increase the effectiveness of HIV prevention (AIDSInfo, 2008). In another study, Van Damme and colleagues (2008) conducted a randomized, double-blind, placebo-controlled trial of cellulose sulfate, an HIV-entry inhibitor formulated as a vaginal gel, involving women at high risk for HIV infection at three African and two Indian sites. A total of 1,398 women were enrolled and randomly assigned to receive cellulose sulfate gel ($n = 706$ participants) or placebo ($n = 692$ participants) and had follow-up HIV tests. The results were 41 newly acquired HIV infections, 25 in the cellulose sulfate group and 16 in the placebo group. The researchers concluded that cellulose sulfate did not prevent HIV infection and may have increased the risk of HIV acquisition.

Sexual Transmission in Women Who have Sex with Women

Myths of lesbian "immunity" or "invulnerabity" with respect to HIV/AIDS are common among both WSW and health care providers. These myths have served to limit targeted and tailored education and prevention efforts for lesbians and bisexual women, negatively influence and affect lesbians' risk perceptions and behaviors, and restrict resources for research on HIV transmission in WSW. Although the CDC (2006b) has noted that there have been no confirmed cases of female-to-female transmission of HIV to date, the risk for HIV infection in WSW may be related to other factors. From a national sample of 1,139 self-identified lesbians, Patsdaughter and colleagues (2003) found that although 83.5% of the sample believed that WSW are at risk for HIV/AIDS, only 15.5% believed that they were personally at risk. However, 64.3% of the sample had taken an HIV test, 11.8% within the past year, with a seroprevalance rate of 0.6%. HIV risks included history of sex with men (74.6%), body piercing (64.7%), tattooing (24.3%), history of sexual abuse (50.7%), rape (27.3%), sex under the influence of drugs or alcohol (36%), contact with menstrual blood during sex (33.3%), and multiple sexual partners during past six months (11.3%). The study found that discrepancies existed between lesbians' perceived personal HIV risk and their perceptions of risk for WSW in general, testing history, and risk factors or behaviors.

From a prevention perspective, the CDC (2006b) has recommended that WSW need to know (1) their own and their partner's serostatus, (2) the risk for exposure through a mucous membrane, and (3) the potential benefits of using condoms during sexual contact with men or when using sex toys. The CDC has also cautioned that the efficacy of barriers such as dental dams during oral sex has not been adequately evaluated.

Heterosexual Transmission in Men

Besides adolescents and college students, sexual health promotion interventions for heterosexuals in the United States have focused primarily on women (Seal & Ehrhardt, 2004). However, as previously mentioned, a consequence of the advent of effective erectile dysfunction (ED) pharmacotherapy is the risk of HIV and other sexually transmitted diseases, especially in the older population (Karlovsky et al., 2004).

Cultural and group values may also globally influence safer-sex practices of heterosexual men. A Brazilian study of heterosexual men found that vulnerability to HIV was related to sexual beliefs and the Hispanic concept of masculinity (Guerriero, Ayres, & Hearst, 2002). Thematic analysis revealed various themes that made the men more vulnerable to HIV, which included: (1) feeling strong and immune to the disease; (2) engaging in impetuous, risky behaviors; (3) inability to refuse a woman; and (4) the belief that men needed sex more than women and that sexual desires cannot be controlled. Other ethnic or cultural sexual beliefs were that men's infidelity is a natural behavior, while women's infidelity is a result of her partner's ineptitude. The men also believed that it was up to the men to make the decision to use or not use condoms and that women can only ask men to use condoms to prevent pregnancy. The men related that refusal to use condoms was related to aesthetical and economical reasons, fear of failing erection, and a loss of sensibility for both men and women. The participants had little knowledge of modes of HIV infection and did not consider themselves vulnerable to HIV or other sexually transmitted diseases (Guerriero et al., 2002).

Extramarital sex, lack of perceived risk for HIV, and risky sexual practices were also found in studies of Hispanic/Latino men from Central and South America. One study of sexually active married or cohabitating men in Mexico City revealed that 15% reported extramarital sex during the past year, usually with coworkers, mistresses, or friends; only 9% reported condom use during last intercourse; and 80% perceived no HIV risk (Pulerwitz, Izazola-Licea, & Gortmaker, 2001). A study in

Bogota, Columbia showed that heterosexual men exhibited more risky sexual behaviors and practices than homosexuals or bisexuals (Miguez-Burbano et al., 2001). Additionally, consistent condom use was reported by only 20% of individuals who practiced anal sex and only 5% among men who had sex with women during menses.

Homosexual Transmission in Men

HIV infection among MSM has been increasing, particularly among communities where there is a stigma against homosexuality. Reports at the 2008 XVII International AIDS Conference in Mexico discussed the challenge of HIV prevention for MSMs. Kevin Frost, CEO of the American Foundation for AIDS Research, stated that "The same kinds of stigma and discrimination and institutionalized homophobia that failed gay men in America is now failing MSM in the rest of the world" (Benin and the Global Fund, 2008, ¶ 1). Richard Wolitski, acting director of the CDC's HIV/AIDS prevention unit, also stated that other factors contributing to the problem included 'prevention fatigue,' confidence in new antiretroviral drugs, the use of methamphetamines, and the arrival of a generation of young men who did not experience the ravages of the 1980s" (Benin and the Global Fund, 2008, ¶ 1).

The National HIV Behavioral Surveillance (NHBS) System was developed in 2002 by the CDC to help health departments monitor selected behaviors of groups at highest risk for HIV infection and to assist in assessing the use of prevention programs and services. HIV testing is considered by the CDC to be a cornerstone of HIV prevention because persons who know their status may reduce risk behaviors and can be referred to appropriate care and treatment. Additional prevention activities in the United States include behavior-change strategies and the provision of both prevention information and prevention materials (e.g., condoms). The NHBS began collecting data from MSM in 17 U.S. metropolitan statistical areas (MSAs) in 2003 and obtained survey data from 25 MSAs in 2005. Sanchez and colleagues (2006) summarized data from approximately 10,000 MSM who participated in the NHBS from November 2003 to April 2005. Over 90% of the participants had ever had an HIV test, 77% within the preceding year. Over half (58%) of the participants reported unprotected anal sex with a primary male partner (e.g., boyfriend, spouse, significant other, or life partner) and over a third (34%) with a casual male partner. While most participants (80%) had received free condoms within the last year, only a few had participated in individual-level HIV prevention programs (15%) and even fewer in group-level interventions (8%). Forty-six percent of the participants reported noninjection drug use during the preceding 12 months, with the most commonly used drugs being marijuana (77%), cocaine (37%), ecstasy (29%), poppers (28%), and stimulants (27%). In addition to male sex partners, 14% of the participants also had had at least one female sex partner in the past year.

Other studies have also noted that gay and nongay identified MSM also have sex with women. For example, a study of African American men in Alabama found that "sneaky sex" (sometimes called "down low" sex) was a high-risk scenario practiced by married or nominally heterosexual men (Lichtenstein, 2000, p. 374). Covert and unprotected sex among bisexually active black men was common, for reasons including the desire to maintain a façade of heterosexuality in homophobic communities. More recently, in a report of a study that included a multiethnic sample of men (i.e., African American, Latino, white, and Asian), Siegel and colleagues (2008) discussed how men who have sex with men and women (MSMW) serve as a "bisexual bridge" for HIV acquisition and transmission (p. 720). Dodge, Jefferies, and Sandfort (2008) called for future HIV prevention intervention efforts to include not only skills building among MSMW but also increased social awareness and acceptance of male homosexuality. These researchers argued that greater support is needed toward "decreasing the secrecy involved in many bisexual men's encounters as well as its consequential risks" (p. 17). Additionally, Dodge and colleagues highlighted the importance of HIV prevention interventions that educate women as well as MSMW.

Several systematic reviews have evaluated the efficacy of behavioral interventions for reducing sexual risk behaviors of MSM. For example, in a meta-analytic review, Herbst and colleagues (2005) concluded that characteristics of successful interventions were that they were based on theoretical models, included interpersonal skills training, incorporated several delivery methods, and were delivered over multiple sessions over a minimum of three weeks. Following a review of behavioral intervention research, Johnson and colleagues (2008) concluded that a variety of behavioral interventions can lead to significant risk reduction in MSM. However, these reviewers also noted that continued research is needed to further identify which behavioral strategies are most effective in reducing HIV transmission as well as which intervention components are most influential, particularly for nonwhite MSM in affluent countries and MSM in resource-limited regions of the world.

Exposure to Blood and Body Fluids

Besides sexual transmission, HIV can be transmitted through blood, body fluids, and other biological products. HIV can be transmitted to patients during blood transfusion, plasma donation, organ transplantation, and artificial insemination (Ganczak & Barss, 2008). HIV can also be transmitted through the use of unsterile or contaminated equipment. Theoretically, this includes any invasive procedure, from an endoscopy in the hospital setting to getting a tattoo or a body piercing. Use of unsterile equipment during a manicure or pedicure where cuticle tissue is clipped or cut is also a potential risk for HIV infection and other blood-borne diseases.

IDUs are at risk for HIV due to the frequency of sharing used needles. Sharing of contaminated needles can also pose an HIV risk for others, such as athletes sharing steroid injections, diabetics sharing insulin syringes, and transgendered persons sharing hormone injections. The common factor is contaminated needles.

Injection Drug Users

IDUs are at risk for HIV due to the frequency of sharing used needles; estimates of incidence rates are between 10 to 50 per 100 person-years (Des Jarlais & Semaan, 2008). Although IDUs account for only 10% of the 4.3 million new cases of HIV infection that are reported on a global basis each year, IDUs account for 30% of new cases outside of sub-Saharan Africa (Des Jarlais & Semaan, 2008). IDUs are a hard-to-reach population from a prevention perspective because of their illegal activities and other lifestyle and structural considerations. However, successes have been reported through community-based outreach, targeted individual- and group-level interventions, access to sterile injection equipment, access to condoms, and simultaneous substance abuse treatment endeavors (Des Jarlais & Semaan, 2008). Most HIV prevention interventions for IDUs follow a harm reduction philosophy.

One method of HIV prevention for this group has been needle exchange programs (NEPs). The first NEP was initiated in Amsterdam, the Netherlands, in 1981 in response to an outbreak of hepatitis B. This is the same year in which AIDS was observed in IDUs (Des Jarlais & Semaan, 2008). Subsequently, NEPs were established in most developed countries and the United States, although not without heated moral and political controversy. One study estimated that an NEP in New York averted four to seven HIV infections per 1,000 clients and reduced HIV treatment costs by $325,000 per prevented case (Belani & Muennig, 2008). However, there has been resistance to implementation of NEPs in resource-limited and transitional countries because of the notion that NEPs pose a threat to the international war on drugs and global drug prohibition (Wodak & Cooney, 2006).

Several countries, including the Netherlands, Switzerland, Germany, Spain, Norway, Luxembourg, Australia, and Canada, have also experimented with safer injection facilities (SIFs), also known as "drug consumption rooms," "safe injection sites," and "consumer rooms" (Kerr et al., 2007; Kerr & Palepu, 2001; Morse, 2008). SIFs provide a safe, clean, and supervised environment for IDUs to inject preobtained drugs. Other services may include emergency response to drug overdose, care for injection-related injuries, assessment and referral to primary health care services, harm reduction education and counseling, needle exchange, and sexual health education with access to condoms and lubricant (Morse, 2008). As with NEPs, there are many legal and ethical issues related to SIFs (Elliott, Malkin, & Gold, 2002). However, SIFs do have the potential to reduce HIV transmission through contaminated needles and equipment.

Contaminated Medical and Cosmetic Equipment

In the United States, strict infection control protocols are in place to prevent blood-borne disease transmission through contaminated equipment. These protocols include the use of one-time use, disposable equipment (e.g., gloves, syringes) and autoclaving for any reusable equipment. However, the strict U.S. protocols may not be available and/or practical in other parts of the world.

Correa and Gisselquist (2006) assessed the variety and frequency of blood exposures in health care and cosmetic services in India by interviewing people living with HIV/AIDS in four districts with a high HIV prevalence rate. Eighty percent reported from 1 to 300 injections in the five years before testing HIV positive. Common lifetime exposures include dental care (31%), surgery (20%), blood tests (100%), and tattooing (47%). When the researchers conducted observations and interviews with physicians, dentists, and others, they found evidence for common to routine reuse of unsterilized equipment for blood tests (e.g., lancets), dental care, tattoos, and surgery.

Blood or Biological Products

In the early 1980s, before HIV transmission was fully understood, the blood therapy industry and its regulators delayed enacting appropriate regulations to protect the nation's blood supply. This delay resulted in HIV infection of persons with hemophilia and blood transfusion recipients around the world, with devastating impact on their quality of life, quality of care, and longevity (Evatt, 2006; Weinberg et al., 2002). Because of public concern about blood-supply decisions made in the 1980s, developed countries in the 1990s adopted diagnostic tests and procedures that improved the safety of the blood supply. However, resource-limited countries still have problems with blood-supply safety issues. It is estimated that up to 10% of HIV infections result from transfusion of blood or blood products in resource-limited countries (Weinberg et al., 2002).

To prevent HIV transmission and protect the safety of the public, HIV remains an absolute exclusion criteria for donation of blood or organs (Gutierrez & Andres, 2007). However, HIV-infected persons can receive blood or organ transplants. HIV infection is also an exclusion for sperm donation. However, new technology such as sperm washing and assisted reproduction techniques has been successfully and safely implemented for HIV serodiscordant couples, resulting in a 70% pregnancy rate in one study (Savasi et al., 2007).

Occupational Exposure for Health Care Providers

Health care workers are at risk for acquisition of HIV and other blood-borne pathogens through occupational exposure to blood and other potentially infectious body fluids (Calfee, 2006). This exposure most frequently results from needle stick injuries, cuts, and splashes from body fluids to mucous membranes or nonintact skin, potentially exposing health care workers to various blood-borne pathogens, including HIV and hepatitis. According to Panlilio and colleagues (2005), "In prospective studies of HCP [health care personnel], the average risk for HIV transmission after a percutaneous exposure to HIV-infected blood has been estimated to be approximately 0.3% . . . and after a mucous membrane exposure, approximately 0.09%" (p. 2). While several thousand health care personnel (e.g., nurses, health aids, physicians) are HIV infected, these infections have largely resulted from nonoccupational exposures to HIV. According to the CDC (2007b), "As of December 2001, occupational exposure to HIV has resulted in 57 documented cases of HIV seroconversion among healthcare personnel (HCP) in the United States."

Using appropriate techniques, personal protective equipment (PPE) and safer "sharp" technology can minimize the risk of these exposures. When exposure does occur, immediate evaluation and initiation of post-exposure prophylaxis (PEP), when indicated, can substantially reduce the risk of transmission of HIV. The U.S. Public Health Service guidelines for management of occupational exposure recommends that priorities for PEP include; (1) adherence to HIV PEP when it is indicated for an expo-sure, (2) expert consultation in management of exposures, (3) follow-up of exposed workers to improve adherence to PEP, and (4) monitoring for adverse events, including seroconversion (Panlilio et al., 2005).

Ganczak and Szych (2007) evaluated self-reported compliance with personal protective equipment (PPE) use among 601 surgical nurses in Poland and factors associated with both compliance and noncompliance. While compliance was high for glove use (83%), it was much lower for protective eyewear (9%). Only 5% of the nurses routinely used gloves, masks, protective eyewear, and gowns when in contact with potentially infective material. The most commonly stated reasons for noncompli-ance were: (1) nonavailability of PPE (37%), (2) the conviction that the source patient was not infected (33%), and (3) staff concern that following locally recommended practices actually interfered with providing good patient care (32%). The researchers recommended wider implementa-tion, evaluation, and improvement of training in infection control, pref-erably combined with practical experience with HIV patients, easier access of PPE, and improved comfort of PPE.

Although infrequent in the United States, HIV infection has occurred as a result of occupational exposure to HIV. Investigation of cases of HIV infection in health care personnel without identified risk factors is coor-dinated by the CDC and state health departments. Documented cases of occupationally acquired HIV/AIDS are those in which HIV serocon-version is temporally related to an exposure to an HIV-positive source and in which the exposed worker has no nonoccupational risk factors for acquisition of HIV. Possible cases of occupationally acquired HIV/AIDS are situations in which a worker is found to be HIV positive; has no nonoccupational risk factors for HIV/AIDS; and has opportunities for occupational exposure to blood, body fluids, or HIV-positive laboratory material. Although seroconversion after exposure was not documented for these personnel, occupational acquisition of their infection might have been possible.

Of the health care personnel for whom case investigations were completed from 1981 through 2006, 57 had documented HIV seroconversion following occupational exposures. Of this group, 24 were nurses. The routes of exposure resulting in infection were: percutaneous (puncture/cut injury) (n = 48), mucocutaneous (mucous membrane and/or skin) (n = 5), combined percutaneous and mucocutaneous (n = 2), and unknown route (n = 2). Forty-nine health care personnel were exposed to HIV-infected blood; three to concentrated virus in a laboratory; one to visibly bloody fluid; and four to an unspecified fluid. In addition, 140 possible cases of HIV infection or AIDS have occurred among health care personnel (CDC, 2007d).

Maternal-Child (Vertical) Transmission

The third way that HIV can be transmitted is from mother to child. HIV-positive mothers can transfer HIV infection to their babies during the birthing process (also see Chapters 13 and 14). Additionally, because HIV is found in breast milk, breast-feeding can result in HIV transmission. Prevention strategies for vertical transmission risk reduction include prenatal HIV counseling and testing, prenatal care, intravenous (IV) zidovudine (AZT) or nevaripine (NVP) during delivery, elective caesarean section for delivery, and avoidance of breast-feeding. The implementation of these strategies has reduced perinatal transmission to less than 2% in the United States (Public Health Service Task Force, 2008). However, perinatal HIV transmission remains a significant concern in all resource-limited countries around the world.

Antiretroviral drugs reduce perinatal transmission by decreasing maternal antepartum viral load and as pre- and postexposure prophylaxis for the infant. Zidovudine (AZT) has been approved by the FDA for the prevention of vertical transmission of HIV from an HIV-infected mother to her fetus. The AZT regimen includes: (1) oral AZT administered to the mother beginning at 14 to 34 weeks of gestation, (2) IV AZT administered to the mother during labor, and (3) oral AZT administered to the neonate for the first six weeks of life.

HIV infection during pregnancy has been associated with increased rates of preterm delivery, low birth weight, and stillbirth (Bartlett & Gallant, 2007). The probability of perinatal transmission is directly related to the mother's HIV viral load at the time of delivery. Factors that reduce perinatal transmission include a reduction of the mother's viral load; use of prenatal, perinatal, and postnatal AZT in developed countries; the use of nevirapine (NVP) in resource-limited countries; and cesarean section.

Although breast-feeding is discouraged among HIV-infected women in developed countries, there is a dilemma in resource-limited countries, where breast-feeding may be the only or best available option. Recent research has suggested that when antiretroviral drugs are given over several weeks to mothers and/or to their newborn infants during the postnatal period, the risk of HIV transmission via breast-feeding can be dramatically reduced (Kumwenda et al, 2008;); moreover, one recent study involving 958 HIV-infected women and their infants in Zambia found that "early, abrupt cessation of breast-feeding by HIV-infected women in a low-resource setting . . . does not improve the rate of HIV-free survival among children born to HIV-infected mothers and is harmful to HIV-infected infants" (Kuhn et al., 2008, p. 130). The risk of HIV transmission with breast-feeding is increased with mastitis, breast abscess, cracked nipples, infant with thrush, primary HIV infection during pregnancy, and prolonged breast-feeding (Bartlett & Gallant, 2007). Researchers are currently studying a nipple shield that can disinfect breast milk. The shield contains a layer of cotton wool soaked in sodium dedecyl sulphate, which deactivates the HIV virus (Breast Milk Purged, 2008).

A priority for prevention of perinatal transmission is preconceptional counseling and care for HIV-infected women of childbearing age. The 2008 Public Health Service Task Force recommendations for reducing perinatal HIV transmission in the United States include:

1 Select effective and appropriate contraceptive methods to reduce the likelihood of unintended pregnancy.
2 Provide preconception counseling on safe sexual practices and elimination of alcohol, illicit drug use, and smoking, which are important both for maternal health as well as for fetal/infant health should the women become pregnant.
3 Choice of an antiretroviral regimen for treatment of HIV-infected women of childbearing potential needs to include consideration of effectiveness for treatment of maternal disease and the drug's potential for teratogenicity should pregnancy occur.
4 Attainment of a stable viral maximally suppressed viral load prior to conception is recommended for HIV-infected women who are on antiretroviral therapy and wish to become pregnant. (Public Health Service Task Force, 2008, p. 8)

HIV PREVENTION INTERVENTIONS
Biomedical Interventions

Research on biomedical interventions poses formidable challenges (Padian et al., 2008). Decades of time and money have been spent in the quest to develop HIV/AIDS vaccines. AIDSinfo (2006) distinguished between: (1) preventive HIV vaccines, which are designed to protect non-infected persons from acquiring HIV infection: and (2) thera-peutic vaccines, which are designed to control the progress of infection in persons who are already HIV positive. To date, there has been no success and many setbacks. Bernstein (2008), executive director of the Global HIV Vaccine Enterprise, has noted several reasons why devel-oping an HIV vaccine has been so difficult:

1   HIV has evolved highly sophisticated ways to evade the immune system. Its extraordinarily high degree of sequence diversity, caused by mutation and recombination, makes it espe-cially challenging to design neutralizing antibodies that recog-nize the broad range of epitopes needed for effective immune protection.
2   HIV wipes out some of the very cells needed to mount an effec-tive immune response. (p. 717)

Bernstein (2008) also noted that part of the problem of developing effec-tive vaccines is the lack of a robust animal model that simulates critical features of both HIV and the human immune system.

About 30 vaccine candidates are currently in trials. Approximately 50 HIV vaccine candidates have been tested in humans; however, only two reached Phase III trials, and both of these were found to be inef-fective. In September 2007, the Merck V520-023 study (also referred to as the STEP study or HVTN 502), which began enrolling participants in December 2004, was called to a halt by an independent Data and Safety Monitoring Board (DSMB) (Clinical Alert, 2007). Preliminary data anal-ysis in this trial showed proportionately more cases of HIV infection in volunteers who received the vaccine versus volunteers who received a placebo.

At the 2008 AIDS Vaccine Conference in Cape Town, South Africa, Bernstein indicated that setbacks in vaccine trials have "forced them [researchers] to look for entirely new ways of creating a defense against the disease" (Henry Kaiser Family Foundation, 2008b). However, it was also noted that the current global economic crisis could further impede future vaccine development and testing Henry Kaiser Family Foundation, 2008a).

Although vaccine research has not been fruitful to date, some progress has been made with other biomedical interventions, although there have been inconsistent levels of evidence. Some studies of male circumcision have demonstrated that circumcision can be protective against HIV acquisition among men; however, this protection against HIV transmission may be greater for men who have sex with women than for men who have sex with men (Millett et al., 2008; Vermund & Qian, 2008). In addition, results from one recent study with HIV-discordant African couples (1,015 men were HIV positive, 770 were married) showed that male circumcision conferred no indirect benefit to the female partners (Vermund & Qian, 2008). Around the world, the proportion of men who are circumcised varies from 5% to 80% by country (on average, an estimated 30 to 40% of adult men worldwide are circumcised) (Gostin & Hankins, 2008). This variation reflects practices with religious and cultural significance as well as hygiene practices (Gostin & Hankins, 2008).

The World Health Organization (WHO) (2008) published its recommendations of priority interventions for HIV/AIDS prevention, treatment, and care in the health sector. WHO's analysis of randomized clinical trials for male circumcision revealed that circumcision reduced the risk of heterosexually acquired HIV in men by about 60%. However, WHO also concluded that there was no definitive evidence that circumcision reduced the risk of HIV transmission from men to women or between men. WHO recommended that male circumcision undertaken by trained health care providers in appropriate clinical settings be considered as part of a comprehensive HIV prevention package. HIV-negative men considering circumcision must be counseled that having sexual relations before complete wound healing occurs could result in an increased risk of acquiring HIV. Therefore, abstention from sexual activity is necessary until the surgical wounds are completely healed.

WHO also advised that because male circumcision does not provide complete protection against HIV, other preventive methods should be continued along with circumcision. These include using male and female condoms, delaying sexual debut, and reducing the number of sexual partners. Additionally, WHO noted that monitoring and evaluating circumcision programs must be maintained to minimize the potential negative gender-related impact of male circumcision programs, such as an increase in unsafe sex or sexual violence. Barriers to circumcision in heterosexual have been noted to include "human rights issues, ethical and legal issues, high cost, fear of pain, safety concerns, availability of surgery services, and sexual risk compensation if men overrate their degree of protection and ongoing risk" (Vermund & Qian, 2008). Given the results of recent research that raise questions about efficacy of circumcision in preventing HIV transmission, cultural and religious factors, and a distrust engendered by colonial exploitation, it appears unlikely that mass circumcision campaigns will be mounted in Africa or in other resource-poor parts of the world (Glenn, 2005).

Another biomedical approach to HIV prevention is the early detection and treatment of STDs. As previously mentioned, the presence of an STD increases the risk of HIV transmission and acquisition. WHO (2008) advised that countries expand the provision of good-quality STD care into primary health care, sexual and reproductive health services, and HIV services. Additionally, WHO recommended that national guidelines based on identified patterns of infection and disease should be developed and disseminated to all providers of STD care.

Lastly, from a biomedical perspective, continued research is needed on the effectiveness of the use of oral and topical antiretroviral compounds to reduce HIV transmission during sexual intercourse. As noted earlier, several vaginal microbicide clinical trials were stopped when they failed to show evidence of protectiveness against HIV infection. However, combinations of different microbicides are being investigated to determine if a combination strategy will be successful in producing an effective vaginal or rectal microbide that will prevent transmission of HIV (AIDSinfo, 2008).

Padian and colleagues (2008) noted some of the challenges with research on biomedical interventions. These include difficulties with product adherence and the possibility of sexual disinhibition, along with the nature of control groups and the effect of adherence on the true effectiveness of the intervention.

Behavioral Strategies

How can behavioral strategies work better to reduce HIV transmission? WHO (2008) noted that behavioral interventions at individual, group, or community levels can generate safer sex behaviors, but interventions must be sustained for behavioral change over long periods of time. Additionally, HIV prevention services around the world have been poorly supported, underresourced, and late in starting. Discussing the challenges of global HIV prevention strategies, Coates, Richter, and Caceres (2008) have defined five key areas relevant to global HIV prevention behavioral strategies:

1 For successful reductions in HIV transmission, the aggregate effect of radical and sustained behavioral changes in a sufficient number of individuals potentially at risk is needed. Combination prevention is essential because HIV prevention is neither simple nor simplistic. Reductions in HIV transmission need widespread and sustained efforts and a mix of communication channels to disseminate messages to motivate people to engage in a range of options to reduce risk.

2 Prevention programs can do better. The effect of behavioral strategies could be increased by aiming for many goals (e.g., delay in onset of first intercourse, reduction in number of sexual partners, increases in condom use) that are achieved by use of multilevel approaches (e.g., couples, families, social and sexual networks, institutions, and entire communities) with populations both uninfected and infected with HIV.

3 Prevention science can do better. Interventions derived from behavioral science have a role in overall HIV-prevention efforts, but they are insufficient when used by themselves to produce substantial and lasting reductions in HIV transmission between individuals or in entire communities.

4 We need to get the simple things right. The fundamentals of HIV prevention need to be agreed on, funded, implemented, measured, and achieved. That, presently, is not the case. (Coates et al., 2008, p. 669)

THE CDC'S PREVENTION RESEARCH SYNTHESIS PROJECT

In 1996, the Prevention Research Branch of the CDC's Division of HIV/AIDS Prevention started the HIV/AIDS Prevention Research Synthesis (PRS) Project. The goals of this initiative were to: (1) systematically review and summarize the U.S.–based HIV behavioral prevention literature and (2) translate scientific evidence into practical information for use by HIV prevention providers and researchers

(CDC, 2007c). A database of over 5,000 articles and reports was reviewed, and over 200 evidence-based prevention interventions met rigorous efficacy review criteria and standards for reducing HIV risk behaviors (Bradley-Springer, 2001). Following efficacy review, PRS has worked on an ongoing basis with the CDC's Replicating Effective Programs (REP) and with the Diffusion of Effective Behavioral Interventions (DEBI) projects to package and translate interventions for use across populations and settings (CDC, 2007c). REP is responsible for working with researchers and community-based partners to develop interventions into ready-to-use packages that include consumer-friendly materials in easy-to-understand language. The DEBI project is responsible for disseminating the intervention packages. Training and technical assistance on the DEBI packages is provided by the Capacity Building Branch (CBB) of the Division of HIV Prevention through the National Network of STD/HIV Prevention Training Centers.

Framework for Classifying HIV Behavioral Interventions

The PRS efficacy review was used to identify and select HIV behavioral prevention interventions. The system used by the CDC for classifying interventions is the tiers of evidence framework. The framework is conceptualized as a multilevel pyramid (see Figure 5.1). At the top of the pyramid are tiers I (i.e., best-evidence) and II (promising-evidence) interventions; the distinction between the two tiers is based on the level of study quality and strength of findings. In the middle are tiers III and IV, which are theory-based interventions that are grounded in behavioral science theory but that do not have enough supporting empirical evidence at this time. At the bottom of the pyramid are unevaluated interventions that represent a multitude of other interventions that have been used but have not been systemically evaluated (CDC, 2007f).

In 1999, the CDC's Division of HIV/AIDS Prevention initiated the HIV/AIDS Prevention Research Synthesis Project (PRS) to review the behavioral intervention literature and make recommendations about what interventions had evidence of reducing sex and drug injection risk behaviors (CDC, 2006a). These recommendations were published in 1999 and updated in 2001 in a document enti-

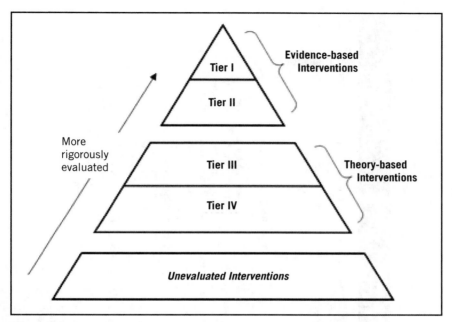

Figure 5.1 Tiers of evidence framework for HIV behavioral interventions.

tled *Compendium of HIV Prevention Interventions with Evidence of Effectiveness.* In 2007, the CDC again updated this compendium and expanded the number of interventions from 24 to 49; additionally, some of the interventions from previous versions were removed due to a lack of sufficient evidence or because they were community based. The 2007 compendium included only individual and group-level interventions, which were classified into best-evidence ($n = 31$) and promising-evidence ($n = 18$) interventions for a variety of target populations, including heterosexual adults, HIV-positive individuals, high-risk youth, MSM, drug users, females, males, and specific racial/ethnic groups (see Tables 5.1 through 5.4). Since its inception, according to Crepaz and colleagues (2003):

> The project has developed standardized guidelines and procedures for systematic review activities; established a cumulative database; performed comprehensive and systematic searches for pertinent HIV prevention intervention studies; implemented thorough activities for selecting and characterizing the studies; and analyzed effectiveness findings.

Table 5.1

BEST-EVIDENCE INDIVIDUAL-LEVEL INTERVENTIONS (ILI)

INTERVENTION	TARGET POPULATION	GOALS	THEORETICAL BASIS	DURATION	DELIVERY METHODS
Choosing Life: Empowerment, Actions, Results (CLEAR)	Young HIV-positive substance abusers	Reduce sexual and substance use risk behaviors Improve mental and physical health	Cognitive behavior therapy Social action theory	Eighteen sessions total (6 sessions per module); each session lasts 1.5 hours	Demonstration Exercise/games Goal setting Lectures Role plays and practice
EXPLORE	HIV-seronegative men who have sex with men (MSM)	Prevent the acquisition of new HIV infection Reduce unprotected anal intercourse, serodiscordant unprotected anal intercourse, and serodiscordant unprotected receptive anal intercourse	Information-motivation-behavior skill model Motivational enhancement Social learning theory	Ten 1-hour core counseling sessions delivered within 4 to 6 months, followed by up to 7 maintenance booster sessions delivered every 3 months up to 45 months; participants also received HIV testing and counseling every 6 months	Counseling Goal setting Motivational interviewing Risk reduction supplies (condoms)
Female- and culturallyspecific negotiation	Inner-city, HIV-negative, heterosexually active, African American female drug injectors and crack cocaine smokers	Reduce HIV risk behaviors among African American women who use crack or inject drugs	Theory of gender and power Theory of planned behavior Theory of reasoned actions Social cognitive theory Transtheoretical model of change	Four 20 to 40 minute sessions delivered over a 3 to 4 week time span	Counseling Develop/plan role plays

Modelo de Intervención Psicomédica (MIP)	Hispanic drug injectors	Reduce injection-related HIV risk behaviors Engage injection drug users in drug treatment and health care Enhance self-efficacy	Miller's motivational interviewing model	Six weekly sessions with ongoing case management	Counseling Case management Demonstrations Goal setting Motivational interviewing Role plays and practice Risk reduction supplies (condoms and needle hygiene materials)
Personalized cognitive risk-reduction counseling	Men who have sex with men (MSM) who are HIV seronegative and have undergone repeat HIV testing	Reduce high-risk sexual behavior (i.e., unprotected anal sex with nonprimary partners of unknown or discordant HIV status)	Gold's model of "on-line" vs. "off-line" self-appraisal of risk behavior Model of relapse prevention	One session that lasts approximately 1 hour	Counseling Goal setting
Project Connect	Minority, inner-city heterosexual couples	Increase safer sex practices among couples (i.e., increasing condom use, decreasing STD transmission, and reducing number of sex partners) Increase relationship communication	AIDS risk reduction model Bronfenbrenner's ecological perspective	Six 2-hour sessions delivered over 6 weeks	Counseling Demonstrations Discussions Exercises Goal setting Practice Risk reduction supplies (male and female condoms) Video

(continued)

Table 5.1

BEST-EVIDENCE INDIVIDUAL-LEVEL INTERVENTIONS (ILI) *continued*

INTERVENTION	TARGET POPULATION	GOALS	THEORETICAL BASIS	DURATION	DELIVERY METHODS
RESPECT: Brief counseling and enhanced counseling	Heterosexual, HIV-negative, STD clinic patients	Eliminate or reduce sex risk behaviors Reduce STD infections	Social cognitive theory Theory of reasoned action	Brief counseling: Two 20-minute sessions (40 minutes total) delivered over 7–10 days Enhanced counseling: One 20-minute and three 60-minute sessions (200 minutes total) delivered over 3–4 consecutive weeks	Counseling Exercise Goal setting Printed Materials Risk reduction supplies (condoms)
START	Young men soon to be released from prison	Eliminate or reduce risk behaviors for HIV, STD, and hepatitis	The intervention did not have an explicit theoretical basis. It was based on behavior change strategies and principles.	The prerelease sessions lasted 60 to 90 minutes and were provided during the 2 weeks prior to release from prison; the postrelease sessions lasted 30 to 60 minutes and were provided approximately 1, 3, 6, and 12 weeks after release from prison, totaling approximately 4–7 hours over a period of 14 weeks.	Counseling Goal setting

| Women's Co-Op | African American women who use crack and are not in drug treatment | Reduce sex risk behaviors (including trading sex for money or drugs and unprotected sex) and drug use (i.e., number of days using crack) Increase employment and housing status | African American feminism Empowerment theory | Four sessions delivered over 6 weeks. Sessions 1 and 2 lasted 30–40 minutes each, and Sessions 3 and 4 lasted 60–90 minutes each. | Counseling Goal setting Printed materials Supplies |

Note: Material adapted from: Centers for Disease Control and Prevention. (2008c). *Best evidence intervention.* Retrieved February 13, 2009, from http://cdc.gov/hiv/topics/research/prs/best-evidence-intervention.htm.

Table 5.2

BEST-EVIDENCE GROUP-LEVEL INTERVENTIONS (GLI)

INTERVENTION	TARGET POPULATION	GOALS	THEORETICAL BASIS	DURATION	DELIVERY METHODS
Becoming a Responsible Teen (BART)	African American adolescents	Increase information and skills to make sound choices Increase abstinence Eliminate or reduce sex risk behaviors	Information Motivation Behavior (IMB) Model Social learning theory	Eight 90–120 minute sessions delivered over 8 weeks	Demonstrations Exercises/games Group discussion Lectures Practice Role plays Video
Be Proud! Be Responsible!	Inner-city African American male adolescents	Increase knowledge and reduce positive attitudes and intentions regarding risky sexual behavior Eliminate or reduce sex risk behaviors	Social cognitive theory Theory of reasoned action Theory of planned behavior	One 5-hour session	Exercises Games Group discussion Lectures Practice Role play Video
Brief group counseling	Homosexual Asian and Pacific Islander (API) men	Increase positive ethnic and sexual identity Increase acknowledgement of HIV risk behaviors Enhance AIDS knowledge, attitudes toward safer sex, safe-sex negotiation skills Eliminate or reduce sex risk behaviors	Health belief model Theory of reasoned action Social cognitive theory	One 3-hour session	Counseling Group discussion Games Role play Exercises

CHOICES	Low-income heterosexually active women	Prevent new sexually transmitted diseases (STDs) Increase use of safer sex strategies such as abstinence, monogamy, and/or condom use	Relapse prevention model	Sixteen weekly 2-hour group sessions	Exercises Goal setting Group discussions Lectures Printed materials
Communal Effectance–AIDS Prevention (CE–AP)	Low income, single, inner-city females attending urban clinics	Reduce HIV transmission risk behaviors and sexually transmitted diseases (STDs) Enhance HIV-preventive psychosocial and structural factors	Social learning theory Conservation of resources (COR) theory Theory of gender and power	Six sessions lasting 1.5 to 2 hours each delivered over 2 to 3 months	Cognitive rehearsal Demonstrations Goal setting Group discussions Lectures Role plays Videos
¡CUÍDATE! (Take Care of Yourself)	Latino youth	Increase skills and self efficacy in negotiating abstinence and condom use Increase abstinence Increase condom use	Social cognitive theory Theory of reasoned action Theory of planned behavior	Six 60-minute modules delivered over two consecutive Saturdays	Demonstrations Group discussion Lecture Video/music Games Practice Role play

(continued)

Table 5.2

BEST-EVIDENCE GROUP-LEVEL INTERVENTIONS (GLI) *continued*

INTERVENTION	TARGET POPULATION	GOALS	THEORETICAL BASIS	DURATION	DELIVERY METHODS
Focus on Kids (FOK) plus ImPACT	High-risk African American youth living in low-income urban community sites	Reduce adolescent truancy, substance abuse, and sexual risk behaviors	Protection motivation theory	Nine intervention sessions (8 for FOK and 1 for ImPACT) approximately 1.5 hours each generally delivered one session per week. ImPACT is delivered to the parents at the beginning of the FOK delivery.	Exercises/Games Group discussion Lectures Role plays Risk-reduction supplies (condoms) Videos
Healthy relationships	People living with HIV	Reduce HIV-transmission risk behaviors	Social cognitive theory	Five 2-hour sessions, with 2 sessions delivered weekly for 2.5 weeks	Exercises Goal setting Group discussions Lectures Printed materials Role plays Video
Health Improvement Project (HIP)	Psychiatric outpatients receiving care for mental illness	Increase HIV-related knowledge, interpersonal skills, and attitudes favoring condom use Avoid unsafe sex practices (including unprotected vaginal sex)	Information-motivation-behavioral skills (IMB) model	Ten sessions delivered twice weekly for 5 weeks	Counseling Exercises/games Group discussion Practice Role plays

Program	Population	Objectives	Theory	Sessions	Methods
Living in Good Health Together ("light")	Sexually active, low-income, inner-city clinic patients at high risk for HIV and STD infection	Eliminate or reduce sex risk behaviors Prevent new STD infections Increase self-efficacy and problem-solving skills for practicing safer sex	Social cognitive theory	Seven 90- to 120-minute sessions conducted twice weekly	Demonstration Exercises Goal setting/plan Role play Practice Video
Project Connect (Couple or woman-alone)	Minority, inner-city heterosexual couples	Increase safer sex practices among couples (i.e., increasing condom use, decreasing STD transmission, and reducing number of sex partners) Increase relationship communication	AIDS risk reduction model Bronfenbrenner's ecological perspective	Six 2-hour sessions delivered over 6 weeks	Counseling Demonstrations Discussions Exercises Goal setting Practice Risk reduction supplies (male and female condoms) Video
Project FIO (The Future Is Ours)	Heterosexual women in family planning clinics	Reduce unsafe sexual encounters (unprotected vaginal or anal sex occasions)	AIDS risk reduction model Social learning theory	Eight 2-hour sessions delivered over 8 weeks, followed by a 2-hour booster session delivered about 7 months after completion of the intervention	Demonstrations Exercises Goal setting Group discussions Lectures Printed materials Role plays Video

(continued)

Table 5.2

BEST-EVIDENCE GROUP-LEVEL INTERVENTIONS (GLI) *continued*

INTERVENTION	TARGET POPULATION	GOALS	THEORETICAL BASIS	DURATION	DELIVERY METHODS
Project SAFE	Mexican American and African American women diagnosed with gonorrhea, chlamydia, syphilis, or trichomonas in public health clinics	Reduce new chlamydia and gonorrhea infections Reduce risky sex behaviors	AIDS risk reduction model	Three 3-hour sessions delivered over 3 weeks. Ongoing STD counseling, testing, and treatment is also provided to everyone.	Counseling Demonstrations Exercises/games Goal setting Group discussions Lectures Printed materials Practice Role plays Video
Self-Help in Eliminating Life-Threatening Diseases (SHIELD)	Low-income, African American drug users	To reduce drug and sex risk behaviors	Active learning theory Cognitive consistency theory Social identity theory Social influence theory Social cognitive theory	Ten 90-minute sessions	Community mobilization Demonstrations Exercises Goal setting Group discussions Outreach Printed materials Role plays and practice Supplies

Sistering, Informing, Healing, Living, and Empowering (SIHLE)	Sexually experienced African American adolescent girls	Reduce sexual risk behaviors Reduce sexually transmitted diseases (STDs) and pregnancy Enhance skills and mediators of HIV preventive behaviors (i.e., HIV knowledge, condom attitudes, barriers, and self-efficacy)	Social cognitive theory Theory of gender and power	Four 4-hour sessions delivered weekly on consecutive Saturdays	Demonstrations Group discussion Lectures Role plays
Sister-to-Sister: Group skills building and one-on-one skills building	Inner-city African American female clinic patients	Eliminate or reduce sex risk behaviors Prevent new STD infections	Social cognitive theory	One session, 200 minutes for the group format and 20 minutes for the one-on-one format	Demonstration Exercises Games Group discussion Lecture/teach Practice Printed materials Role play Video

(continued)

Table 5.2

BEST-EVIDENCE GROUP-LEVEL INTERVENTIONS (GLI) *continued*

INTERVENTION	TARGET POPULATION	GOALS	THEORETICAL BASIS	DURATION	DELIVERY METHODS
Sisters Saving Sisters	Inner-city African American female clinic patients	Eliminate or reduce unprotected sexual intercourse and number of sex partners Prevent new STD infection	Theory of reasoned action Theory of planned behavior Social cognitive theory	One 250-minute session	Demonstrations Exercises Games Group discussions Practice Role play Videos
Seropositive Urban Men's Intervention Trial (SUMIT) enhanced peer-led intervention	HIV-seropositive men who have sex with men (MSM)	Reduce unprotected insertive and receptive anal sex with HIV negative or unknown serostatus partners Reduce unprotected insertive oral sex with HIV-negative or unknown-status partners Increase condom use during insertive anal sex with HIV-negative or unknown-status partners Increase disclosure of HIV status to sex partners	Information-motivation-behavioral skills model Social cognitive theory Theory of planned behavior	6 weekly 3-hour group sessions	Audiotapes Exercises Group discussion Lecture Risk-reduction supplies (condoms) Videos

178

Program	Population	Goals	Theory	Dosage	Methods
Video Opportunities for Innovative Condom Education and Safer Sex (VOICES/VOCES)	African American and Hispanic STD clinic patients	Prevent new STD infections Increase condom use	Health belief model Theory of reasoned action	One 20-minute video followed by one 25-minute group discussion session	Video Group discussion Risk-reduction supplies (condoms) Printed materials
Women's Health Promotion (WHP)	HIV-negative heterosexual Hispanic women	Eliminate or reduce sex risk behavior	Social cognitive theory Theory of reasoned action Health belief model	Twelve 90- to 120-minute sessions delivered over 12 weeks	Exercises Games Group discussions Lectures Practice
Women Involved in Life Learning from Other Women (WiLLOW)	Sexually active, female clinic patients living with HIV	Reduce HIV transmission risk behaviors Reduce sexually transmitted diseases (STDs) Enhance HIV-prevention psychosocial and structural factors	Social cognitive theory Theory of gender and power	Four 4-hour sessions delivered over 4 consecutive weeks	Demonstration Group discussion Lecture

(continued)

Table 5.2

BEST-EVIDENCE GROUP-LEVEL INTERVENTIONS (GLI) *continued*

INTERVENTION	TARGET POPULATION	GOALS	THEORETICAL BASIS	DURATION	DELIVERY METHODS
Women's Co-Op	African American women who use crack and are not in drug treatment	To reduce sex risk behaviors (including trading sex for money or drugs and unprotected sex) and drug use (i.e., number of days using crack) To increase employment and housing status	African American feminism Empowerment theory	Four sessions delivered over 6 weeks. Sessions 1 and 2 last 30–40 minutes each, and Sessions 3 and 4 last 60–90 minutes each.	Counseling Goal setting Printed materials Supplies

Note: Material adapted from: Centers for Disease Control and Prevention. (2008c). *Best evidence intervention.* Retrieved February 13, 2009, from http://cdc.gov/hiv/topics/research/prs/best-evidence-intervention.htm.

Table 5.3

PROMISING EVIDENCE INDIVIDUAL-LEVEL INTERVENTIONS (ILI)

INTERVENTION	TARGET POPULATION	GOALS	THEORETICAL BASIS	DURATION	DELIVERY METHODS
Brief Alcohol Intervention for Needle Exchangers (BRAINE)	Active injection drug users (IDUs) who were also heavy alcohol users	Reduce alcohol use Reduce or eliminate injection-related risk behaviors	Motivational interviewing principles	One 60-minute and one 30-45 minute session delivered 1 month apart	Counseling Goal setting Develop risk-reduction plan Printed materials
Cognitive Behavioral STD/HIV Risk-Reduction	Inner-city African American male adolescents	Increase STD/HIV knowledge Increase decision-making and communication skills Eliminate or reduce STD/HIV risk behaviors Prevent new STD infections	AIDS risk-reduction model (ARRM)	Four 60-minute sessions delivered over 4 consecutive weeks	Video Counseling Practice Risk-reduction supplies (condoms) Develop risk-reduction plan Printed materials
HIV Education and Testing	Inner-city sexually active heterosexual STD clinic patients	Eliminate or reduce sex risk behaviors	None specified	Two sessions approximately 2 weeks apart (one prior to and one after HIV testing)	Counseling Pamphlets Video

(continued)

181

Table 5.3

PROMISING EVIDENCE INDIVIDUAL-LEVEL INTERVENTIONS (ILI) continued

INTERVENTION	TARGET POPULATION	GOALS	THEORETICAL BASIS	DURATION	DELIVERY METHODS
Insights	Heterosexually active, nonmonogamous young women	Increase condom use	Transtheoretical model of behavioral change AIDS risk reduction model Theory of reasoned action	Risk assessment followed by 2 rounds of materials mailed approximately 3 months apart	Printed materials Supplies (condoms)
Partnership for Health (Loss-frame Intervention)	HIV-positive clinic patients	Eliminate or reduce unprotected anal or vaginal sex	Message framing theory Mutual participation Stages of changes	3- to 5-minute session at every clinic visit over 10 to 11 months	Counseling Goal setting Printed materials
RESPECT: Brief Counseling and Enhanced Counseling	Heterosexual, HIV-negative, STD clinic patients	Eliminate or reduce sex risk behaviors Reduce STD infections	Social cognitive theory Theory of reasoned action	Brief counseling: Two 20-minute sessions (40 minutes total) delivered over 7–10 days Enhanced counseling: One 20-minute and three 60-minute sessions (200 minutes total) delivered over 3–4 consecutive weeks	Counseling Exercise Goal setting Printed materials Risk-reduction supplies (condoms)

Intervention	Population	Goals	Theory	Sessions	Methods
Safer Sex	Adolescent females diagnosed with a STD	Prevent recurrence of STDs; Increase condom use; Eliminate or reduce sex risk behaviors	Social cognitive theory; Transtheoretical model of behavioral change; Motivational interviewing	One session, over 30 minutes in length, followed by three booster sessions at 1, 3 and 6 months after randomization	Demonstration; Discussion; Practice; Role play; Video; Risk-reduction supplies (condoms); Printed materials
Safety Counts	Out-of-treatment active crack and injection drug users	Eliminate or reduce sex risk behaviors; Eliminate or reduce drug risk behaviors	Health belief model; Theory of protection motivation; Transtheoretical stages of change model	Nine sessions over a 4–6 month period	Counseling; Exercise; Games; Goal setting/plan; Group discussion; Role play; Video
Sniffer	Intranasal heroin users	Eliminate or reduce noninjection drug use; Prevent transition to injecting drugs	Social Learning Theory	Four 60–90 minute sessions delivered over 2 weeks, plus HIV pre- and posttest counseling	Counseling; Exercises; Group discussion; Lecture; Role play; Risk reduction supplies (condoms); Video

Note: Material adapted from: Centers for Disease Control and Prevention. (2008e). *Promising-evidence interventions.* Retrieved February 12, 2009, from http://cdc.gov/hiv/topics/research/prs/promising-evidence-interventions.htm.

Table 5.4

PROMISING EVIDENCE GROUP-LEVEL INTERVENTIONS (GLI)

INTERVENTION	TARGET POPULATION	GOALS	THEORETICAL BASIS	DURATION	DELIVERY METHODS
Assisting in Rehabilitating Kids (ARK)	Substance-dependent adolescents	Increase abstinence Increase safer sex behaviors Eliminate or reduce sex risk behaviors	Information motivation behavior (IMB) Model extended parallel process model (EPPM)	Twelve 90-minute sessions delivered over 28 days	Games Group discussion Lectures Practice Training
Condom Promotion	Young unmarried college women	Increase intentions to use condoms Increase condom use	Psychosocial model of condom use health belief model	One session lasting 45 minutes	Demonstration Group discussion Lecture Video Practice Risk-reduction supplies (condoms) Role play
Doing Something Different	Inner-city STD clinic patients	Increase condom use Prevent new STD infections	Not reported	One-session	Demonstration Group discussions Practice Printed materials Risk-reduction supplies Role plays Video

Program	Target population	Goals/objectives	Theory	Dosage	Methods
Focus on Kids (FOK)	Low-income, urban African American youth	Increase abstinence Increase condom use	Protection motivation theory	Eight weekly meetings: seven 90-minute sessions and one day-long session Monthly and annual 90-minute booster sessions	Art and crafts Exercises Games Group discussion Lecture Risk reduction supplies (condoms) Role play Social event Storytelling Video
Intensive AIDS Education	Incarcerated, male adolescent drug users	Eliminate or reduce HIV risk behaviors	None reported	Four 1-hour sessions delivered twice a week over a 2-week period	Group discussion Exercises Problem-solving therapy Role play
Nia: A Program of Purpose	Inner-city heterosexually active, African American men	Improve behavioral and communication skills Eliminate or reduce sex risk behaviors	Information-motivation-behavioral (IMB) skills model	Two 3-hour sessions delivered over a week	Demonstration Exercises Group Discussion Practice Risk-reduction supplies (condoms) Role play Video

(continued)

Table 5.4

PROMISING EVIDENCE GROUP-LEVEL INTERVENTIONS (GLI) *continued*

INTERVENTION	TARGET POPULATION	GOALS	THEORETICAL BASIS	DURATION	DELIVERY METHODS
Safety Counts	Out-of-treatment active crack and injection drug users	Eliminate or reduce sex risk behaviors Eliminate or reduce drug risk behaviors	Health belief model Theory of protection motivation Transtheoretical stages of change model	Nine sessions over a 4–6 month period	Counseling Exercise Games Goal setting/plan Group discussion Role play Video
Salud, Educacion, Prevencion y Autocuidado (SEPA)	Low-income, urban, Mexican and Puerto Rican women	Eliminate or reduce sex risk behaviors	Social cognitive theory	Six weekly sessions	Demonstrations Exercises Group discussion Practice Role modeling (educating peers) Role play Video
Sniffer	Intranasal heroin users	Eliminate or reduce noninjection drug use Prevent transition to injecting drugs	Social learning theory	Four 60–90 minute sessions delivered over 2 weeks, plus HIV pre- and posttest counseling	Counseling Exercises Group discussion Lecture Role play Risk reduction supplies (condoms) Video

Street Smart	Runaway youth	Eliminate or reduce sex risk behaviors Eliminate or reduce substance use	Social learning theory	10 sessions (9 small-group and 1 individual) delivered over a 3-week period	Counseling Developing video and art media Exercises/games Goal setting Group discuss Homework Practice Role play Video
Together Learning Choices (TLC)	HIV-positive adolescent and young adult clinic patients	Enhance health behaviors Increase condom use Eliminate or reduce unprotected sex or refuse to have unsafe sex Eliminate or reduce drug and alcohol use	Social action theory	*Stay Healthy* module: 12 sessions, 2 hours each, conducted weekly over 3-month period. *Act Safe* module: 11 sessions, 2 hours each, conducted weekly over 3-month period	Exercises Goal setting Group discussion Practice Role play Video

Note: Material adapted from: Centers for Disease Control and Prevention. (2008e). *Promising-evidence interventions*. Retrieved February 12, 2009, from http://cdc.gov/hiv/topics/research/prs/promising-evidence-interventions.htm.

CDC Evidence-Based Interventions

According to the AIDS Institute (2008) review of 49 evidence-based interventions included in the 2007 CDC compendium, 21 were tailored to women and 28 were tailored to men. Over three-fourths ($n = 38$) were specifically designed for minority populations, including 27 for African Americans and 8 for Hispanics. However, only five interventions were designed to be delivered in Spanish. Despite the continued high incidence of HIV in MSM, only 4 out of the 49 evidence-based interventions were geared toward this population. Nine of the interventions were focused on drug users, and two were targeted to incarcerated populations. Six evidence-based interventions were developed for persons with HIV/AIDS. Over one-fourth of the interventions ($n = 13$) targeted high-risk youth; however, the majority of evidence-based behavioral interventions were aimed at persons age 18 and older. With respect to relationship status, two interventions were designed for women with steady male partners, while three interventions required participants to be either single or in a short-term relationship; one intervention for MSM specifically excluded men who were in a monogamous relationship for two or more years (The AIDS Institute, 2008).

Assessment of the CDC Compendium of Evidence-Based HIV Interventions

The AIDS Institute (2008) conducted an analysis to determine how well the 2007 CDC evidence-based interventions mirrored the populations affected by the HIV epidemic and identified several critical gaps. First, there were no interventions that specifically targeted transgendered individuals, despite the fact that this group is at significantly higher risk for contracting HIV infection compared to other populations. No interventions were identified to specifically target Hispanic men or Native Americans, and only one intervention was intended for Asians/Pacific Islanders. The number of interventions for MSM was woefully inadequate given HIV infection rates in this group, and there were no interventions specifically designed for African American and Hispanic MSM. Although a few interventions were focused on heroin and crack cocaine users, no CDC intervention was geared toward reducing HIV risk related to crystal methamphetamine use, despite the widespread popularity of this recreational drug and association with HIV infection. Furthermore, none of the interventions for drug users was designed to be delivered within the context of needle exchange programs. There were no evidence-based HIV prevention interventions for incarcerated women or older men, despite high rates of HIV in prison populations. There was only one intervention that focused on runaway youth in shelters, but none was designed for other groups of homeless youth. At the other end of the age spectrum, there were only four interventions designed for persons age 50 and older. Although heterosexual transmission of HIV continues to be a problem, relationship status was relatively neglected in behavioral interventions. Likewise, a majority of the interventions had not been adapted to accommodate participants who speak a language other than English. The AIDS Institute (2008) concluded:

> In addition to the groups previously mentioned, the Compendium also fails to include targeted interventions for sex workers, persons over age 50, veterans, and the homeless. These populations are all at high risk of HIV infection and suffer from high and/or growing rates of infections. There is also a strong need for more diversity in regards to intervention settings. For example, there are no interventions for faith-based and rural settings. (p. 3)

On a positive note, The AIDS Institute (2008) commended the CDC's rigor and use of the scientific process for critiquing the evidence and validating the effectiveness of behavioral HIV prevention interventions. The AIDS Institute also challenged the CDC to continue to periodically update and revise the Compendium to assure that best-evidence and positive-evidence interventions reflect the age spectrum and multicultural face of the HIV epidemic in this country.

Subsequently, the CDC (2008a) updated and revised the compendium to include a total of 57 evidenced-based HIV behavioral interventions. Five new interventions were added to the list of best-evidence interventions:

- Healthy Living Project (HLP)
- Living in the Face of Trauma (LIFT)
- Positive Choice: Interactive Video Doctor
- Safe in the City
- Study to Reduce Intravenous Exposures (STRIVE)

Additionally, three interventions were added to the list of promising-evidence interventions:

- Drug Users Intervention Trial (DUIT)
- Options/Opciones Project
- Responsible, Empowered, Aware, Living Men (REAL Men)

PRS continues to conduct efficacy reviews on an ongoing basis. Community-level interventions are currently being reviewed. The CDC evidence-based intervention website will be updated in a timely manner to showcase new information.

FUTURE STRATEGIES— CLINICAL, RESEARCH, AND GLOBAL

Recommendations on HIV prevention strategies for the 21st century have been made by the Global HIV Prevention Working Group. The Working Group is compromised of a panel of experts and consumers affected by HIV/AIDS. The 50-member panel was convened by the Bill and Melinda Gates Foundation and the Henry J. Kaiser Family Foundation. The panel met in August, 2008, and made recommendations on HIV prevention for policy makers, including national authorities, governments, and technical agencies; for international donors; and for members of civil society. The Working Panel also developed recommendations for HIV service providers, which included: (1) tailoring prevention programs to local context; (2) adapting prevention programs to address changes in the social and physical environment of the target population; (3) integrating HIV services with sexual- and reproductive-health services, antenatal settings, and tuberculosis clinical settings; and (4) incorporating HIV risk-reduction counseling, along with access to condoms and other prevention tools, into all HIV treatment programs (Global HIV Prevention Working Group, 2008).

Additionally, the Global Working Group (2008) made recommendations for HIV prevention researchers. The recommendations included an expanded social science focus, with partnerships between ethnographers and prevention-program implementers, to improve understanding of factors that increase vulnerability. Ethnographers were also recommended to conduct formative research needed to identify unique characteristics of the target population and then tailor prevention strategies to the particular population. Additionally, the panel recommended an expanded research focus on studies to assess the effectiveness of HIV prevention in real-world settings. When appropriate, biological end points (e.g., HIV or STD incidence) should be a component of prevention studies. Greater attention should also be paid to identification of contextual issues that may influence risk compensation and evaluation of interventions that minimize risk compensation. Collaboration is needed between social scientists and behavioral scientists to develop and test new prevention interventions that aim to influence the norms and behaviors of social networks and communities and to evaluate structural interventions. Lastly, the panel recommended that for resource-limited settings, researchers need to develop accessible, affordable technologies that can be used for rapid assessment of HIV seroincidence.

HIV prevention is an important component of a global strategy to end the epidemic. The Joint United Nations Programme on HIV/AIDS (UNAIDS) (2008) has summarized some key findings for global HIV prevention strategies. These findings include (UNAIDS, 2008):

1 The global HIV epidemic cannot be reversed without greater progress in reducing the rate of new HIV infections.

2 Prevention programs, particularly in countries with concentrated epidemics, fail to reach many people at risk to HIV exposure, especially MSM and injecting drug users.

3 Young people aged 15 to 24 globally account for 45% of all new HIV infections in adults, but many young people still lack accurate, complete information on how to avoid exposure to the virus.

4 Major progress has been made in reducing mother-to-child transmission of HIV. With continued funding, commitment and strategic action, the incidence of maternal–child transmission of HIV could become rare.

5 Prevention efforts must become more focused on sexual partnerships, especially those that increase HIV risk exposure, including serodiscordant couples and multiple concurrent partners.

6 For optimum effectiveness of prevention programs, effective initiatives are needed that target the social factors that increase risk and vulnerability. These factors include gender inequality, HIV stigma and discrimination, and the social marginalization of those populations most at risk for HIV.

7 Countries need to nurture a "prevention movement" to maintain a strong prevention response. Additionally, countries need to build the human and technical capacity that is necessary to sustain prevention efforts, and must also work to stimulate greater demand for prevention services. (p. 96)

CONCLUSION

In many ways, we have come a long way since Darrow's 1996 reflective concerns regarding HIV prevention (Ojito, 1996). In the 21st century, multiple biomedical, behavioral, and structural interventions have been developed and implemented around the world. Evaluation of primarily behavioral interventions has become more rigorous and systematic, particularly in the United States. However, there is still a long way to go before HIV prevention results in an end to the global epidemic.

In terms of biomedical intervention, microbicides and vaccines theoretically hold the promise for HIV prevention; however, to date, none have been successful. It may be years before an effective microbicide or vaccine model is actually developed and marketed on a widespread basis.

Effective behavioral interventions have been designed and tested, but there are still remaining gaps. For example, although many interventions target urban populations, fewer have been focused to meet the unique needs of rural populations and persons in resource-limited countries. More interventions are needed to meet the diverse characteristics and behaviors of both youth and older adults. Because MSM continue to be the group with high rates of new HIV infection, more interventions need to be specifically targeted for MSM, particularly men of color and MSMW. Additionally, more attention needs to paid to HIV prevention in other sexual minorities such as bisexual individuals, transgender persons, and WSW. Besides concerns with sexual minorities, more interventions need to be focused on heterosexual transmission of HIV, including relational versus individual level interventions. Likewise, interventions must be further designed to educate women of all races and ethnicities in monogamous relationships that their risk for HIV is related to their partner's past and present. For the 21st century, it is imperative that HIV prevention interventions continue to be created and adapted to accommodate widespread cultural, sociodemographic, socioeconomic, and gender-specific factors that mediate risky sexual and drug-related behaviors.

Although a few efforts have emerged, more needs to be done with respect to structural HIV prevention interventions. For example, public health issues need to take precedence over legal and moral roadblocks to providing HIV prevention through needle exchange programs and safer injection facilities to decrease rates of HIV infection among IDUs.

President Obama's promise to "restore science to its rightful place" holds hope that the science of prevention will take precedence over dogma in the next several years. Structural interventions must also address the need for early detection and treatment of STDs.

Much work remains to be done toward preventing new cases of HIV infection on a global basis in the 21st century, including prevention interventions for persons who are already HIV positive. From a nursing perspective, sexual risk assessment and client counseling for all individuals is essential for HIV prevention. Nurses can assume key roles in prevention endeavors in all settings and with diverse populations through practice, research, education, and political action at the local, national, and global levels.

REFERENCES

Adepoju, J. A., Watkins, M. P., & Richardson, A. M. (2007). A quick survey of an HBCU's first year nursing students' perception of the HIV/AIDS phenomenon. *Journal of the National Black Nurses Association, 18*(2), 24–29.

The AIDS Institute. (2008). *An assessment of CDC's HIV prevention interventions portfolio: Identifying the gap.* Retrieved October 20, 2008, from www.theaidsintitute.org.

AIDSInfo. (2006). *Preventive HIV vaccines.* Retrieved November 11, 2008, from www.aidsinfo.nih.gov/ContentFiles/HIVPrevention Vaccines_FS_en.pdf.

AIDSInfo. (2008). HIV/AIDS drug information-carrageenan. Retrieved October 11, 2008, from www.aidsinfo.nih.gov/DrugsNew/DrugDetail NT.aspx?MenuItem=Drugs&Search= On&int_id=400.

Barbosa, R. M., Kalckmann, S., Berquo, E., & Stein, Z. (2007). Notes on the female condom: Experiences in Brazil. *International Journal of STDs and AIDS, 18*(4), 261–266.

Bartlett, J. G., & Gallant, J. E. (2007). *2007 Medical management of HIV infection.* Baltimore: Johns Hopkins Medicine Health Publishing Business Group.

Belani, H. K., & Muennig, P. A. (2008). Cost-effectiveness of needle and syringe exchange for the prevention of HIV in New York City. *Journal of HIV/AIDS and Social Services, 7,* 229–240.

Benin and the Global Fund. (2008). AIDS 2008—*Newspapers examine challenges in HIV prevention among MSM.* Retrieved October 15,

2008, from www.theglobalfund.org/programs/news_summary.aspx? newsid=0&countryid=BE N&lang=en.

Bernstein, A. (2008). AIDS and the next 25 years. *Science, 320,* 717.

Bertens, M. G., Krumeich, A, van den Borne, B., & Schaalma, H. P. (2008). Being and feeling like a woman: Respectability, responsibility, desirability and safe sex among women of Afro-Surinamese and Dutch Antillean descent in the Netherlands. *Culture, Health and Sexuality, 10*(6), 547–561.

Bradley-Springer, L. (2001). Prevention: What works? *American Journal of Nursing, 101*(6), 45–50.

Breast milk purged of HIV virus. (2008). Retrieved November 11, 2008, from http://news.bbcco.uk/2/hi/uk_news/england/cambridgeshire/7629253/stm.

Breslow, R. A., Faden, V. B., & Smothers, B. (2003). Alcohol consumption by elderly Americans. *Journal of Studies Alcohol, 64*(6), 884–892.

Calfee, D. P. (2006). Prevention and management of occupational exposures to human immunodeficiency virus (HIV). *Mount Sinai Journal of Medicine, 73*(6), 852–566.

Camlin, C. S., & Snow, R. C. (2008). Parental investment, club membership, and youth sexual risk behavior in Cape Town. *Health Education and Behavior, 35,* 522–540.

Centers for Disease Control and Prevention. (2006a). *About PRS.* Received October 20, 2008, from www.cdc.gov/hiv/topics/research/prs/about.htm.

Centers for Disease Control and Prevention. (2006b). *HIV/AIDS among women who have sex with women.* Retrieved October 15, 2008, from www.cdc.gov/hiv/topics/women/resources/factsheets/wsw.htm.

Centers for Disease Control and Prevention. (2007a). *HIV and its transmission.* Retrieved October 10, 2008, from www.cdc.gov/hiv/resources/factsheets/transmission.htm.

Centers for Disease Control and Prevention. (2007b). *Preventing occupational HIV transmission to health care personal.* Retrieved February 12, 2009, from www.cdc.gov/hiv/resources/factsheets/print/hcwprev.htm.

Centers for Disease Control and Prevention. (2007c). *PRS, REP, and DEBI.* Retrieved October 20, 2008, from www/cdc/gov/hiv/topics/prs/prs_rep_debi.htm.

Centers for Disease Control and Prevention. (2007d). *Surveillance of occupationally acquired HIV/AIDS in healthcare personnel,* as of December 2006. Retrieved October 10, 2008, from www.cdc.gov/ncidod/dhqp/bp_hcp_w_hiv.html.

Centers for Disease Control and Prevention. (2007e). *The role of STD prevention and treatment in HIV prevention*—CDC fact sheet. Retrieved October 10, 2008, from www.cdc.gov/std/hiv/STDFact-STD&HIV.htm.

Centers for Disease Control and Prevention. (2007f). *Tiers of evidence: A framework for classifying HIV behavioral interventions.* Retrieved October 20, 2008, from www.cdc.gov/hiv/topics/research/pre/tiers-of-evidence.htm.

Centers for Disease Control and Prevention. (2008a). *2008 Compendium of evidence-based HIV prevention interventions.* Retrieved February 8, 2009, from www.cdc.gov/hiv/topics/research/prs/evidence-based-interventions.htm.

Centers for Disease Control and Prevention. (2008b). *Basic information.* Retrieved October 10, 2008, from www.cdc.gov/hiv/topics/basic/index.htm#hi.

Centers for Disease Control and Prevention. (2008c). *Best-evidence intervention.* Retrieved February 13, 2009, from http://cdc.gov/hiv/topics/research/prs/best-evidence-intervention.htm.

Centers for Disease Control and Prevention (2008d). *New HIV incidence estimates: CDC responds.* Retrieved November 11, 2008, from www.cdc.gov/hiv/topics/surveillance/resources/factsheets/print/response.htm.

Centers for Disease Control and Prevention. (2008e). *Promising-evidence interventions.* Retrieved February 12, 2009, from http://cdc.gov/hiv/topics/research/prs/promising-evidence-interventions.htm.

Centers for Disease Control and Prevention. (2008f). *The role of STD detection and treatment in HIV prevention*—CDC fact sheet. Retrieved February 13, 2009, from www.cdc.gov/std/hiv/STDFact-STD&HIV.htm.

Clinical alert: Immunizations are discontinued in two HIV vaccine trials. (2007). Retrieved November 11, 2008, from www.nlm.nih.gov/databases/alerts/hiv_step_study.html.

Coates, T. J., Richter, L., & Caceres, C. (2008). Behavioural strategies to reduce HIV transmission: How to make them work better. *Lancet, 372*(9639), 669–684.

Correa, M., & Gisselquist, D. (2006). Reconnaissance assessment of risks for HIV transmission through health care and cosmetic services in India. *International Journal of STDs and AIDS, 17*(11),743–748.

Crepaz, N., Lyles, C. M., Herbst, J. H., Kay, L. & Britton J. (2003, July 27–30). *Synthesis of HIV Prevention Research: Lessons learned from the CDC's HIV/AIDS Prevention Research Synthesis Project (PRS).*

Paper presented at the National HIV Prevention Conference, Atlanta, GA. Retrieved February 17, 2009, from http://gateway.nlm.nih.gov/MeetingAbstracts/ma?f=102261729.html.

Crosby, R. A., Sanders, S. A., Yarber, W. L., Graham, C. A., & Dodge, B. (2002). Condom use errors and problems among college men. *Sexually Transmitted Diseases, 29*(9), 552–557.

Crosby, R., Yarber, W. L., Sanders, S. A., Graham, C. A., & Arno, J. N. (2008). Slips, breaks and 'falls': Condom errors and problems reported by men attending an STD clinic. *International Journal of STDs and AIDS, 19*(2), 90–93.

Cutler, B., & Justman, J. (2008). Vaginal microbicides and the prevention of HIV transmission, *Lancet Infectious Diseases, 8,* 685–697.

Des Jarlais, D., & Semaan, S. (2008). HIV prevention for injecting drug users: The first 25 years and counting. *Psychosomatic Medicine, 70,* 606–611.

Dodge, B., Jefferies, M. L. IV, & Sandfort, T. G. M. (2008). Beyond the down low: Sexual risk, protection and disclosure among at-risk Black men who have sex with both men and women (MSMW). *Archives of Sexual Behavior, 37,* 683–696.

East, L., Jackson, D., O'Brien, L., & Peters, K. (2007). Use of the male condom by heterosexual adolescents and young people: Literature review. *Journal of Advanced Nursing, 59*(2), 103–110.

Eaton, D. K., Kann, L., Kinchen, S., Shanklin, S., Ross, J., Hawkins, J., et al., and the Centers for Disease Control and Prevention (CDC). (2008, June 6). Youth risk behavior surveillance—United States, 2007. *Morbidity and Mortality Weekly Report Surveillance Summary, 57*(4), 1–131.

Elford, J. (2006). Changing patterns of sexual behaviour in the era of highly active antiretroviral therapy. *Current Opinion Infectious Disease, 19*(1), 26–32.

Elliott, R., Malkin, I., & Gold, J. (2002). *Establishing safe injection facilities in Canada: Legal and ethical issues.* Retrieved November 11, 2008, from www.aidslaw.ca/publications/interfaces/downloadFile.php?ref=776.

Essien, E. J., Meshack, A. F., Peters, R. J., Ogungbade, G. O., & Osemene, N. I. (2005). Strategies to prevent HIV transmission among heterosexual African-American men. *BMC Public Health, 5,* 3.

Evatt, B. (2006). Infectious disease in the blood supply and the public health response. *Seminars in Hematology, 43*(2 Suppl. 3), S4–S9.

Exner, T. M., Dworkin, S. L., Hoffman, S., & Ehrhardt, A. A. (2003). Beyond the male condom: The evolution of gender-specific HIV interventions for women. *Annual Reviews of Sex Research, 14,* 114–136.

Falvo, N., & Norman, S. (2004). Never too old to learn: The impact of an HIV/AIDS education program on older adults' knowledge. *Clinical Gerontologist, 27*(1/2), 103–117.

Food and Drug Administration, U.S. Department of Health and Human Services. (2007). Over-the-counter vaginal contraceptive and spermicide drug products containing nonoxynol 9; Required labeling. Final rule. *Federal Register, 72*(243), 71769–71785.

Ganczak, M., & Barss, P. (2008). Nosocomial HIV infection: Epidemiology and prevention—A global perspective. *AIDS Review, 10*(1), 47–61.

Ganczak, M.. & Szych, Z. (2007). Surgical nurses and compliance with personal protective equipment. *Journal of Hospital Infection, 66*(4), 346–351.

Gillespie-Johnson, M. (2008). HIV/AIDS prevention practices among recent-immigrant Jamaican women. *Ethnicity and Disease, 8*(2 Suppl. 2), S2, 175–178.

Glenn, D. (2005, May 27). Battle over the knife. *Chronicle of Higher Education, 51*(38), A12–A15.

Global HIV Prevention Working Group. (2008). Behavior change and HIV prevention: [Re]considerations for the 21st century. Retrieved October 12, 2008, from www.globalhivprevention.org/pdfs/PWG_behavior%20report_FINAL.pdf.

González-Guarda, R. M., Peragallo, N., & Vasquez, E. P. (2008). HIV risks, substance abuse, and intimate partner violence among Hispanic women and their intimate partners. *Journal of the Association of Nurses in AIDS Care, 19*(4), 252–265.

Gostin, L., & Hankins, C. (2008). Male circumcision as an HIV prevention strategy in sub-Saharan Africa. *Journal of the American Medical Association, 300,* 2539–2541.

Gott, C. M. (2001). Sexual activity and risk-taking in later life. *Health and Social Care in the Community, 9*(2), 72–78.

Graham, C. A., Crosby, R., Yarber, W. L., Sanders, S. A., McBride, K., Milhausen, R. R., et al. (2006). Erection loss in association with condom use among young men attending a public STI clinic: Potential correlates and implications for risk behaviour. *Sexual Health, 3*(4), 255–260.

Graham, J. (2008, December 16). New female condom endorsed by FDA panel. *Chicago Tribune.* Retrieved on February 8, 2009, from

http://archives.chicagotribune.com/2008/dec/16/local/chi-female_
condomdec16.

Guerriero, I., Ayres, J. R., & Hearst, N. (2002). Masculinity and vulnerability to HIV among heterosexual men in Sao Paulo, Brazil. *Revista
de Saúde Pública, 36*(Suppl. 4), 50–60.

Gullette, D. L., & Lyons, M. A. (2006). Sensation seeking, self-esteem,
and unprotected sex in college students. *Journal of the Association of
Nurses in AIDS Care, 17*(5), 23–31.

Gupta, R. N., Wyatt, G. E., Swaminathan, S., Rewari, B. B., Locke, T.
F., Ranganath, V., et al. (2008). Correlates of relationship, psycholog-
ical, and sexual behavioral factors for HIV risk among Indian women.
Cultural Diversity and Ethnic Minority Psychology, 14(3), 256–265.

Gurman, T., & Borzekowski, L. G. (2004). Condom use among Latino
college students. *Journal of American College Health, 52,* 169–178.

Gutierrez, E., & Andres, A. (2007). Selection of donor and organ viability
criteria: Expanding donation criteria. *Journal of Renal Care, 33*(2),
83–88.

Hall, T., Hogben, M., Carlton A. L., Liddon, N., & Koumans, E. H.
(2008). Attitudes toward using condoms and condom use: Difference
between sexually abused and nonabused African American female
adolescents. *Behavioral Medicine, 34*(2), 45–54.

Henry Kaiser Family Foundation. (2008a, October 16). *Kaiser daily HIV/
AIDS report: Researchers at global HIV/AIDS vaccine conference express
concerns about funding levels.* Retrieved November 11, 2008, from www.
kaisernetwork.org/Daily_Reports/rep_index.cfm?DR_ID=55016.

Henry Kaiser Family Foundation. (2008b, October 20). *Kaiser daily HIV/
AIDS report: Researchers at HIV/AIDS vaccine conference discuss new
methods, ongoing trials.* Retrieved November 11, 2008, from www.
kaisernetwork.org/daily_reports/rep_index.cfm?DR_ID=55074.

Herbst, J. H., Sherba, R. T., Crepaz, N., Deluca, J. B., Zohrabyan, L.,
Stall, J. D., et al., and the HIV/AIDS Prevention Research Synthesis
Team. (2005). A meta-analytic review of HIV behavioral interven-
tions for reducing sexual risk behavior of men who have sex with men.
Journal of Acquired Immune Deficiency Syndromes, 39, 228–241.

Hernandez, S. (2003, July 25). Study: Diverse Hispanic groups must
be included in broad battle. *South Florida Sun Sentinel.* Retrieved
October 15, 2008, from www.aegis.com/news/ads/2003/AD031499.
html.

Hillman, J. (2008). Knowledge, attitudes, and experience regarding HIV/
AIDS among older adult inner-city Latinos. *International Journal of
Aging and Human Development, 66*(3), 243–257.

Hodge, D. R. (2008). Sexual trafficking in the United States: A domestic problem with transnational dimensions. *Social Work, 53*(2), 143–152.

Horton, R., & Das, P. (2008). Putting prevention at the forefront of HIV/AIDS. *Lancet, 372*(9637), 421–422.

Jemmott, L. S., Jemmott, J. B. III, & Villarruel, A. M. (2002). Predicting intentions and condom use among Latino college students. *Journal of the Association of Nurses in AIDS Care, 13*(2), 56–69.

Johnson, W. D., Diaz, R. M., Flanders, W. D., Goodman, M., Hill, A. N, Holtgrave, D., et al. (2008). Behavioral interventions to reduce risk for sexual transmission of HIV among men who have sex with men. *Cochrane Database of Systematic Reviews, Issue 3,* Article CD001230.

Jones, S. G., & Messmer, P. R. (2001). The impact of AIDS on the family. In P. L. Munhall & V. M. Fitzsimons (Eds.), *The emergence of family into the 21st century* (pp. 217–236). Boston: Jones & Bartlett.

Jones, S. G., Patsdaughter, C., Farrell, N., Riera, A., Myers, B., & Malow, R. (2007, November). *Health and safer-sex practices of older heterosexual men using prescribed ED drug therapy (Viagra, Levitra & Cialis).* Poster presented at the 20th Annual Association of Nurses in AIDS Care Conference, Orlando, FL.

Jones, S. G., Patsdaughter, C. A., Jorda, M. L., Hamilton, M., & Malow, R. (2008a). SENORITAS: An HIV prevention project for Latina college students at a Hispanic-serving university. *Journal of the Association of Nurses in AIDS Care, 19*(4), 311–319.

Jones, S. G., Patsdaughter, C. A., Martinez Cardenas, V. M., Prado, C., Sanchez, L., & Santiago, V. (2008b, September). *Sexual practices and risk behavior of heterosexual men aged 50 and older using prescribed erectile dysfunction drugs: The FIU Men's Viagra Study.* Paper presented at the U.S. Conference on AIDS, Fort Lauderdale, FL.

Kalmuss, D. (2004). Nonvolitional sex and sexual health. *Archives of Sexual Behavior, 33*(3), 197–209.

Karlovsky, M., Lebed, B., & Mydlo, J. H. (2004). Increasing incidence and importance of HIV/AIDS and gonorrhea among men aged >/= 50 years in the U.S. in the era of erectile dysfunction therapy. *Scandinavian Journal of Urology and Nephrology, 38*(3), 247–252.

Kerr, T., Kimber, J., DeBeck, K., & Wood, E. (2007). The role of safer injection facilities in the response to HIV/AIDS among injection drug users. *Current HIV/AIDS Reports, 4,* 158–164.

Kerr, T., & Palepu, A. (2001). Safe injection facilities in Canada: Is it time? *Canadian Medical Association Journal, 165,* 436–437.

Klein, S. J., Nokes, K. M., Devore, B. S., Holmes, J. M., Wheeler, D. P., & St. Hilaire, M. B. (2001). Age-appropriate HIV prevention messages for older adults: Findings from focus groups in New York state. *Journal of Public Health Management Practice, 7*(3), 11–18.

Kumwenda, N., Hoover, D., Mofenson, L., Thigpen, M., Kafulafula, G., & Qing, L., et al. (2008). Extended antiretroviral prophylaxix to reduce breast-milk HIV-1 transmission. *New England Journal of Medicine, 359,* 119–129.

Kuhn, L., Aldrovandi, G., Sinkala, M., Kankasa, C., Semrau, K., Mwiya, M., et al. (2008). Effects of early, abrupt weaning on HIV-free survival of children in Zambia. *New England Journal of Medicine, 359,* 130–141.

Latka, M. H., Kapadia, F., & Fortin, P. (2008). The female condom: Effectiveness and convenience, not "female control, " valued by U.S. urban adolescents. *AIDS Education and Prevention, 20*(2), 160–170.

Lewis, J. E., Malow, R. M., & Ireland, S. J. (1997). HIV/AIDS risk in heterosexual college students: A review of a decade of literature. *Journal American College of Health, 45*(4), 147–158.

Lichtenstein, B. (2000). Secret encounters: Black men, bisexuality and AIDS in Alabama. *Medical Anthropology Quarterly, 14*(3), 374–393.

Linsk, N. L. (2000). HIV among older adults: Age-specific issues in prevention and treatment. *The AIDS Reader, 10*(7), 430–440.

Longo, B., Camoni, L., Boros, S., & Suligoi, B. (2008). Increasing proportion of AIDS diagnoses among older adults in Italy. *AIDS Patient Care and STDs, 22*(5), 365–371.

Maes, C. A., & Louis, M. (2003). Knowledge of AIDS, perceived risk of AIDS, and at-risk sexual behaviors among older adults. *Journal of the American Academy of Nurse Practitioners, 15*(11), 509–516.

Malinauskas, B. M., Aeby, V. G., Overtone, R. F., Carpenter-Aeby, T., & Barber-Heidal, K. (2007). A survey of energy drink consumption patterns among college students. *Nutrition Journal, 6,* 35.

Marin, B. V. (2003). HIV prevention in the Hispanic community: Sex, culture and empowerment. *Journal of Transcultural Nursing, 14*(3), 186–192.

Merson, M. H., O'Malley J., Serwadda, D., & Apisuk, C. (2008). The history and challenge of HIV prevention. *Lancet, 372*(9637), 475–488.

Miguez-Burbano, M. J., Page, J. B., Angarita, I., Rodriquez, N., Baum, M. K., Burbano, X., et al. (2001). High-risk behaviours in men from

Bogotá, Colombia and the spread of HIV. *International Journal STDs and AIDS, 12*(11), 739–743.

Millett, G., Flores, S., Marks, G., Reed, J., & Herbst, J. (2008). Circumcision status and risk of HIV and sexually transmitted infections among men who have sex with men: A meta analysis. *Journal of the American Medical Association, 300,* 1674–1684.

Moore, S. G., Dahl, D. W., Gorn, G. J., Weinberg, C. B., Park, J., & Jiang, Y. (2008). Condom embarrassment: Coping and consequences for condom use in three countries. *AIDS Care, 20*(5), 553–559.

Moos, R. H., Schutte, K., Brennan, P., & Moos, B. S. (2004). Ten-year patterns of alcohol consumption and drinking problems among older women and men. *Addiction, 99*(7), 829–838.

Morse, P. (2008). *Legal supervised injection facilities.* Retrieved October 11, 2008, from http://sfhiv.org/files/substance/safe_injection_facilities/SIF_factsheet.pdf.

Napierala, S., Kang, M. S., Chipato, T., Padian, N., & van der Straten, A. (2008). Female condom uptake and acceptability in Zimbabwe. *AIDS Education and Prevention, 20*(2), 121–134.

O'Brien, M. C., McCoy, T. P., Rhodes, S. D., Wagoner, A., & Wolfson, M. (2008). Caffeinated cocktails: Energy drink consumption, high-risk drinking, and alcohol-related consequences among college students. *Academy of Emergency Medicine, 15*(50), 453–460.

Office on Women's Health. (2008). *Women and HIV/AIDS gender-specific problems.* Retrieved October 11, 2008 from www.4woman.gov/hiv/gender.

Ojito, M. (1996, July 7). Detective zero. *Tropic Magazine* (Suppl. to the Miami Herald), 6–11, 18–19.

O'Leary, A., & Wingood, G. M. (2000). Interventions for sexually active heterosexual women. In J. L. Peterson & R. J. DiClemente (Eds.), *Handbook of HIV prevention* (pp. 179–200). New York: Kluwer Academic/Plenum.

Opt, S., Loffredo, D., Knowles, L., & Fletcher, C. (2007). College students and HIV/AIDS: A comparison of nontraditional and traditional student perspectives. *Journal of American College Health, 56*(2), 164–174.

O'Sullivan, L. F., Udell, W., & Patel, V. L. (2006). Young urban adults' heterosexual risk encounters and perceived risk and safety: A structured diary study. *Journal of Sex Research, 43*(4), 343–351.

Padian, N. S., Buvé, A., Balkus, J., Serwadda, D., & Cates, W. Jr. (2008). Biomedical interventions to prevent HIV infection: Evidence, challenges, and way forward. *Lancet, 372*(9638), 585–599.

Palmer, L. D. (2000, March 12). Unsafe sex in the age of Viagra; Rising HIV rates show seniors often ignore risks. *The Austin American-Statesman*, A19.

Paniagua, F. A. (1999). Commentary on the possibility that Viagra may contribute to transmission of HIV and other sexual diseases among older adults. *Psychological Reports, 85*(3) (Part 1), 942–944.

Panlilio, A. L., Cardo, D. M., Grohskopf, L. A., Heneine, W., Ross, C. S., and the U.S. Public Health Service. (2005). Updated U.S. Public Health Service guidelines for the management of occupational exposures to HIV and recommendations for postexposure prophylaxis. *Morbidity and Mortality Weekly Report, Recommend Report, 54*(RR-9),1–17.

Patsdaughter, C. A., O'Connor, C. A., Grindel, C. G., Roberts, S. J., & Tarmina, M. S. (2003). The lesbian paradox in HIV risk [Abstract]. *Conference Program of the 16th Annual Association of Nurses in AIDS Care Conference (Spotlight on HIV/AIDS Nursing)*, 70.

Peragallo, N., Deforge, B., O'Campo, P., Lee, S. M., Kim, Y. J., Cianelli, R., et al. (2005). A randomized clinical trial of an HIV-risk-reduction intervention among low-income Latina women. *Nursing Research, 54*, 108–118.

Piot, P., Bartos, M., Larson, H., Zewdie, D., & Mane, P. (2008). Coming to terms with complexity: A call to action for HIV prevention. *Lancet, 372*(9641), 845–859.

Poynten, M., Brown, J. M., Sovero, M., Millwood, I. Y., & Kaldor, J. M. (2008). Microbicide safety and effectiveness: A overview of recent clinical trials. *Current Opinion in HIV and AIDS, 3*, 574–580.

Public Health Service Task Force. (2008). *Recommendations for use of antiretroviral drugs in pregnant HIV-infected women for maternal health and Interventions to reduce perinatal HIV transmission in the United States*. Retrieved October 12, 2008, from http://aidsinfo.nih.gov/contentfiles/PerinatalGL.pdf.

Pulerwitz, J., Izazola-Licea, J. A., & Gortmaker, S. L. (2001). Extra-relational sex among Mexican men and their partners' risk of HIV and other sexually transmitted diseases. *American Journal of Public Health, 91*(10), 1650–1652.

Roberts, S. T., & Kennedy, B. L. (2006). Why are young college women not using condoms? Their perceived risk, drug use, and developmental vulnerability may provide important clues to sexual risk. *Archives in Psychiatric Nursing, 20*(1), 32–40.

Sanchez, T., Finlayson, T., Drake, A., Behel, S., Cribbin, M., DiNenno, E., et al. (2006). Human Immunodeficiency Virus (HIV) risk, prevention, and testing behaviors—United States, National HIV Behavioral

Surveillance System: Men who have sex with men, November 2003–April 2005. *Morbidity and Mortality Weekly Report, Surveillance Summaries, 55*(SS06),1–16.

Sangi-Haghpeykar, H., Posner, S. F., & Pointdexter, A. N. III. (2005). Consistency of condom use among low-income hormonal contraceptive users. *Perspectives in Sexual and Reproductive Health, 37*(4),184–191.

Sarkar, K., Bal, B., Mukherjee, R., Chakraborty, S., Saha, S., Ghosh, A., et al. (2008). Sex-trafficking, violence, negotiating skill, and HIV infection in brothel-based sex workers of eastern India, adjoining Nepal, Bhuta, and Bangladesh. *Journal of Health Population Nutrition, 26*(2), 223–231.

Savasi, V., Ferrazzi, E., Lanzani, C., Oneta, M., Parrilla, B., & Persico, T. (2007). Safety of sperm washing and ART outcome in 741 HIV-1-serodiscordant couples. *Human Reproduction, 22,* 772–777.

Schiffner, T., & Buki, L. P. (2006). Latina college students' sexual health beliefs about papillomavirus infection. *Cultural Diversity and Ethnic Minority Psychology, 12,* 687–696.

Seal, D. W., & Ehrhardt, A. A. (2004). HIV-prevention-related sexual health promotion for heterosexual men: Pitfalls and recommendations. *Archives of Sexual Behavior, 33*(3), 211–222.

Siegel, K., Schrimshaw, E. W., Lekas, H. M., & Parsons, J. T. (2008). Sexual behaviors of non-gay identified non-disclosing men who have sex with men and women. Archives of Sexual Behavior, 37, 720–735.

Simoni-Wastila, L., & Strickler, G. (2004). Risk factors associated with problem use of prescription drugs. *American Journal of Public Health, 94*(2), 266–268.

Trepka, M. J., Kim, S., Pekovic, V., Zamor, P., Velez, E., & Gabaroni, M. V. (2008). High-risk sexual behavior among students of a minority-serving university in a community with a high HIV/AIDS prevalence. *Journal of the American College of Health, 57*(1), 77–84.

United Nations Programme on AIDS (UNAIDS). (2008). 2008 report on the Global AIDS Epidemic. Retrieved October 12, 2008, from www.unaids.org/en/KnowledgeCentre/ HIVData/GlobalReport/ 2008/2008_Global_report.asp.

Van Damme, L., Govinden, R., Mirembe, F. M., Guédou, F., Solomon, S., Becker, M. L., et al., and the CS Study Group. (2008). Lack of effectiveness of cellulose sulfate gel for the prevention of vaginal HIV transmission. *New England Journal of Medicine, 359*(5), 463–472.

Vermund, S., & Qian, H. (2008). Circumcision and HIV protection among men who have sex with men: No final word. *Journal of the American Medical Association, 300,* 1698–1700.

Villarruel, A. M., Jemmott, L. S., & Jemmott, J. B. III. (2005). Designing a culturally based intervention to reduce HIV sexual risk for Latino adolescents. *Journal of the Association of Nurses in AIDS Care, 16*, 23–31.

Weidel, J. J., Provencio-Vasquez, E., & González-Guarda, R. M. (2008). Cultural considerations for intimate partner violence and HIV risks in Hispanics. *Journal of the Association of Nurses in AIDS Care, 19*(4), 247–251.

Weinberg, P. D., Hounshell, J., Sherman, L. A., Godwin, J., Ali, S., Tomori, C., et al. (2002). Legal, financial, and public health consequences of HIV contamination of blood and blood products in the 1980s and 1990s. *Annals of Internal Medicine, 136*(4), 312–319.

Williams, E., & Donnelly, J. (2002). Older Americans and AIDS: Some guidelines for prevention. *Social Work, 47*(2), 105–111.

Wodak, A., & Cooney, A. (2006). Do needle syringe programs reduce HIV infection among injecting drug users? A comparative review of the international evidence. *Substance Use and Misuse, 41*, 777–813.

World Health Organization (WHO). (2008). *Priority interventions: HIV/ AIDS prevention, treatment and care in the health sector.* Retrieved October 12, 2008, from www.who.int/hiv/pub/priority_interventions_ web.pdf.

Yarbel, W. L., Graham, C. A., Sanders, R. A., & Crosby, S. A. (2004). Correlates of condom breakage and slippage among university undergraduates. *International Journal of STDs and AIDS, 15*(7), 467–472.

6

Living with HIV/AIDS

DAVID J. STERKEN

Living with HIV/AIDS is a highly personal journey. Researchers for years have described the journey in terms of laboratory values, drug adherence, and medication side effects (Gray, 2006), long-term sequelae (Kirton, 2008; Sension, 2007), psychological consequences (Kemppainen et al., 2003; Valente, 2003; Van Servellen et al., 2002), symptom management (Chou et al., 2004; Spirig et al., 2005), and quality of life (QOL) (Davis, 2004; Robinson, 2004; Uphold et al., 2007). Such descriptions prove helpful as management strategies for dealing with HIV/AIDS but fall short of actually describing the daily experience of living with HIV/AIDS.

This chapter does not presume to speak for all persons living with HIV (PLWH) worldwide; instead it is an attempt to give a face to the disease of HIV/AIDS. As nurses we have a duty to see the person behind the disease. Our caring demands that we see each patient as an individual and respond according to his or her individual needs.

THE PERSON

The experience of living with HIV/AIDS is highly variable and unique to each individual. Each person living with HIV/AIDS brings to the experience a personal history, beliefs, and values. To understand the impact of the disease on the individual PLWH means that the nurse must look at each person in terms of that individual's personal, social, cultural, and spiritual context. The crisis associated with the diagnosis forces many

205

PLWH to reexamine their own lives. This self-inventory often results, over time, in an inward transformation. Life is no longer about going through unconscious motions but rather about deliberate attempts to find meaning in every circumstance and relationship. What every PLWH fears is being reduced to a disease. Medication side effects and disease progression cause changes in body habitus. The focus of appointments with health care practitioners is often laboratory values and medication compliance, reducing the individual to little more than a "bag of blood" and a "drug cocktail." Who the patient is can get buried underneath the disease, and soon everything in his or her life is interpreted through "HIV-colored glasses." Persons living with HIV can find their passion and purpose in life thwarted unless they become consciously aware that they are more than their disease and view their HIV status as an opportunity rather than obstacle.

The Uncertainty of HIV Infection

Perhaps one of the most distressing factors associated with being HIV-infected is the uncertainty associated with the disease (Brashers et al., 2003; Brashers, Neidig, & Goldsmith, 2004; Cochrane, 2003; Kylmä, Vehviläinen-Julkunen, & Lähdevirta, 2008; Penrod, 2007). Individuals can be infected without their knowledge; and, left unchecked, the virus will ravage their immune systems over time. The ability of HIV to mutate and develop resistance to medication makes medical management a challenge. A person's unique body chemistry and genetic makeup also determine his or her response to HIV and any treatment regimen.

Simple illnesses may create anxiety for PLWH as they imagine the worst—the annihilation of their immune system. Routine laboratory work (e.g., viral load, CD4 count) is often overshadowed by an unconscious fear of disease progression or treatment failure (Kemppainen et al., 2003). Over time this fear may lessen, but it is always present just below the surface. The PLWH anticipates the worst while hoping for the best. A part of that fear is the knowledge that at present no cure exists for HIV/AIDS and that a premature death may be imminent. Some liken this to the sword of Damocles, a foreboding circumstance in which the potential for tragedy hangs by a delicate thread.

The Burden of Being Infected with HIV

The psychological burden of being infected with HIV is difficult to describe and may differ from one person to another, depending on such factors as personal coping skills (Lazarus, 1993; Moskowitz & Wrubel, 2005), resilience (De Santis, 2008; Farber et al., 2003) and presence or absence of support systems (Goldsmith et al., 2007; Siegel, Brown-Bradley, & Lekas, 2004). Fatigue is a frequent complaint of HIV-positive patients (Harmon et al., 2008; Voss et al., 2006, 2007). Many clinicians fail to understand the difference between "being tired" and "fatigued" and automatically associate fatigue with the physical need for sleep. Yet "fatigue" is multidimensional symptom involving physical, mental, emotional, and spiritual energy (Ferrando et al., 1998).

It is safe to say that, for those of us living with HIV, our body is in a constant state of alert on a cellular level. Add to this physical labor the emotional stress (conscious or unconscious) and spiritual challenges, and you have an old-fashioned recipe for fatigue.

We must never forget the "psychic" impact of HIV on our energy level. We might eat a balanced diet, exercise on a regular basis, and get eight hours of sleep every night and yet still suffer from fatigue; however, I would propose that most HIV-related fatigue is related not only to a physical cause but also to multiple psychic (nonphysical) phenomena. Some PLWH refer to this unexplained fatigue as "having an AIDS day." Here are some examples of what I believe causes psychic fatigue:

- Fearing rejection—"People will treat me differently if they know I am HIV positive."
- Lacking physical and emotional love.
- Feeling powerless—"I don't have any choice."
- Fearing relapse—"How long will my treatment keep my HIV under control?"
- Failing to recognize limits and ask for help—Superman/Superwoman complex.
- Feeling undeserving of anything good.
- Being unable to forgive self or others.
- Having an inability to set boundaries.
- Viewing oneself as a "sinner."
- Ignoring one's inner voice.
- "Blaming" the past.

Quality of Life: What Is It Really?

Quality of life: We see this ever-popular phrase in nursing articles describing the lives of people infected with HIV. Yet, I believe that there is a danger in trying to quantify "quality of life" for the purpose of research. Although I would agree that the "quality of life" research has identified many key issues important to PLWH, we must never forget that *quality* is defined differently by each and every individual. *Quality* is defined by Webster as "peculiar and essential character" and "the identifying character." The very definition of the term *quality* takes on a personal nature demanding a level of intimacy between practitioner and patient. Intimacy is seeing more than a physical presence and laboratory values when a practitioner interacts with his or her patient. Intimacy demands that practitioners and the PLWH for whom they care "know" one another on a deeply physical, emotional, mental, and spiritual level.

The nature of the health care system does not foster intimacy; and, as a result, the "quality of life" agenda may be lost in the discovery of a "new combination of drugs." All too often I have seen my fellow sojourners suffer in silence simply because their practitioner allots very little time to develop intimate relationships and thus discover their essential character (quality).

I believe that as patients we are in a unique position not only to add to the body of research that examines quality of life in the HIV-positive population but also to promote patient–practitioner relationships that are more holistic. I am more than my CD4 count and viral load! My life is affected by relationships, job issues, planning for the future, and everyday stressors, all of which affect the quality of my life. Sharing with my health care practitioner the impact psychosocial variables have on my relationships and my ability to live with the disease will enable them to better understand quality of life issues in the HIV population.

The concept of quality of life originated from care of oncology patients (Grimes & Cole, 1996). It developed from the idea that while treatment of disease is often a necessity, a delicate balance must be maintained that allows one to continue to live a life of meaning and purpose. As the result of a national research agenda, initiated by the National Institute for Nursing Research, seeking to identify critical nursing-related areas for HIV research, Larson and Ropka (1990) identified as a priority the need to research the multidimensional problems faced by persons living with HIV infection. Further discussion served to narrow the focus toward identification of psychosocial variables and the impact of these variables on persons with HIV infection, their families, and their loved ones (see related research by D'Cruz, 2004; Gifford et al., 2005; Gore-Felton & Koopman, 2008; Grodeck, 2003; Ironson & Howard, 2008; Menadue, 2003; Nun_es et al., 1995; Palattiyil & Chakrabarti, 2008; WHO, 2005).

Over the past two decades, nurses and other researchers have worked hard to identify how HIV affects quality of life (Burgoyne et al., 2004; Davis, 2004; Eller, 2001; Grossman, Sullivan, & Wu, 2003; Holzemer et al., 2001; Kemppainen, 2001; Phaladze et al., 2005; Robinson, 2004; Uphold et. al., 2007; Webb & Norton, 2004). The following is a list of factors that affect life quality in persons with HIV:

- **Ability to function in daily life activities and roles.** Reliance on others to perform daily activities of living is a disruptive force, which can be mediated by one's enabling skills. Enabling skills are behaviors and skills that are learned as a response to aversive and disruptive events. Thus, the more an individual with HIV disease is involved in self-care and personal, family, and social roles, the greater the perceived level of well being (Grimes & Cole, 1996).
- **Self-transcendence.** Self-transcendence is a developmental characteristic that expands one's boundaries of self to take on broader life perspectives, activities, and purposes that help one discover or make meaning of one's life. Faced with their illness, persons with HIV are able to transform this information from despair to challenge, from psychological crisis to personal growth, from a death sentence to a new meaning and quality of life (Mellors et al., 2001; Mellors, Riley, & Erlen, 1997; Reed, 1991, 2003).
- **Balance.** Achieving a balance is a process in which persons with HIV disease strive to maintain quality as they learn to live with a chronic disease that has a slow, progressive downhill trajectory (Murdaugh, 1998). Bedell (1999) found that those who worked to find and maintain balance in their lives refused to let the clinical aspects of AIDS take control of their daily lives and define how they viewed themselves, or others viewed them, as individuals. Numerous books have been written in recent years that urge people to achieve balance in their lives as a means of achieving the best health possible (see, for example, Singh, 2007).
- **Psychosocial counseling and stress management.** Psychosocial interventions that enhance an individual's sense of control, teach adaptive coping strategies, improve ability to elicit social support, and modify ways that individuals think about stressors may enhance psychological adjustment in HIV-infected individuals, thereby improving the quality of their lives (Carrico & Antoni, 2008; Lutgendorf et al., 1994).

- **Comorbid psychiatric conditions.** Comorbid mood disorders (depression, anxiety or panic attacks) and other psychiatric conditions, such as alcohol abuse and substance dependence, may result in poorer prognosis and response to treatment for persons with HIV (Leserman, 2008; Leserman & Temoshok, 2008; Pence, 2009; Porche & Willis, 2006; Repetto & Petitto, 2008; Sherbourne et al., 2000).

- **Symptom progression.** The trends in a study by Lubeck & Fries (1992) suggest that there is a significant impact on a PLWH's quality of life when he or she has progressed to the stage of having one or more serious opportunistic infections. Cunningham and colleagues (1998) defined symptom progression in terms of "constitutional symptoms" like fever, night sweats, myalgias, fatigue, anorexia (sometimes with nausea and vomiting), and weight loss. They recommended that clinicians should screen the HIV-infected patient regularly for these symptoms so that efforts can be made to treat such complaints before they become detrimental to quality of life. Symptom management by patients and clinicians has been widely discussed in both lay and professional literature (Lorenz et al., 2001; Sousa, Tann, & Kwok, 2006)

- **Will to Live.** Tsevat and colleagues (1999) found that half of the patients interviewed indicated that their life with HIV is better than it was before they contracted HIV. Factors unrelated to health that contributed to health values included spirituality and concern and love for one's children.

- **Social support.** Relationships that provide emotional as well as physical intimacy improve quality of life. Supportive relationships with family, friends, peers, and health care professionals can assist PLWH to develop skills and resources for coping with HIV/AIDS (Friedland, Renwick, & McColl, 1996; Goldsmith et al., 2007).

- **Diet and exercise.** Implementation of a diet and exercise program improved the effects of lipodystrophy and wasting (Arey & Beal, 2002; Reid & Courtney, 2007).

While this list is not comprehensive, it briefly describes some of the key factors that contribute to quality of life in people living with HIV. As PLWH live longer, issues related to quality of life will continue to unfold and prove paramount in the medical management of the disease.

Self-Transcendence: Finding Meaning and Purpose

Self-transcendence and quality of life are concepts that are intimately linked to one another. Self-transcendence is the ability to feel that life has balance even though one might experience significant symptoms associated with an illness (Mellors et al., 1997, 2001; Ramer, Johnson, & Barrett, 2006; Reed, 2003). In short, self-transcendence is a developmental progression toward quality of life, which permits less emotional disruption despite events that heighten one's sense of mortality (Lewis & Galliston, 1989; Reed, 1991).

Coward (1994) examined the concept of self-transcendence from the perspective of both men and women with AIDS. Her findings demonstrate the need to incorporate gender and individual difference when seeking to discover experiences from which PLWH may derive meaning and emotional well-being. Several themes emerged from her research:

Men's Themes

- Experiencing fear: Being rejected by others; experiencing the process of dying; losing connections; not being known/remembered by others after death.
- Taking care of themselves: Taking an active and assertive role in their health care, not giving up the control to someone else.
- Seeking out challenge: Proving one's self and to bolstering self-confidence.
- Creating a legacy: Wanting to be known/remembered by others.
- Accepting that which cannot be changed: Accepting all parts of themselves, including the part with AIDS.
- Connecting with others: Participating in support groups, sharing their knowledge and experience with AIDS, keeping in touch with friends and family.
- Letting go: Decreasing or stopping meaningless activities, work.
- Accepting help: Asking for and accepting help was not always easy.
- Having hope: Seeking ways to live longer, maintaining meaningful personal relationships, continuing to find reason for being through participation in community events.

Women's Themes

- Experiencing fear and aloneness: Overwhelming sense of isolation and abandonment from caring others as well as from God.

- Experiencing uncertainty: Being unable to predict the behavior of others related to their diagnosis; being unable to predict periods of their own illness or wellness.
- Using others as role models: Being motivated by the everyday struggles of others who lived with AIDS.
- Finding inner strength: Seeking therapy, journaling their daily lives.
- Reaching out to receive and to give: Sharing their experience in support groups and individually with other women who have AIDS.
- Making a difference, having purpose: Developing an increased sense of self-worth from believing that their sense of purpose and self-worth, along with their own unique experience, could make a difference.
- Viewing AIDS as an opportunity: Seeing AIDS as providing an opportunity for personal growth.
- Having hope: Expressing hope for living with people who loved them and to whom they could give their love.

In this study, these men and women found meaning in reaching out to relieve their fear and aloneness and in maintaining hope for a cure. Purpose and meaning for the individuals in this study were primarily based on the development and continued maintenance of human relationships rather than the presence or absence of physical symptoms.

The Relationship Challenge

Developing and maintaining intimate relationships is a challenge for the PLWH. Sex is no longer a spontaneous act but rather requires planning and the disclosure of highly personal and potentially volatile information. Many HIV-positive people fear rejection on disclosure of their status to a potential intimate partner. In other cases, where a partner has become infected as a result of a relationship outside of the established relationship, disclosure becomes laden with other emotionally charged issues and may significantly impact intimate relationships (Ortiz, 2007).

Body image often changes significantly with treatment and disease progression. Fat redistribution, loss of muscle mass, and wasting affect self-image and the overall feelings of desirability that are necessary to establish and maintain intimate relationships (Burgoyne et al., 2005; Gagnon & Holmes, 2008; Persson, 2005; Reynolds et al., 2006). Such changes may lead to depression or substance use. Illicit drugs can create an illusion of normalcy and for a period of time create an amnesic effect regarding the reality of the current situation. Unfortunately, once the effects of the substance wear off the reality remains, and the guilt associated with substance use may further perpetuate the depression and low self-esteem.

Shifting the focus of relationships from outward beauty to inward characteristics shines light on the value that a person brings to the world. This shift allows a person to cultivate the gifts that as yet may have remained unexplored. Developing supportive relationships is very important for the long-term mental health of the person with HIV/AIDS.

CONCLUSION

The chronic nature of HIV creates the need to focus on quality of life issues. Although quality of life is personal in nature, research has uncovered themes that will help health care teams to better focus their interventions as they work with PLWH. Care can no longer focus solely on the physical aspects of the disease but must consider the multidimensional aspects of the disease. Many of the quality of life issues identified by researchers focus on the psychosocial impact of the disease, a poignant reminder to practitioners that treatment must be holistic. Treatment must focus on health maintenance and self-care and evolve as PLWH strive to achieve balance and control in their lives following the diagnosis of HIV infection.

REFERENCES

Arey, B., & Beal, M. (2002). The role of exercise in the prevention and treatment of wasting in acquired immune deficiency syndrome. *Journal of the Association of Nurses in AIDS Care, 13*(1), 29–49.

Bedell, G. (1999). Daily life for eight urban gay men with HIV/AIDS. *The American Journal of Occupational Therapy, 54,* 197–206.

Brashers, D., Neidig, J., & Goldsmith, D. (2004). Social support and the management of uncertainty for people living with HIV or AIDS. *Health Communication, 16,* 305–331.

Brashers, D., Neidig, J., Russell, J., Cardillo, L., Haas, S., Dobbs, L., et al. (2003). The medical, personal, and social causes of uncertainty in HIV illness. *Issues in Mental Health Nursing, 24,* 497–522.

Burgoyne, R., Collins, E., Wagner, C., Abbey, S., Halman, M., Nur, M., et al. (2005). The relationship between lipodystrophy-associated body changes and measures of quality of life and mental health for HIV-positive adults. *Quality of Life Research, 14*, 981–990.

Burgoyne, R., Rourke, S., Behrens, D., & Salit, I. (2004). Long-term quality-of-life outcomes among adults living with HIV in the HAART era: The interplay of changes in clinical factors and symptom profile. *AIDS Behavior, 8*, 151–163.

Carrico, A., & Antoni, M. (2008). Effects of psychological interventions on neuroendocrine hormone regulation and immune status in HIV-positive persons: A review of randomized controlled trials. *Psychosomatic Medicine, 70*, 575–584.

Chou F., Holzemer, W., Portillo, C., & Slaughter, R. (2004). Self-care strategies and sources of information for HIV/AIDS symptom management. *Nursing Research, 53*, 332–339.

Cochrane, J. (2003). The experience of uncertainty for individuals with HIV/AIDS and the palliative care paradigm. *International Journal of Palliative Nursing, 9*, 382–388.

Coward, D. (1994). Meaning and purpose in the lives of persons with AIDS. *Public Health Nursing, 11*, 331–336.

Cunningham, W., Shapiro, M., Hays, R., Dixon, W., Visscher, B., George, W., et al. (1998). Constitutional symptoms and health-related quality of life in patients with symptomatic HIV disease. *American Journal of Medicine, 104*, 129–136.

Davis, S. (2004). Clinical sequelae affecting quality of life in the HIV-infected patient. *Journal of the Association of Nurses in AIDS Care, 15* (5S), 28S–33S.

D'Cruz, P. (2004). *Family care in HIV/AIDS. Exploring lived experience.* New Delhi: Sage.

De Santis, J. (2008). Exploring the concepts of vulnerability and resilience in the context of HIV infection. *Research & Theory for Nursing Practice, 22*, 273–287.

Eller, L. (2001). Quality of life in persons with HIV. *Clinical Nursing Research, 10*, 401–423.

Farber, E., Mairsalimi, H., Williams, K., & McDaniel. (2003). Meaning of illness and psychological adjustment to HIV/AIDS. *Psychosomatics, 44*, 485–491.

Ferrando, S., Evans, S., Goggin, K., Sewell, M., Fishman, B., & Rabkin, J. (1998). Fatigue in HIV illness: Relationship to depression, physical limitations, and disability. *Psychosomatic Medicine, 60*(6), 759–764.

Friedland, J., Renwick, R., & McColl, M. (1996). Coping and social support as determinants of quality of life in HIV/AIDS. *AIDS Care, 8*, 15–31.

Gagnon, M., & Holmes, D. (2008). Moving beyond biomedical understanding of lipodystrophy in people living with HIV/AIDS. *Research & Theory for Nursing Practice, 22*, 228–240.

Gifford, A., Lorig, K., Laurent, D., & Gonzalez, V. (2005). *Living well with HIV & AIDS.* Boulder, CO: Bull Publishing Company.

Goldsmith, D., Brashers, D., Kosenko, K., & O'Keefe, D. (2007). Social support and living with HIV: Findings from qualitative studies. In T. Edgar, V. Freimuth & S. Noar (Eds.), *Communication Perspectives on HIV/AIDS for the 21st Century* (pp. 101–136). Philadelphia: Lawrence Erlbaum Associates.

Gore-Felton, C., & Koopman, C. (2008). Behavioral mediation of the relationship between psychosocial factors and HIV disease progression. *Psychosomatic Medicine, 70*, 569–574.

Gray, J. (2006). Becoming adherent: Experiences of persons living with HIV/AIDS. *Journal of the Association of Nurses in AIDS Care. 17*(3), 47–54.

Grimes, D., & Cole, F. (1996). Self-help and quality of life in persons with HIV disease. *AIDS Care, 8*, 691–699.

Grodeck, B. (2003). *The first year: HIV: An essential guide for the newly diagnosed.* New York: Marlowe and Company.

Grossman, H., Sullivan, P., & Wu, A. (2003). Quality of life and HIV: Current assessment tools and future directions for clinical practice. *AIDS Reader, 13*, 583–597.

Harmon, J., Barroso, J., Pence, B., Leserman J., & Salahuddin, N. (2008). Demographic and illness-related variables associated with HIV-related fatigue. *Journal of the Association of Nurses in AIDS Care, 19*(2), 90–97.

Holzemer, W., Hudson, A., Kirksey, K., Hamilton, M., & Bakken. (2001). The revised sign and symptom checklist for HIV. *Journal of the Association of Nurses in AIDS Care, 12*(5), 60–70.

Ironson, G., & Hayward, H. (2008). Do positive psychosocial factors predict disease progression in HIV? A review of the evidence. *Psychosomatic Medicine, 70*, 546–554.

Kemppainen, J. (2001). Predictors of quality of life in AIDS patients. *Journal of the Association of Nurses in AIDS Care, 12*(2), 61–70.

Kemppainen, J., Holzemer, W., Nokes, K., Eller, L., Corless, I., Bunch, E., et al. (2003). Self-care and management of anxiety and fear in HIV disease. *Journal of the Association of Nurses in AIDS Care, 14*(2), 21–29.

Kirton, C. (2008). Managing long-term complications of HIV infection. *Nursing 2008, 38*(8), 44–51.

Kylmä, J., Vehviläinen-Julkunen, K., & Lähdevirta, J. (2008). Hope, despair and hopelessness in living with HIV/AIDS: A grounded theory study. *Journal of Advanced Nursing, 33,* 764–775.

Larson, E., & Ropka, M. E. (1990). HIV epidemic: Nursing research in HIV infection: Prevention and care. National nursing research agenda. Developing knowledge for practice: Challenges and opportunities. Washington, DC: United States Department of Health and Human Services, Government Printing Office.

Lazarus, R. (1993). Coping theory and research: Past, present, and future. *Psychosomatic Medicine, 55,* 34–247.

Leserman, J. (2008). Role of depression, stress, and trauma in HIV disease progression. *Psychosomatic Medicine, 70,* 539–545.

Leserman, J., & Temoshok, L. (2008). A road well traveled (although not yet a super highway). *Psychosomatic Medicine, 70,* 521–522.

Lewis, S., & Galliston, M. (1989). Family functioning study (technical paper). Seattle: University of Washington.

Lorenz, C., Shapiro, M., Asch, S., Bozette, S., & Hays, R. (2001). Association of symptoms and health-related quality of life: Findings from a national study of persons with HIV infection. *Annals of Internal Medicine, 134,* 854–860.

Lubeck, D., & Fries, J. (1992). Changes in quality of life among persons with HIV infection. *Quality of Life Research, 1,* 359–366.

Lutgendorf, S., Antoni, M., Schneiderman, N., & Fletcher, M. (1994). Psychosocial counseling to improve quality of life in HIV infection. *Patient Education and Counseling, 24,* 217–235.

Mellors, M., Erlen, J., Coontz, P., & Lucke, K. (2001). Transcending the suffering of AIDS. *Journal of Community Health Nursing, 18,* 235–246.

Mellors, M., Riley, T., & Erlen, J. (1997). HIV, self-transcendence, and quality of life. *Journal Association of Nurses in AIDS Care, 8,* 59–69.

Menadue, D. (2003) *Positive: Living with HIV/AIDS.* Crows Nest NSW, Australia: Allen & Unwin.

Moskowitz, J., & Wrubel, J. (2005). Coping with HIV as a chronic illness: A longitudinal analysis of illness appraisals. *Psychology and Health, 20,* 509–532.

Murdaugh, C. (1998). Health-related quality of life in HIV disease: Achieving a balance. *Journal Association of Nurses in AIDS Care, 9*(6), 59–71.

Nuñes, J., Raymond, S., Nicholas, P., Leuner, J., & Webster, A. (1995). Social support, quality of life, immune function, and health in persons living with HIV. *Journal of Holistic Nursing, 13,* 174–198.

Ortiz, M. (2007). HIV, AIDS, and sexuality. *Nursing Clinics of North America, 42,* 639–653.

Palattiyil, G., & Chakrabarti, M. (2008). Coping strategies of families in HIV/AIDS care: Some exploratory data from two developmental contexts. *AIDS Care, 20,* 881–885.

Pence, B. (2009). The impact of mental health and traumatic life experiences on antiretroviral treatment outcomes for people living with HIV/AIDS. *Journal of Antimicrobial Chemotherapy, 63.* Advance Access published on January 18, 2009; doi: doi:10.1093/jac/dkp006.

Penrod, J. (2007). Living with uncertainty: Concept advancement. *Journal of Advanced Nursing, 57,* 658–667.

Persson, A. (2005). Facing HIV: Body shape change and the (in)visibility of illness. *Medical Anthropology, 24,* 237–264.

Phaladze, N., Human. S., Dlamini, S., Hulela, E., Mahlubi Hadebe, I., Sukati, N., et al. (2005). Quality of life and the concept of "living well" with HIV/AIDS in sub-Saharan Africa. *Journal of Nursing Scholarship, 37*(2), 120–126.

Porche, D., & Willis, D. (2006). Depression in HIV-infected men. *Issues in Mental Health Nursing, 27,* 391–401.

Ramer, L., Johnson, D., & Barrett. M. (2006). The effect of HIV/AIDS disease progression on spirituality and self-transcendence in a multicultural population. *Journal of Transcultural Nursing, 17,* 280–289.

Reed, P. (1991). Toward a nursing theory of self-transcendence: Deductive reformulation using developmental theories. *Advances in Nursing Science, 13,* 64–77.

Reed, P. (2003). The theory of self-transcendence. In M. J. Smith & P. R. Liehr (Eds.), *Middle range theory for nursing* (pp. 145–165). New York: Springer.

Reid, C., & Courtney, M. (2007). A randomized clinical trial to evaluate the effect of diet on quality of life and mood of people with HIV lipodystrophy. *Journal of the Association of Nurses in AIDS Care, 18*(4), 3–11.

Repetto, M., & Petitto, J. (2008). Psychopharmacology in HIV-infected patients. *Psychosomatic Medicine, 70,* 585–592.

Reynolds, N., Neidig, J., Wu, A., Gifford, A., & Holmes, W. (2006). Balancing disfigurement and fear of disease progression: Patient perceptions of HIV body fat redistribution. *AIDS Care, 18,* 663–673.

Robinson, P. (2004). Measurement of quality of life in HIV disease. *Journal of the Association of Nurses in AIDS Care, 15*(5), 14S–19S.

Sension, M. (2007). Long-term suppression of HIV infection: Benefits and limitations of current treatment options. *Journal of the Association of Nurses in AIDS Care, 18*(1S), S2-10, S23-6.

Sherbourne, C., Hays, R., Fleishman, J., Vitiello, B., Magruder, K. Bing, E., et al. (2000). Impact of psychiatric conditions on health-related quality of life in persons with HIV infection. *American Journal of Psychiatry, 157,* 248–254.

Siegel, K., Brown-Bradley, C. J., & Lekas, H. M. (2004). Strategies for coping with fatigue among HIV-positive individuals fifty years and older. *AIDS Patient Care & Studies, 18*(5), 275–288.

Sousa, K., Tann, S., & Kwok, O. (2006). Reconsidering the assessment of symptom status in HIV/AIDS care. *Journal of the Association of Nurses in AIDS Care, 17*(2), 36–46.

Singh, S. (2007). *Achieving a healthy balanced life.* Lincoln, NE: iUniverse.

Spirig, R., Moody, K., Battegay, M., & DeGeest. (2005). Symptom management in HIV/AIDS. *Advances in Nursing Science, 28,* 333–344.

Tsevat, J., Sherman, S., McElwee, J., Mandell, K., Simbartl, L., Sonnenberg, F., et al. (1999). The will to live among HIV-infected patients. *Annals of Internal Medicine, 131,* 194–198.

Uphold, C., Holmes, W., Reid, K., Findley, K., & Parada, J. (2007). Healthy lifestyles and health-related quality of life among men living with HIV infection. *Journal of the Association of Nurses in AIDS Care, 18*(6), 54–66.

Valente, S. (2003). Depression and HIV disease. *Journal of the Association of Nurses in AIDS Care, 14*(2), 41–51.

van Servellen, G, Aguirre, M., Sarna, L., & Brecht, M. (2002). Differential predictors of emotional distress in HIV-infected men and women. *Western Journal of Nursing Research, 24,* 49–72.

Voss, J., Sukati, N., Seboni, N., Makoae, L., Moleko, S., & Human, S. (2007). Symptom burden of fatigue in men and women living with HIV/AIDS in southern Africa. *Journal of the Association of Nurses in AIDS Care, 18*(4), 22–31.

Voss, J., Dodd, M., Portillo, C., & Holzemer, W. (2006). Theories of fatigue: Application in HIV/AIDS. *Journal of the Association of Nurses in AIDS Care, 17,* 37–50.

Webb, A., & Norton, M. (2004). Clinical assessment of symptom-focused health-related quality of life in HIV/AIDS. *Journal of the Association of Nurses in AIDS Care, 15*(2), 67–81.

World Health Organization. (2005). What is the impact of HIV on families? Copenhagen: WHO Regional Office for Europe. Retrieved January 30, 2009, from www.euro.who.int/Document/E87762.pdf.

7

The Medical Management of HIV Disease

JAMES L. RAPER

As the world enters the third decade of the HIV/AIDS pandemic, millions of adults and children around the globe are living with HIV/AIDS (Hall et al., 2008). (HIV/AIDS epidemiologic data are presented in Chapter 1.) Millions more are infected with HIV but are unaware of their infection. During the almost three decades of the epidemic, better approaches to the diagnosis and medical treatment of HIV/AIDS and related conditions have emerged. As a result of earlier diagnosis and improved treatments, HIV/AIDS is increasingly manageable as a chronic condition. Persons living with HIV/AIDS (PLWH) who have access to expert medical care can now live a longer and better-quality life than PLWH even a decade ago.

In general, AIDS is diagnosed when the CD4 count is below 200/mL and is characterized by the appearance of opportunistic infections. Most recently, in an unprecedented move, the Centers for Disease Control (CDC) recalculated their estimates of the number of new HIV infections (Centers for Disease Control [CDC], 2008), sharing that there are 40% more new infections than once believed. The estimate of 40,000 new cases each year was increased to 56,000 new cases. The CDC reported that the change in estimates was due to new methods of surveillance and testing that pinpoint the time of infection within a few months. While HIV infection and AIDS continue to cause illness and death, medical treatment has dramatically improved survival rates, especially since the introduction of highly active antiretroviral therapy (HAART) in 1995 (Delgado et al., 2003).

Antiretroviral therapy (ART) for treatment of HIV continues to improve since the advent of combination therapy in 1996. New medicines offer new mechanisms of action, better potency, dosing convenience, and improved safety profiles. Some earlier medicines have been removed from the market, and others are being used less often. Resistance testing is used more frequently in clinical practice, and drug–drug (medication) interactions between antiretroviral and other medicines are more complex.

The objective of this chapter is to provide nurses with an abridged up-to-date framework for the medical care of patients living with HIV. The primary subject areas included are: (1) standards of HIV medical care for the treatment for HIV disease and common concomitant illnesses; (2) issues related to adherence to antiretroviral medication and engagement with health care services; (3) medication and food interactions; (4) adverse medication effects; (5) medication resistance; 6) nonpharmacological treatment approaches; (7) immune reconstitution; (8) organ transplantation; and (9) factors associated with HIV disease prognosis. This framework outlines the current understanding of how clinicians should use antiretroviral medications to treat adults and adolescents infected with HIV-1. However, because the science and understanding of HIV rapidly evolves, the appropriate use of available new medicines and new clinical data may rapidly change treatment options and preferences. The most current treatment guidelines are available at http://aidsinfo.nih.gov/guidelines. The author enthusiastically encourages readers to review the most current recommendations.

The importance of coupling the information contained in this chapter and other references with expertise in the clinical care of patients with HIV cannot be overemphasized. Multiple studies demonstrate that better patient outcomes occur when care is rendered by an HIV experienced clinician who: (1) provides HIV primary care to at least 50 HIV-infected patients and (2) participates in ongoing continuing education on HIV-related topics (Delgado et al., 2003; Hecht et al., 1999; Kitahata et al., 1996, 2003; Laine et al., 1998). Expert care can result in decreased mortality, decreased rates of hospitalization, improved adherence with treatment guidelines, lower cost of care, and improved medication adherence.

STANDARDS OF HIV MEDICAL CARE
Assessment

Assessment is the basis on which all health care is rendered; thus a comprehensive baseline evaluation must be performed and maintained

Table 7.1

INITIAL ASSESSMENT

HIV antibody testing (if previous laboratory confirmation is not available)

Assessment of comorbidities, economic factors, mental illness, social support, substance abuse, and other factors that are known to impair the ability to adhere to treatment and to alter outcomes

BUN and creatinine

CD4 T-cell count

Chemistry profile

Chest X-ray, if clinically indicated

Complete blood count

Fasting blood glucose and serum lipids

Genotypic resistance testing, regardless of whether therapy will be initiated immediately

Hepatitis A, B, and C serologies

PAP smear, cervical

Plasma HIV RNA

RPR or VDRL

Screening for *Chlamydia trachomatis* and *Neisseria gonorrhoeae* to identify high-risk behavior and the need for sexually transmitted disease (STD) therapy—screen specific to exposure: oral, genital, and/or rectal

Toxoplasma gondii IgG

Transaminase levels

Tuberculin skin test (TST) or interferon-_ release assay (IGRA) (unless a history of prior tuberculosis or positive TST or IGRA)

Urinalysis

throughout the care of a patient with HIV. A complete medical history, physical examination, and laboratory evaluation should be performed for every patient entering care to confirm the presence and stage of HIV infection, determine the presence of coinfections, and assess the overall health status as recommended by the primary care guidelines for the management of HIV-infected patients (Aberg et al., 2004). The laboratory tests displayed in Table 7.1 should be performed for all new patients during the initial patient encounter.

Although all these laboratory tests are important in evaluating a patient's health status, the CD4 T-cell count and plasma HIV RNA (viral load) greatly determine both when to initiate HIV treatment and the effectiveness of the treatment. Furthermore, genotypic resistance testing is used to guide the selection of the antiretroviral medications in both treatment-naïve and -experienced patients. While not included as a part of the initial laboratory studies, a viral tropism assay should be performed prior to initiation of CCR5 antagonist medications and HLA-B*5701 testing should be performed prior to initiation of antiretroviral therapy with the nucleoside analog reverse transcriptase inhibitor (NRTI) abacavir because patients who possess the HLA-B*5701 allele have an increased risk for hypersensitivity reactions (HSR) to abacavir (Mallal et al., 2008; Saag et al., 2008). Hypersensitivity reaction is the main side effect of abacavir. It can be severe and, in rare cases, fatal. Genetic testing can indicate whether a person will be hypersensitive; over 90% of patients can safely take abacavir.

Goals of Treatment

Goals of treatment with antiretroviral (ART) medication are listed in Table 7.2. The most important goals are to: (1) achieve maximal suppression of plasma viral load for as long as possible, (2) delay the development of medication resistance, (3) preserve CD4 T-cell numbers, and (4) confer substantial clinical benefits. These goals are achieved by

Table 7.2

HIV TREATMENT GOALS
Improve quality of life
Maximally and durably suppress viral load
Prevent vertical HIV transmission
Prolong survival
Reduce HIV-related morbidity
Restore and preserve immunologic function

reducing HIV-related morbidity and mortality, improving quality of life, and restoring and preserve immunologic function in persons infected with (Moyle et al., 2008).

Unfortunately, complete eradication of HIV infection is not possible with the available antiretroviral medications because latently infected CD4 T-cells that are established during the earliest stages of acute HIV infection (Chun et al., 1998) persist with a long half-life in spite of prolonged suppression of HIV plasma viremia (Chun et al., 1997; Finzi et al., 1997, 1999; Wong et al., 1997).

Clinicians who follow approved treatment guidelines and strategies recognize substantial reductions in HIV-related morbidity and mortality (Mocroft et al., 1998; Palella et al., 1998; Vittinghoff et al., 1999) and reduced vertical transmission from infected mother to infant (Garcia et al., 1999; Mofenson et al., 1999). Higher HIV plasma viral loads are associated with more rapid disease progression (Mellors et al., 1996), while other factors such as heightened T-cell activation with cellular turnover and expression of immune activation markers probably contribute as well to clinical disease progression the rate of CD4 T-cell decline (Rodriguez et al., 2006).

The goal of maximal viral suppression with initial ART may be difficult in some HIV-infected patients who have preexisting medication resistance. To be successful, ART regimens need to contain at least two, and preferably three, active medicines from multiple medication classes. If maximal initial suppression below the level of HIV detection (<50 copies/mL) is not achieved or is lost, it is important to change medication regimens to include at least two active medicines to achieve the maximal suppression goal. If it is not possible to achieve the HIV RNA <50 copies/mL goal in a clinically and immunologically stable patient, a time period of persistent detectable viremia may be acceptable while waiting for the availability of new medicine.

In general, viral load reduction to <50 copies/mL in most treatment-naïve patient occurs within the first 12 to 24 weeks of therapy. Predictors of virologic success are presented in Table 7.3. Virologic suppression is always observed. Viral suppression rates in clinical practice may be lower than the 80 to 90% seen in clinical trials. However, the use of current easier-to-take, coformulated, and potent ART regimens probably decrease the differences in outcomes between clinical trials and clinical practice (Moore et al., 2005). To achieve treatment goals, clinicians and patients must work together to define priorities, investigate options, and mutually determine the best treatment plan.

Table 7.3

PREDICTORS OF VIROLOGIC SUCCESS

Excellent adherence to treatment regimen

High potency of antiretroviral medication regimen

Higher baseline CD4 T cell count

Low baseline viral load

Reduce HIV-related morbidity

Rapid (i.e., ≥ 1 $\log_{10}$ in 1 to 4 months) reduction of viral load in response to treatment

Selecting

Selecting the initial combination ART regimen is extremely important. Today, there are more than 20 FDA-approved antiretroviral medicines from six mechanistic classes from which to design combination ART regimens. HIV medications are always used in combination to reduce the amount of HIV in the blood (plasma viral load) by helping to block or "inhibit" certain steps during the HIV replication process.

The recommended treatment for HIV infection is a combination of three or more medications from two different classes. The six different mechanistic classes or "families" of HIV antiretroviral medications include nucleoside reverse transcriptase inhibitors (NRTIs), also called "nukes"; nonnucleoside reverse transcriptase inhibitors (NNRTIs), also called "nonnukes"; protease inhibitors (PIs); fusion inhibitors (FIs), also called "entry inhibitors"; integrase inhibitors (IIs); and CCR5 antagonists. Each class of HIV medications fights HIV infection in a different way. The primary difference among the classes is the stage of HIV replication that the medications target.

The main mechanism of action of NRTIs is the inhibition of replication of retroviruses, including HIV, by interfering with viral RNA-directed DNA polymerase (reverse transcriptase). NNRTIs also inhibit replication of HIV by acting as a specific, noncompetitive, reverse transcriptase inhibitor and by disrupting the catalytic site of the enzyme. PIs are selective and competitive inhibitors of HIV protease. PIs play an essential role to prevent cleavage of protein precursors essential for HIV maturation, infection of new cells, and replication. FIs work by blocking an important step in the process of HIV entry into CD4 cells known as fusion. By blocking fusion,

FIs may prevent HIV from entering and infecting CD4 cells. Integrase inhibitors (IIs) work by blocking the integrase enzyme that HIV needs to make more virus. CCR5 antagonists work by blocking a molecule called CCR5 that is found on the surface of CD4 cells so HIV cannot enter.

The most extensively studied combination ART regimens for treatment-naïve patients includes either (1) one NNRTI with two NRTIs or (2) one PI (with or without ritonavir-boosting) with two NRTIs. The potent inhibitory effect of ritonavir on metabolism of the cytochrome P450 3A4 isoenzyme allows the addition of low-dose ritonavir to other PIs (except nelfinavir) as a pharmacokinetic booster to increase medication levels and prolong plasma half-lives of the active PIs. This "boosting" allows for reduced dosing frequency and/or pill burden, which may improve overall adherence to the ART regimen. The increased trough concentration (Cmin) may improve the antiretroviral activity of the active Pis, which can be beneficial when the patient harbors HIV-resistant strains to Pis (Dragsted et al., 2003, 2005; Shulman et al., 2002). The potential for increased risk of hyperlipidemia and drug–drug interactions is the major drawback associated with ritonavir boosting.

Both NNRTI- and PI-based regimens result in suppression of HIV RNA levels and CD4 T-cell increases in a large majority of patients (Gallant et al., 2004; Gulick et al., 2006; Riddler et al., 2006; Squires et al., 2004; Staszewski et al., 1999). A list of several preferred and alternative ART regimens is available from which to choose (see Table 7.4). ART regimens vary in efficacy, pill burden, and potential side effects. A patient-specific individualized regimen that maximizes adherence may be more successful in achieving full viral suppression. Many patient-specific characteristics are considered in the selection of ART regimen. These characteristics include:

■ Comorbid conditions (e.g., cardiovascular disease, chemical dependency, liver disease, psychiatric disease, pregnancy, renal diseases, or tuberculosis);
■ Convenience (e.g., pill burden, dosing frequency, and food and fluid considerations);
■ Gender and pretreatment CD4 T-cell count if considering nevirapine;
■ Genotypic drug resistance testing;
■ HLA B*5701 testing if considering abacavir;
■ Patient adherence potential;
■ Potential adverse drug effects;
■ Potential drug interactions with other medications; and
■ Pregnancy potential.

Table 7.4

ART MEDICATIONS AND TREATMENT STRATEGIES, NAÏVE PATIENTS

	COLUMN 1 (NNRTI OR PI OPTIONS – IN ALPHABETICAL ORDER)			COLUMN 2 (DUAL-NRTI OPTIONS)
Preferred Components	NNRTI efavirenz[1]	or	Protease Inhibitor • atazanavir + ritonavir • fosamprenavir + ritonavir (2x/day) • lopinavir/ritonavir[2] (2x/day) (coformulated)	Preferred Components • tenofovir/emtricitabine[3] (coformulated)
Alternative to Preferred Components	NNRTI nevirapine[4]	or	Protease Inhibitor • atazanavir[5] • fosamprenavir • fosamprenavir + ritonavir (1x/day) • lopinavir/ritonavir (1x/day) (coformulated) • saquinavir + ritonavir	Alternative to Preferred Components (order of preference) • abacavir/lamivudine[3] (for patients who test negative for HLAB*5701) (co-formulated); • zidovudine/lamivudine[3] (coformulated); or • didanosine + (emtricitabine or lamivudine)

The middle column header "PLUS" connects Column 1 and Column 2.

[1] Efavirenz is not recommended for use in the first trimester of pregnancy or in sexually active women with childbearing potential who are not using effective contraception.

[2] The pivotal study that led to the recommendation of lopinavir/ritonavir as a preferred PI component was based on twice-daily dosing. A smaller study has shown similar efficacy with once-daily dosing but also showed a higher incidence of moderate to severe diarrhea with the once-daily regimen (16% vs. 5%). In addition, once-daily dosing may be insufficient for those with viral loads >100,000 copies/mL.

[3] Emtricitabine may be used in place of lamivudine and vice versa.

[4] Nevirapine should not be initiated the following treatment-naïve patients: women with CD4 count >250 cells/μL or in men with CD4 count >400 cells/μL because of increased risk for symptomatic hepatic events in these patients.

[5] Atazanavir must be boosted with ritonavir if used in combination with efavirenz or tenofovir.

Initiation

Initiation of ART in the chronically HIV-infected patient is guided by clinical evidence and expert recommendations (Panel on Antiretroviral Guidelines for Adults and Adolescents, 2008). Current guidelines advise that persons presenting with an AIDS-defining illness or severe symptoms be treated, regardless of their CD4 cell count or viral load. Although there are important new findings that support earlier treatment for HIV at higher CD4 cell counts (Kitahata et al., 2009; Sterne et al., 2009) current guidelines do not reflect these recommendations. See Table 7.5 for current patient specific criteria and treatment recommendations. See Table 7.6 for a list of currently available ART agents. Considerations for ART in special patient populations such as acute HIV infection, HIV-infected adolescents, injection drug users, HIV-infected women of reproductive age and pregnant women, hepatitis B/HIV coinfection, hepatitis C/HIV coinfection, mycobacterium tuberculosis disease, or latent tuberculosis infection with HIV coinfection is beyond the scope of this chapter and are not reflected in the tables herein. Nurses who work with these populations are encouraged to refer to other references for patient population specific ART-related information.

Table 7.5

CRITERIA FOR INITIATING ART FOR THE CHRONICALLY HIV-1 INFECTED PATIENT

CLINICAL CONDITION AND/OR CD4 COUNT	RECOMMENDATIONS
• History of AIDS-defining illness • CD4 count <200 cells/µL • CD4 count 200-350 cells/µL • Pregnant women • Patients with HIV-associated nephropathy • Patients coinfected with hepatitis B virus (HBV), when HBV treatment is indicated (Treatment with fully suppressive antiviral drugs active against both HIV and HBV is recommended.)	ART should be initiated.
Patients with CD4 count >350 cells/µL who do not meet any of the specific conditions listed above.	The optimal time to initiate therapy in asymptomatic patients with CD4 count >350 cells/µL is not well defined. Patient scenarios and comorbidities should be taken into consideration.

Table 7.6

ANTIRETROVIRAL MEDICATIONS AND USUAL ADULT DOSING BY MECHANISTIC CLASS

GENERIC NAME	TRADE NAME	USUAL ADULT DOSE
Nucleoside reverse transcriptase inhibitors (NRTIs)		
Abacavir (ABC)	Ziagen	300 mg bid or 600mg daily
Abacavir/Lamivudine (ABC/3TC)	Epzicom	600/300 mg daily
Abacavir/Lamivudine/Zidovudine (ABA/AZT/3TC)	Trizivir	300/150/300 mg bid
Didanosine (ddI)	Videx	400 mg EC daily if >60kg or 250 mg EC daily if <60 kg
Emtricitabine (FTC)	Emtriva	200 mg daily
Emtricitabine/Tenofovir (FTC/TDF)	Truvada	200/300 mg daily
Lamivudine (3TC)	Epivir	150 mg bid or 300 mg daily
Lamivudine/Zidovudine (ZDV/3TC)	Combivir	300/150 mg bid
Stavudine (d4T)	Zerit	40 mg bid if >60 kg or 30 mg bid if <60 kg
Tenofovir (TDF)	Viread	300 mg daily
Zidovudine (ZDV)	Retrovir	300 mg bid
Nonnucleoside reverse transcriptase inhibitors (NNRTIs)		
Efavirenz (EFV)	Sustiva	600 mg daily at bedtime
Etravirine (ETV)	Intelence	200 mg BID with a meal
Nevirapine (NVP)	Viramune	200 mg bid—dose is initiated at 200 mg daily for 14 days to reduce rash risk
Protease inhibitors (PIs)		
Atazanavir (ATV)	Reyataz	400 mg daily or 300 mg daily + 100mg RTV daily
Darunavir (DRV)	Prezista	600 mg bid + 100mg RTV bid or 800 mg daily + 100mg RTV daily
Fosamprenavir (FPV)	Lexiva	PI exp: 700 mg bid + RTV 100 mg bid Naïve: 1400 mg BID or 1400 mg daily +100 mg RTV daily or 700 mg bid + 100 mg RTV bid

Table 7.6

ANTIRETROVIRAL MEDICATIONS AND USUAL ADULT DOSING BY MECHANISTIC CLASS *continued*

GENERIC NAME	*TRADE NAME*	USUAL ADULT DOSE
Protease inhibitors (PIs) *continued*		
Indinavir (IDV)	*Crixivan*	800 mg q8h *or* 800 mg BID + 100–200 mg RTV bid
Lopinavir/ Ritonavir (LPVr)	*Kaletra*	400/100 mg bid *or* as 600/150 mg bid if given in combination w/ NVP or EFV
Nelfinavir (NFV)	*Viracept*	1,250 mg bid
Ritonavir (RTV)	*Norvir*	600 mg bid—dose is gradually increased over <10 days *or* 100–200 mg daily or bid when given as a "minidose" to boost other PIs
Saquinavir Mesylate (SQV)	*Invirase*	1,000 mg bid + RTV 100 mg bid
Tipranavir (TPV)	*Aptivus*	500 mg bid with RTV 200 mg bid
Fusion inhibitors (FIs)		
Enfuviritide (T-20)	*Fuzeon*	90 mg by subcutaneous injection bid—Refrigerate *after* reconstituted w/ sterile water
CCR5 antagonists		
Maraviroc (MVC)	*Selzentry*	150–600 mg bid depending on coadministration with CYP3A inhibitors or CYP3A inducers
Integrase inhibitors (IIs)		
Raltegravir (RAL)	*Isentress*	400 mg bid

ADHERENCE TO ANTIRETROVIRAL MEDICATION AND ENGAGEMENT WITH HEALTH CARE SERVICES

As discussed previously, the primary goals of ART are to improve and/or preserve the immune system and decrease HIV-associated morbidity and mortality. As a secondary benefit, by decreasing HIV-RNA levels in blood and semen, effective ART probably decreases HIV transmission related to continued high-risk behaviors (Porco et al., 2004; Vernazza et al., 1997, 2000; Zhang et al., 1998). However, an analysis by Wilson and colleagues (2008) suggests that the risk of HIV transmission in heterosexual partnerships in the presence of effective treatment is low but not zero and that the transmission risk in male homosexual partnerships is high over repeated exposures. If the claim of noninfectiousness in effectively treated patients was widely accepted, and condom use subsequently declined, the potential exists for substantial increases in the incidence of HIV.

Regardless of baseline CD4 T-cell count (Gras et al., 2007; Mocroft et al., 2007) effective ART, with maximal viral suppression, can increase CD4 T-cell count in the most patients. With appropriate use of ART, sustained viral suppression is possible for many years. However, clinicians must be aware that immediate viral rebound followed by decreases in CD4 T-cell count occurs in most patients whenever ART is interrupted. Therefore, except for serious adverse events or concurrent medical conditions that preclude oral therapy, once the decision is made to start ART, treatment should be continued without interruption.

Adherence

Adherence to ART is important to achieve maximal treatment response. Many factors lead to less than complete adherence. The factors include complexity of medication regimens, such as the number of pills; side effects; frequency of administration; food restrictions or requirements; refrigeration requirements; patient factors, such as active substance abuse and depression; poor health literacy; limited finances; nonreadiness to change health care–related behaviors; and health system issues, including interruptions in medication access and inadequate treatment education and social support. Conditions that promote adherence should be maximized before initiating ART (See "Adherence" section of Panel on Antiretroviral Guidelines for Adults and Adolescents, 2008).

Patient counseling and education should be conducted before starting ART. The patient should understand the potential benefits and risks of ART (see Table 7.7), including adverse medication effects and the need for long-term adherence to the prescribed ART regimen.

Whereas adherence to ART is a major determinant for starting therapy, patient readiness to start ART is a key factor in future adherence (Ammassari et al., 2002). Depression and substance abuse may negatively affect adher-

Table 7.7

POTENTIAL BENEFITS AND RISKS OF ART

POTENTIAL BENEFITS OF EARLY THERAPY

- Maintenance of a higher CD4 T-cell count and prevention of potentially irreversible damage to the immune system

- Decreased risk for HIV-associated complications that can sometimes occur at CD4 counts >350 cells/μL, including tuberculosis, non-Hodgkin lymphoma, Kaposi's sarcoma, peripheral neuropathy, HPV-associated malignancies, and HIV-associated cognitive impairment

- Decreased risk of non-opportunistic medical conditions, including cardiovascular disease, renal disease, liver disease, and non–AIDS-associated malignancies and infections

- Decreased risk of HIV transmission to others, which will have positive public health implications

POTENTIAL RISKS OF EARLY THERAPY

- Treatment-related side effects and toxicities

- Viral resistance to medications because of incomplete viral suppression, resulting in loss of future treatment options

- Less time for the patient to learn about HIV and its treatment and less time to prepare for the need for adherence to ART

- Increased total time exposed to medication, with greater chance of treatment fatigue

- Premature use of ART before the development of more effective, less toxic, and/or better studied combinations of antiretroviral medications

- Transmission of medication-resistant virus in patients who do not maintain full viral suppression

ence and response to ART. Both conditions must be addressed, whenever possible, before ART is started. However, no patient should automatically be denied ART simply because the clinician unilaterally judges that the patient exhibits behaviors or characteristics that potentially affect adherence. Instead, clinicians should discuss in detail the necessity for long-term adherence to medications before starting ART. Clinicians should employ every available strategy to assess and improve ART adherence.

High rates of ART adherence are associated with HIV viral suppression, reduced rates of medication resistance (Bangsberg, Moss, & Deeks, 2004; Sethi et al., 2003) and improved survival (Wood et al., 2003). Lifelong commitment to therapy requires a commitment from both the patient who takes the medication and the health care team that supports the patient in the many aspects of ART, including medication selection, acquisition, and monitoring; management of side effects; and social support and encouragement.

Maintaining lifelong adherence to ART is challenging for patients, particularly when they start ART before developing any HIV-related signs and symptoms. However, the efficacy of ART to increase life expectancy for people living with HIV is well worth the challenge.

Adherence to ART has been thoroughly studied; however, the determinants, measurements, and effective interventions to achieve maximal adherence are insufficiently characterized and not well understood. While various strategies can be used and are associated with improvements in adherence, measuring adherence is difficult. While there are no established standards for measuring adherence, it is clear that both patient self-report of complete adherence and clinician estimates of likelihood of a patient's adherence are unreliable predictors of patient adherence. On the other hand, patient estimates of suboptimal adherence is a strong predictor and should be taken seriously (Cheever, 1999; Crespo-Fierro, 1997; Greenberg, 1984).

Achieving long-term adherence success is primarily dependent on (1) negotiating a treatment plan to which the patient will commit and (2) ongoing assessment of adherence (Fowler, 1998; Williams & Friedland, 1997). Prior to writing the first medication prescription, clinicians must assess their patient's readiness to take medication. Patients need to understand that the first ART regimen is the best chance for long-term success (CDC, 1998). Equally important to adherence is the existence of trusting relationships among the patient, clinicians, and other members of the health care team, including nurses, case managers, social workers, pharmacists, nutritionists, and others. Establishing a trusting relationship is the basis for effective communication that makes quality treatment outcomes possible. However, developing trusting relationships can take repeated interactions during several office visits and the patience of clinicians not to rush starting ART before a patient develops a willingness to do so. Some patients will develop a readiness state for ART, with less preparation, more quickly than others.

Given that medications are consistently available through a variety of means (including the patient's insurance provider, personal resources, and governmental and pharmaceutical companies' patient assistant programs), successful clinicians use a variety of resources to facilitate their patients' best adherence outcomes. Adherence counseling and assessment should be done during every clinical encounter. Early detection of nonadherence (e.g., failure to achieve or loss of viral suppression, patient report of poor adherence, pharmacy reports of prolonged dispensing intervals that do not support patient's assertion of adherence) and prompt intervention can greatly reduce the chance of virologic failure and development of viral resistance. When necessary, patient-specific interventions can also be employed to assist in identifying adherence educational needs and strategies to overcome less than optimal adherence. Examples include use of educational aids, adherence support groups, adherence counselors, behavioral interventions (McPherson-Baker et al., 2000), and use of clinic- or community-based case managers and peer educators/navigators.

The most common reasons for nonadherence to initiation of ART are complexity and pill burden. Fortunately, greatly simplified and highly potent ART regimens are now available. Nurses can use the following interventions to help patients achieve maximal adherence:

- Provide an accessible, trusting health care team.
- Verify patient readiness to start ART.
- Use a team approach with prescribing providers, nurses, nutritionists, mental health personnel, pharmacists, and peer counselors.
- Tailor regimens to individual lifestyles.
- Simplify regimens, including dosing and food requirements.
- Clarify the regimen (e.g., provide a dosing schedule with clear direction for the times to take each medication).
- Provide education related to medication self-administration and dosing.
- Anticipate and treat side effects.
- Review potential side effects.
- Identify and remove personal barriers to adherence.
- Engage family, friends, and other available sources of social support.
- Use educational aids, including pictures, personal diaries, pillboxes, and calendars.
- Ask the patient to self-monitor adherence.

MEDICATION AND FOOD INTERACTIONS

Potential drug–drug and/or drug–food interactions are important considerations in ART. Beginning with selection of an antiretroviral regimen, clinicians use their knowledge of these interactions in designing an ART regimen that minimizes undesirable interactions and takes advantage of established pharmacodynamics (PD) and pharmacokinetics (PK). Clinicians should know that pharmacodynamics are the relationships between the dose or concentration of medication in the body (exposure) and measured effects and that PK is the time course of a medicine in humans. Drug–drug interactions occur when either the PK or the PD of one medicine is altered by another. Specifically, the interactions are a source of variability in medication response and are graded responses that are dependent on the concentration of the interacting species and on dose and time. Drug–drug interactions may affect absorption rate, availability, distribution, and hepatic or renal clearance and may be antagonistic, synergistic, or additive. A review of potential drug–drug interactions should be done when any new medication, including over-the-counter agents, is added to an existing ART regimen. Factors that affect PK and PD are presented in Table 7.8.

Most drug interactions with antiretroviral medications are mediated through the inhibition or induction of hepatic drug metabolism (Piscitelli & Gallicano, 2001). All PIs and NNRTIs are metabolized in the liver by the cytochrome (CYP) system, particularly by the CYP3A4 isoenzyme. Cytochromes use a multitude of both exogenous and endogenous compounds as substrates in enzymatic reactions. All PIs are substrates of CYP3A4, so their metabolic rate may be changed in the presence of CYP inducers or inhibitors. Adding to the complexity of drug–drug interactions, some PIs may also be inducers or inhibitors of other CYP isoenzymes and of P-glycoprotein.

Unlike PIs and NNRTIs, NRTIs do not undergo hepatic transformation through the CYP metabolic pathway. However, some NRTIs have other routes of hepatic metabolism. Significant PD interactions of NRTIs and other drugs have been reported. No clinically significant drug–drug interaction has been identified with the FI, enfuvirtide. Raltegravir, the sole II strand transfer inhibitor currently available, is primarily eliminated by glucuronidation mediated by the enzyme UDP-glucuronosyltransferases (UGT1A1). Maraviroc, the first FDA-approved CCR5 antagonist, is a substrate of CYP3A enzymes. It can be significantly

Table 7.8

FACTORS AFFECTING PHARMACOKINETICS (PK) AND PHARMACODYNAMICS (PD) VARIABILITY

Age

Drug formulation

Drug–disease interactions—altered gastrointestinal, renal, and hepatic function

Drug–drug interactions

Drug–food interactions—when the food is eaten and when the medication is taken
- Food can speed up or slow down the action of a medication
- Impaired absorption of vitamins and minerals in the body
- Stimulation or suppression of the appetite
- Drugs may alter how nutrients are used in the body
- Herbs may interact with anesthesia, beta-blockers, and anticoagulants

Genetic differences

HIV virus genotype and phenotype

Host immunologic status

Individual PD characteristics of E_{max}, EC_{50}

Individual PK characteristics of absorption, distribution, metabolism, and excretion (ADME)

PK in healthy volunteers v HIV-infected individuals

Pregnancy

Sex differences

increased in the presence of strong CYP3A inhibitors like ritonavir and other PIs and is reduced when used with CYP3A inducers like efavirenz or rifampin. Dose adjustment is necessary when used in combination with these inhibiting and inducing agents.

The list of medicines that may have significant interactions with PIs or NNRTIs is extensive. Some examples of these medicines include medications commonly prescribed in HIV patients for non-HIV medical conditions, such as anticonvulsants, azole antifungals, benzodiazepines, calcium channel blockers, erectile dysfunction agents (such as sildenafil), ergot derivatives, immunosuppressants (such as cyclosporine and tacrolimus), lipid-lowering agents (statins), macrolides, methadone, oral contraceptives, and rifamycin.

The use of medical herbs in the Western world and the co-use of modern and traditional therapies is common. Unfortunately, using these agents creates the potential for both PK and PD herb–drug interactions. For example, CYP may be particularly vulnerable to modulation by the multiple active constituents of herbs because the CYPs are subject to induction and inhibition by exposure to a wide variety of xenobiotics. Thus, unapproved medical therapies, such as St. John's wort, can cause troublesome interactions because they influence the CYP system. The use of these unapproved therapies should be avoided.

While it is beyond the scope of this text to present a comprehensive listing of all the known drug–drug interactions that relate to the medical care of patients with HIV, readers are encouraged to visit www.aidsinfo.nih.gov for a current listing of well-described drug interactions with different antiretroviral agents and suggested recommendations on contraindication, dose modification, and alternative agents.

ADVERSE MEDICATION EFFECTS
Side Effects

Side effects occur with virtually all antiretroviral medicines and are among the most common reasons for switching or discontinuation of ART and for medication nonadherence (O'Brien et al., 2003). Both clinical and laboratory adverse events (AE) are common (Fellay et al., 2001). The spectrum of AEs includes potentially life-threatening and serious toxicities that may lead to long-term consequences. Additionally, AEs that present as clinical symptoms may affect overall quality of life or may have an impact on overall medication adherence. Unfortunately, AEs may result in major morbidity and even mortality. While some common AEs were observed during premarketing clinical trials, some less frequent toxicities (e.g., lactic acidosis with hepatic steatosis and progressive ascending neuromuscular weakness syndrome) and some long-term complications (e.g., dyslipidemia and fat maldistribution) were not recognized until after the medicines were used in the general HIV-infected population for a longer period of time. See Table 7.9 for a comprehensive presentation of ART associated AEs.

Table 7.9

ANTIRETROVIRAL MEDICATION ASSOCIATED ADVERSE EFFECTS

ADVERSE EFFECTS	CAUSATIVE ARVS	ONSET/CLINICAL MANIFESTATION	ESTIMATED FREQUENCY	RISK FACTORS	PREVENTION/ MONITORING	MANAGEMENT
Acute hepatic failure	NVP	Onset: Greatest risk within first few weeks of therapy; can occur through 18 weeks Symptoms: Abrupt onset of flulike symptoms (nausea, vomiting, myalgia, fatigue), abdominal pain, jaundice, or fever with or without skin rash; may progress to fulminant hepatic failure with encephalopathy Approximately 1/2 of the cases have accompanying skin rash. Some may present as part of DRESS syndrome (drug rash with eosinophilia and systemic symptoms).	Symptomatic hepatic events: • 4% overall (2.5%–11% from different trials) • In women: 11% in those w/ pre-NVP CD4 >250 cells/μL vs. 0.9% w/ CD4 <250 cells/μL • In men: 6.3% w/ pre-NVP CD4 >400 cells/μL vs. 2.3% w/ CD4 <400 cells/μL	• Treatment-naïve patients with higher CD4 count at initiation (>250 cells/μL in women and >400 cells/μL in men) • Female gender (including pregnant women) • HIV (-) individuals when NVP is used for postexposure prophylaxis • High NVP concentration	• Avoid initiation of NVP in women w/ CD4 >250 cells/μL or men w/ CD4 >400 cells/μL unless the benefit clearly outweighs the risk. • Counsel patients re: signs and symptoms of hepatitis; stop NVP and seek medical attention if signs and symptoms of hepatitis, severe skin rash, or hypersensitivity reactions appear • Monitoring of ALT and AST (every 2 weeks x first month, then monthly x 3 months, then every 3 months) • Obtain AST and ALT in patients with rash. • 2-week dose escalation may reduce incidence of hepatic events.	• Discontinue ARV including NVP (caution should be taken in discontinuation of 3TC, FTC, or TDF in HBV-coinfected patients). • Discontinue all other hepatotoxic agents if possible. • Rule out other causes of hepatitis. • Aggressive supportive care as indicated. *Note:* Hepatic injury may progress despite treatment discontinuation. Careful monitoring should continue until symptom resolution. *Do not rechallenge patient with NVP.* The safety of other NNRTIs (EFV, ETR, or DLV) in patients who experienced significant hepatic event from NVP is unknown—use with caution.

(continued)

239

Table 7.9

ANTIRETROVIRAL MEDICATION ASSOCIATED ADVERSE EFFECTS *continued*

ADVERSE EFFECTS	CAUSATIVE ARVS	ONSET/CLINICAL MANIFESTATION	ESTIMATED FREQUENCY	RISK FACTORS	PREVENTION/ MONITORING	MANAGEMENT
Bleeding events	TPV/r: reports of intracranial hemorrhage (ICH) PIs: Increased bleeding in hemophiliac patients	Median time to ICH event: 525 days on TPV/r therapy Hemophiliac patients: Increased spontaneous bleeding tendency—in joints, muscles, soft tissues, and hematuria	In 2006, 13 cases of ICH reported, with TPV/r use, including 8 fatalities. For hemophilia: frequency unknown.	For ICH: • Patients with CNS lesions, head trauma, recent neurosurgery, coagulopathy, hypertension, alcohol abuse, or receiving anticoagulant or antiplatelet agents. For hemophiliac patients: • PI use	For ICH: • Avoid use of TPV/r in patients at risk for ICH. For hemophiliac patients: • Consider using NNRTI-based regimen. • Monitor for spontaneous bleeding.	For ICH: • Discontinue TPV/r; manage ICH with supportive care. For hemophiliac patients: • May require increased use of factor VIII products.
Bone marrow suppression	ZDV	Onset: few weeks to months Laboratory abnormalities: • Anemia • Neutropenia Symptoms: fatigue because of anemia; potential for increase of bacterial infections because of neutropenia	Severe Anemia (Hgb < 7 g/dL): 1.1%–4% Severe Neutropenia (ANC <500 cells/µL): 1.8%–8%	• Advanced HIV • High dose • Preexisting anemia or neutropenia. • Concomitant use of bone marrow suppressants (such as cotrimoxazole, ribavirin, ganciclovir, etc.).	• Avoid use in patients at risk. • Avoid other bone marrow suppressants if possible. • Monitor CBC with differential at least every three months (more frequently in patients at risk).	• Switch to another NRTI if there is an alternative option. • Discontinue concomitant bone marrow suppressant if there is an alternative option. Otherwise: For neutropenia: • Identify and treat other causes. • Consider treatment with filgrastim. For anemia: • Identify and treat other causes of anemia (if present). • Blood transfusion if indicated. • Consider erythropoietin therapy.

| Cardiovascular effects | Possibly PIs and other ARVs with unfavorable effects on lipids (e.g. EFV, d4T) | Onset: months to years after beginning of therapy. Presentation: premature coronary artery disease | 3–6 per 1,000 patient-years | Other risk factors for cardiovascular disease such as smoking, age, hyperlipidemia, hypertension, diabetes mellitus, family history of premature coronary artery disease, and personal history of coronary artery disease. | • Assess each patient's cardiac risk factors.
• Consider non-PI- based regimen.
• Monitor and identify patients with hyperlipidemia or hyperglycemia.
• Counseling for life style modification: smoking cessation, diet, and exercise. | • Early diagnosis, prevention, and pharmacologic management of other cardiovascular risk factors such as hyperlipidemia, hypertension, and insulin resistance/diabetes mellitus.
• Assess cardiac risk factors.
• Lifestyle modifications: diet, exercise, and/or smoking cessation.
• Switch to agents with less propensity for increasing cardiovascular risk factors, i.e., NNRTI- or ATV-based regimen and avoid d4T use. |

(continued)

241

Table 7.9

ANTIRETROVIRAL MEDICATION ASSOCIATED ADVERSE EFFECTS *continued*

ADVERSE EFFECTS	CAUSATIVE ARVS	ONSET/CLINICAL MANIFESTATION	ESTIMATED FREQUENCY	RISK FACTORS	PREVENTION/ MONITORING	MANAGEMENT
Central nervous system effects	EFV	Onset: begin with first few doses Symptoms: may include one or more of the following: drowsiness, somnolence, insomnia, abnormal dreams, dizziness, impaired concentration and attention span, depression, hallucination; exacerbation of psychiatric disorders; psychosis; suicidal ideation Most symptoms subside or diminish after 2–4 weeks	>50% of patients may have some symptoms.	• Preexisting or unstable psychiatric illnesses. • Use of concomitant drugs with CNS effects. • Rates in African Americans may be higher due to genetic predisposition of slower clearance.	• Take at bedtime or 2–3 hours before bedtime. • Take on an empty stomach to reduce drug concentration and CNS effects. • Warn patients regarding restriction of risky activities such as operating heavy machinery during the 1st 2–4 weeks of therapy.	• Symptoms usually diminish or disappear after 2–4 weeks. • May consider discontinuing therapy if symptoms persist and cause significant impairment in daily function or exacerbation of psychiatric illness.
Fat maldistribution	PIs, thymidine analogs – d4T > ZDV	Onset: gradual—months after initiation of therapy Symptoms: • Lipoatrophy—peripheral fat loss manifested as facial thinning, thinning of extremities and buttocks (d4T) • Increase in abdominal girth, breast size, and dorsocervical fat pad (buffalo hump)	High—exact frequency uncertain; increases with duration on offending agents	• Lipoatrophy—low baseline body mass index.	Lipoatrophy: avoid thymidine nucleosides or switch from ZDV or d4T to ABC or TDF.	• Switching to other agents—may slow or halt progression; however, may not reverse effects. • Injectable poly-L-lactic acid for treatment of facial lipoatrophy.

| Hepato-toxicity (clinical hepatitis or asymptomatic serum transaminase elevation) | All NNRTIs; All PIs; Most NRTIs; Maraviroc | Onset:
NNRTI: for NVP—2/3 within 1st 12 weeks
NRTI: over months to years
PI: generally after weeks to months
Symptoms/findings:
NNRTI:
• Asymptomatic to nonspecific symptoms such as anorexia, weight loss, or fatigue. Approximately ⅓ of patients with NVP-associated symptomatic hepatic events present with skin rash.
NRTI:
• ZDV, ddI, d4T: may cause hepatotoxicity associated with lactic acidosis with microvesicular or macrovesicular hepatic steatosis because of mitochondrial toxicity.
• 3TC, FTC, or TDF: HBV coinfected patients may develop severe hepatic flare when these drugs are withdrawn or when resistance develops.
PI:
• Clinical hepatitis and hepatic decompensation have been reported with TPV/RTV and DRV/RTV, but also other PIs to varying degrees. Underlying liver disease increases risk.
• Generally asymptomatic, some with anorexia, weight loss, jaundice, etc. | Varies with the different agents | • Hepatitis B or C coinfection
• Alcoholism
• Concomitant hepatotoxic drugs
• Elevated ALT and/or AST at baseline
• For NVP-associated hepatic events—female w/ pre-NVP CD4 >250 cells/μL or male w/ pre-NVP CD4 >400 cells/μL | • NVP: monitor liver associated Enzymes at baseline, 2 and 4 weeks, then monthly for 1st 3 months; then every 3 months.
• TPV/RTV: contraindicated in patients with moderate to severe hepatic insufficiency; for other patients follow frequently during treatment.
• Other agents: monitor liver associated enzymes at least every 3–4 months or more frequently in patients at risk. | • Rule out other causes of hepatotoxicity—alcoholism, viral hepatitis, chronic HBV w/ 3TC, FTC, or TDF withdrawal, or HBV resistance, etc.
For symptomatic patients:
• Discontinue all ARVs (with caution in patients with chronic HBV infection treated w/ 3TC, FTC, and/or TDF) and other potential hepatotoxic agents.
• After symptoms subside and serum transaminases returned to normal, construct a new ARV regimen without the potential offending agent(s).
For asymptomatic patients:
• If ALT >5–10x ULN, some may consider discontinuing ARVs, others may continue therapy with close monitoring.
• After serum transaminases return to normal, construct a new ARV regimen without the potential offending agent(s)
Note: Please refer to information regarding NVP-associated symptomatic hepatic events and NRTI-associated lactic acidosis with hepatic steatosis in this table. |

(continued)

Table 7.9

ANTIRETROVIRAL MEDICATION ASSOCIATED ADVERSE EFFECTS *continued*

ADVERSE EFFECTS	CAUSATIVE ARVS	ONSET/CLINICAL MANIFESTATION	ESTIMATED FREQUENCY	RISK FACTORS	PREVENTION/ MONITORING	MANAGEMENT
Hypersensitivity reaction (HSR)	ABC	Onset of 1st reaction: median onset—9 days; approximately 90% within 1st 6 weeks. Onset of rechallenge reactions: within hours of rechallenge dose. Symptoms: acute onset of symptoms (in descending frequency): high fever, diffuse skin rash, malaise, nausea, headache, myalgia, chills, diarrhea, vomiting, abdominal pain, dyspnea, arthralgia, respiratory symptoms (pharyngitis, dyspnea, tachypnea) With continuation of ABC, symptoms may worsen to include: hypotension, respiratory distress, vascular collapse. Rechallenge reactions: generally greater intensity than 1st reaction, can mimic anaphylaxis.	Clinically suspected ≈ 8% in clinical trial (2%–9%); 5% in retrospective analysis; significantly reduced with pretreatment HLA screening	• HLA-B*5701, HLA-DR7, HLADQ3 (from Australian data). • Higher incidence of grade 3 or 4 HSR with 600mg once daily dose than 300mg twice-daily dose in one study (5% vs. 2%).	• HLA B*5701 screening prior to initiation of ABC. • Those patients tested (+) for HLA B*5701 should be labeled as allergic to abacavir in medical records. • Educate patients about potential signs and symptoms of HSR and need for reporting of symptoms promptly. • Wallet card with warning information for patients.	• Discontinue ABC and other ARVs. • Rule out other causes of symptoms (e.g., intercurrent illnesses such as viral syndromes and other causes of skin rash, etc.). • Most signs and symptoms resolve 48 hours after discontinuation of ABC. *More severe cases:* • Symptomatic support—antipyretic, fluid resuscitation, pressure support (if necessary). • *Do not rechallenge patients with ABC after suspected HSR*

Hyperlipidemia	All PIs (except unboosted ATV); d4T; EFV (to a lesser extent)	Onset: weeks to months after beginning of therapy. Presentation: All PIs except ATV: Increase in LDL and total cholesterol (TC) and triglyceride (TG), decrease in HDL LPV/r and RTV: disproportionate increase in TG d4T: mostly increase in TG; may also have increase in LDL and total cholesterol (TC) EFV or NVP: increase in HDL, slight increase TG.	Varies with different agents. Swiss Cohort: Increase TC and TG – 1.7–2.3x higher in patients receiving (non-ATV) PI	• Underlying hyperlipidemia. • Risk based on ARV therapy PI: LPV/r & RTV - boosted PIs > NFV & APV > IDV > ATV; NNRTI: EFV more common than NVP NRTI: d4T most common	• Use non-PI, non-d4T based regimen • Use ATV-based regimen • Fasting lipid profile at baseline, 3–6 months after starting new regimen, then annually or more frequently if indicated (in high-risk patients, or patients with abnormal baseline levels).	• Follow guidelines for management. • Assess cardiac risk factor. • Lifestyle modification: diet, exercise, and/or smoking cessation. • Switching to agents with less propensity for causing hyperlipidemia. Pharmacologic management: • Increase total cholesterol, LDL, TG 200–500mg/dL: "statins"— pravastatin or atorvastatin (Consider drug interaction information). • TG >500mg/dL: gemfibrozil or micronized fenofibrate.

(continued)

Table 7.9

ANTIRETROVIRAL MEDICATION ASSOCIATED ADVERSE EFFECTS *continued*

ADVERSE EFFECTS	CAUSATIVE ARVS	ONSET/CLINICAL MANIFESTATION	ESTIMATED FREQUENCY	RISK FACTORS	PREVENTION/ MONITORING	MANAGEMENT
Injection site reactions	T20	Onset: Within first few doses. Symptoms: pain, pruritus, erythema, ecchymosis, warmth, nodules, rarely injection site infection.	98%	• All patients.	• Educate patients regarding use of sterile technique, ensure solution at room temperature before injection, rotate injection sites, avoid injection into sites with little subcutaneous fat or sites of existing or previous reactions.	• Massaging area after injection may reduce pain. • Wear loose clothing—especially around the injection site areas or areas of previous reactions. • Rarely, warm compact or analgesics may be necessary.
Insulin resistance/ diabetes mellitus	All PIs	Onset: weeks to months after beginning of therapy Presentation: Polyuria, polydipsia, polyphagia, fatigue, weakness; exacerbation of hyperglycemia in patients with underlying diabetes.	Up to 3%–5% of patients developed diabetes in some series.	• Underlying hyperglycemia, family history of diabetes mellitus.	• Use PI-sparing regimens. • Fasting blood glucose 1–3 months after starting new regimen, then at least every 3–6 months.	• Diet and exercise. • Consider switching to an NNRTI-based regimen. • Metformin. • "Glitazones." • Sulfonylurea. • Insulin.

| Lactic acidosis/hepatic steatosis +/- pancreatitis (severe mitochondrial toxicities) | NRTIs, esp. d4T, ddI, ZDV | Onset: months after initiation of NRTIs
Symptoms:
• Insidious onset with nonspecific gastrointestinal prodrome (nausea, anorexia, abdominal pain, vomiting, weight loss, and fatigue.
• Subsequent symptoms may be rapidly progressive with tachycardia, tachypnea, hyperventilation, jaundice, muscular weakness, mental status changes, or respiratory distress.
• Some may present with multiorgan failure (hepatic failure, acute pancreatitis, encephalopathy, and respiratory failure).
Laboratory findings:
• Increased lactate (often >5 mmole).
• Low arterial pH (some as low as <7.0).
• Low serum bicarbonate
• Increased anion gap
• Elevated serum transaminases, prothrombin time, bilirubin
• Low serum albumin
• Increase serum amylase and lipase in patients with pancreatitis
• Histologic findings of the liver—microvesicular or macrovesicular steatosis | Rare:
One estimate 0.85 cases per 1,000 patient years. Mortality up to 50% in some case series (esp. in patients with serum lactate >10 mmole).
• d4T + ddI
• d4T, ZDV, ddI use (d4T most frequently implicated).
• Long duration of NRTI use.
• Female gender.
• Obesity.
• Pregnancy (esp. with d4T+ddI).
• ddI + hydroxyurea or ribavirin.
• High baseline body mass index. | • Routine monitoring of lactic acid is not recommended.
• Consider obtaining lactate levels in patients with low serum bicarbonate or high anion gap and with complaints consistent with lactic acidosis.
• Appropriate phlebotomy technique for obtaining lactate level should be used. | • Discontinue all ARVs if this syndrome is highly suspected (diagnosis is established by clinical correlations, drug history, and lactate level).
• Symptomatic support with fluid hydration.
• Some patients may require IV bicarbonate infusion, hemodialysis or hemofiltration, parenteral nutrition, or mechanical ventilation.
• IV thiamine and/or riboflavin —resulted in rapid resolution of hyperlactatemia in some case reports
Note:
• Interpretation of high lactate level should be done in the context of clinical findings
• The implication of asymptomatic hyperlactatemia is unknown at this point.
ARV treatment options:
• Use NRTIs with less propensity of mitochondrial toxicities - (e.g., ABC, TDF, 3TC, FTC) - should not be introduced until lactate returns to normal).
• Recommend close monitoring of serum bicarbonate or lactate after restarting NRTIs.
• Consider NRTI-sparing regimens. |

(continued)

Table 7.9

ANTIRETROVIRAL MEDICATION ASSOCIATED ADVERSE EFFECTS *continued*

ADVERSE EFFECTS	CAUSATIVE ARVS	ONSET/CLINICAL MANIFESTATION	ESTIMATED FREQUENCY	RISK FACTORS	PREVENTION/ MONITORING	MANAGEMENT
Lactic acidosis/ rapidly progressive ascending neuromuscular weakness	Most frequently implicated ARV: d4T	Onset: months after initiation of ARV, then dramatic motor weakness occurring within days to weeks. Symptoms: very rapidly progressive ascending demyelinating polyneuropathy, may mimic Guillain-Barré syndrome; some patients may develop respiratory paralysis requiring mechanical ventilation; resulted in deaths in some patients. Laboratory findings may include: • Low arterial pH • Increased lactate • Low serum bicarbonate • Increased anion gap • Markedly increased creatinine Phosphokinase	Rare	• Prolonged d4T use (found in 61 of 69 [88%] cases in one report)	• Early recognition and discontinuation of ARVs may avoid further progression.	Discontinuation of ARVs. • Supportive care, including mechanical ventilation if needed (as in cases of lactic acidosis listed previously). • Other measures attempted with variable success: plasmapheresis, high-dose corticosteroid, intravenous immunoglobulin, carnitine, acetylcarnitine. • Recovery often takes months—ranging from complete recovery to substantial residual deficits. • Symptoms may be irreversible in some patients. *Do not rechallenge patient with offending agent.*

Nephro-lithiasis/ urolithiasis/ crystalluria	IDV: most frequent; Reports with ATV	Onset: any time after beginning of therapy, especially at times of reduced fluid intake. Laboratory abnormalities: pyuria, hematuria, crystalluria; rarely, rise in serum creatinine and acute renal failure Symptoms: flank pain and/or abdominal pain (can be severe), dysuria, frequency.	12.4% of nephrolithia-sis reported in clinical trials (4.7%–34.4% in different trials)	• History of nephrolithia-sis. • Patients un-able to main-tain adequate fluid intake. • High peak IDV concentration. • Increase duration of exposure.	• Increase hydration. • Pain control. • May consider switching to alternative agent or therapeutic drug monitoring if treatment option is limited. • Stent placement may be required.
Nephro-toxicity	IDV, TDF	Onset: IDV: months after therapy TDF: weeks to months after therapy Laboratory and other findings: IDV: increase serum creatinine, pyuria; hydronephrosis or renal atrophy TDF: increase serum creatinine, proteinuria, hypophosphatemia, glycosuria, hypokalemia, nonunion gap metabolic acidosis Symptoms: IDV: asymptomatic; rarely develop to end-stage renal disease TDF: asymptomatic to signs of nephrogenic diabetes insipidus, Fanconi syndrome	Severe toxic-ity is rare.	• History of renal disease. • Concomitant use of nephro-toxic drugs.	• Stop offending agent, generally reversible. • Supportive care. • Avoid use of other nephrotoxic drugs. • Adequate hydration if on IDV therapy. • Monitor serum cre-atinine, urinalysis, serum potassium and phosphorus in patients at risk. • Electrolyte replace-ment as indicated.

(continued)

Table 7.9

ANTIRETROVIRAL MEDICATION ASSOCIATED ADVERSE EFFECTS *continued*

ADVERSE EFFECTS	CAUSATIVE ARVS	ONSET/CLINICAL MANIFESTATION	ESTIMATED FREQUENCY	RISK FACTORS	PREVENTION/ MONITORING	MANAGEMENT
Osteone-crosis	All PIs	Clinical Presentation (generally similar to non-HIV population): • Insidious in onset, with subtle symptoms of mild to moderate periarticular pain. • 85% of the cases involving one or both femoral heads, but other bones may also be affected. • Pain may be triggered by weight bearing or movement.	Reported incidence on the rise. Symptomatic osteonecrosis: 0.08%–1.33%; Asymptomatic osteonecrosis: 4% from MRI reports	• Diabetes. • Prior steroid use. • Old age. • Alcohol use. • Hyperlipidemia. • Role of ARVs and osteonecrosis— still controversial.	• Risk reduction (e.g., limit steroid and alcohol use). • Asymptomatic cases w/ <15% bony head involvement; follow with MRI every 3–6 months x 1 yr, then every 6 months x 1 yr, then annually—to assess for disease progression.	Conservative management: • Decrease weight bearing on affected joint. • Remove or reduce risk factors. • Analgesics as needed. Surgical Intervention: • Core decompression +/- bone grafting— for early stages of disease. • For more severe and debilitating disease— total joint arthroplasty.
Pancre-atitis	ddI alone; ddI + d4T; ddI + hydroxyurea (HU), ribavirin (RBV), or TDF	Onset: usually weeks to months Laboratory abnormalities: increased serum amylase and lipase Symptoms: postprandial abdominal pain, nausea, vomiting	ddI alone: 1%–7% ddI with HU: increase by 4–5 fold ddI with RBV, d4T, or TDF: increase frequency	• High intracellular and/or serum ddI concentrations. • History of pancreatitis. • Alcoholism. • Hypertriglyceridemia. • Concomitant use of ddI with d4T, HU, or RBV. • Use of ddI + TDF without ddI dose reduction.	• ddI should not be used in patients with history of pancreatitis. • Avoid concomitant use of ddI with d4T, TDF, HU, or RBV. • Reduce ddI dose when used with TDF. • Monitoring of amylase/lipase in asymptomatic patients is generally not recommended.	• Discontinue offending agent(s). • Symptomatic management of pancreatitis: bowel rest, IV hydration, pain control, then gradual resumption of oral intake. • Parenteral nutrition may be necessary in patients with recurrent symptoms on resumption of oral intake.

Peripheral neuro-pathy	ddI, d4T, ddC	Onset: weeks to months after initiation of therapy (may be sooner in patients with preexisting neuropathy) Symptoms: • Begins with numbness and paresthesia of toes and feet • May progress to painful neuropathy of feet and calf • Upper extremities less frequently involved • Can be debilitating for some patients • May be irreversible despite discontinuation of offending agent(s)	ddI: 12%–34% in clinical trials d4T: 52% in monotherapy trial ddC: 22%–35% in clinical trials Incidence increases with prolonged exposure	• Preexisting peripheral neuropathy. • Combined use of these NRTIs or concomitant use of other drugs that may cause neuropathy. • Advanced HIV disease. • High dose or concomitant use of drugs that may increase ddI intracellular activities (e.g., HU or RBV).	• Avoid using these agents in patients at risk if possible. • Avoid combined use of these agents. • Patient query at each encounter. • May consider discontinuing offending agent before pain becomes disabling; may halt further progression, but symptoms may be irreversible. Pharmacological management (with variable successes). • Gabapentin (most experience), tricyclic antidepressants, lamotrigine, oxycarbamazepine (potential for CYP interactions), topiramate, tramadol. • Narcotic analgesics. • Capsaicin cream. • Topical lidocaine.

(continued)

Table 7.9

ANTIRETROVIRAL MEDICATION ASSOCIATED ADVERSE EFFECTS *continued*

ADVERSE EFFECTS	CAUSATIVE ARVS	ONSET/CLINICAL MANIFESTATION	ESTIMATED FREQUENCY	RISK FACTORS	PREVENTION/ MONITORING	MANAGEMENT
Stevens-Johnson syndrome (SJS)/ toxic epidermal necrosis (TEN)	NVP > EFV, DLV, ETR Also reported with: APV, FPV, ABC, DRV, ZDV, ddl, IDV, LPV/r, ATV	Onset: first few days to weeks after initiation of therapy **Symptoms:** Cutaneous involvement: • Skin eruption with mucosal ulcerations (may involve orogingival mucosa, conjunctiva, anogenital area) • Can rapidly evolve with blister or bullae formation • May eventually evolve to epidermal detachment and/or necrosis • For NVP, may occur with hepatic toxicity *Systemic Symptoms:* fever, tachycardia, malaise, myalgia, arthralgia *Complications:* ↓ oral intake → fluid depletion; bacterial or fungal superinfection; multiorgan failure	NVP: 0.3%–1% DLV & EFV: 0.1%, ETR <0.1% 1–2 case reports for ABC, FPV, ddl, ZDV, IDV, LPV/r, ATV, DRV	• NVP: Female, black, Asian, Hispanic	• For NVP: 2-week lead in period with 200mg once daily, then escalate to 200mg twice daily. • Educate patients to report symptoms as soon as they appear. • Avoid use of corticosteroid during NVP dose escalation; may increase incidence of rash.	• Discontinue all ARVs and any other possible agent(s) (e.g., cotrimoxazole). Aggressive symptomatic support may include: • Intensive care support. • Aggressive local wound care (e.g., in a burn unit). • Intravenous hydration. • Parenteral nutrition, if necessary. • Pain management. • Antipyretics. • Empiric broad-spectrum antimicrobial therapy if superinfection is suspected. Controversial management strategies: • Corticosteroid. • Intravenous immunoglobulin. *Do not rechallenge patient with offending agent.* • It is unknown whether patients who experienced SJS while on one NNRTI are more susceptible to SJS from another NNRTI; most experts would suggest avoiding use of this class unless no other options are available.

Various factors contribute to the occurrence of AEs. For instance, patient-specific characteristics, such as being female, may predispose patients to develop Stevens-Johnson syndrome and symptomatic hepatic events from nevirapine (Baylor & Johann-Liang, 2004) or lactic acidosis from NRTIs (Moyle et al., 2002). Similarly, possessing the HLA-B*5701 allele increases the risk for hypersensitivity reactions to abacavir (Mallal et al., 2008; Saag et al., 2008). Other AE-associated factors include use of concomitant antiretroviral medications with overlapping and additive toxicities; comorbid conditions like alcoholism (Dieterich et al., 2004); coinfection with hepatitis B or C that may increase risk of hepatotoxicity (den Brinker et al., 2000); drug–drug interactions that may lead to an increase in dose-related toxicities like concomitant use of hydroxyurea or the combination of ribavirin and didanosine that may increase didanosine-associated toxicities (Lafeuillade, Hittinger, & Chadapaud, 2001; Moore et al., 2000).

AE-related profiles of the PI-based versus NNRTI-based regimens differ. PI-based ART regimens are generally associated with more gastrointestinal symptoms (e.g., nausea, vomiting, and diarrhea) and lipid abnormalities. NNRTI-based regimens are more commonly associated with rash and central nervous system side effects (efavirenz). Both types of ART regimens may cause elevations in hepatic transaminases. In one major clinical trial, lipoatrophy (>20% loss of limb fat by DEXA scan) was observed more frequently with efavirenz (NRTI)-based ART than in the lopinavir/ritonavir (PI)-based ART. Higher rates of lipoatrophy were seen when stavudine and, to a lesser degree, zidovudine were part of the regimens (Riddler et al., 2008).

MEDICATION RESISTANCE
Antiretroviral

Antiretroviral medication resistance occurs when HIV replicates while the patient is taking an antiretroviral medicine. The replication may be the result of poor patient adherence to the ART regimen or possible drug–drug or drug–food interactions that interfere with absorption, distribution, metabolism, or excretion of the medicine, resulting in uncontrolled HIV replication and genetic mutational changes. These changes confer medication resistance. The first sign of HIV resistance to ART is the presence of detectible plasma viral RNA on two separate viral load measurements. Various assays are used to determine the nature of HIV medication resistance. The most commonly used resistance assays are phenotypic assays and genotypic assays.

Phenotype assays are used to measure sensitivity to various antiretroviral medicines. The assay reports HIV sensitivity in terms of a ratio above the normal or wild-type IC_{50}. In other words, it is the half maximal (50%) inhibitory concentration (IC) of a medicine (50% IC, or IC_{50}). This information allows a clinician to determine the relative extent of resistance. Genotype assays are used to identify the presence of specific resistance mutations of the HIV genes known to be associated with resistance to specific antiretroviral agents (see Table 7.10).

Table 7.10

RESISTANCE MUTATIONS TO ANTIRETROVIRAL MEDICINE

ANTIRETROVIRAL MEDICINE	CODON MUTATION
Mutation in reverse transcriptase gene associated with resistance to NRTIs	
Nucleoside reverse transcriptase inhibitors (NRTIs)	
Multi-NRTI resistance: 69 insertion complex (affects all NRTIs)	
	M41L, A62V, 69, K70R, L210W, T215Y/F, K219O/E
Multi-NRTI resistance: 151 insertion complex (affects all NRTIs)	
	A62V, V75I, F77L, F116Y, Q151M
Multi-NRTI resistance: Thymidine analogue-associated mutations (TAMS; affects all NRTIs)	
	M41L, D67N, K70R, L210W, T215Y/F, K219O/E
Abacavir (ABC)	K65R, L74V, Y115F, M184V
Didanosine (ddl)	K65R, L74V
Emtricitabine (FTC)	K65R, M184V
Lamivudine (3TC)	K65R, M184V
Stavudine (d4T)	M41L, D67N, K70R, L210W, T215Y/F, K219Q/E
Tenofovir (TDF)	K65R, K70E
Zidovudine (ZDV)	M41L, D67N, K60R, L210W, T215Y/F, K219Q/E
Nonnucleoside reverse transcriptase inhibitors (NNRTIs)	
Efavirenz (EFV)	L100I, K103N, V106M, V108I, Y181C/I, Y188L, G190S/A, P225H
Etravirine (ETV)	V90I, A98G, L100I, K101E/P,V106I, V179D/E/T, Y181C/I/V, G190S/A
Nevirapine (NVP)	L100I, K103N, V106M, V108I, Y181C/I, Y188L, G190S/A

Table 7.10

RESISTANCE MUTATIONS TO ANTIRETROVIRAL MEDICINE *continued*

ANTIRETROVIRAL MEDICINE		CODON MUTATION

Mutation in the protease gene associated with resistance to protease inhibitors (PIs)

PIs	Critical	Secondary
Atazanavir (ATV)	I50L, I84V, N88S	L10I/F/V/C, G16E, K20R/M/I/T/V, L24I, V32I, L33I/F/V, E34Q, M36I/L/V, M46I/L, G48V, F53L/Y, I54L/V/M/T/A, D60E, I62V, I64L/M/V, A71V/I/T/L, G73C/S/T/A, V82A/T/F/I, I85V, L90M, I93L/M
Darunavir (DRV)	I50V, I54M/L, L76V, I84V	V11I, V32I, L33F, I47V, G73S, L89V
Fosamprenavir (FPV)	I50V, I84V	L10F/I/R/V, V32I, M46I/L, I54L/V/M, G73S, L76V, V82A/F/S/T, L90M
Indinavir/ Ritonavir (IDVr)	M46I/L, V82A/F/T, I84V,	L10I/R/V, K20M/R, L24I, V32I, M36I, I54V, A71V/T, G73S/A, L76V, V77I, L90M
Lopinavir/ Ritonavir (LPVr)	V32I, I47V/A, V82A/F/T/S	L10F/I/R/V, K20M/R, L24I, L33F, M46I/L, I50V, F53L, I54V/L/A/M/T/S, L63P, A71V/T, G73S, L76V, I84V, L90M
Nelfinavir (NFV)	D30N, L90M	L10F/I, M36I, M46I/L, A71V/T, V77I, V82A/F/T/S, I84V, N88D/S
Saquinavir (SQV)	G48V, L90M	L10I/R/V, L24I, I54V/L, I62V, A71V/T, G73S, V77I, V82A/F/T/S, I84V
Tipranavir (TPV)	L33F, I47V, Q58E, T74P, V82L/T, I84V	L10V, I13V, K20M/R, F35G, M36I, K43T, M46L, I54A/M/V, H69K, N83D, L90M

Mutations in the envelope gene associated with resistance to fusion inhibitors (FIs) and CCR5 antagonists

Enfuviritide (T-20)   G36D, I37V, V38A/M/E, Q39R, Q40H, N42T, N43D

Maraviroc (MVC)   Activity limited to CCR5 virus only. CXCR4-CCR5 mixed and CXCR4 viruses do not respond.

Mutations in the integrase gene associated with resistance to integrase inhibitors (IIs)

Raltegravir (RAL)   Y143R/H/C, Q148H/K/R, N155H

Adapted from Johnson et al., 2008.

Genotype testing identifies viral mutations on the reverse transcriptase (RT), protease (PR), envelope, and integrase genes. Notation of the specific mutations is standardized by identifying the first letter of the usual amino acid, the location on the gene (number) followed by the first letter of the amino acid change related to the mutation. For example, the M184V mutation conveys that on the 184 position of the RT enzyme the methionine amino acid residue was replaced with a valine amino acid residue. This is one of the most commonly associated cytosine analog-resistant mutations to confer high-level resistance to medications such as emtricitabine and lamivudine. Other RT gene mutation, like M41L, D67N, K70R, L210W, T215Y/F and K219O/E, are more commonly known as thymidine analog mutation or TAMs. The presence of these mutations affects all NRTIs. K65R reduces viral sensitivity to abacavir, didanosine, emtricitabine, lamivudine, and tenofovir. K103N, a major RT mutation, renders cross resistance to efavirenz and nevirapine.

PR gene mutations are classified as critical and secondary. When present, PR mutations render HIV resistant to various PI agents. As the number of mutations emerges, HIV develops increasingly high-grade resistance whereby mutation can prevent the PI from binding to the catalytic site of action, allowing the normal gag-pol protein to be cleaved and form new virus. Like some RT mutations, some PR mutations confer broad, PI class cross-resistance to multiple medicines. L90M and I50L are two examples of very significant critical PR cross-resistance mutations.

Medication resistance to most PIs requires multiple mutations in the HIV protease and seldom develops following early virologic failure, especially when ritonavir boosting is used. However, medication resistance to efavirenz or nevirapine is conferred by a single mutation in reverse transcriptase and develops rapidly following virologic failure (Hirsch et al., 2003).

Pretreatment

Pretreatment HIV medication resistance occurs between 6 and 16% in ART-naïve patients. The presence of transmitted medication-resistant viruses, particularly those with nonnucleoside reverse transcriptase inhibitor (NNRTI) mutations, may be responsible for not achieving the treatment goal of HIV suppression of <50 copies/mL (Wheeler, Mahle, & Bodnar, 2007). Therefore, pretreatment HIV genotypic resistance testing should be considered in selection the best ART regimen.

Although covered by most insurance providers, resistance assays are expensive. Nurses should be familiar with the important considerations and limitations associated with HIV resistance testing (see Table 7.11) and be able to explain these to the patient. It is critical that collection of blood for resistance testing should be performed when the patient is taking ART whenever possible or within 4 weeks of stopping antiretroviral medicine. Resistance testing is not recommended when VL is less than 1,000 copies/mL.

Virologic Failure

Virologic failure, defined as the failure to achieve or maintain suppression of viral replication to less than 50 copies/mL, may be categorized as either (1) incomplete virologic response (as when two consecutive HIV RNA are greater than 400 copies/mL after 24 weeks or when HIV RNA is greater than 50 copies/mL by 48 weeks in a treatment-naïve patient who is initiating ART) or (2) virologic rebound (when HIV RNA is repeatedly detected at greater than 50 copies/mL after virologic suppression).

Table 7.11

HIV RESISTANCE TESTING: IMPORTANT CONSIDERATIONS AND LIMITATIONS

- Biologic cutoffs based on normal distribution of susceptibility to drug for wild-type strain from treatment-naïve patients.

- Clinical cutoffs based on data from clinical trials or cohort studies to determine change in susceptibility that results in reduced virologic response.

- Clinical phenotypic cutoff values include diminished versus no response; partial activity may be useful when treatment options are limited. Analysis complicated by prior drug exposure and activity of other drugs in salvage regimen.

- Consider phenotyping over genotyping when treatment history complex and/or significant resistance is expected.

- May detect resistance only in species that make up >10 to 20% of viral population.

- Measures susceptibility to individual medicines, not medication combinations.

- Phenotypic resistance reported as fold change in IC50 for the test strain versus reference wild-type strain.

- Testing should be performed on therapy whenever possible or within 4 weeks of stopping antiretroviral medicines and is not recommended when VL is less than 1,000 copies/mL.

Baseline HIV RNA affects the time course of suppression. Some patients take longer than others to suppress HIV RNA levels. The timing, pattern, and/or slope of HIV RNA decrease may predict ultimate virologic response (Weverling et al., 1998). Unfortunately, there is no consensus on the optimal time to change ART when virologic failure occurs. The more aggressive approach is to change the medication regimen for any repeated detectable viremia after suppression to less than 50 copies/mL in a patient taking ART. Again, an assessment of adherence is essential. Other approaches for when to change ART allow for detectable viremia up to an arbitrary level (e.g., 1,000 to 5,000 copies/mL when resistance testing can more easily be performed). However, ongoing viral replication in the presence of antiretroviral medicines promotes the selection of drug resistance mutations (Barbour et al., 2002) and may limit future ART options. Isolated episodes of viremia ("blips," e.g., single levels of 51 to 1,000 copies/mL) may simply represent laboratory variation (Nettles et al., 2005) and are not usually associated with subsequent virologic failure. Rebound to higher viral load levels or more frequent episodes of viremia increase the risk of failure (Greub et al., 2002).

Causes of ART Failure

While ART is highly successful, it is not without failure. Many factors are associated with an increased risk of ART treatment failure (see Table 7.12). Suboptimal adherence and toxicity may account for 28 to 40% of treatment failure and regimen discontinuations (d'Arminio Monforte et al., 2000). Multiple risk factors for treatment failure can occur simultaneously. Factors not associated with treatment failure include gender, pregnancy, and history of past substance use.

When ART failure occurs it is essential to determine the cause(s). Candid conversation with the patient and his or her family member(s) coupled with investigation of pharmacy records allows the clinician to explore the various risk factors for ART failure (see Table 7.13). In assessing ART failure, it is important to identify as many contributing factors as possible. Careful identification of reasons for failure allows the clinician to address patient needs more effectively and reduces the potential for subsequent ART failure.

Other circumstances should be considered when assessing for virologic failure and planning for optimal patient outcomes. In some patients with extensive prior treatment and drug resistance (e.g., when new ART that contains at least two fully active agents cannot be identified), viral suppression below 50 copies/mL is difficult to achieve.

Table 7.12

FACTORS ASSOCIATED WITH ART FAILURE

- Patient factors at baseline:
  - AIDS diagnosis
  - Comorbid conditions (e.g., affective mental health disorders and active substance use)
  - Earlier calendar year of starting ART when less potent regimens or less well-tolerated antiretroviral medicines were used
  - Higher pretreatment HIV RNA level (regimen-specific)
  - Lower pretreatment or nadir CD4 T-cell count
  - Pretreatment drug-resistant virus
  - Prior ART failure, with development of drug resistance or cross resistance

- Nonadherence to ART and clinic appointments

- ART side effects and toxicity

- Suboptimal pharmacokinetics caused by variable absorption, metabolism, and/or penetration into HIV reservoirs, food or fasting requirements, adverse drug–drug interactions with concomitant medications and foods

- Suboptimal potency of the antiretroviral regimen

- Unknown reasons

When maximal virologic suppression cannot be achieved, the goals are to preserve immunologic function and to prevent clinical progression. Even partial virologic suppression of HIV RNA $>0.5 \log_{10}$ copies/mL from baseline is associated with clinical benefits (Murray et al., 1999). However, these marginal benefits must be balanced with the ongoing risk for accumulating additional resistance mutations. It is reasonable to maintain a patient on the same regimen, rather than changing the regimen, depending on the stage of HIV disease.

Discontinuation or Interruption of ART

Discontinuation or interruption of ART is associated with HIV viral rebound, immune decompensation, and clinical progression. Similarly, discontinuation of ART regimens containing emtricitabine, lamivudine, or tenofovir in patients with hepatitis B coinfection may experience an exacerbation of hepatitis on ART discontinuation (Bessesen et al., 1999). Nonetheless, unplanned interruption of ART may become necessary for a number of reasons. Severe drug toxicity, concurrent illness, surgery that precludes oral therapy, and antiretroviral medication nonavailability are

Table 7.13

PATIENT CHALLENGES, ASSOCIATED FACTORS, AND STRATEGIES FOR OVERCOMING ART FAILURE

PROBLEM/ CHALLENGE	KEY ASSOCIATED FACTORS	STRATEGIES FOR SUCCESS
Adherence to ART	Access to medications Affective mental disorders Active substance use	Address barriers to access • Copays • Transportation • Enrollment in public assistance and patient assistance programs for medication acquisition • Mental heath and substance abuse referral Simplify the regimen (if possible) • Decrease pill count • Decrease dosing frequency
Medication Intolerance	Side effects	Counsel regarding likely duration of some side effects (e.g., the limited duration of gastrointestinal symptoms with some regimens) Implement strategies for intolerance: • Treat symptoms with antidiarrheals and antiemetics • Exchange one drug to another within drug class to avoid gastrointestinal symptoms, anemia, or central nervous system symptoms
Pharmaco-kinetic Issues	Assess for recent history of vomiting or diarrhea to assess the likelihood of short-term malabsorption	Review concomitant medications and dietary supplements for possible adverse drug–drug interactions Substitute antiretroviral agents and/or concomitant medications, if possible
Suspected Drug Resistance	Obtain resistance testing while the patient is taking the failing regimen or within four weeks after regimen discontinuation	Design ART with at least two, and prefer-ably three, fully active medicines on the basis of drug history, resistance testing, or new mechanistic class
Prior Treat-ment with No Resistance Identified	Consider the timing of the drug resistance test to determine if the patient was not taking ART and/or was nonadherent	Consider resuming the same ART or start-ing a new regimen and then repeating genotypic testing early (e.g., in 2–4 weeks) to determine whether a resistant viral strain emerges Consider intensifying with one drug like te-nofovir or pharmacokinetic enhancement by using ritonavir boosting of an unboosted PI

Table 7.13

PATIENT CHALLENGES, ASSOCIATED FACTORS, AND STRATEGIES FOR OVERCOMING ART FAILURE *continued*		
PROBLEM/ CHALLENGE	**KEY ASSOCIATED FACTORS**	**STRATEGIES FOR SUCCESS**
Prior Treatment and Drug Resistance	Consider changing ART sooner, rather than later, to minimize continued selection of resistance mutations	Discontinue an NNRTI with ongoing viremia and evidence of NNRTI resistance to decrease the risk of selecting additional NNRTI-resistance mutations New ART should include at least two, and preferably three, fully active agents

but a few of the common reasons why patients discontinue ART. Potential risks and benefits of interruption vary according to a number of factors, including the clinical and immunologic status of the patient, the reason for the interruption, the type and duration of the interruption, and the presence or absence of resistant HIV at the time of interruption.

NONPHARMACOLOGICAL TREATMENT APPROACHES

Despite the effectiveness of available ART in suppressing HIV progression, many HIV-positive people report using complementary and alternative medicine (CAM) to manage HIV symptoms and side effects of conventional HIV medication (see Table 7.14). CAM refers to a group of diverse medical and health care systems, therapies, and products (e.g., nutritional supplements, herbal remedies, acupuncture, meditation, and so on) that are not considered a part of medical training or practice in countries where allopathic medicine forms the basis of the national health care system. As many as 60% of HIV-infected patients use CAM to treat HIV-related health concerns (Duggan et al., 2001; Mikhail et al., 2004). In the context of conventional HIV care, where survival depends on proper use of and adherence to ART (Lohse et al., 2007), the potential for CAM use to interfere with the success of ART is an important concern. Uncertain CAM interactions and side effects may compromise the efficacy of ART (Ernst, 2002; Hennessy et al., 2002). The potential for adverse outcomes may be amplified when HIV-infected patients do not disclose their CAM use to their primary HIV care providers or when patients' preferences for CAM interfere with acceptance of conventional HIV treatments (Gold & Ridge, 2001; Kremer et al., 2006).

CAM use is more common among HIV-infected patients with greater education and financial resources. CAM users are more likely to have experienced symptoms of HIV disease progression and to have longer disease duration. Findings with respect to the association of CAM use with depressive symptoms and the use of active coping strategies are mixed. Littlewood and Vanable (2008) identified five major themes that emerged from a synthesis of available CAM studies. They found that HIV-infected patients use CAM primarily for the following reasons: (1) to promote health or to improve or maintain quality of life; (2) to treat nutritional deficiencies, fatigue, and nausea; to alleviate pain related to peripheral neuropathy progression; and to augment the effects of conventional HIV treatments; (3) to prevent or ameliorate side effects (e.g., gastrointestinal and dermatological problems, fatigue, neuropathy, and lipodystrophy); (4) to provide a safe alternative to conventional ART as a way of responding to or counteracting the potential long-term adverse effects of ART and CAM in congruence with patient's culture or health beliefs; and (5) to achieve a way of being more actively involved in one's health care and treatment decisions.

Unfortunately, although limited, there is some reported association between CAM use and ART nonadherence. Jernewall and colleagues (2005) found that (1) users of "Latino CAM" (i.e., traditional healing practices in Latino culture such as Curanderismo, Espiritismo, and Santeria) were less likely to attend medical appointments and had lower rates of ART adherence, and (2) users of plant-based remedies had lower rates of adherence to ART. More recently, HIV-infected women who reported using oral CAM (primarily vitamins and immunity boosters) to treat their HIV were more likely to report missing at least one dose of ART in the past 30 days (Owen-Smith, Diclemente, & Wingood, 2007).

Many HIV-infected patients view CAM as an important part of their care. As such, providers should strive to incorporate routine assessment of CAM use as a means of informing treatment planning and maximizing long-term health outcomes for their HIV-positive patients. The major reasons why HIV clinicians should be concerned about the use of CAM include: (1) the potential for CAM use to interfere with use of and adherence to conventional ART and (2) nondisclosure of CAM use to medical care providers. A patient's beliefs about ART may influence whether CAM is used as an adjunct or alternative to conventional medications. Disclosure of CAM use to HIV care providers is clearly the first step toward ensuring patient safety. Clinicians are encouraged to regularly and systematically assess patient use of CAM. At a minimum, clinicians

Table 7.14

COMPLEMENTARY AND ALTERNATIVE MEDICINE (CAM)

"Asian" CAM	Ginseng-based supplements	Nutritional supplements
"Latino" CAM	Glutamine	Oils or incense
Activities	Herbal medicine	Pharmacologic or biologic
Acupuncture/ acupressure	Herbal products	Physical/body–mind
Alternative medical systems	Herbal remedies	Plant-based
Antioxidants	Herbal teas	Practitioners
B-complex stress formula	Herbal therapy	Prayer
Bioelectromagnetic (e.g., crystals)	High-dose megavitamins	Protein powder preparation
Biological-based therapies	Holy water	Psychic healing
Body work	Homeopathic remedies	Psychotherapy
Candles	Homeopathy	Recreational drug
Cannabis	Humor	Reflexology
Chinese herbs	Imagery	Religious activities
Chiropractic care	Imagery & Meditation	Religious healing
Chiropractor	Immune-enhancement agents	Self-help
Consult spiritualist	Immunity boosters	Special diet
Diet	Lifestyle change	Special foods
Dietary modifications	Manipulative and body-based	Spiritual
Dietary supplements	Marijuana	Structural or energetic
Energy healing	Massage	Supplements
Energy therapies	Meditation	Support groups
Exercise	Mega-dose vitamins	Supportive counseling
Exercise/Yoga/Tai Chi	Mind–body	Tactile therapies
Faith healing	Mineral supplements	Touch Therapies
Folk remedy	Naturopathic products	Traditional medicine
Food supplements	Nonprescribed prescription medication	Unlicensed drugs
Garlic		Vitamins
		Yoga

should document the types, sources, and expected benefits of CAM, as well as the patient's experiences with each type of CAM, including the duration and frequency of use and perceived effects of CAM.

Clinicians who understand their patients' reasons for using CAM may be in a better position to address the potential risks associated with CAM use, such as poor adherence to ART. CAM use and nondisclosure of CAM use may stem from mistrust of the health care system and, by proxy, the clinicians. Alternatively, CAM use may signal a desire for increased involvement in one's health care, misperceptions concerning conventional treatment, or idiosyncratic health and religious beliefs. Assessment of CAM use provides clinicians an opportunity to provide accurate and unbiased information on CAM and to work collaboratively with CAM-using patients to develop treatment plans that optimize adherence to prescribed treatments, satisfaction with care, and health outcomes.

IMMUNE RECONSTITUTION

The introduction of ART has resulted in significant declines in the incidence of AIDS-associated opportunistic illness (OI) mediated through adequate immune reconstitution. Despite satisfactory control of HIV replication and improvements in CD4 lymphocyte counts, some patients initiating ART experience clinical deterioration and unique reactions to opportunistic pathogens during immune recovery (Murdoch et al., 2008). When clinical deterioration occurs during immune recovery and is associated with the host inflammatory response to pathogens, the clinical presentation is called immune reconstitution inflammatory syndrome (IRIS). The symptoms are the result of an exuberant inflammatory response or "dysregulation" of the immune system to a variety of previously diagnosed or incubating opportunistic pathogens, as well as responses to other as yet undefined antigens. A variety of manifestations of IRIS have been described. IRIS may be targeted at viable infective antigens, dead or dying infective antigens, host antigens, tumor antigens, and other antigens, giving rise to a heterogeneous range of clinical manifestations. The most common infections associated with IRIS mycobacterial infections (e.g., Mycobacterium avium complex and tuberculosis), fungi, and herpes viruses. Noninfectious conditions associated with IRIS include autoimmune diseases (e.g., systemic lupus erythematosus and rheumatoid arthritis) and malignancies (e.g., Kaposi sarcoma, lymphoma, and lung cancer) (Dhasmana et al., 2008).

While IRIS is an increasingly recognized phenomenon of paradoxical worsening of patients with AIDS on initiation of ART, treatment for this disorder includes continuation of primary therapy against the offending pathogen to decrease the antigenic load, continuation of effective ART, and judicious use of anti-inflammatory agents. Studies report 17 to 32% of patients initiating ART will develop IRIS (Shelburne & Hamill, 2003). The syndrome usually occurs within the first 90 days of ART and mainly affects patients with lower baseline CD4 cell counts (< 100 cells/μL). Although the clinical manifestations of IRIS are sometimes dramatic and result in substantial morbidity, the fact that these patients are capable of generating an inflammatory response allows many of them ultimately to discontinue secondary prophylaxis for the offending pathogen. Hospitalization and increased resources may be required for up to one-quarter of patients with IRIS, but the majority of patients recover without significant intervention, and ART may be safely continued in most cases.

ORGAN TRANSPLANTATION

Although the initial experience of Stock and colleagues (2003) detailing the experience of 10 kidney transplant patients receiving cyclosporin A (CSA)/mycophenolate mofetil (MMF)/prednisone maintenance therapy without induction was favorable with regard to patient and graft survival, control of HIV replication, and lack of AIDS-defining infections, acute rejection (AR) occurred in half the patients, with 60% of those requiring antilymphocyte antibody treatment. Additionally, two patients developed wound infections, and there were three cases of significant bacterial or viral infection. Thus, HIV infection remains an absolute contraindication to renal transplantation in most transplant centers. Only four programs (University of Pittsburgh Medical Center, University of California at San Francisco [UCSF], University of Barcelona, Drexel University College of Medicine and Hahnemann University Hospital) reported their single-center results (Gruber et al., 2008).

More recently, the UCSF group reported much more favorable results based on their experience with eight patients while employing three modifications of the UCSF regimen: (1) adding an anti-interleukin (IL)-2 receptor antibody for induction; (2) increasing CSA target trough levels; and (3) monitoring predose mycophenolic acid (MPA) concentrations from 2 to 4 weeks to 6 months posttransplant (Gruber et al., 2008).

They reported a preliminary experience with focusing on the endpoints of patient and graft survival; acute rejection; renal function; and cytomegalovirus (CMV) and other infections. The results of their pilot study suggest that appropriately selected HIV-positive patients on ART can undergo successful renal transplantation with a low incidence of both AR and AIDS-associated and non–AIDS-associated infections, despite the presence of multiple other high-risk factors. While their preliminary results are promising, they concluded that using IL-2 receptor inhibitor induction therapy in combination with increased CSA target trough levels and both surveillance and as-needed predose MPA concentration monitoring in the early posttransplant period will need to be verified in larger numbers of HIV-positive renal allograft recipients with longer follow-up.

OPPORTUNISTIC INFECTIONS AND OTHER COMMON CONCOMITANT ILLNESSES

In 1993 the CDC defined the following conditions the AIDS surveillance case definition:

- Candidiasis of bronchi, trachea, or lungs
- Candidiasis, esophageal
- Cervical cancer, invasive
- Coccidioidomycosis, disseminated or extrapulmonary
- Cryptococcosis, extrapulmonary
- Cryptosporidiosis, chronic intestinal (greater than one month's duration)
- Cytomegalovirus disease (other than liver, spleen, or nodes)
- Cytomegalovirus retinitis (with loss of vision)
- Encephalopathy, HIV-related
- Herpes simplex: chronic ulcer(s) (greater than one month's duration); or bronchitis, pneumonitis, or esophagitis
- Histoplasmosis, disseminated or extrapulmonary
- Isosporiasis, chronic intestinal (greater than one month's duration)
- Kaposi's sarcoma
- Lymphoma, Burkitt's (or equivalent term)
- Lymphoma, immunoblastic (or equivalent term)
- Lymphoma, primary, of brain
- Mycobacterium avium complex or M. kansasii, disseminated or extrapulmonary

- Mycobacterium tuberculosis, any site (pulmonary or extrapulmonary)
- Mycobacterium, other species or unidentified species, disseminated or extrapulmonary
- *Pneumocystis jirovecii* Pneumonia
- Pneumonia, recurrent
- Progressive multifocal leukoencephalopathy
- Salmonella septicemia, recurrent
- Toxoplasmosis of brain
- Wasting syndrome due to HIV

While hospitalizations and deaths have decreased dramatically due to ART in the United States and other industrialized nations (Palella et al., 2006), opportunistic infections (OIs) continue to cause mortality and morbidity, especially in resource-limited areas of the world. These infections occur because many patients are unaware of their HIV infection until they present with an initial OI. Some patients are aware of their HIV infection but do not take ART because of psychosocial or economic factors. And, while some patients take ART, they fail to attain or maintain appropriate virologic and immunologic response due to issues of poor adherence, pharmacokinetics, or unexplained biologic factors (Jones et al., 1999; Palacios et al., 2006; Perbost et al., 2005). Thus, to provide comprehensive high-quality care clinicians must be knowledgeable about optimal means for the prevention and management of OIs for these patients.

The relationship between OIs and HIV infection is bidirectional. HIV causes immunosuppression that allows OIs to develop. OIs and other coinfections common in PLWH such as sexually transmitted infections and hepatitis can adversely affect the natural history of HIV infection. Some OIs are associated with reversible increases in HIV plasma viral load. These increases in plasma HIV viral load may possibly lead to accelerated HIV progression or increased HIV transmission (Quinn, 2000). Thus, while chemoprophylaxis and vaccination for the prevention of OIs directly prevent OI-related morbidity and mortality, they may also contribute to reduced rate of progression of HIV disease.

Prevention and Treatment of Opportunistic Infections

Nurses providing care to PLWH must possess comprehensive awareness of the multidimensional aspects of prevention and treatment of

OIs. Fortunately, this information is readily available for each OI. The depth and breadth of the information cover the following broad categories: (1) prevention of exposure to opportunistic pathogens, (2) prevention of disease, (3) discontinuation of primary prophylaxis after immune reconstitution, (4) treatment of disease, (5) monitoring for adverse effects (including IRIS), (6) management of treatment failure, (7) prevention of disease recurrence (commonly referred to as "secondary prophylaxis" or chronic maintenance therapy), (8) discontinuation of secondary prophylaxis after immune reconstitution, and (9) special considerations during pregnancy.

Chemoprophylaxis against OIs aims either to prevent a first episode of an OI (primary prophylaxis) or the recurrence of an OI (secondary prophylaxis). Most commonly chemoprophylaxis is recommended to prevent three major OIs: pneumocystis (jirovecii) pneumonia (PCP), *mycobacterium avium* complex (MAC), and toxoplasmosis. Prophylaxis also is recommended to prevent tuberculosis (TB) in patients with latent mycobacterium tuberculosis infection. In some situations, prophylaxis against other OIs may be considered; see the OI prevention guidelines of the U.S. Public Health Service and the Infectious Diseases Society of America, available at http://AIDSinfo.nih.gov.

Pneumocystis jirovecii Pneumonia

PCP remains the most common life-threatening infection in the United States for people living with AIDS. Primary prophylaxis is indicated for all HIV-infected patients with a CD4 count of <200 cells/μL or a history of oral thrush. PCP prophylaxis may also be indicated in patients with CD4 counts of >200 cells/μL in the presence of a CD4 percentage of <14%, other OIs, or fever >100°F that persists for >2 weeks. When a patient's CD4 count is declining toward 200 cells/μL, the CD4 count should be monitored closely. PCP prophylaxis should be considered for patients with a CD4 count between 200 and 250 cells/μL if monitoring of the CD4 will not be possible within three months.

Recommended Regimens for PCP Prophylaxis

The most commonly recommended regimen is trimethoprim-sulfamethoxazole (TMP-SMX) (also called cotrimoxazole, Bactrim, or Septra), one *double*-strength tablet daily. An alternative dosage is TMP-SMX, one *single*-strength tablet daily, although the lower dosage may not be as effective. These PCP TMP-SMX prophylaxis regimens also are effective in preventing toxoplasmosis. However, many patients cannot tolerate sulfa medications. Severe reactions include persistent neutropenia; rash, including severe erythroderma; and Stevens-Johnson syndrome. Some patients with milder sulfa reactions, like rash without fevers or systemic symptoms, may undergo desensitization. Desensitization is done cautiously and requires diligence from the patient and careful management by the provider. A variety of rapid versus slow sulfa desensitization schedules are available.

Other PCP prophylaxis regimens include:

- Dapsone 100 mg orally daily or 50 mg orally twice daily. These regimens do not prevent toxoplasmosis.
- Dapsone 50 mg orally daily plus pyrimethamine 50 mg orally once per week plus leucovorin 25 mg orally once per week. This regimen is effective in reducing the risk of toxoplasmosis.
- Dapsone 200 mg orally plus pyrimethamine 75 mg plus leucovorin 25 mg, all once per week, also effective in reducing the risk of toxoplasmosis. Of special concern is the finding that G6PD deficiency occurs in approximately 10% of African American males, and in 1 to 2% of males of Mediterranean, Indian, and Asian descent. Glucose-6-phosphate dehydrogenase (G6PD) deficiency can increase the risk of hemolytic anemia or methemoglobinemia in patients receiving dapsone (also see Lashley, 2000.) Thus, screening for G6PD deficiency before starting dapsone should be considered.
- Aerosolized pentamidine (AP) 300 mg once per month, via Respirgard II nebulizer. However, this regimen does not prevent toxoplasmosis. Aerosolized pentamidine may increase the risk of extrapulmonary pneumocystosis, pneumothorax, and bronchospasm. It increases the risk of TB transmission if the patient has active pulmonary tubercular disease, unless ventilation (negative pressurized facility with outside venting) is provided. AP should not be given in patients in whom TB is suspected. The availability of treatment facilities offering AP may be limited due to the necessity for special equipment and negative pressurized treatment facilities.
- Atovaquone suspension 1,500 mg daily. This drug reduces the risk of toxoplasmosis. Atovaquone is much more expensive than dapsone. It should be taken with high-fat meals for optimal absorption.
- TMP-SMX 1 double-strength tablet orally three times per week (e.g., Monday, Wednesday, Friday).

Secondary PCP Prophylaxis

Prophylaxis should be given to all patients with a history of PCP.

Discontinuing PCP Prophylaxis

Primary or secondary prophylaxis can be discontinued if the CD4 count increases to >200 cells/µL for at least three months in response to effective ART, with the following cautions:

- If the patient had PCP and the episode of PCP occurred at a CD4 count of >200 cells/µL, it may be prudent to continue PCP prophylaxis for life, regardless of how high the CD4 count rises as a consequence of ART.
- If PCP prophylaxis is discontinued, the patient's clinical status and CD4 count must be observed closely to determine the necessity of resuming prophylaxis.
- PCP prophylaxis should be reinitiated if the CD4 count decreases to <200 cells/µL or the patient meets other criteria as indicated above.

Mycobacterium avium Complex (MAC)—*Disseminated*

MAC is common in patients with AIDS and occurs when the CD4 count is <50 cells/µL. Primary prophylaxis is indicated for all PLWH with CD4 counts of <50 cells/µL. Before starting prophylaxis, providers rule out active MAC infection by clinical assessment and, if warranted, by acid-fast bacilli (AFB) blood cultures.

Recommendations for primary MAC prophylaxis:

- Azithromycin 1,200 mg weekly or clarithromycin 500 mg orally twice a day. However, clarithromycin is not recommended during pregnancy, and it can have significant interactions with efavirenz and other drugs. If breakthrough disseminated MAC occurs, it may be macrolide class resistant.

Alternative MAC prophylaxis includes:

- Rifabutin 300 mg daily, or azithromycin 1,200 mg daily plus rifabutin 300 mg daily. Again, Rifabutin significantly interacts with many drugs, such as certain nonnucleoside reverse transcriptase inhibitors and protease inhibitors, along with many other medi-cations. Thus, it be should be avoided or dose adjusted if used with rifabutin.

Secondary MAC prophylaxis should be continued indefinitely as chronic maintenance therapy, unless immune reconstitution occurs in response to ART. The two most common secondary-treatment regimens include:

- Clarithromycin 500 mg twice daily plus ethambutol 15 mg/kg once daily or
- Azithromycin 500 to 600 mg once daily plus ethambutol 15 mg/kg once daily

Discontinuing Primary MAC Prophylaxis

Primary MAC prophylaxis can be discontinued if responses to effective ART result in sustained increases in CD4 counts to >100 cells/µL for at least three months. Careful observation and monitoring are required, and prophylaxis should be reinstituted if the CD4 count decreases to <50 to 100 cells/µL.

Discontinuing Secondary MAC Prophylaxis

Secondary MAC prophylaxis can be discontinued after at least 12 months of treatment for MAC if the patient is asymptomatic and has a sustained CD4 counts of >100 cells/µL during ART for at least six months.

Toxoplasmosis

Toxoplasmic encephalitis (TE) remains relatively common in patients with AIDS. It is usually caused by reactivation of latent *Toxoplasma gondii* infection in patients with advanced immunosuppression with CD4 counts of <100 cells/µL. It is recommended that all HIV-infected patients be tested for toxoplasmosis immunoglobulin G (IgG) antibody soon after the diagnosis of HIV infection (see Table 7.1). Toxoplasmosis IgG-negative patients should be counseled to avoid sources of infection such as contact with animals (e.g., veterinary work and employment in pet stores, farms, or slaughterhouses) that may pose a risk of infection. The available data are insufficient to justify a recommendation against work in such settings. Primary prophylaxis should be administered to all HIV-infected patients with CD4 counts of <100 cells/µL who are seropositive for Toxoplasma. IgG-negative patients should avoid exposure to *Toxoplasma*. Recommendations for primary *toxoplasmosis* prophylaxis:

- TMP-SMX 1 double-strength tablet daily that is also effective for PCP prophylaxis.

Other toxoplasmosis prophylaxis regimens include the following, which are also effective in preventing PCP:

- TMP-SMX, one single-strength tablet daily.
- Dapsone 50 mg daily plus pyrimethamine 50 mg weekly plus folinic acid 25 mg weekly.
- Dapsone 200 mg weekly plus pyrimethamine 75 mg weekly plus folinic acid 25 mg orally weekly (see warnings above related to dapsone and G6PD deficiency).
- Atovaquone 1,500 mg orally daily, with or without pyrimethamine 25 mg daily plus folinic acid 10 mg daily. Unfortunately, this alternative is quite expensive.

(Neither AP nor dapsone alone provides protection against TE.)

Secondary toxoplasmosis prophylaxis should be continued indefinitely as chronic maintenance therapy, unless immune reconstitution occurs in response to ART. The most common chronic maintenance therapies include:

- Pyrimethamine 25 to 50 mg orally once daily plus sulfadiazine 500 to 1,000 mg orally every six hours plus folinic acid 10 mg orally once daily (also effective as PCP prophylaxis).
- Pyrimethamine 25 to 50 mg orally once daily plus clindamycin 300 to 450 mg orally every six to eight hours plus folinic acid 10 mg orally once daily.
- Pyrimethamine 25 to 50 mg orally once daily plus atovaquone 1,500 mg orally once daily plus folinic acid 10 mg orally once daily (also effective as PCP prophylaxis).

Primary prophylaxis for TE can be discontinued in response to effective ART with CD4 counts of >200 cells/µL for at least three months. CD4 counts should be monitored carefully, and prophylaxis should be reinstituted if CD4 counts decrease to <200 cells/µL.

Secondary TE prophylaxis may be discontinued when signs and symptoms resolve with treatment and with CD4 counts of >200 cells/µL for at least six months during ART.

Patient Education Related to Opportunistic Infections

By effectively providing patients with OI-related knowledge, nurses play a vital role in the prevention of OIs and their recurrence. Comprehensive patient education should include instruction related to:

- Adherence (potentially for life) to reduce the risk of the OI.
- Adverse effects of the selected medication(s) and recommended patient responses in the event of rashes, diarrhea, and other adverse events.
- Avoidance of clarithromycin for women of childbearing potential, emphasizing the need for effective contraception to avoid potential teratogenic effects of clarithromycin.
- Avoidance of exposure to *toxoplasma* for *toxoplasma* IgG-negative patients by avoiding eating raw or undercooked meat, especially pork, lamb, game, and venison. Patients should wash hands after handling raw meat and after gardening or contact with soil. Encourage patients not to adopt or handle stray cats, and, if they own cats, to wash hands thoroughly after cleaning litter boxes.
- Notification of provider if illness occurs.
- Purpose of each medication, with special emphasis on dosage and frequency of administration.
- Relative frequency of OIs despite prophylaxis.

(See Lashley and Durham [2007], for additional precautions for immunodeficiency precautions.)

The causes, associated signs and symptoms, diagnostic evaluation, and treatment of the most common HIV associated OIs can be found in Table 7.15. In 2008, the National Institutes of Health (NIH), the CDC, and the HIV Medicine Association of the Infectious Diseases Society of America (HIVMA/IDSA) proposed new comprehensive guidelines for treating OIs among HIV-infected adults and adolescents. Companion guidelines are available for HIV-infected children. The most recent guidelines are available at http://AIDSinfo.nih.gov. The guidelines are intended for clinicians, other health care providers, HIV-infected patients, and policy makers residing in the United States. The guidelines pertinent to other regions of the world, especially resource-limited countries, may differ with respect to the spectrum of OIs of interest and diagnostic and therapeutic capacity.

Table 7.15

IDEOLOGICAL CAUSES, ASSOCIATED SIGNS AND SYMPTOMS, DIAGNOSTIC EVALUATION AND TREATMENT OF COMMON HIV-ASSOCIATED OPPORTUNISTIC INFECTIONS (OIS)

MICROBE THAT CAUSES INFECTION, BODY PART AFFECTED, AND SYMPTOMS	HOW INFECTION IS DIAGNOSED	TREATMENT
Candida albicans (fungus) Mouth (thrush) Vagina (yeast infection) Esophagus (only AIDS-defining OI) Loss of taste and appetite, vaginal discharge, difficulty swallowing	Stains and cultures Endoscopy	**Oropharyngeal candidiasis: Initial episodes (7–14 day treatment):** • Fluconazole 100 mg PO daily; or • Clotrimazole troches 10 mg PO 5 times daily • Nystatin suspension 4–6 mL QID or 1–2 flavored pastilles 4–5 times daily **Esophageal candidiasis (14–21 days):** • Fluconazole 100 mg (up to 400mg) PO or IV daily (AI) **Uncomplicated vulvovaginal candidiasis:** • Oral fluconazole 150 mg for 1 dose • Topical azoles (clotrimazole, butoconazole, miconazole, tioconazole, or terconazole) for 3–7 days **Fluconazole-refractory oropharyngeal candidiasis:** • Itraconazole oral solution ≥200 mg PO daily • Posaconazole oral solution 400 mg PO BID • Amphotericin B deoxycholate 0.3 mg/kg IV daily • Anidulafungin 100 mg IV x 1, then 50 mg IV daily • Caspofungin 50 mg IV daily • Micafungin 150 mg IV daily • Voriconazole 200 mg PO or IV BID • Amphotericin B suspension 100 mg/mL (not available in U.S.)—1 mL PO QID **Fluconazole-refractory esophageal candidiasis:** • Posaconazole oral solution 400 mg PO BID x 28 days • Amphotericin B deoxycholate 0.3–0.7 mg/kg IV daily • Lipid formulation of amphotericin B 3–5 mg/kg IV daily • Anidulafungin 100 mg IV x 1, then 50 mg IV daily • Micafungin 150 mg IV daily • Caspofungin 50 mg daily • Voriconazole 200 mg PO or IV BID

Cryptococcus neoformans ("Crypto") (fungus) Brain: Meningitis Fever, headache, lack of stiff neck (stiff neck is caused by bacterial meningitis)	Lumbar puncture for examination of CSF Serum cryptococcal antigen	<u>Preferred induction therapy:</u> Amphotericin B deoxycholate 0.7 mg/kg IV daily plus flucytosine 100 mg/kg PO daily in 4 divided doses for at least 2 weeks; or Lipid formulation Amphotericin B 4–6 mg/kg IV daily (consider for persons who develop renal dysfunction on therapy or have high likelihood of renal failure) plus flucytosine 100 mg/kg PO daily in 4 divided doses for at least 2 weeks • Preferred consolidation therapy (after at least 2 weeks of successful induction—defined as significant clinical improvement & negative CSF culture): • Fluconazole 400 mg PO daily for 8 weeks <u>Preferred maintenance therapy:</u> Fluconazole 200 mg PO daily lifelong or until CD4+ count ≥200 cells/μL for >6 months as a result of ART
Cryptosporidiosis and **Microsporidiosis** (protozoa) GI tract Diarrhea, often watery without high fever, cramps	Stool cultures, GI colonoscopy with biopsy	Initiate or optimize ART for immune restoration Symptomatic treatment of diarrhea plus Aggressive oral or IV hydration and replacement of electrolyte loss

(continued)

Table 7.15

IDEOLOGICAL CAUSES, ASSOCIATED SIGNS AND SYMPTOMS, DIAGNOSTIC EVALUATION AND TREATMENT OF COMMON HIV-ASSOCIATED OPPORTUNISTIC INFECTIONS (OIS) *continued*

MICROBE THAT CAUSES INFECTION, BODY PART AFFECTED, AND SYMPTOMS	HOW INFECTION IS DIAGNOSED	TREATMENT
Cytomegalovirus (CMV) (virus) Eyes, GI tract, brain and central nervous system, lungs Blurry vision, diarrhea and abdominal pain, fever, chills	Direct ophthalmoscopic exam Biopsy of gut tissue, stains of sputum	<u>Preferred therapy for CMV retinitis:</u> For immediate sight-threatening lesions: Ganciclovir intraocular implant + valganciclovir 900 mg PO (BID for 14–21 days, then once daily) • One dose of intravitreal ganciclovir may be given immediately after diagnosis until ganciclovir implant can be placed. • For small peripheral lesions: Valganciclovir 900mg PO BID for 14–21 days, then 900 mg PO daily • Chronic maintenance therapy (Secondary prophylaxis): Valganciclovir 900 mg PO daily (AI); or • Ganciclovir Implant (may be replaced every 6–8 months if CD4+ count remains <100 cells/µL) + valganciclovir 900 mg PO daily until immune recovery. <u>CMV esophagitis or colitis:</u> Ganciclovir IV or Foscarnet IV for 21–28 days or until resolution of signs and symptoms. Oral valganciclovir may be used if symptoms are not severe enough to interfere with oral absorption. • Maintenance therapy is generally not necessary, but should be considered after relapses. <u>CMV pneumonitis:</u> Treatment should be considered in patients with histologic evidence of CMV pneumonitis and who do not respond to treatment of other pathogens. • The role of maintenance therapy has not been established. <u>CMV neurological disease:</u> Treatment should be initiated promptly: Combination of ganciclovir IV + foscarnet IV to stabilize disease and maximize response, continue until symptomatic improvement. • Maintenance therapy (with valganciclovir PO + IV foscarnet) should be continued for life unless there is evidence of immune recovery

Organism	Diagnostics	Treatment
Mycobacterium tuberculosis (TB)	Sputum stains and tests, cultures, X-rays	Empiric treatment should be initiated and continued in HIV-infected persons in whom TB is suspected until all diagnostic work-up is complete
Lungs, bone marrow, liver, lungs, GI tract, virtually anywhere		Treatment of drug-susceptible active TB disease:
		Initial phase (2 months): Isoniazid (INH)* + [rifampin (RIF) or rifabutin (RFB)] + Pyrazinamide (PZA) + Ethambutol (EMB); if drug susceptibility report shows sensitivity to INH & RIF, and PZA, then EMB may be discontinued before 2 months of treatment
Fever, chills, flulike aches and pains, anemia, weakness, cough, weight loss		• Continuation phase: INH + (RIF or RFB) daily or TIW (AIII) or BIW (if CD4+ count >100/µL)
		• Duration of therapy: *Pulmonary TB*—6 months, *Pulmonary TB w/ cavitary lung lesions & (+) culture after 2 months of TB treatment*—9 months
		• *Extrapulmonary TB w/ CNS, bone, or joint infections*—9–12 months
		• *Extrapulmonary TB in other sites*—6–9 months
		* All patients receiving INH should receive pyridoxine 25–50 mg PO daily
Mycobacterium avium Complex (MAC)	Blood cultures	Preferred therapy for disseminated MAC:
		At least 2 drugs as initial therapy with:
Disseminated through the bone marrow (seen also in liver, lungs)		Clarithromycin 500mg PO BID + ethambutol 15 mg/kg PO daily
		• Addition of rifabutin may also be considered: Rifabutin 300mg PO daily (dosage adjusted may be necessary based on drug–drug interactions)
Fever, chills, flulike aches and pains, anemia, weakness		• Chronic maintenance therapy/secondary prophylaxis: Same as treatment drugs and regimens
		• Duration (chronic maintenance therapy): Lifelong therapy, unless in patients with sustained immune recovery on ART

(continued)

Table 7.15

IDEOLOGICAL CAUSES, ASSOCIATED SIGNS AND SYMPTOMS, DIAGNOSTIC EVALUATION AND TREATMENT OF COMMON HIV-ASSOCIATED OPPORTUNISTIC INFECTIONS (OIS) *continued*

MICROBE THAT CAUSES INFECTION, BODY PART AFFECTED, AND SYMPTOMS	HOW INFECTION IS DIAGNOSED	TREATMENT
Pneumocystis jirovecii Pneumonia (PCP) Lungs. Rarely ear, skin, and other internal organs Shortness of breath, cough (usually dry), fever	Chest X-ray, sputum for silver stain, BAL (bronchoalveolar lavage), rarely lung biopsy	<u>Preferred treatment for moderate to severe PCP:</u> • Trimethoprim-sulfamethoxazole (TMP-SMX): [15–20 mg TMP and 75–100 mg SMX]/kg/day IV given q6h or q8h, may switch to PO after clinical improvement <u>Preferred treatment for mild to moderate PCP:</u> • Same daily dose of TMP-SMX as above, given PO in 3 divided doses; or • TMP-SMX (160 mg/800 mg or DS) 2 tablets TID • Duration of therapy: 21 days <u>Preferred secondary prophylaxis:</u> • TMP-SMX (160 mg/800 mg or DS) tablet PO daily or • TMP-SMX (80 mg/400 mg or SS) tablet PO daily
Progressive multifocal leukoencephalopathy (PML) caused by JC virus Brain Personality change, loss of various body functions, progressive	MRI of brain, CNS PCR for JC Virus	Initiate antiretroviral therapy in ART-naïve patients Optimize ART in patients who develop PML in phase of HIV viremia on antiretroviral therapy

Toxoplasma gondii encephalitis

Brain: Encephalitis

Fever, confusion, local neurologic deficits, seizures

CT scan of brain
Serum toxo titer

- Pyrimethamine 200 mg PO x 1, then 50mg (<60 kg) to 75 mg (≥60 kg) PO daily plus Sulfadiazine 1,000 (<60 kg) to 1,500 mg (≥60 kg) PO q6h plus Leucovorin 10–25 mg PO daily (can increase up to 50 mg or higher)
- Duration for acute therapy:
- At least 6 weeks; longer duration if clinical or radiologic disease is extensive or response is incomplete at 6 weeks
- Preferred chronic maintenance therapy:
- Pyrimethamine 25–50 mg PO daily plus Sulfadiazine 2,000–4,000 mg PO daily (in two to four divided doses) plus Leucovorin 10–25 mg PO daily

FACTORS ASSOCIATED WITH HIV DISEASE PROGNOSIS

ART has led to significant increases in survival and quality of life (Lima et al., 2007). However, the effect of ART on life expectancy is not well understood. In a recent study published by the Antiretroviral Therapy Cohort Collaboration (2008) the investigators used data from a multinational collaboration of HIV cohort studies in Europe and North America to explore the effect of ART on life expectancy. Patients were included in the analysis if they were aged 16 years or over and ART-naïve when initiating treatment. Abridged life tables were constructed to estimate life expectancies for individuals on ART in calendar year intervals of 1996–99, 2000–02, and 2003–05, and stratified by sex, baseline CD4 cell count, and history of injecting drug use. The average number of years remaining to be lived by those treated with ART at 20 and 35 years of age was then estimated. Potential years of life lost from 20 to 64 years of age and crude mortality rates were also calculated.

The investigators reported that 18,587, 13,914, and 10,854 eligible patients initiated ART in 1996–99, 2000–02, and 2003–05, respectively. A total of 2,056 (4.7%) deaths were observed during the study period, with crude mortality rates decreasing from 16.3 deaths per 1,000 person-years in 1996–99 to 10.0 deaths/1,000 person-years in 2003–05. Potential years of life lost per 1,000 person-years also decreased over the same time, from 366 to 189 years. Life expectancy at age 20 years increased from 36.1 (SE 0.6) years to 49.4 (0.5) years. Women had higher life expectancies than men. Patients with presumed HIV infection from transmission via injection drug use had lower life expectancies than did those from other transmission groups (32.6 [1.1] years versus 44.7 [0.3] years in 2003–05). Life expectancy was lower in patients with lower baseline CD4 cell counts than in those with higher baseline counts (32.4 [1.1] years for CD4 cell counts below 100 cells/μL vs. 50.4 [0.4] years for counts of 200 cells/μL or more). Their conclusion was that the average number of years remaining to be lived at age 20 years was about two-thirds of that in the general population in these countries.

CONCLUSION

Fortunately, since nearly the beginning of the epidemic, intense scientific efforts and funding have been available and focused on controlling

HIV. Over the past two decades the evolution of successful therapeutic antiretroviral options has made it possible to manage HIV infection as a chronic disease for all stages of HIV infection and disease. New antiretroviral medications may turn out to be a knockout that will have great influence on the course of HIV treatment and patient survival. As we look forward to the promising benefits of newer drugs, it is remarkable to reflect on the incredible progress made with every passing year.

In this chapter we reviewed several key areas of importance related to the medical management of HIV. These topics included: (1) standards of HIV medical care for the treatment for HIV disease and common concomitant illnesses; (2) issues related to adherence to antiretroviral medication and engagement with health care services; (3) medication and food interactions; (4) adverse medication effects; (5) medication resistance; (6) nonpharmacological treatment approaches; (7) immune reconstitution; (8) organ transplantation; and (9) factors associated with HIV disease prognosis. However, because the science and understanding of HIV rapidly evolves, the appropriate use of available new medicines and new clinical data may rapidly change treatment options and preferences. The author highly suggests that nurses review the most current treatment recommendations which are available at http://aidsinfo.nih.gov/guidelines. The importance of coupling the information contained in this chapter and other references with expertise in the clinical care of patients with HIV cannot be overemphasized.

REFERENCES

Aberg, J. A., Gallant, J. E., Anderson, J., Oleske, J. M., Libman, H., & Currier, J. S. (2004). Primary care guidelines for the management of persons infected with human immunodeficiency virus: Recommendations of the HIV Medicine Association of the Infectious Diseases Society of America. *Clinical Infectious Diseases, 39,* 609–629.

Ammassari, A., Trotta, M. P., Murri, R., Castelli, F., Narciso, P., Noto, P., et al. (2002). Correlates and predictors of adherence to highly active antiretroviral therapy: Overview of published literature. *Journal of Acquired Immune Deficiency Syndrome, 31*(Suppl. 3), S123–127.

Antiretroviral Therapy Cohort Collaboration. (2008). Life expectancy of individuals on combination antiretroviral therapy in high-income countries: A collaborative analysis of 14 cohort studies. *Lancet, 372,* 293–299.

Bangsberg, D. R., Moss, A. R., & Deeks, S. G. (2004). Paradoxes of adherence and drug resistance to HIV antiretroviral therapy. *Journal of Antimicrobial Chemotherapy, 53,* 696–699.

Barbour, J. D., Wrin, T., Grant, R. M., Martin, J. N., Segal, M. R., Petropoulos, C. J., et al. (2002). Evolution of phenotypic drug susceptibility and viral replication capacity during long-term virologic failure of protease inhibitor therapy in human immunodeficiency virus-infected adults. *Journal of Virology, 76,* 11104–11112.

Baylor, M. S., & Johann-Liang, R. (2004). Hepatotoxicity associated with nevirapine use. *Journal of Acquired Immune Deficiency Syndrome, 35,* 538–539.

Bessesen, M., Ives, D., Condreay, L., Lawrence, S., & Sherman, K. E. (1999). Chronic active hepatitis B exacerbations in human immunodeficiency virus-infected patients following development of resistance to or withdrawal of lamivudine. *Clinical Infectious Diseases, 28,* 1032–1035.

Centers for Disease Control. (1998). Report of the NIH panel to define principles of therapy of HIV infection and guidelines for the use of antiretroviral agents in HIV-infected adults and adolescents. *Morbidity and Mortality Weekly Report, 47*(RR-5), 1–41.

Centers for Disease Control. (2008). *Adult prevention and treatment of opportunistic infections guidelines working group. Guidelines for prevention and treatment of opportunistic infections in HIV-infected adults and adolescents* [DRAFT]. Retrieved September 27, 2008, from http://aidsinfo.nih.gov/contentfiles/Adult_OI.pdf.

Cheever, L. (1999). *What do we know about adherence levels in different populations? Adherence to HIV therapy: Building a bridge to success.* Retrieved September 2008 from Forum for Collaborative HIV Research Web site, www.hivforum.org.

Chun, T. W., Engel, D., Berrey, M. M., Shea, T., Corey, L., & Fauci, A. S. (1998). Early establishment of a pool of latently infected, resting CD4(+) T cells during primary HIV-1 infection. *Proceedings of the National Academy of Sciences USA, 95,* 8869–8873.

Chun, T. W., Stuyver, L., Mizell, S. B., Ehler, L. A., Mican, J. A., & Baseler, M. (1997). Presence of an inducible HIV-1 latent reservoir during highly active antiretroviral therapy. *Proceedings of the National Academy of Sciences USA, 94,* 13193–13197.

Crespo-Fierro, M. (1997). Compliance/adherence and care management in HIV disease. *Journal of the Association of Nurses in AIDS Care, 8,* 43–54.

d'Arminio Monforte, A., Lepri, A. C., Rezza, G., Pezzotti, P., Antinori, A., Phillips, A. N., et al. (2000). Insights into the reasons for discontinuation of the first highly active antiretroviral therapy (HAART) regimen in a cohort of antiretroviral naïve patients. I.CO.N.A. Study Group. Italian Cohort of Antiretroviral-Naïve Patients. *AIDS, 14,* 499–507.

Delgado, J., Heath, K. V., Yip, B., Marion, S., Alfonso, V., Montaner, J. S., et al. (2003). Highly active antiretroviral therapy: Physician experience and enhanced adherence to prescription refill. *Antiviral Therapy, 8*(5), 471–478.

den Brinker, M., Wit, F. W., Wertheim-van Dillen, P. M., Jurriaans, S., Weel, J., van Leeuwen, R., et al. (2000). Hepatitis B and C virus co-infection and the risk for hepatotoxicity of highly active antiretroviral therapy in HIV-1 infection. *AIDS, 14,* 2895–2902.

Dhasmana, D. J., Dhadak, K., Raven, P., Wilkinson, R. J., & Meintjes, G. (2008). Immune reconstitution inflammatory syndrome in HIV-infected patients receiving antiretroviral therapy: Pathogenesis, clinical manifestations and management. *Drugs, 68,* 191–208.

Dieterich, D. T., Robinson, P. A., Love, J., & Stern, J. O. (2004). Drug-induced liver injury associated with the use of nonnucleoside reverse-transcriptase inhibitors. *Clinical Infectious Diseases, 38* (Suppl. 2), S80–89.

Dragsted, U. B., Gerstoft, J., Pedersen, C., Peters, B., Duran, A., Obel, N., et al. (2003). Randomized trial to evaluate indinavir/ritonavir versus saquinavir/ritonavir in human immunodeficiency virus type 1-infected patients: The MaxCmin1 Trial. *Journal of Infectious Diseases, 188,* 635–642.

Dragsted, U. B., Gerstoft, J., Youle, M., Fox, Z., Losso, M., Benetucci, J., et al. (2005). A randomized trial to evaluate lopinavir/ritonavir versus saquinavir/ritonavir in HIV-1-infected patients: The MaxCmin2 trial. *Antiviral Therapy, 10,* 735–743.

Duggan, J. Peterson, W. S., Schutz, M., Khuder, S., & Charkraborty, J. (2001). Use of complementary and alternative therapies in HIV-infected patients. *AIDS Patient Care STDS, 15*(3), 159–167.

Ernst, E. (2002). The dark side of complementary and alternative medicine. *International Journal of STD and AIDS, 13*(12), 797–800.

Fellay, J., Boubaker, K., Ledergerber, B., Bernasconi, E., Furrer, H., Battegay, M., et al. (2001). Prevalence of adverse events associated with potent antiretroviral treatment: Swiss HIV Cohort Study. *Lancet, 358,* 1322–1327.

Finzi, D., Blankson, J., Siciliano, J. D., Margolick, J. B., Chadwick, K., & Pierson, T. (1999). Latent infection of CD4+ T cells provides a mechanism for lifelong persistence of HIV-1, even in patients on effective combination therapy. *Nature Medicine, 5*, 512–517.

Finzi, D., Hermankova, M., Pierson, T., Carruth, L. M., Buck, C., Chaissond R. E., et al. (1997). Identification of a reservoir for HIV-1 in patients on highly active antiretroviral therapy. *Science, 278*, 1295–1300.

Fowler, M. E. (1998). Recognizing the phenomenon of readiness: Concept analysis and case study. *Journal of the Association of Nurses in AIDS Care, 9*, 72–76.

Gallant, J. E., Staszewski, S., Pozniak, A. L., DeJesus, E., Suleiman, J. M., Miller, M. D., et al. (2004). Efficacy and safety of tenofovir DF vs. stavudine in combination therapy in antiretroviral-naive patients: A 3-year randomized trial. *Journal of the American Medical Association, 292*, 191–201.

Garcia, P. M., Kalish, L. A., Pitt, J., Minkoff, H., Quinn, T. C., Burchett, S. K., et al. (1999). Maternal levels of plasma human immunodeficiency virus type 1 RNA and the risk of perinatal transmission. Women and Infants Transmission Study Group. *New England Journal of Medicine, 341*, 394–402.

Gold, R. S., & Ridge, D. T. (2001). "I will start treatment when I think the time is right": HIV-positive gay men talk about their decision not to access antiretroviral therapy. *AIDS Care, 13*(6), 693–708.

Gras, L., Kesselring, A. M., Griffin, J. T., van Sighem, A. I., Fraser, C., Ghani, A. C., et al. (2007). CD4 cell counts of 800 cells/mm3 or greater after 7 years of highly active antiretroviral therapy are feasible in most patients starting with 350 cells/mm3 or greater. *Journal of Acquired Immune Deficiency Syndrome, 45*, 183–192.

Greenberg, R. N. (1984). Overview of patient compliance with medication dosing: A literature review. *Clinical Therapy, 6*, 592–599.

Greub, G., Cozzi-Lepri, A., Ledergerber, B., Staszewski, S., Perrin, L., Miller, V., et al. (2002). Intermittent and sustained low-level HIV viral rebound in patients receiving potent antiretroviral therapy. *AIDS, 16*, 1967–1069.

Gruber, S. A., Doshi, M. D., Cincotta, E., Brown, K. L., Singh, A., Morawski, K., et al. (2008). Preliminary experience with renal transplantation in HIV+ recipients: Low acute rejection and infection rates. *Transplantation, 86*, 269–274.

Gulick, R. M., Ribaudo, H. J., Shikuma, C. M., Lalama, C., Schackman, B. R., Meyer, W. A. III, et al. (2006). Three- vs. four-drug antiretroviral regimens for the initial treatment of HIV-1 infection: A randomized controlled trial. *Journal of the American Medical Association, 296,* 769–781.

Hall, H. I., Song, R., Rhodes, P., Prejean, J., An, Q., Lee, L. M., et al. (2008). Estimation of HIV Incidence in the United States. *Journal of the American Medical Association, 300,* 520–529.

Hecht, F. M., Wilson, I. B., Wu, A. W., Cook, R. L., & Turner, B. J. (1999). Optimizing care for persons with HIV infection. Society of General Internal Medicine AIDS Task Force. *Annals of Internal Medicine, 131,* 136–143.

Hennessy, M., Kelleher, D., Spiers, J. P., Barry, M., Kavanaugh, P., Back, D., et al. (2002). St. Johns wort increases expression of P-glycoprotein: Implications for drug interactions. *British Journal of Clinical Pharmacology, 53*(1), 75–82.

Hirsch, M. S., Brun-Vézinet, F., Clotet, B., Conway, B., Kuritzkes, D. R., D'Aquila, R. T., et al. (2003). Antiretroviral drug resistance testing in adults infected with human immunodeficiency virus type 1: 2003 recommendations of an International AIDS Society-USA Panel. *Clinical Infectious Diseases, 37,* 113–128.

Jernewall, N., Zea, M. C., Reisen, C. A., & Poppen, P. J. (2005). Complementary and alternative medicine and adherence to care among HIV-positive Latino gay and bisexual men. *AIDS Care, 17*(5), 601–609.

Jones, J. L., Hanson, D. L., Dworkin, M. S., Alderton, D. L., Fleming, P. L., Kaplan, J. E., et al. (1999). Surveillance for AIDS-defining opportunistic illnesses, 1992–1997. *Morbidity and Mortality Weekly Report CDC Surveillance Summaries, 48,* 1–22.

Johnson, V. A., Brun-Vezinet, F., Clotet, B., Gunthard, H. F., Kuritzkes, D. R., Pillay, D., et al. (2008). Update of the Drug Resistance Mutations in HIV-1: December 2008. *Topics in HIV Medicine, 16,* 138–145.

Kitahata, M. M., Koepsell, T. D., Deyo, R. A., Maxwell, C. L., Dodge, W. T., & Wagner, E. H. (1996). Physicians' experience with the acquired immunodeficiency syndrome as a factor in patients' survival. *New England Journal of Medicine, 334,* 701–706.

Kitahata, M. M., Van Rompaey, S. E., Dillingham, P. W., Koepsell, T. D., Deyo, R. A., & Dodge, W. (2003). Primary care delivery is associated with greater physician experience and improved survival among persons with AIDS. *Journal of General Internal Medicine, 18,* 95–103.

Kitahata, M.M., Gange, S.J., Abraham, A.G., Merriman, B., Saag, M.S., Justice, A.C. et al. (2009). Effect of early versus deferred antiretroviral therapy for HIV on survival. *New England Journal of Medicine, 360,* 1815–1826.

Kremer, H., Ironson, G., Schneiderman, N., & Hautzinger, M. (2006). To take or not to take: Decision-making about antiretroviral treatment in people living with HIV/AIDS. *AIDS Patient Care STDS, 20*(5), 335–349.

Lafeuillade, A., Hittinger, G., & Chadapaud, S. (2001). Increased mitochondrial toxicity with ribavirin in HIV/HCV coinfection. *Lancet, 357,* 280–281.

Laine, C., Markson, L. E., McKee, L. J., Hauck, W. W., Fanning, T. R., & Turner, B. J. (1998). The relationship of clinic experience with advanced HIV and survival of women with AIDS. *AIDS, 12,* 417–424.

Lashley, F.R. (2000). Genetics in nursing education. *Nurs Clin North Am, 35,* 795–805.

Lashley, F.R., & Durham, J.D. (2007). *Emerging infectious diseases.* New York: Springer.

Lima, V. D., Hogg, R. S., Harrigan, P. R., Moore, D., Yip, B., Wood, E., et al. (2007). Continued improvement in survival among HIV-infected individuals with newer forms of highly active antiretroviral therapy. *AIDS, 21,* 685–692.

Littlewood, R. A., & Vanable, P. A. (2008). Complementary and alternative medicine use among HIV-positive people: Research synthesis and implications for HIV care. *AIDS Care, 20*(8), 1002–1018.

Lohse, N., Hansen, A. B., Pedersen, G., Kronborg, G., Gerstoft, J., Sørensen, H. T., et al. (2007). Survival of persons with and without HIV infection in Denmark, 1995–2005. *Annals of Internal Medicine, 146*(2), 87–95.

Mallal, S., Phillips, E., Carosi, G., Molina, J. M., Workman, C., & Tomazic, J. (2008). HLA-B*5701 screening for hypersensitivity to abacavir. *New England Journal of Medicine, 358,* 568–579.

McPherson-Baker, S., Malow, R. M., Penedo, F., Jones, D. L., Schneiderman, N., & Klimas, N. G. (2000). Enhancing adherence to combination antiretroviral therapy in non-adherent HIV-positive men. *AIDS Care, 12,* 399–404.

Mellors, J. W., Rinaldo, C. R. Jr., Gupta, P., White, R. M., Todd, J. A., & Kingsley, L. A. (1996). Prognosis in HIV-1 infection predicted by the quantity of virus in plasma. *Science, 272,* 1167–1170.

Mikhail, I. S., DiClemente, R., Person, S., Davies, S., Elliott, E., Wingood, G., et al. (2004). Association of complementary and alternative medicines with HIV clinical disease among a cohort of women living with HIV/AIDS. *Journal of Acquired Immune Deficiency Syndrome, 37*(3), 1415–1422.

Mocroft, A., Phillips, A. N., Gatell, J., Ledergerber, B., Fisher, M., Clumeck, N., et al. (2007). Normalisation of CD4 counts in patients with HIV-1 infection and maximum virological suppression who are taking combination antiretroviral therapy: An observational cohort study. *Lancet, 370,* 407–413.

Mocroft, A., Vella, S., Benfield, T. L., Chiesi, A., Miller, V., & Gargalianos, P. (1998). Changing patterns of mortality across Europe in patients infected with HIV-1. EuroSIDA Study Group. *Lancet, 352,* 1725–1730.

Mofenson, L. M., Lambert, J. S., Stiehm, E. R., Bethel, J., Meyer, W. A., & Whitehouse, J. (1999). Risk factors for perinatal transmission of human immunodeficiency virus type 1 in women treated with zidovudine. Pediatric AIDS Clinical Trials Group Study 185 Team. *New England Journal of Medicine, 341,* 385–393.

Moore, R. D., Keruly, J. C., Gebo, K. A., & Lucas, G. M. (2005). An improvement in virologic response to highly active antiretroviral therapy in clinical practice from 1996 through 2002. *Journal of Acquired Immune Deficiency Syndrome, 39,* 195–198.

Moore, R. D., Wong, W. M., Keruly, J. C., & McArthur, J. C. (2000). Incidence of neuropathy in HIV-infected patients on monotherapy versus those on combination therapy with didanosine, stavudine and hydroxyurea. *AIDS, 14,* 273–278.

Moyle, G., Gatell, J., Perno, C. F., Ratanasuwan, W., Schechter, M., & Tsoukas, C. (2008). Potential for new antiretrovirals to address unmet needs in the management of HIV-1 infection. *AIDS Patient Care STDS, 22,* 459–471.

Moyle, G. J., Datta, D., Mandalia, S., Morlese, J., Asboe, D., & Gazzard, B. G. (2002). Hyperlactataemia and lactic acidosis during antiretroviral therapy: Relevance, reproducibility and possible risk factors. *AIDS, 16,* 1341–1349.

Murdoch, D. M., Venter, W. D., Feldman, C., & Van Rie A. (2008). Incidence and risk factors for the immune reconstitution inflammatory syndrome in HIV patients in South Africa: A prospective study. *AIDS, 22,* 601–610.

Murray, J. S., Elashoff, M. R., Iacono-Connors, L. C., Cvetkovich, T. A., & Struble, K. A. (1999). The use of plasma HIV RNA as a study endpoint in efficacy trials of antiretroviral drugs. *AIDS, 13,* 797–804.

Nettles, R. E., Kieffer, T. L., Kwon, P., Monie, D., Han, Y., Parsons, T., et al. (2005). Intermittent HIV-1 viremia (Blips) and drug resistance in patients receiving HAART. *Journal of the American Medical Association, 293,* 817–829.

O'Brien, M. E., Clark, R. A., Besch, C. L., Myers, L., & Kissinger, P. (2003). Patterns and correlates of discontinuation of the initial HAART regimen in an urban outpatient cohort. *Journal of Acquired Immune Deficiency Syndrome, 34,* 407–414.

Owen-Smith, A., Diclemente, R., & Wingwood, G. (2007). Complementary and alternative medicine use decreases adherence to HAART in HIV-positive women. *AIDS Care, 19*(5), 589–593.

Palacios, R., Hidalgo, A., Reina, C., de la Torre, M., Márquez. M., & Santos, J. (2006). Effect of antiretroviral therapy on admissions of HIV-infected patients to an intensive care unit. *HIV Medicine, 7,* 193–196.

Palella, F. J. Jr., Baker, R. K., Moorman, A. C., Chmiel, J. S., Wood, K. C., Brooks, J. T., et al. (2006). HIV Outpatient Study Investigators, mortality in the highly active antiretroviral therapy era: Changing causes of death and disease in the HIV outpatient study. *Journal of Acquired Immune Deficiency Syndrome, 43,* 27–34.

Palella, F. J., Delaney, K. M., Moorman, A. C., Loveless, M. O., Fuhrer, J., & Satten, G. A. (1998). Declining morbidity and mortality among patients with advanced human immunodeficiency virus infection. HIV Outpatient Study Investigators. *New England Journal of Medicine, 338,* 853–860.

Panel on Antiretroviral Guidelines for Adults and Adolescents. (2008). *Guidelines for use of antiretroviral agents in HIV-1-infected adults and adolescents.* Retrieved February 7, 2009, from http://aidsinfo.nih.gov/contentfiles/AdultandAdolescentGL.pdf.

Perbost, I., Malafronte, B., Pradier, C., Santo, L. D., Dunais, B., Counillon, E., et al. (2005). In the era of highly active antiretroviral therapy, why are HIV-infected patients still admitted to hospital for an inaugural opportunistic infection? *HIV Medicine, 6,* 232–239.

Piscitelli, S. C., & Gallicano, K. D. (2001). Interactions among drugs for HIV and opportunistic infections. *New England Journal of Medicine, 344,* 984–996.

Porco, T. C., Martin, J. N., Page-Shafer, K. A., Cheng, A., Charlebois, E., Grant, R. M., et al. (2004). Decline in HIV infectivity following the introduction of highly active antiretroviral therapy. *AIDS, 18,* 81–88.

Quinn, T. C., Wawer, M. J., Sewankambo, N., Serwadda, D., Li, C., Wabwire-Mangen, F., et al. (2000). Viral load and heterosexual transmission of human immunodeficiency virus type 1. *New England Journal of Medicine, 342,* 921–929.

Riddler, S. A., Haubrich, R., DiRienzo, A. G., Peeples, L., Powderly, W. G., Klingman, K. L., et al. (2006, August). A prospective, randomized, Phase III trial of NRTI-, PI-, and NNRTI-sparing regimens for initial treatment of HIV-1 infection - ACTG 5142 [Abstract THLB0204]. *XVI International AIDS Conference,* Toronto, Canada.

Riddler, S. A., Haubrich, R., DiRienzo, A. G., Peeples, L., Powderly, W. G., Klingman, K. L., et al. (2008). Class-sparing regimens for initial treatment of HIV-1 infection. *New England Journal of Medicine, 358,* 2095–2106.

Rodriguez, B., Sethi, A. K., Cheruvu, V. K., Mackay, W., Bosch, R. J., Kitahata, M., et al. (2006). Predictive value of plasma HIV RNA level on rate of CD4 T-cell decline in untreated HIV infection. *Journal of the American Medical Association, 296,* 1498–1506.

Saag, M., Balu, R., Phillips, E., Brachman, P., Martorell, C., & Burman, W. (2008). High sensitivity of human leukocyte antigen-b*5701 as a marker for immunologically confirmed abacavir hypersensitivity in white and black patients. *Clinical Infectious Diseases, 46,* 1111–1118.

Sethi, A. K., Celentano, D. D., Gange, S. J., Moore, R. D., & Gallant, J. E. (2003). Association between adherence to antiretroviral therapy and human immunodeficiency virus drug resistance. *Clinical Infectious Diseases, 37,* 1112–1118.

Shelburne, S. A. III, & Hamill, R. J. (2003). The immune reconstitution inflammatory syndrome. *AIDS, 5,* 67–79.

Shulman, N., Zolopa, A., Havlir, D., Hsu, A., Renz, C., Boller, S., et al. (2002). Virtual inhibitory quotient predicts response to ritonavir boosting of indinavir-based therapy in human immunodeficiency virus-infected patients with ongoing viremia. *Antimicrobial Agents & Chemotherapy, 46,* 3907–3916.

Squires, K., Lazzarin, A., Gatell, J. M., Powderly, W. G., Pokrovskiy, V., Delfraissy, J. F., et al. (2004). Comparison of once-daily atazanavir with efavirenz, each in combination with fixed-dose zidovudine and lamivudine, as initial therapy for patients infected with HIV. *Journal of Acquired Immune Deficiency Syndrome, 36,* 1011–1019.

Staszewski, S., Morales-Ramirez, J., Tashima, K. T., Rachlis, A., Skiest, D., Stanford, J., et al. (1999). Efavirenz plus zidovudine and lamivudine, efavirenz plus indinavir, and indinavir plus zidovudine and lamivudine in the treatment of HIV-1 infection in adults. *New England Journal of Medicine, 341,* 1865–1873.

Sterne, J.A., May, M., Costagliola, D., de Wolf, F., Phillips, A.N., Harris, R. et al. (2009). Timing of initiation of antiretroviral therapy in AIDS-free HIV-1-infected patients: a collaborative analysis of 18 HIV cohort studies. *Lancet, 373,* 1352–1363.

Stock, P. G., Roland, M. E., Carlson, L., Freise, C. E., Roberts, J. P., Hirose, R., et al. (2003). Kidney and liver transplantation in human immunodeficiency virus-infected patients: A pilot safety and efficacy study. *Transplantation, 76,* 370–375.

Vernazza, P. L., Gilliam, B. L., Dyer, J., Fiscus, S. A., Eron, J. J., Frank, A. C., et al. (1997). Quantification of HIV in semen: Correlation with antiviral treatment and immune status. *AIDS, 11,* 987–993.

Vernazza, P. L., Troiani, L., Flepp, M. J., Cone, R. W., Schock, J., Roth, F., et al. (2000). Potent antiretroviral treatment of HIV-infection results in suppression of the seminal shedding of HIV. *AIDS, 14,* 117–121.

Vittinghoff, E., Scheer, S., O'Malley, P., Colfax, G., Holmberg, S. D., & Buchbinder, S. P. (1999). Combination antiretroviral therapy and recent declines in AIDS incidence and mortality. *Journal of Infectious Diseases, 179,* 717–720.

Weverling, G. J., Lange, J. M., Jurriaans, S., Prins, J. M., Lukashov, V. V., Notermans, D. W., et al. (1998). Alternative multidrug regimen provides improved suppression of HIV-1 replication over triple therapy. *AIDS, 12,* F117–122.

Wheeler, W., Mahle, K., & Bodnar, U. (2007, February). *Antiretroviral drug-resistance mutations and subtypes in drug-naive persons newly diagnosed with HIV-1 infection.* Poster session presented at the annual meeting of the Conference on Retroviruses and Opportunistic Infections, Los Angeles, CA.

Williams, A., & Friedland, G. (1997). Adherence, compliance, and HAART. *AIDS Clinical Care, 9,* 51–54, 58.

Wilson, D. P., Law, M. G., Grulich, A. E., Cooper, D. A., & Kaldor, J. M. (2008). Relation between HIV viral load and infectiousness: A model-based analysis. *Lancet, 372,* 270–271.

Wong, J. K., Hezareh, M., Günthard, H. F., Havlir, D. V., Ignacio, C. C., & Spina, C. A. (1997). Recovery of replication-competent HIV despite prolonged suppression of plasma viremia. *Science, 278,* 1291–1295.

Wood, E., Hogg, R. S., Yip, B., Harrigan, P. R., O'Shaughnessy, M. V., & Montaner, J. S. (2003). Is there a baseline CD4 cell count that precludes a survival response to modern antiretroviral therapy? *AIDS, 17,* 711–720.

Zhang, H., Dornadula, G., Beumont, M., Livornese, L. Jr., Van Uitert, B., Henning, K., et al. (1998). Human immunodeficiency virus type 1 in the semen of men receiving highly active antiretroviral therapy. *New England Journal of Medicine, 339,* 1803–1809.

8

Managing Symptoms in HIV Disease

MICHAEL K. KLEBERT

This chapter explores nursing and patient evidence-based management of selected HIV-related symptoms commonly encountered in an outpatient setting. Because of improvements in the treatment, HIV disease is increasingly considered to be a chronic illness. Symptom management in the context of various chronic illnesses is a burgeoning field. A well-established knowledge base of symptom management literature exists for palliative and cancer care, and symptom-management research relative to HIV is ever growing. The *Journal of Pain and Symptom Management*, once the near-exclusive domain of cancer and palliative care literature, has increasingly focused in the last five years on HIV-related topics. The University of California at San Francisco (UCSF) School of Nursing has developed an interdepartmental and multidisciplinary center, the International Center for HIV/AIDS Research and Clinical Training in Nursing, committed to research, education, and care of persons with HIV, including research related to symptoms, adherence, and self-care.

In the early years of the HIV epidemic prior to the introduction of antiretroviral therapy (ART), symptoms were widespread and often dramatic (Hench et al., 1995). Symptoms could be intractable in the face of less-than-optimal treatments for HIV. Symptom palliation was often patients' and their caregivers' best hope. The HIV Cost and Services Utilization Study (HCSUS) (Mathews et al., 2000), a multistage nationally representative probability sample of 4042 HIV-infected adults, established, among other outcomes, overall prevalence rates of 14 HIV-related symptoms. For instance, the prevalence of symptoms in people with HIV and/or

AIDS is about 50%. Of that number, about 50% reported two to seven symptoms each (Hench et al., 1995; Holzemer et al., 1999a; Justiceet al., 1999; Sousa et al., 1999). Widespread availability of highly active antiretroviral treatments (HAART), at least in resource-rich countries, brought swift and dramatic decreases in opportunistic illnesses (OIs). The number and severity of symptoms associated with both OIs and advanced HIV infection also decreased for many patients. Medication adherence was recognized early on as an essential component of any successful treatment regimen (see Chapter 7). The interest in symptom management waned somewhat as understanding and enhancing adherence became dominant. The recognition that effective symptom management is critical in achieving and maintaining medication adherence has led to a resurgence of interest in HIV-related symptom management.

Symptoms are a perceived deviation from the normal healthy state of the individual. Symptoms may appear early with acute HIV infection but are often overlooked by patients and providers as flulike. Kelley, Barbour, and Hecht (2007) noted in their study that 80% of 120 recent seroconverters reported symptoms. Nearly one-third (30%) of these patients reported fatigue, malaise, headache, fever, night sweats, pharyngitis, anorexia, arthralgias, and myalgias (Kelley et al., 2007).

SYMPTOM MANAGEMENT: THEORETICAL BACKGROUND

Faculty and students at the UCSF School of Nursing developed a symptom-management model (Dodd et al., 2001). This model (see Figure 8.1) provides the Nursing Center for Symptom Management with a basis for a discipline of symptom management to bridge all disease states and engage collaborative interactions between and among health care providers and patients by stimulating research in symptom management.

On initial examination the UCSF model appears complex, but one can quickly grasp that any attempt at effective symptom management must acknowledge three domains: (1) the person experiencing the symptom or symptoms, (2) the environment in which the person lives, and (3) basic issues of health and illness. These three dimensions are interrelated. These dimensions (the patient's symptom experience and how they perceive, appraise, and respond to symptoms) interact with symptom-management components, and these in turn interact to result

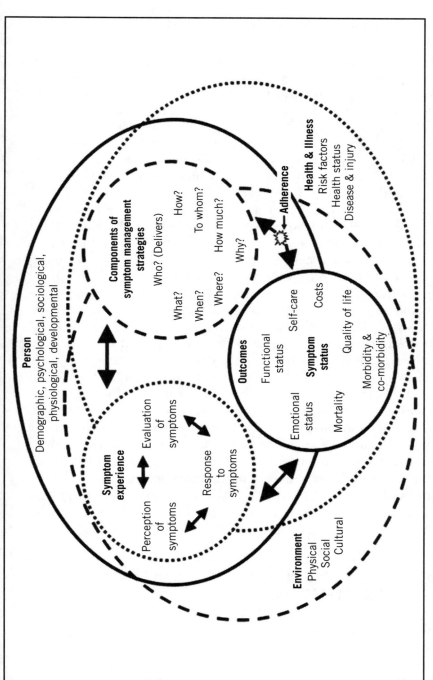

Figure 8.1 UCSF Symptom management model. Source: University of California, San Francisco (UCSF) School of Nursing Center for Symptom Management (Dodd et al., 2001).

in symptom status. The UCSF model is evidence based (Chou, 2004; Dodd et al., 2001) and provides a basis on which to design research studies and to facilitate discussion between caregivers and patients. Spirig and colleagues (2005) emphasized the role of social support in an alternative model rooted in self-regulatory theory. These models serve to inform practitioners and researchers about the multidimensional character of symptoms, ultimately improving management strategies.

Once HIV infection is established, individuals may live for long periods before developing symptoms of advancing illness or opportunistic disease. When the HIV diagnosis is determined, it is important to document a baseline against which to gauge future symptoms. In patients who immediately begin HAART, symptom management is often targeted at controlling and minimizing side effects of the new regimen while also establishing optimal adherence patterns. This period may be complicated by the patient's realization that he or she is experiencing a new and potentially life-threatening diagnosis. Patients are often overwhelmed and experience anger, depression, anxiety, and fear. In this context, symptoms, particularly those that are less problematic or obvious, may be ignored as more pressing problems are addressed. The focus of early clinic visits after initiation of HAART may be solely focused on what is needed to get the patient adjusted to the new regimen, possibly resulting in providers underestimating symptoms in their patients. Thus, symptoms may be overlooked and not addressed in a timely manner. Patients may be left to confront and manage these symptoms at home while remaining adherent to their medication regimen (Ferrando, 1998) and managing their day-to-day lives, often in the context of poverty. Kilbourne and colleagues (2002) reported that patients with public or HMO insurance may be less likely to receive treatment for their symptoms. While current treatment regimens are now simpler to take and are better tolerated, patients who are in their second and third regimens are often managing complex treatment regimens that are more likely to be associated with symptoms.

WHAT DO WE KNOW ABOUT HIV-RELATED SYMPTOMS?

The presence of HIV-related symptoms is negatively linked to patient appraisal and adjustment to chronic illness (Bova, 2001). HIV-infected women with symptoms have a significantly more negative outlook towards life when compared to asymptomatic women and even women with AIDS diagnosis. Symptoms account for about a third of the adjustment to illness (Bova, 2001). The presence of symptoms related to side effects of antiretroviral agents also negatively affects adherence to medical regimens. Heath and colleagues (2002) reported in a cross-sectional, voluntary annual survey of 638 patients that intentional nonadherence to antiretroviral therapy is common among persons experiencing therapy-related side effects. They also concluded that any perceived symptom may result in intentional nonadherence to antiretroviral medications, and this happened whether or not the symptoms were clinically related to the underlying medication regimen. The subjects in this study reported an average of 12 therapy-related symptoms, and most subjects experienced at least one symptom that they perceived as severe. The researchers concluded that patients perceived symptoms, and those that clinicians do not generally consider as reasons to change or end treatment may have been underestimated. HIV-related symptoms are associated with decreased quality of life (Hughes et al., 2004; Siddiqui et al., 2007; Yengopal & Naidoo, 2008). In a nationally representative study of 2,267 adults interviewed on two occasions just as the HAART era began, oral white patches, anorexia/nausea, cough or difficulty breathing, and weight loss were associated with more disability days and worse quality of life (Lorenz et al., 2001). In addition, headache, oral lesions, and complaints were associated with worse overall health.

A patient's social support system has a large impact on symptom severity and self-management. Ashton and colleagues (2005) determined that social support helps buffer symptoms and improves coping with the symptoms. Brashers, Neidig, and Goldsmith (2004) noted that uncertainty and lack of support affects the self-management of chronic HIV.

There may be a relationship between HAART and symptoms. In an online survey aimed at assessing the prevalence of symptoms, their burden, and the association with use of highly active antiretroviral therapy (HAART), 347 self-identified gay men also reported age, CD4 cell count, HIV viral load, year of diagnosis, and HAART use and completed a symptom-assessment scale. Men on HAART reported more symptoms (14 on average) than those who were not on HAART, even when controlling for age, CD4, and viral load. Mean distress indices were higher for those receiving HAART treatment with respect to both global and physical distress. The researchers also found that symptoms of psychological distress were common in both those on HAART ($n = 210$) and those not receiving HAART (Harding et al., 2006).

HIV-infected persons may experience multiple and frequent symptoms. Data collected in the era after the availability of HAART (Mathews et al., 2000) identified that oral and gastrointestinal symptoms as well as pain, dyspnea, and weight loss were present in 24 to 51% of 2,864 HIV infected patients. Batterham, Garsia, and Greenop (2002) affirmed that weight loss was still common in the HAART era. HIV-related symptoms are also associated with increased disability and worse perceptions of health and quality of life (Lorenz et al., 2001).

HCSUS provides some of the best information about the prevalence, severity, and range of symptoms (Mathews et al., 2000). The most common symptoms in this study of 4,042 HIV-infected adults receiving medical care were fever or night sweats, 51.1%; diarrhea, 51%; nausea and anorexia, 49.8%; numbness and tingling, 48.9%; severe headache, 39.3%; and, in women, vaginal symptoms, 35.6%. Symptom number and "bothersomeness" varied significantly by teaching status of care setting, exposure/risk group, educational achievement, sex, annual income, employment, and insurance category, with symptoms being greatest in women and injection drug users, as well as in persons with lower educational levels, lower income, and Medicare enrollment or those who were followed up at teaching hospitals. The researchers concluded that the prevalence and bothersomeness of HIV-related symptoms are substantial and vary by setting of care and patient characteristics.

A more current understanding of common symptoms has is derived from recent work of national and international settings where access to HAART is only now becoming widespread and quantifying symptoms are a focus. In one study of 200 newly diagnosed Nigerian individuals, researchers noted that weight loss (65.5% of subjects) was by far the most common symptom, followed by fever (41.5%), chronic cough (38.5%), diarrhea (32%), and pruritis and rash (13 and 12.5% respectively) (Akolo et al., 2008). This study also quantified signs (a departure from typical symptom discussion in the literature) with pallor (25% of subjects), thrush (20.5%), wasting (20%), lipodystrophy (18%), dermatitis (16%), and nail and skin hyperpigmentation (13.5%) (Akolo et al., 2008). In patients who are more seriously ill, symptoms are often multiple and severe. In a study of 117 patients in palliative programs, researchers found that patients experienced more than 10 symptoms on average, and many felt that their symptoms were not being treated (Karus et al., 2005). Researchers have found that oral lesions were less prevalent in antiretroviral regiments containing efavirenz than those that are protease inhibitor based (Akolo et al., 2008; Aquino-Garcia et al., 2008). The most common oral symptoms where candidiasis, herpes labialis, necrotizing periodontitis, xerostoma, and oral hairy leukoplakia.

Falco, Crespo, and Ribera (2003) identified a constellation of symptoms associated with lactic acidosis, which is most often associated with thymidine drugs, stavudine. These symptoms were insidious in appearance and included nausea, vomiting, abdominal pain, fatigue, and weight loss. Stavudine usage has dropped off precipitously as a result. The research findings briefly presented above point to two conclusions worth highlighting. First, symptoms can and often do occur in clusters, requiring that the nurse elicit a careful history. Second, the patient history must include all medications, prescription and otherwise, that the patient is using.

SYMPTOM ASSESSMENT

It is critical to understand that symptoms are subjective, that is, they are "perceived" from each patient's perspective. In HIV care, patient reports of symptoms have been shown to be more sensitive than provider reports, irrespective of symptom severity (Justiceet al., 2001a). Patient symptom reports are also more sensitive than provider reports with regard to the patient's physical state and health-related quality of life (Justice et al., 1999, 2001a). Nurses must listen carefully to patients when they describe symptoms and attribute the causes of these symptoms Johnson and colleagues (2003) determined that patients make distinctions between symptoms that they attribute to disease and those they believe are related to side effects of medications. Symptoms thought to be related to underlying HIV infection predicted how these patients felt about their general health state. Despite current treatment advances, persons living with HIV disease are likely to experience a range of symptoms over the course of their illness. When the nurse becomes aware of a symptom, she or he should:

- Evaluate each symptom fully, ascertaining symptom characteristics such as:
  - Duration: How long has the symptom been present?
  - Periodicity: Is the symptom constant, or does it recur at intervals?
  - Severity/intensity: How bad is this symptom?
  - Exacerbating and ameliorating factors: What makes this symptom worse? What makes it better?

- ◆ Past history of similar symptoms: Has this ever happened before?
- ◆ Self-care strategies that the patient has employed: What has the patient tried and how did it work?
- ■ In collaboration with the provider team and patient, the nurse should formulate interventions with the following principles in mind:
  - ◆ Identify underlying mechanisms where possible.
  - ◆ Choose treatment or management strategies that have the optimal likelihood of success in the context of the patient's social and personal environment.
  - ◆ Involve, where possible, social supports in the management of the symptom.
  - ◆ Maximize patient ability to recognize and self-manage the symptom(s).
  - ◆ Minimize the impact on patient health care status.
  - ◆ Maintain or improve quality of life.

SYMPTOM ASSESSMENT INSTRUMENTS

Symptom assessment should be explicit and active rather than passive (Lorenz et al., 2001). The nurse should not expect the patient to volunteer symptoms. Patient-completed symptom checklists are one strategy for identifying and establishing a basis for a discussion about symptoms (Justice et al., 2001a). When patients are first seen in any setting, a baseline inventory of symptoms and symptom severity should be obtained.

Several symptom inventories are in use today. Justice and colleagues (2001b) developed and validated the "Symptoms Distress Module" in the NIAID-sponsored AIDS Clinical Trials Group (ACTG). This self-report checklist seeks to capture the presence and degree of bother across 20 common HIV symptoms over the last four weeks. It is still in use today in ACTGs but not widely available. Foremost and best supported by the literature is the "Revised Sign and Symptom Check-List for Persons with HIV Disease" (SSC-HIVrev) developed by Holzemer and associates (Holzemer et al., 2001). The SSC-HIVrev consists of 53 questions, including eight questions related to gynecological symptoms in women. On the day that the patient completes the questionnaire, he or she rates the symptoms on a four-point Likert-type scale as "mild," "moderate," or "severe." If the patient is experiencing the symptom, he or she records it as "0," mild "1," moderate "2," and severe "3." The items are summed for a scale score. Higher scores reflect worse symptoms. The instrument is comprehensive, is easy to understand, takes a relatively short time to complete, and can guide further clinical assessment. Originally validated in domestic populations, the instrument has also been validated internationally (Holzemer et al., 1999b, 2001; Sousa, Tann, & Kwok, 2006; Sukati et al., 2005; Tsai, Hsiung, & Holzemer, 2003).

SELECTED SYMPTOMS

The physical symptoms discussed below remain persistent in persons living with HIV disease in spite of advances in HIV treatment. This review includes fatigue, oral complaints, diarrhea, and sexual dysfunction.

Fatigue

Fatigue is a common symptom of HIV that is frequently overlooked, ignored (Jenkin, Koch, & Kralik, 2006), and inadequately treated (Siegel, Brown-Bradley, & Lekas, 2004). Most persons with HIV disease experience fatigue, sometimes severe, at some point in their illness, usually increasing as the disease progresses. Fatigue has been the focus of much research across many disease states. Achieving consensus on a theoretical model of fatigue has not been possible (Voss et al., 2006). In general, however, there is consensus that fatigue is a complex symptom with many potential causes (Lee, Portillo, & Miramontes, 2001). Physiological causes of fatigue in HIV typically include anemia, infection, nutritional deficiencies (e.g., B12), dehydration, diarrhea, loss of muscle mass as seen with wasting, sleep disorders (Lee et al., 2001), and low testosterone levels (Evans & Lambert, 2007). Fatigue has also been linked to medication side effects and to depression and anxiety (Ferrando et al., 1998; Voss et al., 2007).

Assessment Strategies

- Because fatigue is frequently ignored, the nurse should acknowledge that the symptom is valid.
- Assess the impact of fatigue: When is it present, how bad is it, what brings it on, what relieves it?

- Assess what interventions the patient has and their effectiveness.
- Elicit a thorough medical history and review of medications that could contribute to anemia/fatigue.
- Conduct a full physical examination.
- Assess for depression and anxiety.
- Check complete blood count, testosterone and B12 levels, and other tests to rule out infection.
- Review dietary history and practices.
- Assess hydration status and body shape.
- Take a careful sleep history that includes sleep patterns and sleep hygiene.
- Refer for sleep studies if indicated.

Nursing and Self-Care Strategies

The goal of these strategies is to assist the patient to minimize or eliminate fatigue:

- Treat underlying infection.
- Treat anemia or modify medications.
- Control diarrhea and maintain hydration.
- Plan with patient best times to engage in strenuous activities and track these in a diary.
- Start a progressive exercise program, yoga, or qigong.
- Consider acupuncture and massage.
- Assure adequate rest and sleep.
- Suggest prayer, which many have used, when appropriate (Coleman et al., 2006).
- Enlist support of social group or family (Eller et al., 2005).
- Engage with a support group(s) (Eller et al., 2005).

Fever

Fever is an alteration in the normal body temperature that is brought about by host defence mechanisms in response to infectious organisms or endogenous pyrogens. Cytokines are considered responsible for temperature elevations through the increased synthesis of hypothalamic E group prostaglandins (PGE), resulting in a higher-temperature set point. This response can be considered an adaptive response (Kluger et al., 1998; Wang et al., 1998)

Fever is common with bacterial (most common cause), viral, and fungal opportunistic illnesses; cancers; drug reactions; and noninfectious processes, including some medications used to treat OI and HIV. Fever is also seen in untreated HIV infection. Immune reconstitution syndrome (IRIS) has recently been recognized as another cause of fever as the immune system "wakes up" from profound HIV assault and begins to rebuild itself. Once the immune system begins to return to a normal state, inflammatory processes also return as the immune system is reconstituted, and this stronger immune system can now sense and respond to "onboard" infectious organisms. These organisms include the Pneumocystis jirovecii, herpes infections, cytomegalovirus, and Mycobacterium tuberculosis and require the same aggressive treatment they would otherwise receive. IRIS is rare but has the potential of life-threatening severity.

Assessment Strategies

- Elicit a thorough medical history, including review of new medications, recent immunizations, recent travel, level of exposure to animals, recent dining out, water supply.
- Assess body temperature and hydration status.
- Conduct a full physical examination to identify or exclude potential causes of infection.

Nursing and Self-Care Strategies

The goal of these strategies is to promote patient comfort and avoid or reduce the complications of fever:

- Be sure the patient has a working, readable thermometer and train and encourage him or her in its use. Based on the history, encourage the patient keep a log of these temperatures, realizing that taking a temperature at anything less than four-hour intervals may not be adequate for identifying febrile episodes (Henker & Carlson, 2007; O'Grady et al., 1998).
- Educate the patient that temperatures approaching 40.5°C are dangerous and should be reported to the health care team as soon as possible.
- Maintain hydration to counter the effects of sweating and hyperventilation with fever.
- Avoid chilling by maintaining thermal comfort. After sweating episodes, warm and dry clothes will help control chilling.

Oral Symptoms

Oral manifestations of HIV are common and may be the first clinical features of the disease noted by the patient and/or health care provider (Greenspan & Greenspan, 1997). The frequency of the symptoms has decreased as much as 30% with the availability of HAART (Ceballos-Salobrena et al., 2000). Common causes of oral symptoms include infectious diseases such as *Candida albicans* (oral thrush), bacterial infections associated with gingivitis and periodontal disease, and viral disease such as Epstein–Barr (oral hairy leukoplakia), herpes simplex, herpes zoster, papilloma, and, less commonly, cytomegalovirus virus. Kaposi sarcoma lesions can sometimes present in the oral cavity. Aphthous ulcers have also been noted.

Common fungal infections, including angular cheilitis, erythematous (atrophic) candidiasis, and pseudomembranous candidiasis, are common findings in HIV-infected individuals. Angular cheilitis is often underdiagnosed in people with HIV because it may also be present in people who do not have HIV disease and is usually associated with oral fungal disease (Patton, 2000). Oral fungal infections are more likely in women infected with HIV (Campisi, et al., 2001) and in current smokers who have HIV (Palacio et al., 1997).

The presentation of linear gingival erythema (LGE) can be one of the early signs of HIV infection. LGE has a distinct clinical appearance manifesting as a distinctive red line (1 to 3 mm wide) at the free gingival margin with or without punctate erythema of the alveolar gingiva. Frustratingly, LGE can appear despite good oral hygiene practices in HIV-infected people. Periodontitis in the presence of HIV is more severe, progresses more rapidly, and is often much more painful than periodontitis in a non–HIV-infected person.

Epstein–Barr virus (EBV) causes oral hairy leukoplakia (OHL). EBV may be spread from B lymphocytes to monocytes, which then enter the epithelium and initiate productive viral infection of keratinocytes (Tugizov et al., 2007). OHL typically presents either on one or on both sides of the tongue but can also be located on the buccal or labial mucosa floor of the mouth and even on the palate and oropharyngeal tissues. OHL appears as a discrete, hairy-appearing white patch on the lateral borders of the tongue. OHL can also present variously as corrugated, smooth, flat, or papular in appearance in contrast to fungal white patches. These lesions cannot be wiped off, thereby differentiating them from pseudomembranous candidiasis lesions that can be wiped off and leave a red and sometimes bleeding surface. OHL is usually asymptomatic, but the lesion may cause discomfort and, especially when superinfected with candida, present a cosmetic problem. Diagnosis of OHL is extremely important and remains a good predictor of HIV disease progression.

Aphthous ulcerations (RAU [recurrent aphthous ulcer], "canker sore," "aphthous ulcer," and "recurrent stomatitis") are characterized by recurrent ulcers of the nonkeratinized oral mucosa and oropharynx (Reznik, 2005). The most common areas of aphthous formation include the labial and buccal mucosa, tongue, and floor of the mouth. Three types of lesions are found in patients with recurrent aphthous ulcers. In non–HIV-infected patients, minor aphthous ulcers are the most common; in HIV-infected patients, herpetiform and major-type lesions appear most often. In RAU-disposed individuals, the condition seems to be exacerbated after infection with HIV. Though aphthous ulcers can be seen in any patient, they are more prevalent in some populations: Women are affected slightly more than men, and smokers less frequently than nonsmokers (Palacio et al., 1997). Although the etiology of RAU is unknown, precipitating factors often include trauma, stress, and certain food products. There is usually a prodromal stage, experienced as a burning sensation, and, when the ulcer is established, pain may become intense.

Human papillomavirus (HPV) oral infection has not dramatically declined since the introduction of HAART (Cameron & Hagensee, 2008). Oral warts caused by HPV may appear as cauliflower-like, spiky, or slightly raised with a flat surface (Greenspan & Greenspan, 1997).

Assessment Strategies

■ The nurse should conduct a thorough medical history that includes a review of current HIV viral load and CD4 count, new or changed medications, and a review of symptoms, including odd patches or lesions in the lips, gums, palate, and oropharynx, specifically asking about oral pain, spontaneous bleeding, or bleeding when brushing, flossing, or eating.
■ Assess oral self-care behaviours of flossing, brushing, and oral rinses.
■ Assess frequency, duration, and type of tobacco use.
■ Thoroughly examine the entire oral cavity, starting with a close look at the head, face, and neck. Attention should be paid to the submandibular lymph nodes along the cervical chain into the clavicular area, looking for swelling and tenderness.

- Examine the lips and junction of the lips.
- In the oral cavity, check the palate, buccal mucosa, gingiva, and sublingual area for leukoplakia, erythroplakia, ulcerations, or any other abnormalities. Examine all surfaces of the tongue. Getting at the posterior lateral borders can be difficult to assess. Using 2x2 gauze, grasp the tip of the patient's tongue and carefully pull it to one side, then the other, to facilitate a careful examination.
- Examine the soft palate, pillar and trigone area, and retropharyngeal area. Finally, examine the patient's dentition and periodontal structures.

Nursing and Self-Care Strategies

The goal of these strategies is to promote patient oral health through education, self-assessment, and self-care:

- Encourage and facilitate twice-yearly dental examinations by a dentist who is aware of the patient's HIV diagnosis.
- Instruct and review oral self-exam and oral hygiene.
- Encourage the use of chlorhexadine mouth rinses to potentially reduce the severity and pain of ulceration.
- Consider the use of oral antiviral agents (e.g., acyclovir) to reduce the duration of pain and time to healing for a first attack of herpes labialis.
- Recall that the cure of oral candidiasis is similar with both topical antifungal treatment (itraconazole, miconazole) and oral antifungal treatment (fluconazole, ketoconazole).
- Know that oral warts are most effectively removed via surgical or laser excision, but recurrence is common. Treatment may, therefore, be reserved for lesions that interfere with function or are esthetically disturbing to the patient.

Diarrhea

Diarrhea is an alteration in normal bowel function. Definitions of diarrhea are variable but typically can include loose, poorly formed stools to completely liquid. Acute diarrhea is usually associated with infection and is, as the term suggests, acute. Defining chronic diarrhea is more variable, yet several essential attributes of chronic noninfectious diarrhea can be readily identified. These include increased frequency, decreased consistency, extended duration, urgency, and cramping and/or nausea and/or abdominal pain and incontinence. *Diarrhea is a common symptom associated with HIV among persons with HIV and AIDS,* affecting 50 to 60% of persons living with HIV disease at some point during their illness (Asch et al., 1998; Barroso, 1999; Coleman & Holzemer, 1999; Hench et al., 1995; Mathews et al., 2000; Simon, 1998; Turner et al., 2004).

A cause or causes for diarrhea cannot be established in about half of cases (Navin et al., 1999). Causes of diarrhea are multifactorial and include the use of medications to treat HIV, undiagnosed opportunistic infections, and enteropathy specific to HIV (Bjarnason et al., 1996; Grohmann et al., 1993; Kotler, 1999; Kotler et al., 1984, 1995; Murphy et al., 1999; Navin et al., 1999; Sharpstone et al., 1999; Simon, Kotler, & Brandt, 1996; Wanke et al., 1998; Weber et al., 1992, 1999). People living with HIV disease with chronic diarrhea use more medical resources, have more outpatient visits, use more medications, and miss more work than do people with HIV and/or AIDS without diarrhea (Lubeck et al., 1993). Chronic diarrhea can be debilitating, affecting social life and causing worry about a spiral toward death, often termed the "beginning of the end" (Snijders et al., 1998) The Swiss Cohort Study ($n = 1,933$) established that chronic diarrhea negatively predicts survival (Navin et al., 1999).

Providers typically prescribe sequential prescription and nonprescription medications for treatment of chronic nonbloody diarrhea (CND) with the knowledge that 55% of people with HIV and/or AIDS may experience complete resolution of diarrhea (Gazzard & Sharpstone, 1995; Wilcox, 1997). However, there remains sizable proportion of people with HIV disease for whom treatments are not effective to cope with diarrhea, a bothersome symptom that can last from 2 to 37 months (Gazzard & Sharpstone, 1995).

In describing diarrhea it is important to assess the number of stools a day, characteristics of the stool (poorly formed, loose, watery), and overall duration of the diarrhea, as excess loss of liquid can result in dehydration and electrolyte imbalance. Patients tend to manage diarrhea at home unless it threatens their ability to function either socially or physically.

Infectious causes of diarrhea include common parasites such as giardia, salmonella, and shigella; bacterial diseases like clostridium difficile; and fungal infections such as cryptococcosis, isosporiasis, and microsporidiosis. Noninfectious causes are typically medication related, especially some components of HAART regimens or other medications used to treat and prevent OI. However, many patients have chronic diarrhea for long periods of time that cannot be definitively linked to medications.

Assessment Strategies

- Conduct a medical history review to establish onset, duration, and contributing medical and pharmacological factors, including new or changed medications (e.g., antiretroviral medications, antibiotics, and over-the-counter or alternative preparations), dietary changes, sexual habits (especially oral anal contacts), travel or relocation.
- Assess weight for loss from prior visits or changes from usual weight.
- Perform a physical examination to determine hydration status and abdominal abnormalities.
- Encourage patient report to establish CND onset, frequency, periodicity, consistency, stool type, incontinence, and nocturnal events over a set period. The patient report is enhanced by the use of a patient diary.
- Obtain stool cultures to establish or exclude infectious causes. The standard methodology is three sets of ova and parasite cultures that the patient collects at home and returns. The ideal specimen is taken to the laboratory within an hour or two hours of collection. This collection method requires careful patient teaching about hygiene, collection, transport, and support. Providing a stool "hat" as well as collection containers and paper or plastic bags and gloves will be very helpful to the patient and ease collection.
- Observe stool characteristics and record stool frequency and stool weights over a 24-hour period (in-patient setting).

Arrange for and support mechanical and radiological visualization of the colon. There are few very well-validated instruments to assist clinicians in assessing diarrhea. Tinmouth and colleagues (2007) reviewed numerous assessment tools but discovered that only one was validated in the setting of HIV diarrhea. The authors then demonstrated a prospective measure of stool frequency and form and found that in some settings the measure might have value. Further research is needed in this area.

Nursing and Patient Self-Management Strategies

Treating the underlying infection, particularly in the context of HAART, will often result in resolution of the diarrhea. Diarrhea from HAART or OI treatment medications will require careful observation. Often the symptoms are self-limiting and resolve as either the patient gets used to the medications, the illness resolves, or the medication is discontinued. Because any HAART medications cause diarrhea at least in the short term, the offending medication can usually be replaced with a better-tolerated agent. However, because the first one to two months are usually the worst in terms of new symptoms, treating diarrhea through the early medication period with antidiarrheal medications (either prescription or over the counter) may allow the patient to become accustomed to the medication and preserve the treatment option. Antidiarrheal medications include opioid tincture, paregoric, or absorbents like kaopectate. Probably one of the most common over-the-counter medications used by patients with chronic diarrhea is loperamide that is titrated to control diarrhea. Probiotics have been advanced as a possible treatment for diarrhea with varying levels of success. Recently, Anukam and colleagues (2008) used probiotic-enhanced yogurt to combat diarrhea in Nigerian women with diarrhea. In the small study of 24 women, all 12 women who received probiotic-enhanced yogurt responded compared to only two of the control group receiving only yogurt. Further research is indicated, however. In another study conducted in Nigeria with 30 subjects, researchers used bovine colostrum (ColoPlus) to decrease stool frequency from 7 to 1 stool a day (Floren et al., 2006). This intervention also decreased fatigue and increased CD4 in an uncontrolled trial to 30 patients with severe diarrhea. Further better-controlled research into this agent is warranted.

Anastasi and colleagues (2006) explored the use of normal foods, close food intake monitoring, and support in the management of chronic diarrhea. In this study of 75 men and women reporting at least three diarrhea stools a day over the preceding 3 months, 28% reported decreased stool frequency, while 20% reported improved stool consistency. While several groups have determined some success with zinc supplements in young children, the authors all call for further study (Bhandari et al., 2005; Brooks et al., 2005; Patel, Dhande, & Rawat, 2005; Shamir et al., 2005). Canani and colleagues (2007) determined in a blind study in adults that zinc supplements were not helpful. More study is warranted.

Sexual Dysfunction

In a study of 101 women, Bova (2001) reported that 90% of women remain sexually active after learning of their HIV status, 60% report that they are monogamous, and about half use condoms with each act of intercourse. About 60% had measurable viral loads with a mean CD4 count of 392. In a French study of 1,812 sexually active HIV-positive persons (at least two partners in the last 12 months), a full third of both men and women noted sexual dysfunction, which was more frequent in those less sexually active (Bouhnik et al., 2008). Men and women with HIV remain sexually active when possible but encounter sexual dysfunction. Sexual dysfunction has been linked to decreases in medication adherence (Richardson et al., 2006; Trotta et al., 2008), poor body image, and depression (Sharma et al., 2007).

Asboe and colleagues (2007) noted in a cross-sectional European study of 668 men that 35% reported erectile dysfunction, graded as being of mild to moderate severity, and another 24% had dysfunction graded moderate to severe. Sexual dysfunction was associated with increased age, heterosexuality, not consuming alcohol, depression or the use of antidepressants or antipsychotics, and antiretroviral therapy. Low sexual desire was associated with age, depression, and African American race. While ED was associated with long-term HIV treatment, it was not associated with specific antiretroviral medications (Asboe et al., 2007). Body image and mental health status were associated with sexual dysfunction in 357 sexually active men (Guaroldi et al., 2007). Testosterone levels and HAART were not associated with sexual function among these men (Guaroldi et al., 2007).

Causes of sexual dysfunction in men and women are multifactoral. They include psychogenic causes like depression and anxiety, as well as vascular and neurological disease, hormonal imbalances, postsurgical procedures, and injury. Numerous medications, including antihypertensives, anxiolytics, antidepressants, antipsychotics, and chemotherapeutics can contribute to sexual dysfunction.

Assessment Strategies

- Open-ended questions and general questions are usually indicated to start the conversation and convey permission and openness to the discussion.
  - Ask about desire and arousal, quality, strength, duration of erection in men, and whether they get morning erection and can achieve orgasm.
  - Ask about desire and arousal, lubrication, orgasm satisfaction, and pain in women.
- Review the medical history to establish onset, duration, and contributing medical and pharmacological factors, including new or changed medications.

- Conduct a physical examination.
- Assess for depression and anxiety.
- Assess blood pressure and lab and hormonal tests as indicated.

Nursing and Patient Self-Management Strategies

- Encourage men to limit or stop smoking, using alcohol, and abusing drugs.
- Several oral medications are on the market for ED. Sildenafil, vardenafil, and tadalafil have been shown to be effective. Alprostadil, either intraurethral or intercavernosal, may also be also effective.
- Ginseng, penile prosthesis, vacuum devices, and psychosexual counseling may help men.
- Explore ways to make sexual encounters more arousing and intimate: sensual massage, fantasy play, erotic talk, sex toys, and varied setting for intercourse.
- Counsel patients regarding lubrication, mutual masturbation, and oral–genital stimulation.

SELF-MANAGEMENT OF SYMPTOMS

Investigators and clinicians understand that HIV has evolved into a chronic disease. Self-care practices are essential to maintain the highest level of health possible for persons living with HIV disease. Gifford and Groessl (2002) offered an early model of self-care focused on not only medication adherence but also symptom management, goal setting, communication, and gaining access to resources and services. Chou and colleagues (2004) categorized eight types of self–care strategies that individuals use to manage symptoms. In a secondary analysis, 359 patients reported 776 unique self-management strategies. The eight categories were: (1) medications (23.45%); (2) self-comforting (15.21%); (3) complementary treatment (14.69%); (4) daily thoughts and activities (12.89%); (5) diet changing (10.95%); (6) help seeking (9.28%); (7) spiritual care (6.83%); and (8) exercise (6.70%). This study also elicited sources of information for these strategies, and the majority of the patients' information came from themselves (34%), their personal network (19%), or their community (18%).

Recently, investigators conducted a study comparing an HIV/AIDS symptom manual providing self-management strategies for 21 basic HIV symptoms to a basic nutrition manual given to patients (Wantland et al.,

2008). The goal was to determine whether symptom frequency and severity would be decreased. This large study was comprised of 775 individuals and was conducted over three months in 12 different sites in the United States and abroad. There were significant decreases in symptom frequency and severity among subjects in the experimental group compared to those in the control group. Three factors predicted increased symptom severity: (1) using protease inhibitors, (2) having another illness, and (3) being Hispanic and receiving care in the United States. This study illustrates that providing appropriate information can assist patients in managing their symptoms.

CONCLUSION

Nurses play an important role in symptom recognition, symptom management, and patient teaching and support aimed at promoting self-care. Readers are encouraged to consult the growing body of research and literature, including the forthcoming third edition of the Association of Nurses in AIDS Care's (ANAC) *Core Curriculum for HIV/AIDS Nursing,* to update their knowledge of symptom management in the care of persons with HIV disease.

REFERENCES

Akolo, C., Ukoli, C. O., Ladep, G. N., & Idoko, J. A. (2008). The clinical features of HIV/AIDS at presentation at the Jos University Teaching Hospital. *Nigerian Journal of Medicine: Journal of the National Association of Resident Doctors of Nigeria, 17*(1), 83–87.

Anastasi, J. K., Capili, B., Kim, A. G., McMahon, D., & Heitkemper, M. M. (2006). Symptom management of HIV-related diarrhea by using normal foods: A randomized controlled clinical trial. *Journal of the Association of Nurses in AIDS Care, 17*(2), 47–57.

Anukam, K. C., Osazuwa, E. O., Osadolor, H. B., Bruce, A. W., & Reid, G. (2008). Yogurt containing probiotic Lactobacillus rhamnosus GR-1 and L. reuteri RC-14 helps resolve moderate diarrhea and increases CD4 count in HIV/AIDS patients. *Journal of Clinical Gastroenterology, 42*(3), 239–243.

Aquino-Garcia, S. I., Rivas, M. A., Ceballos-Salobrena, A., Acosta-Gio, A. E., & Gaitan-Cepeda, L. A. (2008). Short communication: Oral lesions in HIV/AIDS patients undergoing HAART including efavirenz. *AIDS Research & Human Retroviruses, 24*(6), 815–820.

Asboe, D., Catalan, J., Mandalia, S., Dedes, N., Florence, E., Schrooten, W., et al. (2007). Sexual dysfunction in HIV-positive men is multifactorial: A study of prevalence and associated factors. *AIDS Care, 19*(8), 955–965.

Asch, S., Turner, B. J., Bozzette, S. A., McCutchan, J. A., Gifford, A. L., Shapiro, M. F., et al. (1998, June 28–July 3). *Quality of medical care for three common HIV-related symptoms in a nationally representative sample of HIV+ persons in care in the US.* International AIDS Conference, Geneva, Switzerland.

Ashton, E., Vosvick, M., Chesney, M., Gore-Felton, C., Koopman, C., O'Shea, K., et al. (2005). Social support and maladaptive coping as predictors of the change in physical health symptoms among persons living with HIV/AIDS. *AIDS Patient Care & STDs, 19*(9), 587–598.

Barroso, J. (1999). A review of fatigue in people with HIV infection. *Journal of the Association of Nurses in AIDS Care, 10*(5), 42–49.

Batterham, M. J., Garsia, R., & Greenop, P. (2002). Prevalence and predictors of HIV-associated weight loss in the era of highly active antiretroviral therapy. *International Journal of STD & AIDS, 13*(11), 744–747.

Bhandari, N., Mazumder, S., Taneja, S., Dube, B., Black, R. E., Fontaine, O., et al. (2005). A pilot test of the addition of zinc to the current case management package of diarrhea in a primary health care setting. *Journal of Pediatric Gastroenterology & Nutrition, 41*(5), 685–687.

Bjarnason, I., Sharpstone, D. R., Francis, N., Marker, A., Taylor, C., Barrett, M., et al. (1996). Intestinal inflammation, ileal structure and function in HIV. *AIDS, 10*(12), 1385–1391.

Bouhnik, A. D., Preau, M., Schiltz, M. A., Obadia, Y., Spire, B., & the VESPA Group (2008). Sexual difficulties in people living with HIV in France--results from a large representative sample of outpatients attending French hospitals (ANRS-EN12-VESPA). *AIDS & Behavior, 12*(4), 670–676.

Bova, C. (2001). Adjustment to chronic illness among HIV-infected women. *Journal of Nursing Scholarship, 33*(3), 217–223.

Brashers, D. E., Neidig, J. L., & Goldsmith, D. J. (2004). Social support and the management of uncertainty for people living with HIV or AIDS. *Health Communication, 16*(3), 305–331.

Brooks, W. A., Santosham, M., Roy, S. K., Faruque, A. S., Wahed, M. A., Nahar, K., et al. (2005). Efficacy of zinc in young infants with acute watery diarrhea. *American Journal of Clinical Nutrition, 82*(3), 605–610.

Cameron, J. E., & Hagensee, M. E. (2008). Oral HPV complications in HIV-infected patients. *Current HIV/AIDS Reports, 5*(3), 126–131.

Campisi, G., Pizzo, G., Mancuso, S., & Margiotta, V. (2001). Gender differences in human immunodeficiency virus-related oral lesions: An Italian study. *Oral Surgery Oral Medicine Oral Pathology Oral Radiology & Endodontics, 91*(5), 546–551.

Canani, R. B., Ruotolo, S., Buccigrossi, V., Passariello, A., Porcaro, F., Siani, M. C., et al. (2007). Zinc fights diarrhoea in HIV-1-infected children: In-vitro evidence to link clinical data and pathophysiological mechanism. *AIDS, 21*(1), 108–110.

Ceballos-Salobrena, A., Gaitan-Cepeda, L. A., Ceballos-Garcia, L., & Lezama-Del Valle, D. (2000). Oral lesions in HIV/AIDS patients undergoing highly active antiretroviral treatment including protease inhibitors: A new face of oral AIDS? *AIDS Patient Care & STDs, 14*(12), 627–635.

Chou, F. Y. (2004). Testing a predictive model of the use of HIV/AIDS symptom self-care strategies. *AIDS Patient Care & STDs, 18*(2), 109–117.

Chou, F. Y., Holzemer, W. L., Portillo, C. J., & Slaughter, R. (2004). Self-care strategies and sources of information for HIV/AIDS symptom management. *Nursing Research, 53*(5), 332–339.

Coleman, C. L., Eller, L. S., Nokes, K. M., Bunch, E., Reynolds, N. R., Corless, I. B., et al. (2006). Prayer as a complementary health strategy for managing HIV-related symptoms among ethnically diverse patients. *Holistic Nursing Practice, 20*(2), 65–72.

Coleman, C. L., & Holzemer, W. L. (1999). Spirituality, psychological well-being, and HIV symptoms for African Americans living with HIV disease. *Journal of the Association of Nurses in AIDS Care, 10*(1), 42–50.

Dodd, M., Janson, S., Facione, N., Faucett, J., Froelicher, E. S., Humphreys, J., et al. (2001). Advancing the science of symptom management. *Journal of Advanced Nursing, 33*(5), 668–676.

Eller, L. S., Corless, I., Bunch, E. H., Kemppainen, J., Holzemer, W., Nokes, K., et al. (2005). Self-care strategies for depressive symptoms in people with HIV disease. *Journal of Advanced Nursing, 51*(2), 119–130.

Evans, W. J., & Lambert, C. P. (2007). Physiological basis of fatigue. *American Journal of Physical Medicine & Rehabilitation, 86* (Suppl.1), S29–46.

Falco, V., Crespo, M., & Ribera, E. (2003). Lactic acidosis related to nucleoside therapy in HIV-infected patients. *Expert Opinion on Pharmacotherapy, 4*(8), 1321–1329.

Ferrando, S. (1998). Behavioral research on AIDS—protease inhibitors and the new millennium: Comment on Kelly, Otto-Salaj, Sikkema, Pinkerton, and Bloom (1998). *Health Psychology, 17*(4), 307–309.

Ferrando, S., Evans, S., Goggin, K., Sewell, M., Fishman, B., & Rabkin, J. (1998). Fatigue in HIV illness: Relationship to depression, physical limitations, and disability. *Psychosomatic Medicine, 60*(6), 759–764.

Floren, C. H., Chinenye, S., Elfstrand, L., Hagman, C., & Ihse, I. (2006). ColoPlus, a new product based on bovine colostrum, alleviates HIV-associated diarrhoea. *Scandinavian Journal of Gastroenterology, 41*(6), 682–686.

Gazzard, B. G., & Sharpstone, D. (1995). Management of diarrhoea in HIV infection. *AIDS, 9* (Suppl. A), S213–219.

Gifford, A. L., & Groessl, E. J. (2002). Chronic disease self-management and adherence to HIV medications. *Journal of Acquired Immune Deficiency Syndromes, 31* (Suppl. 3), S163–166.

Greenspan, D., & Greenspan, J. S. (1997). Oral manifestations of HIV infection. *AIDS Clinical Care, 9*(4), 29–33.

Grohmann, G. S., Glass, R. I., Pereira, H. G., Monroe, S. S., Hightower, A. W., Weber, R., et al. (1993). Enteric viruses and diarrhea in HIV-infected patients. Enteric Opportunistic Infections Working Group. *New England Journal of Medicine, 329*(1), 14–20.

Guaroldi, G., Luzi, K., Murri, R., Granata, A., De Paola, M., Orlando, G., et al. (2007). Sexual dysfunction in HIV-infected men: Role of antiretroviral therapy, hypogonadism and lipodystrophy. *Antiviral Therapy, 12*(7), 1059–1065.

Harding, R., Molloy, T., Easterbrook, P., Frame, K... & Higginson, I. J. (2006). Is antiretroviral therapy associated with symptom prevalence and burden? *International Journal of STD & AIDS, 17*(6), 400–405.

Heath, K. V., Singer, J., O'Shaughnessy, M. V., Montaner, J. S., & Hogg, R. S. (2002). Intentional nonadherence due to adverse symptoms associated with antiretroviral therapy. *Journal of Acquired Immune Deficiency Syndromes, 31*(2), 211–217.

Hench, K., Anderson, R., Grady, C., & Ropka, M. (1995). Investigating chronic symptoms in HIV: An opportunity for collaborative nursing research. *Journal of the Association of Nurses in AIDS Care, 6*(3), 13–17.

Henker, R., & Carlson, K. K. (2007). Fever: Applying research to bedside practice. *AACN Advanced Critical Care, 18*(1), 76–87.

Holzemer, W. L., Corless, I. B., Nokes, K. M., Turner, J. G., Brown, M. A., Powell-Cope, G. M., et al. (1999a). Predictors of self-reported adherence in persons living with HIV disease. *AIDS Patient Care & STDs, 13*(3), 185–197.

Holzemer, W. L., Henry, S. B., Nokes, K. M., Corless, I. B., Brown, M. A., Powell-Cope, G. M., et al. (1999b). Validation of the Sign and Symptom Check-List for Persons with HIV Disease (SSC-HIV). *Journal of Advanced Nursing, 30*(5), 1041–1049.

Holzemer, W. L., Hudson, A., Kirksey, K. M., Hamilton, M. J., & Bakken, S. (2001). The revised Sign and Symptom Check-List for HIV (SSC-HIVrev). *Journal of the Association of Nurses in AIDS Care, 12*(5), 60–70.

Hughes, J., Jelsma, J., Maclean, E., Darder, M., & Tinise, X. (2004). The health-related quality of life of people living with HIV/AIDS. *Disability & Rehabilitation, 26*(6), 371–376.

Jenkin, P., Koch, T., & Kralik, D. (2006). The experience of fatigue for adults living with HIV. *Journal of Clinical Nursing, 15*(9), 1123–1131.

Johnson, M. O., Catz, S. L., Remien, R. H., Rotheram-Borus, M. J., Morin, S. F., Charlebois, E., et al. (2003). Theory-guided, empirically supported avenues for intervention on HIV medication nonadherence: Findings from the Healthy Living Project. *AIDS Patient Care & STDs, 17*(12), 645–656.

Justice, A. C., Chang, C. H., Rabeneck, L., & Zackin, R. (2001a). Clinical importance of provider-reported HIV symptoms compared with patient-report. *Medical Care, 39*(4), 397–408.

Justice, A. C., Holmes, W., Gifford, A. L., Rabeneck, L., Zackin, R., Sinclair, G., et al. (2001b). Development and validation of a self-completed HIV symptom index. *Journal of Clinical Epidemiology, 54*(Suppl. 1), S77–90.

Justice, A. C., Rabeneck, L., Hays, R. D., Wu, A. W., & Bozzette, S. A. (1999). Sensitivity, specificity, reliability, and clinical validity of provider-reported symptoms: A comparison with self-reported symptoms. Outcomes Committee of the AIDS Clinical Trials Group. *Journal of Acquired Immune Deficiency Syndromes, 21*(2), 126–133.

Karus, D., Raveis, V. H., Alexander, C., Hanna, B., Selwyn, P., Marconi, K., et al. (2005). Patient reports of symptoms and their treatment at three palliative care projects servicing individuals with HIV/AIDS. *Journal of Pain & Symptom Management, 30*(5), 408–417.

Kelley, C. F., Barbour, J. D., & Hecht, F. M. (2007). The relation between symptoms, viral load, and viral load set point in primary HIV infection. *Journal of Acquired Immune Deficiency Syndromes, 45*(4), 445–448.

Kilbourne, A. M., Andersen, R. M., Asch, S., Nakazono, T., Crystal, S., Stein, M., et al. (2002). Response to symptoms among a U.S. national probability sample of adults infected with human immunodeficiency virus. *Medical Care Research & Review, 59*(1), 36–58.

Kluger, M. J., Kozak, W., Conn, C. A., Leon, L. R., & Soszynski, D. (1998). Role of fever in disease. *Annals of the New York Academy of Sciences, 856,* 224–233.

Kotler, D. P. (1999). Characterization of intestinal disease associated with human immunodeficiency virus infection and response to anti-retroviral therapy. *Journal of Infectious Diseases, 179* (Suppl. 3), S454–456.

Kotler, D. P., Gaetz, H. P., Lange, M., Klein, E. B., & Holt, P. R. (1984). Enteropathy associated with the acquired immunodeficiency syndrome. *Annals of Internal Medicine, 101*(4), 421–428.

Kotler, D. P., Giang, T. T., Thiim, M., Nataro, J. P., Sordillo, E. M., & Orenstein, J. M. (1995). Chronic bacterial enteropathy in patients with AIDS. *Journal of Infectious Diseases, 171*(3), 552–558.

Lee, K. A., Portillo, C. J., & Miramontes, H. (2001). The influence of sleep and activity patterns on fatigue in women with HIV/AIDS. *Journal of the Association of Nurses in AIDS Care, 12* (Suppl.), 19–27.

Lorenz, K. A., Shapiro, M. F., Asch, S. M., Bozzette, S. A., & Hays, R. D. (2001). Associations of symptoms and health-related quality of life: Findings from a national study of persons with HIV infection. *Annals of Internal Medicine, 134*(9 Pt. 2), 854–860.

Lubeck, D. P., Bennett, C. L., Mazonson, P. D., Fifer, S. K., & Fries, J. F. (1993). Quality of life and health service use among HIV-infected patients with chronic diarrhea. *Journal of Acquired Immune Deficiency Syndromes, 6*(5), 478–484.

Mathews, W. C., McCutchan, J. A., Asch, S., Turner, B. J., Gifford, A. L., Kuromiya, K., et al. (2000). National estimates of HIV-related symptom prevalence from the HIV Cost and Services Utilization Study. *Medical Care, 38*(7), 750–762.

Murphy, B., Taylor, C., Crane, R., Okong, P., & Bjarnason, I. (1999). Comparison of intestinal function in human immunodeficiency virus-seropositive patients in Kampala and London. *Scandinavian Journal of Gastroenterology, 34*(5), 491–495.

Navin, T. R., Weber, R., Vugia, D. J., Rimland, D., Roberts, J. M., Addiss, D. G., et al. (1999). Declining CD4+ T-lymphocyte counts are associated with increased risk of enteric parasitosis and chronic diarrhea: Results of a 3-year longitudinal study. *Journal of Acquired Immune Deficiency Syndromes & Human Retrovirology, 20*(2), 154–159.

O'Grady, N. P., Barie, P. S., Bartlett, J. G., Bleck, T., Garvey, G., Jacobi, J., et al. (1998). Practice guidelines for evaluating new fever in critically ill adult patients.Task Force of the Society of Critical Care Medicine and the Infectious Diseases Society of America. *Clinical Infectious Diseases, 26*(5), 1042–1059.

Palacio, H., Hilton, J. F., Canchola, A. J., & Greenspan, D. (1997). Effect of cigarette smoking on HIV-related oral lesions. *Journal of Acquired Immune Deficiency Syndromes & Human Retrovirology, 14*(4), 338–342.

Patel, A. B., Dhande, L. A., & Rawat, M. S. (2005). Therapeutic evaluation of zinc and copper supplementation in acute diarrhea in children: Double blind randomized trial. *Indian Pediatrics, 42*(5), 433–442.

Patton, L. L. (2000). Sensitivity, specificity, and positive predictive value of oral opportunistic infections in adults with HIV/AIDS as markers of immune suppression and viral burden. *Oral Surgery Oral Medicine Oral Pathology Oral Radiology & Endodontics, 90*(2), 182–188.

Reznik, D. A. (2005). Oral manifestations of HIV disease. *Topics in HIV Medicine, 13*(5), 143–148.

Richardson, D., Lamba, H., Goldmeier, D., Nalabanda, A., & Harris, J. R. (2006). Factors associated with sexual dysfunction in men with HIV infection. *International Journal of STD & AIDS, 17*(11), 764–767.

Shamir, R., Makhoul, I. R., Etzioni, A., & Shehadeh, N. (2005). Evaluation of a diet containing probiotics and zinc for the treatment of mild diarrheal illness in children younger than one year of age. *Journal of the American College of Nutrition, 24*(5), 370–375.

Sharma, A., Howard, A. A., Klein, R. S., Schoenbaum, E. E., Buono, D., & Webber, M. P. (2007). Body image in older men with or at-risk for HIV infection. *AIDS Care, 19*(2), 235–241.

Sharpstone, D., Neild, P., Crane, R., Taylor, C., Hodgson, C., Sherwood, R., et al. (1999). Small intestinal transit, absorption, and permeability in patients with AIDS with and without diarrhoea. *Gut, 45*(1), 70–76.

Siddiqui, U., Bini, E. J., Chandarana, K., Leong, J., Ramsetty, S., Schiliro, D., et al. (2007). Prevalence and impact of diarrhea on health-related quality of life in HIV-infected patients in the era of highly active antiretroviral therapy. *Journal of Clinical Gastroenterology, 41*(5), 484–490.

Siegel, K., Brown-Bradley, C. J., & Lekas, H. M. (2004). Strategies for coping with fatigue among HIV-positive individuals fifty years and older. *AIDS Patient Care & STDs, 18*(5), 275–288.

Simon, D. (1998). Evaluation of diarrhea in HIV-infected patients. *Gastrointestinal Endoscopy Clinics of North America, 8*(4), 857–867.

Simon, D., Kotler, D. P., & Brandt, L. J. (1996). Chronic unexplained diarrhea in human immunodeficiency virus infection: Determination of the best diagnostic approach. *Gastroenterology, 111*(1), 269–271.

Snijders, F., de Boer, J. B., Steenbergen, B., Schouten, M., Danner, S. A., & van Dam, F. S. (1998). Impact of diarrhoea and faecal incontinence on the daily life of HIV-infected patients. *AIDS Care, 10*(5), 629–637.

Sousa, K. H., Holzemer, W. L., Henry, S. B., & Slaughter, R. (1999). Dimensions of health-related quality of life in persons living with HIV disease. *Journal of Advanced Nursing, 29*(1), 178–187.

Sousa, K. H., Tann, S. S., & Kwok, O. M. (2006). Reconsidering the assessment of symptom status in HIV/AIDS care. *Journal of the Association of Nurses in AIDS Care, 17*(2), 36–46.

Spirig, R., Moody, K., Battegay, M., & De Geest, S. (2005). Symptom management in HIV/AIDS: Advancing the conceptualization. *Advances in Nursing Science, 28*(4), 333–344.

Sukati, N. A., Mndebele, S. C., Makoa, E. T., Ramukumba, T. S., Makoae, L. N., Seboni, N. M., et al. (2005). HIV/AIDS symptom management in Southern Africa. *Journal of Pain & Symptom Management, 29*(2), 185–192.

Tinmouth, J., Kandel, G., Tomlinson, G., Walmsley, S., Steinhart, H. A., & Glazier, R. (2007). Systematic review of strategies to measure HIV-related diarrhea. *HIV Clinical Trials, 8*(3), 155–163.

Trotta, M. P., Ammassari, A., Murri, R., Marconi, P., Zaccarelli, M., Cozzi-Lepri, A., et al. (2008). Self-reported sexual dysfunction is frequent among HIV-infected persons and is associated with suboptimal adherence to antiretrovirals. *AIDS Patient Care & STDs, 22*(4), 291–299.

Tsai, Y. F., Hsiung, P. C., & Holzemer, W. L. (2003). Validation of a Chinese version of the sign and symptom checklist for persons with HIV diseases. *Journal of Pain & Symptom Management, 25*(4), 363–368.

Tugizov, S., Herrera, R., Veluppillai, P., Greenspan, J., Greenspan, D., & Palefsky, J. M. (2007). Epstein-Barr virus (EBV)-infected monocytes facilitate dissemination of EBV within the oral mucosal epithelium. *Journal of Virology, 81*(11), 5484–5496.

Turner, M. J., Angel, J. B., Woodend, K., & Giguere, P. (2004). The efficacy of calcium carbonate in the treatment of protease inhibitor-induced persistent diarrhea in HIV-infected patients. *HIV Clinical Trials, 5*(1), 19–24.

Voss, J., Portillo, C. J., Holzemer, W. L., & Dodd, M. J. (2007). Symptom cluster of fatigue and depression in HIV/AIDS. *Journal of Prevention & Intervention in the Community, 33*(1–2), 19–34.

Voss, J. G., Dodd, M., Portillo, C., & Holzemer, W. (2006). Theories of fatigue: Application in HIV/AIDS. *Journal of the Association of Nurses in AIDS Care, 17*(1), 37–50.

Wang, W. C., Goldman, L. M., Schleider, D. M., Appenheimer, M. M., Subjeck, J. R., Repasky, E. A., et al. (1998). Fever-range hyperthermia enhances L-selectin-dependent adhesion of lymphocytes to vascular endothelium. *Journal of Immunology, 160*(2), 961–969.

Wanke, C. A., Mayer, H., Weber, R., Zbinden, R., Watson, D. A., & Acheson, D. (1998). Enteroaggregative Escherichia coli as a potential cause of diarrheal disease in adults infected with human immunodeficiency virus. *Journal of Infectious Diseases, 178*(1), 185–190.

Wantland, D. J., Holzemer, W. L., Moezzi, S., Willard, S. S., Arudo, J., Kirksey, K. M., et al. (2008). A randomized controlled trial testing the efficacy of an HIV/AIDS symptom management manual. *Journal of Pain & Symptom Management, 36*(3), 235–246.

Weber, R., Bryan, R. T., Owen, R. L., Wilcox, C. M., Gorelkin, L., & Visvesvara, G. S. (1992). Improved light-microscopical detection of microsporidia spores in stool and duodenal aspirates. The Enteric Opportunistic Infections Working Group. *New England Journal of Medicine, 326*(3), 161–166.

Weber, R., Ledergerber, B., Zbinden, R., Altwegg, M., Pfyffer, G. E., Spycher, M. A., et al. (1999). Enteric infections and diarrhea in human immunodeficiency virus-infected persons: Prospective community-based cohort study. *Swiss HIV Cohort Study. Archives of Internal Medicine, 159*(13), 1473–1480.

Wilcox, C. M. (1997). Chronic unexplained diarrhea in AIDS: Approach to diagnosis and management. *AIDS Patient Care & STDs, 11*(1), 13–17.

Yengopal, V., & Naidoo, S. (2008). Do oral lesions associated with HIV affect quality of life? *Oral Surgery Oral Medicine Oral Pathology Oral Radiology & Endodontics, 106*(1), 890–897.

9

HIV/AIDS Nursing Case Management Within the Global Community

DEBORAH GRITZMACHER
RICHARD L. SOWELL

The Joint United Nations Programme on HIV/AIDS (UNAIDS) of the World Health Organization (WHO) has reported that

> globally, less than one person in five at risk of HIV has access to basic HIV prevention services. Only 31% of people who needed HIV-related treatment had access to it by end 2007. The UNAIDS Secretariat along with their partner organizations, have undertaken consultations to define the concept and a framework for universal access to HIV/AIDS prevention, treatment and care by 2010. (WHO, 2008)

HIV/AIDS requires a comprehensive approach that coordinates all aspects of care and eliminates the fragmentation that has historically existed as a result of conflicts between prevention and treatment advocates. Prevention, treatment, and care efforts are complementary initiatives that require coordination.

Case management offers a useful framework for coordinating HIV/AIDS services. However, the evolution of HIV/AIDS treatments, the chronic nature of HIV/AIDS, the diverse populations requiring HIV/AIDS services, and the global impact of HIV/AIDS require a reconceptualization of case management. Additionally, the paramount role of treatment and care management in HIV/AIDS service delivery underscores the importance of a wide range of health care professionals in the delivery, coordination, treatment, and care of persons living with HIV/AIDS (PLWH). HIV prevention initiatives are also a key aspect of case management. A cost-effective use of resources, maximizing access

321

to care, and seeking the most optimal outcomes of care form the basic principles underpinning case management. The successful case manager needs to implement these principles in consideration of individual clients, norms of specific populations, and the availability of resources in widely varying environments. The work of case management is bounded by existing advantages, constraints, and beliefs or values. The right to have access to health care and to live without stigma and discrimination are basic human rights of persons with HIV infection (Greef et al., 2008) and serve as an important consideration in case management.

CASE MANAGEMENT

The need to provide cost-effective, evidence-based, comprehensive services to a diverse global population of PLWH is a significant challenge to health care providers and HIV/AIDS service organizations. Case management, which provides an organized approach to address these challenges, needs to be flexible enough to be useful both in resource-rich and resource-limited settings. Advances in medical treatment and physiological status monitoring that have made HIV/AIDS a chronic disease in Western countries may not be available in many remote regions and/ or in resource-limited countries. Yet, the case management approach can offer significant benefits in all settings by managing available care, linking individuals to available services, and serving as a tool for community development.

Historical Perspective

Case management is not a new concept. An early version of case management can be identified in the total care management approach of physicians and nurses in rural America. Early American physicians and nurses who were members of communities cared for their neighbors in the context of their local community and available resources. These community-based health care providers often went beyond strict medical treatment and/or nursing care to link clients to community resources or, when resources were not available, to create needed resources. In addition, formal community service coordination can be traced to the turn of the 20th century in public health nursing and social work (Fuszard et al., 1988). Nurses, from the beginning of the profession, have planned care by working with the patient, families, and communities and acting as purveyors of health care services to meet the needs of the patient and to facilitate collaboration. This coordinated approach is consistent with commonly accepted components of case management, including: case finding and screening, conducting comprehensive assessments, identifying problems (diagnosis), planning care, implementing and monitoring plans of care, and evaluating outcomes or reassessment (Porsche, 2000).

Case management, in concept, has been a part of nursing care for patients long before the HIV/AIDS pandemic. Nursing case management has been defined by the American Nurses Credentialing Center, a subsidiary of the American Nurses Association (ANA) (n.d.):

> [A] dynamic and systemic collaborative approach to provide and coordinate healthcare services to a defined population. Nurse case managers continually evaluate each individual's health plan and specific challenges and then seek to overcome obstacles that affect outcomes. A nurse case manager uses a framework that includes interaction, assessment, planning, implementation, and evaluation. . . . The nurse case manager may fulfill the roles of advocate, collaborator, facilitator, risk manage, educator, mentor, liaison, negotiator, consultant, coordinator, evaluator, and/or researcher.

This definition of case management is consistent with other definitions of case management. For example, the Case Management Society of America (CMSA) (2008) states that "Case Management is a collaborative process of assessment, planning, facilitation and advocacy for options and services to meet an individual's health needs through communications and available resources to promote quality cost-effective outcomes."

By definition, nurses are the ideal case managers for individuals who have chronic disease requiring both treatment and care management. The nursing process, according to the American Nurses Association (2008), is based on a tradition of assessment, nursing diagnosis, planning, implementation, and evaluation, all elements of case management. Job descriptions for case managers may demand basic licensure and/or certification as an advanced practice nurse, but master's-prepared social workers or experienced case workers with a history of providing care for families can also assume the title of case manager. (Qualified nurses may be certified as a case management nurse by the American Nurses Credentialing Center.) As HIV has evolved into a chronic condition, HIV case management includes the disease management model (i.e., the management of care from wellness through acute illness, rehabilitation, and wellness again). Nurse practitioners with special knowledge of the care needs of PLWH have been identified as health care professionals who can provide medical case management for this population (Kirton, Ferri, & Eleftherakis, 1999).

Existing case management models fall into four broad categories: the hospital model, the traditional model, the direct care model, and the gap-filling model (Porsche, 2000). The hospital model of case management has a primary focus on discharge planning. This approach to case management is short term and acute care oriented. Often the focus of this model is on containing costs by getting clients out of the hospital or finding placement for clients who do not need acute care but do not have home situations that allow discharge. The traditional case management model uses case managers to assess client needs and monitor them over a longer term, linking them to appropriate services that are available in the community. Ideally, the case manager is able to follow clients during hospital episodes as well as in the community. The traditional model might be viewed as resource identification and linkage. In many community-based case management programs, social workers have been effective case managers, especially when there is a high need for clients to gain access to social services such as housing assistance, transportation, and legal support (Sowell & Grier, 1995; Sowell & Meadows, 1994). The direct-care case management model is distinguished by the direct-care provider serving as the case manager or as a care manager. Clients who have complex treatment or direct-care needs that require careful coordination can most benefit from this approach to case management. The gap-filling model of case management is similar to the traditional model, with the additional authority for the case manager to purchase additional needed services or supportive resources for the client and/or family. Case management models observed in field situations are likely to contain elements of one or more of the four basic case management models. These models should be evaluated on the basis of the outcomes that they achieve for clients, measured both by cost containment and enhancement of quality of life.

HIV/AIDS Case Management

While the concept of case management continued to evolve in the 1960s and 1970s as a response to increasing health care cost and fragmentation, the advent of HIV/AIDS in the 1980s sparked a renewed interest in case management. The lack of infrastructure needed to respond to HIV/

AIDS, combined with the absence of HIV-related services in some rural communities, demanded a new approach to case management. HIV/AIDS case managers often not only had to help clients to access services but also had to create community services that were lacking and needed by their clients. Early HIV/AIDS case managers recognized the unique service needs of persons with HIV/AIDS and worked as advocates for them to gain access to existing health and social services.

HIV/AIDS-specific case management can be traced to the multisite HIV/AIDS demonstration projects funded by the Robert Wood Johnson Foundation, the Health Resources and Services Administration (HRSA), and the United States Public Health Service (USPHS) in 1986. These demonstration projects received funds to support care delivery and coordination programs in nine cities (Fleishman, Mor, & Laliberte, 1995). Based on the outcomes of these demonstration projects, HIV/AIDS case management was later formalized by federal legislation with the passage of the Ryan White Comprehensive AIDS Resources Emergency (CARE) Act of 1990. Many of the case management models resulting from the Ryan White CARE Act were community-based models using social workers to link clients to services in a community. In many instances, community case management and medical management remained completely separate and were poorly coordinated with little opportunity to interact or maintain a comprehensive record of the client's medical status and social situation as the client moved between acute treatment and the community.

The core processes of HIV/AIDS case management have remained essentially the same over the past 25 years, with client assessment, need identification, care planning, linkage to services, and ongoing evaluation of client outcomes and needs forming the foundation of the process. However, the evolution of HIV as a pandemic affecting diverse populations has led to changes in client needs, especially in light of the expansion of treatment options. Combating rejection and gaining access to experimental drug therapies were paramount issues for gay men who were first identified as having HIV/AIDS; groups becoming infected with HIV needed basic assistance such as drug treatment, food and housing, and child care. The hallmarks of HIV/AIDS case management have been flexibility and the ability to balance the needs of vastly diverse groups; however, all affected individuals and groups need assistance and advocacy in efforts to combat the stigma and discrimination that may prevent their full access to services and resources (Rao et al., 2008). (Also see Chapter 11.) Unfortunately, even with dramatic advancements in treatment and a more mainstream approach to HIV/AIDS treatment and care, significant challenges remain in combating HIV-related stigma and discrimination. These challenges require case managers to continue to serve as educators for the general public and as advocates for persons with HIV/AIDS (Mykhalovskiy et al., 2009).

There is growing recognition that the increasing complexity of treatment regimens and the chronic nature of HIV infection demand a rethinking of HIV/AIDS case management in which treatment management, provision of social services, and prevention efforts become more closely integrated into a comprehensive model of service delivery. Such a model may benefit from an interdisciplinary team approach in which health care, social service professionals, and community advocates form a comprehensive team able to address a wide range of client needs (Akerjordet & Severinsson, 2008; Clarke & Aiken, 2008). However, the successful management of HIV as a chronic disease with complex treatment regimens underscores the need for skilled nurses to serve in a leadership role in any case management model or team. While health care providers may believe that structure (Jeffrey, Xia, & Craig, 2007) and defined protocols (Hughes, Barber, & Nelson, 2008) assure confidence in the delivery of treatment, case managers require assessment skills that facilitate flexible and adaptable treatment and care interventions applicable to specific situations and clients with the goal of achieving acceptable outcomes using available and/or appropriate resources (Knebel et al., 2008).

The "prevention with positives" approach advocated by the President's Emergency Plan for AIDS Relief (PEPFAR) (2008), along with efforts by the Centers for Disease Control and Prevention (CDC) (2006), provide strategies to reduce new HIV infections using education and counseling of HIV-infected clients by health care providers. These strategies serve as driving forces for the reconceptualization of AIDS case management models. There is a need for a new model of case management that provides a comprehensive framework for the delivery and coordination of HIV/AIDS treatment, social services, and prevention education. Such a new model will require nurses, especially advanced-practice nurses, to take on greater responsibility as case managers to integrate treatment and care management with education and social service coordination. For such a case management model to be useful in the wider global community, it must be applied in light of the diversity of clients served and the availability of resources, including health professionals.

GLOBAL HIV/AIDS NURSING CASE MANAGEMENT MODEL

The Global HIV/AIDS Nursing Case Management Model developed by the authors and presented in Figure 9.1 provides a new or expanded conceptualization of case management. The Global Model provides a framework for HIV/AIDS treatment and service delivery coordination in a wide range of health care environments with various resource availabilities.

The case manager, in the role of primary provider, is responsible for designing and evaluating care so that the patient has cost-effective comprehensive services. The services are based on evidence from research and tradition in the patient's medical culture so that the resulting outcomes approximate the standards of care and meet the needs of the patient and family. This unique case manager–patient relationship takes into account client diversity and the case manager's role. Mutual respect of the client and case manager roles allows for optimal functioning and understanding during care. This model is fluid and overlapping to represent the ever-changing environment of HIV/AIDS.

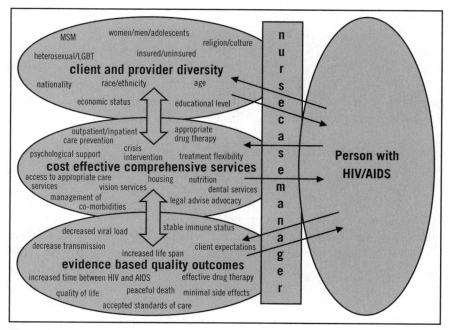

Figure 9.1 Global HIV/AIDS nursing case management model.

The Global HIV/AIDS Nursing Case Management Model recognizes and acknowledges the goals of case management used successfully in the United States and links those goals to a global perspective of the pandemic. In this model case managers conjoin HIV/AIDS patients with cost-effective comprehensive services and evidence-based quality outcomes while respecting not only the diversity of the patients (i.e., culture, sexual preference, and so on) but also the professional diversity of the case manager and the availability of resources. The model offers a revised framework that builds on a variety of previously identified case management models for the delivery of HIV/AIDS case management services. It underscores the need for adaptive practitioners to accommodate the needs and availability of services in diverse situations and regions. Additionally, the model acknowledges that individuals available to serve as case managers in different regions of the world may vary significantly. While Western medicine practitioners perceive an organized and coordinated system in a U.S. urban area, a rural resource-limited country will likely have a very different system of delivery. The goal of the case manager is to provide patients in the specific system with the best treatment and care management available at that place and time. As previously noted in this chapter, the increasing complexity of managing advanced drug therapies in the context of a physically and mentally devastating chronic disease requires a level of skill most notably found among advanced-practice nurses. In resource-limited regions where nurses provide a significant portion of treatment to persons with HIV/AIDS, the advanced-practice nurse may be the backbone of care and treatment coordination (case management) (Guberski, 2007). However, many regions and communities have no professional nurses, and lay or traditional healers provide treatment. The Global Model proposed here provides a broad enough framework to allow adaptation to such care delivery realities. While the advanced-practice nurse or physician is the preferred coordinator of treatment, these individuals must often work with local constituents and health care delivery systems to fully use the available resources such as local healers, tribal leaders, and support groups (Wools-Kaloustian & Kimaiyo, 2006). In many regions of the world, some of the most effective support for persons with HIV/AIDS has resulted from local community groups that have developed and coordinated community services, provided HIV/AIDS education, and advocated for the rights of HIV-infected individuals and their families (Gopalen & Pinsky, 2008). These activities supported PLWH long before drug therapies were available. The proposed case management model acknowledges the need to incorporate community-developed services into any care coordination system, even when drug therapies and professional providers become available. Additionally, the model's underpinnings acknowledge that advanced drug therapies and professional health care providers may not be readily available in many regions of the world (Wainberg & Jeang, 2008). Therefore, an important tenet of the model is the belief that all persons with HIV/AIDS deserve the best care coordination possible, thus requiring flexibility to build the local system on available services and personnel while continuing to strive for cost-effective care and services that produce quality outcomes.

Cost-Effective Comprehensive Services

Little evidence exits concerning direct costs for the case management of PLWH (Kumaranayake, 2008). Gilman and Green (2008) propose that efficient use of staff and shared affiliations save money and provide a cost savings with early intervention. These savings, however, rest more on patient characteristics and the time of entry into the system of care than on the treatment provided. In general, the highest costs result from the most complicated needs and more sophisticated treatments, which are more often linked to minority and indigent patients. However, some research supports the assertion that case management can decrease cost and increase the quality of care and service provided to clients (Leenerts, Koehler, & Neil, 1996; Sowell et al., 1992).

HIV infection rates continue to increase in many populations, and there are concerns that the required care will overwhelm the existing health care delivery systems serving these populations. It has been argued that providing appropriate levels of treatment and care to all persons with HIV/AIDS will destroy the health care system in many countries with a high incidence of HIV/AIDS (Lewis, 2005). Perhaps HIV/AIDS is underscoring the weaknesses or nonexistence of health care delivery in resource-limited countries. If it is accepted that health and adequate health care are basic rights (Castro & Farmer, 2005; Daniels, 1985) then developing new approaches to health care delivery and coordination of services is a mandate throughout the world. In those regions most affected by HIV/AIDS, the existence of other life-threatening diseases already requires attention to health care delivery and coordination. Malaria and tuberculosis (TB), for example, are copandemics with HIV/AIDS in many regions. Case managers are required to address these diseases in developing and implementing plans of care for persons with

HIV/AIDS (Farrington, 2008). The need to manage clients who may be dually infected with or at risk for more than one life-threatening disease adds to the complexity of treatment and care coordination. Additionally, the contagious nature of TB, as well as the resistance to treatment of some strains of TB, requires new approaches to care delivery and coordination (Farrington, 2008). In recent years, there has been growing recognition that any comprehensive approach to addressing HIV/AIDS in many regions of the globe will require inclusion of treatment for malaria and TB (Swaminathan et al., 2008). Rather than fragment the cost of care delivery for these overlapping pandemics, a more effective and cost-responsible model of health care delivery will bring treatment and care coordination for HIV/AIDS, malaria, and TB together in one system that fully uses limited resources.

A paramount consideration for health care providers and care coordinators is the problem of drug resistance and adherence to prescribed therapy (McPherson-Baker et al., 2005). If patients fail to adhere to prescribed therapy, HIV can mutate and become drug resistant (Harrigan et al., 2004), leading to less effective therapy and the potential of transmitting mutated virus. Theoretically, a person newly infected with mutated HIV could have drug-resistant virus, leading to challenges in prescribing an effective drug regimen and the earlier progression to AIDS. This situation makes adherence to drug therapy a critical issue in HIV/AIDS treatment. (See Chapter 7.)

The literature is replete with research seeking effective interventions to support drug therapy adherence (Osterberg & Blaschke, 2005; Safren et al., 2001; Shelton et al., 2006). While there has not been a definitive approach to achieving adherence to drug therapy, available research suggests that best results are achieved when the client receives support that assists him or her in identifying and overcoming barriers to adherence over time (Stirratt & Gordon, 2008); thus the development of a supportive relationship between a client and case manager offers a potentially effective strategy to support increased drug adherence. The provision of effective case management services should assist in identifying and addressing clients' other needs or concerns that can affect adherence to therapy. Case management has been associated with improved antiretroviral adherence (Katz et al., 2001; Kushel et al., 2006)

Drug side effects accompany all antiretroviral drug therapies. The most common are lipodystrophy, wasting, hyperlipidemia, fatigue, anemia, peripheral neuropathy, nausea, diarrhea, and hepatotoxicity

(AIDS Meds, 2007; Montessori et al., 2004). (See Chapter 7.) Case managers, working with primary health care providers, can assist clients in managing adverse side effects and developing strategies to maximize their quality of life while continuing to adhere to drug therapy. One important role for the case manager may be to assist the client in reporting to the primary health care provider the adverse effects drug therapy is having on his or her life situation and advocate for adjustment of therapy rather than discontinuing or not adhering to prescribed drug therapy.

HIV/AIDS PREVENTION AND CASE MANAGEMENT

According to a recent UNAIDS report, "The global HIV/AIDS pandemic shows no signs of being controlled, and gains in expanding treatment access may not be sustainable without greater progress in reducing the rate of new HIV infections (UNAIDS Global Report, 2008, p. 1)." The most cost-effective approach to HIV/AIDS is the prevention of HIV infection. In the United States, it is estimated that HIV/AIDS costs more than $500,000 from diagnosis to death (Schackman et al., 2006). Resources expended to prevent infection can have tremendous returns. However, prevention efforts are not maximized if these efforts are implemented as a separate strategy that does not include treatment and care efforts (Cohen, 2008).

HIV/AIDS prevention case management is a primary consideration both in decreasing the number of new HIV infections and in achieving cost-effective comprehensive services for persons with HIV/AIDS and their family. The goal of prevention case management is to provide the education and support needed by individuals to avoid or refrain from engaging in behaviors that increase the risk for HIV transmission; therefore, prevention case management targets both HIV-negative and HIV-positive individuals. Aspects of prevention case management include education, advocacy, psychological support, and treatment strategies.

In the United States, the primary health care provider is expected to furnish counseling about safer sexual practices and testing to every patient and the family or significant other of that patient (CDC, 2006). This initiative is built on the assumption that known HIV-infected persons and PLWH receiving care are more easily accessible than the uninfected population. However, management of the disease, including immune status monitoring, drug regimen alternations, and physical assessments, is often a primary focus of physicians and other primary care providers. Effective treatment is targeted at decreasing viral load so that HIV-infected individuals have less chance of transmitting the virus. Medical management of HIV/AIDS may leave little time for education and ongoing support needed to facilitate risk behavior change. Prevention case managers work, over time, with HIV-infected clients to increase knowledge and decrease risk behaviors that can result in a lower risk of transmitting HIV.

HIV testing is not mandatory in the United States, but the value of individuals knowing their HIV serostatus is widely viewed as a key component of HIV/AIDS prevention. (See Chapters 2 and 5.) Prevention case managers play an important role in providing information to clients who have not been tested for HIV infection or who previously tested HIV negative. Those clients who are at increased risk for infection but resist being tested can be offered counseling and made aware that early treatment may decrease viral load, which lessens the chance of infecting a partner and may preserve immune function (Capiluppi et al., 2000). Additionally, induction-maintenance therapy can reduce overall costs of HIV/AIDS treatment and care (Curlin, Wilkin, & Mittler, 2008). (Induction regimens [often using three drugs] reduce therapy-resistant pathogens to levels that can be controlled using a maintenance regimen.)

Prevention of mother-to-baby transmission of HIV infection as result of early identification and treatment of women who are HIV infected has resulted in substantial cost saving and decrease in morbidity in the United States (Sansom et al., 2007). (See Chapter 13.) Routine HIV testing is offered and encouraged for all pregnant women, both in the prenatal period and during labor and delivery in the United States (CDC, 2003). Prevention case management offers an effective strategy for decreasing perinatal transmission of HIV by providing a mechanism for a case manager to work with HIV-infected women or women at high risk to address their medical and psychosocial needs. This work facilitates adherence to drug therapies by HIV-infected women and the monitoring of HIV serostatus during pregnancy if not initially infected.

Worldwide perinatal prevention interventions have been much more difficult. The powerlessness of women in a male-dominated society leaves many women susceptible to infection. It is unlikely that women in many parts of the world can request condom use. Rape of women is not uncommon (Mardorossian, 2002). In addition, women often have limited access to drug therapy and medical care.

The case manager, whether a health care provider such as a registered nurse or a nonprofessional health worker, has a significant role to play in achieving cost-effective care coordination that reaches established outcome goals. Regardless of the care delivery setting, the case manager will need to do a thorough health assessment of the client, including identification of psychological and sociologic needs. This assessment becomes the basis for the delivery of cost-effective services to the client. Table 9.1 provides a list of key questions that will assist the case manager to obtain necessary care and service planning information. With answers to these essential questions, case managers can more effectively complete the task of developing and implementing a plan that supports cost-effective comprehensive services to all clients.

Evidence-Based Quality Outcomes

Increasingly, international health advocacy groups and organizations have developed standards of care and treatment for PLWH (WHO, 2004). These standards of treatment and care provide case managers worldwide with guidelines for establishing and obtaining appropriate case management and care outcomes. The case manager's role includes identification

Table 9.1

QUESTIONS USED TO OBTAIN COMPREHENSIVE CARE PLANNING DATA

1 What are the immediate needs of the patient?

2 What resources are available in the environment?

3 Is the case manager delivering direct treatment and care?

4 What patient characteristics must be considered when planning care?

5 What other personnel or groups are assisting with the treatment and care of the client?

6 Does the client have, or is he or she at risk for, other life-threatening conditions?

7 What community and cultural norms must be considered?

8 What outcomes do the client and family identify and expect?

9 How are collaborative relationships initiated and maintained to provide care for the client?

10 How can the case management system provide help with the resources that are not currently available in the client?

11 What is the client's level of HIV prevention knowledge, and what prevention strategies are in place and being used?

12 Are there needed services that are not available but could be developed?

of appropriate goals of service delivery and the determination of specific strategies to reach these goals within the practice environment.

Evidence-based quality outcomes for U.S. PLWH may encompass decreased viral loads, improved immunity, increased time between HIV diagnosis and progression to AIDS, and effective drug therapy with minimal side effects. In resource-limited countries, outcomes may be limited to assistance with nutrition, treating symptoms, safety, and helping to minimize stigma and discrimination. An essential part of providing case management in any practice environment is recognizing and deploying those services that are attainable without denigrating the efforts of other caregivers, including nontraditional caregivers. A number of different systems of case management have been effective in responding to clients' needs in the context of available resources and acceptable cultural traditions.

Evidence-based practice is designed to meet the needs of clients and families by achieving quality outcomes that are established from empirical research that is accepted and respected by current practitioners through professional organizations. Standards of care or practice are most often established by professional organizations, review panels, and oversight boards based on the evidence from controlled trials and published research that is translated into clinical procedures, methods, and/or outcomes. Evidence-based practices may be identified in consultation with other practitioners or may be based on the clinical experience from a specific practice (Melnyk & Fineout-Overholt, 2005). A key to evidence-based outcomes is that the practitioner's interventions are accepted principles in particular situations, and the practitioner has a reasonable expectation that a given outcome will result from an intervention.

Within the context of the Global HIV/AIDS Nursing Case Management Model, a quality outcome requires that it be established in collaboration with the client. Many health care providers have great difficulty relinquishing treatment or outcome control to the client and family, who may have specific expectations or needs. The practitioner's goal may be to fix the problem; however, the education and experience of that practitioner influences the ability to let go if the client's decisions do not coincide with what the practitioner thinks is best (Alexander, 2008). "Best care" as identified by health care providers and PLWH (Laschinger et al., 2004) involves "communication, collaboration, compassion, respect, and support" (p. 40) and encompasses both practitioner and the team involved in providing care, as well as the client, significant other, and/or family. When direct-care providers serve as case managers, it may be especially important for all aspects of practitioner–client interaction to be based on these principles.

It is essential that case manager and administrators of case management systems establish standards of care and service from which clear outcomes, expectations, or goals can be derived and evaluated. Such standards serve as a necessary road map to achieving quality outcomes (Grier & Sowell, 1993; Sowell & Grier, 1995). Quality outcomes of case management for persons with HIV/AIDS can include clinical outcomes, psychological outcomes, sociological outcomes, and spiritual outcomes. While nurse case managers may be most comfortable focusing on clinical outcomes, the delivery of comprehensive services requires attention to all aspects of the client. Failing to address issues that fall into the psychological or social domains can result in exacerbation of clinical issues that result in increased cost and poor client outcomes. Nurse case managers working in more acute settings need to keep in mind that the role of the case manager is to collaborate and refer clients to insure they receive the care and services needed.

Yet another source for standards of service and acceptable case management outcomes is found in the law. The legal issues surrounding HIV/AIDS will differ according to the laws of the country where care is rendered; thus case managers need to be familiar with the law in their country as they develop plans of care for clients or prepare to advocate to services for specific groups of clients. In many regions, women and children have few rights, and failure to understand the impact of codified or common law that affects these clients can adversely affect clients' safety and well-being (Gaillard et al., 2002). In developed countries such as the United States, case managers must be familiar with any state requirements specific to their practice and aware of the patient's rights, responsibilities, and available assistance. Table 9.2 provides a list of life situations that can qualify a person with HIV/AIDS to obtain legal assistance.

Diversity

HIV/AIDS infects individuals without regard to race, age, income, sex, sexual preference, social standing, or any other demographic descriptor. Rather than being a punishment for evil or being possessed by spirits, a belief of some cultures and religions, HIV infection is the result of human behaviors commonly found across cultures and groups that place an individual in intimate contact with HIV-infected body fluids. The causative agent of AIDS and modes of HIV transmission have

Table 9.2

EXAMPLES OF QUALIFYING SITUATIONS FOR LEGAL ASSISTANCE

If an individual is HIV positive, the Legal Aid Society can help if the client:

- Cannot take care of a child
- Needs help with distribution of property
- Needs help handling money or property
- Needs help with medical decisions and advanced directives
- Is unable to pay hospital bills
- Needs bankruptcy advice
- Needs help with a current job and rights as an employee
- Needs help with Medicare Part B coinsurance
- Needs help with COBRA
- Needs help with debt collectors
- Needs help with assistance programs
- Was denied Social Security
- Is dealing with unauthorized HIV status disclosure
- Was denied Medicaid, Medicare, or food stamps

Source: John Warchol, Esq. and Marcus Johns, Esq., Atlanta Legal Aid Society.

been clearly established in science. However, the diversity represented in those infected with and affected by HIV/AIDS makes appropriate response efforts to the pandemic challenging because of wide variations in education, treatment, and care delivery strategies. Cultural norms and traditions, attitudes and beliefs about disease, and existing approaches to health care and symptom management will influence, among different groups, those strategies that will be accepted and effective in responding to the many issues surrounding HIV/AIDS. How diversity is accepted and interpreted by case managers can profoundly affect all interactions with and understanding by an HIV-positive patient.

Case managers must understand diversity, whether that diversity is lifestyle choice, sexual preference, race, culture, knowledge level, material wealth, or nationality, among a vast list of diversities, and learn to respond to the need of the patient without bias. A best practice is exhibited when case managers are aware and understand that working with diverse clients requires a conscious effort. Case managers must never assume that because a protocol has been established, it covers every patient (Alexander, 2008). Misunderstanding on the part of the provider or the patient can lead to mistrust and nonadherence to treatment. A trusting relationship between the case manager and the patient serves as a key component of effective case management.

Case managers need to strive to understand bias and respect the diversity of each individual and cultural group requiring HIV/AIDS care to provide appropriate care within the bounds of a patient's needs and wishes. However, within these bounds the case managers need to remain cognizant of their role in providing cost-effective care that is based on established standards of care and outcomes goals. This mandate may be a particular challenge for case managers who engage clients whose cultural expectations and/or group traditions are in direct conflict with established standards of care or equitable allocation of resources to the overall client group being served. The challenge for the case manager is to maintain as much flexibility as possible in supporting the individual clients while continuing to meet established outcome expectation of the case management system.

Just as there is diversity in the global HIV/AIDS client population, there can be great diversity among case managers. In the United States alone, case managers may come from diverse cultural, ethnic, and educational backgrounds. Additionally, case managers can represent a number of professional disciplines, including nursing, advanced-practice nursing, social work, ministry, and allied health. Globally, case managers may be lay healers or shamans, traditional medicine providers, or essentially anyone who is willing to provide care. This diversity in both potential case management clients and potential case managers supports the need for a global model of HIV/AIDS case management that acknowledges and embraces this diversity while providing a framework to organize key components of the case management process.

In the United States, members of ethnic minority groups have felt a disproportionate impact from the HIV/AIDS epidemic. Addressing U.S. minorities, case managers are warned that "the lack of culturally competent service providers . . . challenges receiving quality healthcare . . . and may result in . . . cultural mistrust" (Adimora et al., 2008, p. 117). Mistrust can lead to misperceptions of patients by health care providers and patient nonadherence to treatment, placing HIV-infected patients at a distinct disadvantage. All case managers need to know that cultural misunderstanding can severely affect a patient's care but can be avoided with reflection and continued learning (Alexander, 2008).

Another approach to understanding diversity and developing cultural competence is immersion in different cultures. Whether one is a student or a new case manager unfamiliar with the client base, observing how people with different perceptions interact in daily life is a valued teaching tool (Haack, 2008). Caceres, Aggleton, and Galea (2008) looked at the attitude in most countries permitting "social exclusion" of men who have sex with men and transgender individuals. However, the inequality extends to other subcultures with political practices that favor those in power and exclude other groups. In many countries, women are powerless and are vulnerable in societies where their partners' extramarital sex is not seen as a problem (Benefo, 2008). Case managers need to be aware of how accepted behaviors can have an impact on risk. Reconciling services to accommodate diverse cultures, beliefs, religions, lifestyles, ages, and income and education levels remains a challenge to effective case managers.

CONCLUSION

Case management has a long history rooted in the coordination of care provided by nurses and other health professionals in both the community and care delivery systems. The primary goal of case management is to coordinate care and services for clients in a way that supports high-quality outcomes and the cost-effective use of available resources. HIV/AIDS-specific case management evolved out of the need to address the lack of or fragmentation of care and services provided to persons with HIV/ AIDS. HIV/AIDS case managers initially sprang from affected communities with the additional role of advocating for needed care and services for a population facing rejection, stigma, and discrimination. Even though advances in drug therapy, treatment modalities, and access to care have extended the lives of HIV-infected persons in more developed countries, case management continues to be critical for care and treatment coordination that supports the appropriate use of health care and social services. Linking clients to appropriate levels of care and service with the goal of managing cost of care remains a central focus of case management efforts. The concept of comprehensive, cost-effective services in HIV/AIDS now includes education and prevention initiatives as part of case management.

HIV/AIDS is a global pandemic affecting all regions and groups. The growing complexity of HIV/AIDS treatment, the increasing diversity of those individuals and groups affected by HIV infection, and the disparity of accessible resources requires a rethinking of current models of care coordination. The need to prescribe and monitor drug therapies, evaluate immune markers, and identify potential side effects of prescribed therapy across the stages of a chronic illness underscore the value of having nurses, especially advanced practice nurses, serve as care coordinators or case managers. Because the scope of the potential needs of persons with HIV/AIDS and their significant others is broad, nurse case managers must work with an interdisciplinary team whose skills and knowledge can be applied to achieve desired case management outcomes. In resource-limited regions, this team may include community elders, traditional care providers, and religious leaders who work in collaboration with professionally trained health care and social service workers.

The HIV/AIDS Nursing Case Management Model that has been proposed in this chapter provides an expanded view of HIV/AIDS case management that can serve as a framework for delivery and coordination of services to individuals with HIV/AIDS in the global community. The model acknowledges the diversity of individuals affected by HIV/AIDS, as well as disparities in services and resources available to address the needs of persons with HIV/AIDS. However, the model provides a useful tool conceptualizing the organization of available resources, as well as considering what standards of care and outcome goals are culturally acceptable and appropriate in the context of the environment. The model offers a fluid approach to care and service organization and delivery that acknowledges that the actual case management content and process may look quite different in different regions and communities based on a variety of variables such as availability of health care providers, cultural norms and traditions, and attitudes and expectations of clients. Yet the core components outlined in the HIV/AIDS Nursing Case Management Model are essential elements of any successful approach to care coordination and/or case management systems.

REFERENCES

Adimora, A., Britton, C., Caine, V., Carter, G., Clark, M., Fraser-Howze, et al. (2008). Consensus report of the National Medical Association:

Addressing the HIV/AAIDS crisis in the African American community: Fact, fiction, and policy HIV/AIDS consensus panel. *Journal of the National Medical Association, 100*(1), 117–129.

AIDS Meds. (n.d.) *Currently approved drugs for HIV: A comparative chart.* Retrieved May 11, 2007, from www.aidsmeds.com/articles/DrugChart_10632.shtml.

Akerjordet, K., & Severinsson, E. (2008). Emotionally intelligent nurse leadership: A literature review study. *Journal of Nursing Management, 16*(5), 565–577.

Alexander, G. (2008). Cultural competence models in nursing. *Critical Care Nursing Clinics of North America, 20*(4), 415–421.

American Nurses Association (2008). *The nursing process: A common thread amongst all nurses.* Retrieved November 15, 2008, from www.nursingworld.org/EspeciallyForYou/StudentNurses/Thenursingprocess.aspx.

American Nurses Credentialing Center. (n.d.). *Nursing case management.* Retrieved November 15, 2008, from www.nursecredentialing.org/Documents/Certification/Application/NursingSpecialty/CaseManagementApplication.aspx.

Benefo, K. (2008). Determinants of Zambian men's extra marital sex: A multi-level analysis. *Archives of Sexual Behavior, 37*(4), 517–529.

Caceres, C., Aggleton, P., & Galea, J. (2008). Social diversity, social inclusion, and HIV/AIDS. *AIDS, 22* (Suppl 2), 45–55.

Capiluppi, B., Cuiffreda, D., Quinzan, G. P., Sciandra, M., Marroni, M., Morandini, B., et al. (2000). Four drug-HAART in primary HIV-1 infection: Clinical benefits and virologic parameters. *Journal of Biological Regulators Homeostatic Agents, 14*(1), 58–62.

Case Management Society of America (2008). Retrieved November 15, 2008, from www.cmsa.org/Home/CSMA/WhatisaCaseManager/tabid/224/Default.aspx.

Castro, A., & Farmer, P. (2005). Understanding and addressing AIDS-related stigma: From anthropological theory to clinical practice in Haiti. *American Journal of Public Health, 95*(1), 53–59.

Centers for Disease Control and Prevention. (2003). Advancing HIV prevention: New strategies for a changing epidemic. *Morbidity and Mortality Weekly Report, 52*(15), 339–332.

Centers for Disease Control and Prevention. (2006). Revised recommendations for HIV testing of adults, adolescents, and pregnant women in health care settings. *Morbidity and Mortality Weekly Report, 55*(RR-14), 1–17.

Clarke, S., & Aiken, L. (2008). An international hospital outcomes research agenda focused on nursing: Lessons from a decade of collaboration. *Journal of Clinical Nursing, 17*(24), 3317–3323.

Cohen, J. (2008). Treatment and prevention exchange vows at international conference. *Science, 321*(5891), 902–903.

Curlin, M., Wilkin, T., & Mittler, J. (2008). Induction-maintenance therapy for HIV-1 infection. *Future HIV Therapy, 2*(2), 175–185.

Daniels, N. (1985). *Just health care.* London: Cambridge University Press.

Farrington, A. (2008). Partnerships to support global health. *Microbe, 3*(8), 367–369.

Fleishman, J., Mor, V., & Laliberte, L. (1995). Longitudinal patterns of medical service use and costs among people with AIDS. *Health Services Research, 30*(3), 403–424.

Fuszard, B., Bowman, R., Howell, H., Malioski, A. Morrison, C., & Wahlstedt, P. (1988). *Nursing case management.* Washington, DC: American Nurses Association.

Gaillard, P., Melis, R., Mwanyumba, F., Claeys, P., Muigai, E., Mandaliya, K., et al. (2002). Vulnerability of women in African setting: Lessons for mother-to-child HIV transmission prevention programmes. *AIDS, 16*(6), 937–939.

Gilman, B., & Green, J. (2008). Understanding the variation in cost among HIV primary care providers. *AIDS care—Psychological and socio-medical aspects of AIDS/HIV, 20*(9), 1050–1056.

Gopalen, P., & Pinsky, B. (2008). African housing organizations respond to the HIV and AIDS crisis. *Open House International, 33*(4), 8–15.

Greef, M., Uys, L., Holzemer, W., Makoae, L., Diamini, P., Kohi, T., et al. (2008). Experiences of HIV/AIDS stigma of persons living with HIV/AIDS and nurses involved in their care from five African countries. *African Journal of Nursing and Midwifery, 10*(1), 78–108.

Grier, J., & Sowell, R. (1993). Standards and evaluation in community-based case management. *Journal of the Association of Nurses in AIDS Care, 4*(1), 32–33.

Guberski, T. (2007). Nurse practitioners, HIV/AIDS, and nursing in resource-limited settings. *Journal for Nurse Practitioners, 3*(10), 695–702.

Haack, S. (2008). Engaging pharmacy students with diverse populations to improve cultural competence. *American Journal of Pharmaceutical Education, 72*(5), 1–6.

Harrigan, P. R., Hogg, R. S., Dong, W. W., Yip, B., Wynhoven, B., Woodward, J., et al. (2004). Predictors of HIV drug-resistance mutations in a large antiretroviral-naïve cohort initiating triple antiretroviral therapy. *The Journal of Infectious Diseases, 191*(3), 339–347.

Hughes, A., Barber, T., & Nelson, M. (2008). New treatment options for HIV salvage patients: An overview of second generation PIs, NNRTIs, integrase inhibitors, and CCR5 antagonists. *Journal of Infection, 57*(1), 1–10.

Jeffrey, A., Xia, X., & Craig, I. (2007). Structured treatment interruptions: A control mathematical approach to protocol design. *Journal of Process Control, 17*(1), 586–590.

Katz, M., Cunningham, W., Fleishman, J., Andersen, R., Kellogg, T, Bozzette, S., et al. (2001). Effect of case management on unmet needs and utilization of medical care and medications among HIV-infected persons. *Annals of Internal Medicine, 135*, 557–565.

Kirton, C., Ferri, R., & Eleftherakis, V. (1999). Primary care and case management of persons with HIV/AIDS. *Nursing Clinics of North America, 34*, 71–94.

Knebel, E., Puttkammer, N., Demes, A., Devirois, R., & Prismy, M. (2008). Developing a competency-based curriculum in HIV for nursing schools in Haiti. *Human Resources for Health*, 6–17.

Kumaranayake, L. (2008). The economics of scaling up: Cost estimation for HIV/AIDS interventions. *AIDS, 22* (Suppl. 1), 23–33.

Kushel, M., Colfax, G., Ragland, K., Heineman, A., Palacio, H., & Bangsberg, D. (2006). Case management is associated with improved antiretroviral adherence and CD4+ cell counts in homeless and marginally housed individuals with HIV infection. *Clinical Infectious Diseases, 43*, 234–242.

Laschinger, S., Van Manen, L., Stevenson, T., & Fothergill-Bourbonnais, F. (2004). Health care providers' and patients' perspectives on care in HIV ambulatory clinics across Ontario. *Journal of the Association of Nurses in AIDS Care, 16*(1), 37–48.

Leenerts, M., Koehler, J., & Neil, R. (1996). Nursing care models increase care quality while reducing costs. *Journal of the Association of Nurses in AIDS Care, 7*(4), 37–49.

Lewis, M. (2005, April). Addressing the challenge of HIV/AIDS: Macroeconomic, fiscal and institutional issues. Retrieved November 2008 from http://ssrn.com/abstract=997375.

Mardorossian, C. (2002). Toward a new feminist theory of rape. *Journal of Women in Culture and Society, 27*(3), 743–776.

McPherson-Baker, S., Jones, D., Duran, R., Kilmas, N., & Schniederman, N. (2005). Development and implementation of a medication adherence training instrument for persons living with HIV. *Behavior Modification, 29*(2), 286–317.

Melnyk, B., & Fineout-Overholt, E. (2005). *Evidence-based practice in nursing and healthcare.* New York: Lippincott Williams & Wilkins.

Montessori, V., Press, N., Harris, M., Akagi, L., & Montaner, J. S. (2004). Adverse effects of antiretroviral therapy for HIV infection. *Canadian Medical Association Journal, 170*(2), 229–238.

Mykhalovskiy, E., Patten, S., Sanders, C., Bailey, M., & Taylor, D. (2009). Beyond buzzwords: Toward a community-based model of the integration of HIV treatment and prevention. *AIDS Care—Psychological and Socio-Medical Aspects of AIDS/HIV, 21*(1), 25–30.

Osterberg, L., & Blaschke, T. (2005). Adherence to medication. *The New England Journal of Medicine, 353*(5), 487–497.

Porsche, D. (2000). Principles of HIV case management. In J. Durham & F. Lashley (Eds.), *The person with HIV/AIDS: Nursing perspectives* (pp. 387–400). New York: Springer Publishing.

President's Emergency Plan for AIDS Relief (PEPFAR). (2008). *PEPFAR: A commitment renewed.* Retrieved November 2008 from www.PEPFAR.gov.

Rao, D., Pryor, J. B., Gaddist, B. W., & Mayer, R. (2008). Stigma, secrecy, and discrimination: Ethnic/racial differences in the concerns of people living with HIV/AIDS. *AIDS and Behavior, 12*(2), 265–271.

Ryan White Comprehensive AIDS Resources Emergency ACT (2006). Retrieved November 2008 from http://hab.hrsa.gov/law.htm.

Safren, S., Otto, M., Worth, J., Salomon, E., Johnson, W., Mayer, K., et al. (2001). Two strategies to increase adherence to HIV antiretroviral medication: Life-Steps and medication monitoring. *Behavior Research and Therapy, 39*(10), 1151–1162.

Sansom, S., Harris, N., Sadek, R., Lampe, M., Ruffo, N., & Fowler, M. (2007). Towards elimination of perinatal human immunodeficiency virus transmission in the United States: Effectiveness of funded prevention programs, 1999–2001. *American Journal of Obstetrics and Gynecology, 197* (Suppl. 3), S90–S95.

Schackman, B. R., Gebo, K. A., Walensky, R. P., Losina, E., Muccio, T., Sax, P. E., et al. (2006). The lifetime cost of current human immunodeficiency virus care in the united states. *Medical Care, 44*(11), 990–997.

Shelton, R. C., Golin, C. E., Smith, S. R., Eng, E., & Kaplan, A. (2006). Role of the HIV/AIDS case manager: Analysis of a case management adherence training and coordination program in North Carolina. *AIDS Patient Care and STDs, 20*(3), 193–204.

Sowell, R., & Grier, J. (1995). Integrated case management: The AID Atlanta model. *Journal of Case Management, 4*(1), 15–21.

Sowell, R., Gueldner, S., Killeen, M., Lowenstein, A., Fuszard, B., & Swansburg, R. (1992). Impact of case management on hospital charges of PWAs in Georgia. *Journal of Nurses in AIDS Care, 3*(2), 24–31.

Sowell, R., & Meadows, T. (1994). An integrated case management model: Developing standards, evaluation, and outcome criteria. *Nursing Administration Quarterly, 18*(2), 53–64.

Stirratt, M. J., & Gordon, C. M. (2008). Adherence to biomedical HIV prevention methods: Considerations drawn from HIV treatment adherence research. *Current HIV/AIDS Reports, 5*(4), 186–192.

Swaminathan, S., Hanna, L., Sundaramurthi, J., Lenord, A., Angayarkanni, B., Francis, A., et al. (2008). Prevalence and pattern of cross-reaching antibodies to HIV in patients with tuberculosis. *AIDS Research and Human Retroviruses, 24*(7), 941–946.

UNAIDS Global Report (2008). Preventing new HIV infections: The key to reversing the epidemic. Retrieved November 2008 from http://data.unaids.org/pub/GlobalReport/ 2008/jc1510_2008_global_report_pp95_128_en.pdf.

Wainberg, M. A., & Jeang, K. (2008). *25 years of HIV-1 research - progress and perspectives.* BMC Medicine, 6, 31–31. Retrieved February 25, 2009, from Cinahl Plus with Full Text databases.

Warchol, J., & Marcus, J. (2008). *Aid Atlanta on . . . HIV and the law* [Abstract]. Atlanta, GA: Atlanta Legal Aid Society.

Wools-Kaloustian, K, & Kimaiyo, S. (2006). Extending HIV care in resource-limited settings. *Current HIV/AIDS Reports, 3*(4), 182–186.

World Health Organization (WHO). (2004). *Standards for quality HIV care: A tool for quality assessment, improvement, and accreditation.* Retrieved November 2008 from www.emro.who.int/aiecf/web94.pdf.

World Health Organization (WHO). (2008). *Towards Universal Access.* Geneva: Author. Retrieved February 15, 2009, from www.who.int/hiv/pub/towards_universal_access_report_2008.pdf.

Special Populations

SECTION
III

10 Caregivers of People Living with HIV Disease: Core Concerns and Issues

JOAN S. GRANT
NORMAN L. KELTNER
JAMES L. RAPER

Formal and informal caregivers encounter significant challenges in meeting demands of caregiving to persons living with HIV/AIDS (PLWH) (UNAIDS, 2008; Sheriff, 2009). This chapter discusses stigma, caregiver burden, and grief related to loss as these relate to caregivers of PLWH. Global strategies for addressing these caregiving issues include: (1) identifying important caregiving problems and skills, (2) developing effective coping strategies, and (3) using community resources to assist caregivers.

Because medical treatment has dramatically improved survival rates in persons living with HIV (PLWH), especially since the introduction of highly active antiretroviral therapy (HAART) in 1995 (Delgado et al., 2003), many people now live with this chronic long-term disease. (Global epidemiologic data for HIV/AIDS are presented in Chapter 1.) Knowing the global impact of HIV/AIDS assists heath professionals to better appreciate the importance of caregiving as it relates to PLWH.

American populations most affected by HIV/AIDS are increasingly poor, marginalized, and uninsured or publicly insured. African Americans and Latinos now represent the majority of new AIDS cases and PLWH in the United States. Women and youth also are experiencing rapid increases in rates of HIV infection. HIV incidence remains high among men who have sex with men (MSM) and injection drug users, with young African American MSM experiencing particularly high rates of new infections. Of significance importance, approximately 56,300 people were newly infected with HIV in 2006, the most recent year for which data are available (CDC, 2008). Over half (53%) of these new infections occurred in gay

347

and bisexual men. African American men and women also were affected significantly and are estimated to have an incidence rate that was seven times greater than the incidence rate among whites.

CAREGIVERS AND THE CHALLENGES THEY FACE

Essentially there are two groups of caregivers that provide clinical care and supportive services to PLWH, formal and informal caregivers. Formal caregivers include nurses and medical professionals, behavioral health specialists, and social workers, all of whom are trained and compensated for their caregiving activities. Formal caregivers face many pressures as they struggle to keep pace with rapidly changing standards of HIV care, limited resources, dwindling reimbursement, and increased numbers of HIV-infected patients.

Strategies for counteracting burnout among formal caregivers must address individual and situational factors. Formal caregivers may be able to change the ways in which they deal with stressors by developing a greater awareness of their own personalities, values, and coping styles and strategies. However, their efforts will be only partially effective if negative policies and practices in the workplace remain unchanged. Mounting administrative and bureaucratic requirements, such as insurance precertifications, prior authorizations, grant writing, and mandatory service reporting have a negative impact on the professional milieu of providing care to PLWH. Finding ways to enhance the work environment may ultimately prove more effective in preventing burnout than teaching these formal caregivers how to manage stress.

Over time, improved medical treatments, concerns about costs of inpatient hospital care, and patient preferences have shifted HIV care from hospitals to home and community-based settings (London et al., 2001; Wrubel & Folkman, 1997). While modern family and medical ideologies of the mid-1900s argued the wisdom of greater reliance on health care professionals and medical institutions, the emergence of chronic illnesses such as HIV/AIDS has led to a reassertion of the importance of families in caring for the sick.

Family structures of PLWH are consistent with the diverse nature of families within society (Moodyet al., 2007; Prachakul et al.,2009). Both traditional and nontraditional family structures support PLWH. Because HIV/AIDS is a chronic disease, people from these traditional and nontraditional family structures often become their primary informal caregivers (Moody et al.; Prachakul & Grant, 2003; Prachakul et al., 2009). This shift places intense demands on relatives, spouses or partners, and friends who serve as informal caregivers for PLWH, many of whom have limited knowledge of HIV management or available resources.

Many strategies recommended in the caregiving literature assume caregivers are middle income, fairly well educated, and surrounded by family and friends who are willing to help care recipients. As HIV continues to penetrate poor and marginalized communities, new or modified approaches are needed to help caregivers manage stress and maintain good physical and mental health. These strategies will require family-centered case management and integrated primary care and behavioral health services for PLWH and their caregivers. As caregivers, these families deal with many difficult issues. This chapter will discuss some of these issues, such as facing stigma, dealing with caregiver psychological burden, and managing the grief related to loss. Global strategies for addressing these issues include identifying important caregiving skills, developing effective coping strategies, and using community resources to assist caregivers.

STIGMA

Unlike some other caregivers, informal caregivers of PLWH often experience social stigma (Wight et al., 2007). This phenomenon is generally referred to as "secondary stigma," or stigma by association. Parents of PLWH may be held responsible for the "bad" behavior that led to the HIV infection of their children (Ogden & Nyblade, 2005). For example, in examining problems and needs of 48 PLWH and their primary family caregivers, Wacharasin and Homchampa (2008) reported fear of stigmatization as a primary concern of caregivers. Wight and colleagues (2006) also examined perceived HIV stigma in 135 AIDS caregiving dyads in the United States. Dyadic stigma was influenced by the caregiver's HIV status, dyad ethnic composition, caregiving duration, and household income. Those who do acknowledge their caregiving status may find it difficult to obtain support from familial or social networks. Rather than face stigmatization, caregivers may try to conceal their caregiving activities by withdrawing from social relationships. In clinical practice, family caregivers may exacerbate demands of caregiving by driving long distances to avoid community awareness of their care recipient's HIV status. Some informal caregivers even avoid employing the professional services of home health care, infusion therapy, and hospice providers in their attempts to avoid HIV/AIDS disclosure within their communities. Nurses working with informal caregivers fearful of HIV disclosure must be sensitive to the family caregiver's fear of discrimination and stigma. Nurses, knowledgeable of "HIV-friendly" referral agencies with well-established histories of providing confidential services, can play a key role in meeting the need for professional home-centered services and bringing solace to an informal caregiver fearful of HIV stigmatization.

Caregivers of HIV-infected children also face stigma. For example, Thampanichawat (2008) found primary caregivers ($n = 27$) of children with HIV infection dealt with the stigma of AIDS while managing their anxiety and fear of loss, bore much burden of care, and faced many difficulties because of limited resources. Similar studies report increased financial difficulties, problems in child care and support, and compromised help-seeking due to stigma. These findings emphasize the need to develop interventions to enable caregivers to seek out and identify financial resources and child care and to support and empower caregivers to deal with stigma (Joseph & Bhatti, 2004). Whereas caregivers for family members with other chronic diseases may be recognized by others for their commitment to care recipients, these studies underscore the perception that family caregivers of PLWH may be stigmatized.

Health care providers also may fear stigmatization in their work with HIV-positive patients (Durham, 1994). Caregivers, whether formal or informal, risk what Goffman (1963) called "courtesy stigma," in which they experience stigma from their association with HIV/AIDS and PLWH. This stigma may influence their willingness to work with PLWH or make their work more difficult (Snyder, Omoto, & Crain, 1999). (See Chapter 11 for a fuller discussion of stigma.)

CAREGIVER BURDEN

Many factors contribute to the physical, financial, emotional, and social challenges associated with caregiving (Kipp & Nkosi, 2008; Pakenham & Dadds, 1995; Stetz & Brown, 2004). Caregiver burden can be assessed in terms of the objective and subjective impact upon caregivers' lives. The term *objective burden* relates to the extent to which caregiving disrupts daily routines and social relationships and negatively affects available resources. *Subjective burden* relates to caregivers' perceptions of and reactions to demands of caregiving. Caregivers with high levels of subjective psychological burden may report they feel "trapped," "nervous," or "depressed" about their relationships with care recipients or "resent" caregiving tasks, even when objective caregiving burden is low. Depending on specific needs of care recipients, caregiving responsibilities may include many different types of tasks, such as lifting, bathing, dressing, and feeding; listening, talking, and providing emotional support; completing household chores, including changing bed linen and laundry and shopping; arranging for health care and interfacing with the health care system; providing around-the-clock supervision of the care recipient; supervising medication schedules; giving telephone reassurance; and providing transportation.

Many informal caregivers of PLWH suffer severe economic hardships. In a report of 283 Early Intervention Services providers of the Ryan White Comprehensive AIDS Resource Emergency (CARE) Act (Title III) providing primary care to PLWH during 2002 and 2003, Gilman & Green (2008) revealed that about 12% of served patients were privately insured, 12% were covered by Medicare, 34% were enrolled in Medicaid, 6% had other public insurance, and almost 30% were uninsured. The mean cost of providing their care was $2,956 annually.

When a key wage earner is forced to reduce work hours or leave paid employment to care for a sick relative or partner, the consequences can be devastating. As unpaid bills accumulate, basic needs may become jeopardized or go unmet. This loss of income may also interfere with caregivers' access to such resources as home health, infusion therapy, drug rehabilitation and respite care, and other services that could make the caregiver role more manageable. Helping informal caregivers to better use a variety of support mechanisms during difficult times can be nurses' most powerful intervention for a family in distress over caring for someone with HIV disease.

Emotional issues surrounding caregiving also are significant. Caregiving usually comes unrepentantly and represents a role for which most people are neither socialized nor prepared to fulfill. To meet the demands of caregiving, caregivers must restructure their preexisting obligations and social activities and the ways in which they relate to care recipients. Interpersonal strains commonly intensify as caregivers and care recipients attempt to resolve issues of autonomy and reciprocity within the context of an increasingly unidirectional giving relationship. Progressive expansion of the caregiver role may be necessary over the course of illness. This increasing dependence on the caregiver may require significant adjustments in family, work, and social commitments.

Emotional stressors for caregivers include:

■ Changes in household roles, such as household financial management, meal preparation, and keeping in touch with friends and relatives;
■ Concerns over the care recipient's health and safety;
■ Fears (on the part of (HIV-infected caregivers) of being left alone in the future with no one to provide care;
■ Feelings of anger and resentment about changes in their loved one and the caregiving role;
■ Feelings of guilt about wanting personal time or about feeling angry when their loved one needs care;
■ Loss of friends and supports due to increased time needed for caregiving;
■ Negative effects on caregivers' health due to the demands of caregiving;
■ Changes in personal identity from the addition of a caregiving role and reductions in employment due to caregiving; and
■ Feelings of depression.

Although depression has been linked to caregiving for a PLWH (Pirraglia et al., 2005), caregiver psychological burden (CPB) has received less attention in the literature. Prachakul and Grant (2003) reported that CPB resulting from role overload was positively correlated with poor health in both HIV-positive and HIV-negative caregivers. Furthermore, they found that CPB was significantly associated with depression, that is, depression contributes to CPB and increased CPB may lead to depression.

Several variables are thought to inflict greater CPB, such as quality of the PLWH–caregiver dyad relationship. Miller and colleagues (2007) assessed 176 of these dyads. Seventeen to 66 percent of these dyads reported difficulty in their relationships, often related to caregiver depression and CPB. Other variables affecting the relationship include physical functioning, HIV medication adherence, and HIV patient depression. These results suggest that relationships are impaired in many PLWH–caregiver dyads and that this impairment is exacerbated by caregiver depression and CPB.

Characteristics such as coping style also likely influence CPB. Some studies have examined the relationship of coping with CPB among caregivers of PLWH. Individuals who use emotion-oriented coping incorporate strategies to regulate their emotions, while those who use avoidance-oriented coping strategies use either distraction or other people to avoid specific situations. Akintola (2008) noted that family members of PLWH commonly used ineffective emotion-focused coping strategies such as denial, concealment, anger, and impatience. People who use task-oriented coping use interventions such as problem-solving to address concerns. Task-oriented coping seems to be more adaptive than either emotion- or avoidance-oriented coping (McCausland & Pakenham, 2003). These findings emphasize the need to develop and test the usefulness of programs to develop task-oriented skills to address caregiving problems.

Similarly, Martin and colleagues (2004) examined coping strategies among families of HIV-infected children. Passive coping and spiritual support were coping techniques used most often, while social support was used least often. Nonbiological caregivers sought out more community resources and support than biological caregivers, suggesting a need to target families least likely to use resources and to teach them to effectively seek out and benefit from social and community supports.

REWARDS OF CAREGIVING

Although studies of caregiving tend to focus on the "burden" of caring, there also are many rewards. Positive aspects of providing care to PLWH include the ability to:

- Bring a mission and purpose to one's life;
- Increase an appreciation for one's own health and well-being;
- Develop empathy and self-knowledge;
- Enhance personal and spiritual growth;
- Experience positive feelings associated with loving, caring, and feeling needed;
- Feel closeness and love, share humor and fun, and experience the pleasure of knowing someone more fully;
- Grow closer together as a couple and fulfill a commitment to care for one's partner "in sickness and in health";
- Improve relationships with other family members who share in the caregiving;
- Connect with other caregivers; and
- Make a difference in the life of someone in need.

GRIEF RELATED TO LOSS

Caregivers of PLWH often go through bereavement and reconstruct their lives on the death of their loved one. For example, Cadell, & Marshall (2007) explored gay or transsexual bereaved caregivers after they had lost a partner from HIV/AIDS. Caregivers found the death of their partner and loss of the caregiving role removed a large part of their identity. On the death of their partner, caregivers went through a process of "restorying." They no longer viewed themselves as caregivers but reconstructed this previous role by finding meaning in the caregiving experience with their deceased partner. This reconstruction allowed many of the caregivers to acknowledge they were good caregivers. Therefore, health professionals need to develop strategies to facilitate restorying by caregivers to potentially allow them to move forward with their life.

Some literature suggests PLWH often trust and depend on their caregivers for their health and well-being, excluding help from other friends and family. For example, Munro and Edward (2008) reported that gay men caregivers of PLWH in Australia experienced several challenges before the actual death of their loved ones who had AIDS. Caregivers had to become very knowledgeable and vigilant regarding management of opportunistic infections. PLWH wanted their caregivers to provide total care and to limit access to other sources of community support, often as a strategy to deal with their stigma. These findings emphasize the need to assist both PLWH and their caregivers to ensure quality of time together, while recognizing that both need time for themselves.

GLOBAL STRATEGIES FOR ADDRESSING CAREGIVER ISSUES

Moroney and colleagues (1998) presented a conceptual model of care that depicts the complex and often reciprocal nature of the care relationship. Their model, which takes into account the strengths and needs of all care partners, features a triadic relationship among the informal caregiver, the care recipient, and the formal (professional) caregiver. All three roles are acknowledged and valued in terms of associated responsibilities and needs. Each party brings a dedication to participate as a respectful and valuable care team member. Their model allows for more than one informal or formal caregiver's involvement in care coordination and/or provision. The care triad functions within a complex system of variables that influence provision of support or services to caregivers and care recipients to address problems.

IDENTIFYING IMPORTANT CAREGIVING PROBLEMS AND SKILLS

A few studies have examined problems experienced by caregivers of PLWH. Studies using other populations cite common caregiving problems. For example, caregivers may assume responsibilities previously assumed by care recipients. Caregivers require assistance in managing activities of daily living (ADLs) and instrumental support such as respite, transportation, and financial assistance (Bakas et al., 2002; Ploeg et al., 2001; Stewart et al., 1998). Subsequently, caregivers experience a loss of independence and inadequate time to manage these multiple roles and responsibilities, citing problems in maintaining their own physical health, resulting in fatigue (Stewart et al., 1998). As a result, caregivers may have inadequate time for themselves (Ploeg et al., 2001; van den Heuvel et al., 2001) and restrictions in their social life. Relationships with caregivers' families and friends may also change as a result of the caregiver role (Ploeg et al., 2001; Thommessen et al., 2001; van den Heuvel et al., 2001).

Pakenham, Dadds, and Lennon (2002) identified other problems experienced by caregivers of PLWH. In descending order of frequency, problems included relationship difficulties (e.g., communication problems and disclosure of HIV status concerns), health or infection control concerns (e.g., care recipients' declining health and cross-infection concerns), care recipients' own problems (e.g., drug/alcohol use and mood changes), emotional distress (e.g., helplessness and emotional exhaustion or burnout), existential concerns (e.g., finding meaning for the future and concerns about death), social difficulties (e.g., stigma and dealing with health professionals), grief and bereavement, and competing caregiving and employment demands.

Dementia associated with HIV, if present, places additional demands on caregivers. In managing dementia, caregivers often maintain constant vigilance over activities of daily living to ensure the safety of their loved ones and that of others (Meadows, Le Maréchal, & Catalán, 1999; Munro & Edwards, 2008). Other investigators have cited behaviors associated with dementia such as lack of motivation, memory loss, mood swings, and incontinence that increase caregiving burnout and fatigue (Bakas et al., 2002). These studies emphasize the need for health providers to work with caregivers so they become more knowledgeable in managing these problems while also allocating time for themselves. Other studies also emphasize the need for interventions to strengthen knowledge (Maneesriwongul et al., 2004) and accessibility to assistance, while also focusing on programs and interventions that encourage PLWH to allow assistance from family and friends other than the primary caregiver to lessen caregiver burnout or burden (Joseph & Bhatti, 2004; Wacharasin & Homchampa, 2008).

In summary, there are limited studies that examine problems experienced by caregivers of PLWH and skills to assist them. Health care professionals play an important role in helping these caregivers to develop strategies to manage problems they encounter and to cope more effectively with the potential negative effects associated with HIV caregiving. Handouts and booklets that are easy to read and that provide short, concise suggestions for managing problems (e.g., ADLs or managing cognitive, behavioral, and emotional changes) are important for caregivers who are often tired and overwhelmed with daily medical regimens. For example, strategies for dealing with specific problems (e.g., impaired memory), such as posting reminders of important tasks (e.g., taking specific medication, medical appointments, and the like), setting short-term goals, and providing positive reinforcement for goals accomplished by these caregivers are important.

COPING STRATEGIES

Caregivers of PLWH deal with many issues, including coping with day-to-day living, their loved one's denial of illness, and managing various treatment appointments and medical regimens. Because dementia may be a consequence of HIV, caregivers need to observe the daily activities of PLWH (Meadows et al., 1999; Munro and Edwards, 2008).

Resilience seems to be a major strategy for coping with the demands of caregiving (Munro and Edwards, 2008). Using humor, providing caring environments, having faith, reframing negative experiences, and feeling hope all enhance resilience (Garmezy, 1993; McCausland & Pakenham, 2003; Werner, 1993). Support networks also seem to be essential in developing resilience. These support networks facilitate caregivers' talking, laughing, crying, and relating to PLWH, thereby enhancing resilience.

Poindexter and Shippy (2008) explored how support networks enhanced resilience when network members were HIV positive. These networks included members of a caring community that provided safety, support, mentoring, and inspiration. Participants in this study demonstrated that living with HIV changed one's network because people die of HIV; new friends are made when one seeks services; and HIV-positive networks replace those lost through stigma and rejection. Resilience also forms from dealing with exposure to caregiving risks and successful negotiation through effective problem-solving skills (Edward, 2005; Palattiyil, & Chakrabarti, 2008).

Engler and associates (2006) examined the role of active-approach (task), blame-withdrawal (emotion), and distancing (avoidance) coping on caregiver burden among a heterogeneous group of 176 caregivers of persons living with HIV. After controlling for demographic variables and caregiver depression, active-approach (task) coping and distancing (avoidance) coping independently moderated the relationship between perceived severity of HIV-related symptoms (stress) and caregiver burden, suggesting that coping lessens the effect of stress on burden. These findings suggest the potential value of developing psychosocial interventions designed to strengthen active-approach or task-oriented coping and lessen avoidance coping.

In developing psychosocial interventions, some research indicates that up to eight sessions may be needed to develop effective adaptive coping skills, such as problem solving (Grant et al., 2002). In one study, Fife and colleagues (2008) evaluated an intervention to facilitate adaptive coping by 84 PLWH, with participation by their cohabiting partners. The psychosocial educational intervention used four two-hour sessions, focusing on communication, stress appraisal, adaptive coping strategies, and building social support over six months. Both members of the dyad were included in each session. The comparison control included four supportive phone calls to the PLWH. Results suggested this educational intervention is a potentially effective model for managing stress in PLWH. Studies using other populations suggest effective adaptive coping skills may be taught using the telephone (Grant et al., 2002). The limited extant research on caregivers of PLWH suggests that psychosocial interventions may facilitate coping and improve caregiver burden and other outcomes. Other research suggests that dyadic interventions may be more useful than individual interventions, but additional research needs to be conducted before drawing this conclusion (Pakenham et al., 2002).

COMMUNITY RESOURCES TO ASSIST CAREGIVERS

A number of community resources are available to assist caregivers. As noted above, resiliency is bolstered by support and knowing that one is not alone. For example, the Family Caregiver Alliance (Toseland, 2004) has identified five "best practices" caregiver education and support programs to assist caregivers of frail older persons. Many elements of these programs are applicable to the caregivers of PLWH. In addition, the Caregiver Community Action Network is comprised of current or former family caregivers who understand the caregiver's experience. The NFCA also provides information regarding caregiver organizations; information, advocacy, and support resources; caregiver-specific websites; end-of-life planning, hospice, and bereavement information; advocacy assistance; home care agencies; assisted living, nursing homes, and residential care; medical transport and hospitality housing; respite resources; and training for family caregivers (National Family Caregivers Association, 2008b). The National Family Caregivers Association (2008a) also offers some useful suggestions for caregivers:

1 Take control of life and avoid letting a loved one's illness or disability always take center stage. Balance life so that both the loved one's and the caregiver's needs are met. Caregivers have to meet their own needs to be able to best meet the needs of PLWH.

2 Allocate personal time, time for the loved one, and time for other important people and things in their lives. Take advantage of other family, friends, and respite resources who can offer assistance. Caregivers need to make a concerted effort to allow themselves personal time (e.g., a short break to shop, read, or enjoy a movie). They also need longer breaks (e.g., two weeks) away from caregiving that offer physical and psychosocial rest and enjoyment, leaving caregivers refreshed and better able to meet their caregiving demands.

3 Recognize potential signs and symptoms of depression (e.g., difficulty sleeping, poor appetite, feeling sad, and the like) and obtain professional help promptly.

4 Understand circumstances, choices, and abilities change throughout the caregiving experience. Set goals regarding what can realistically be achieved. When people offer assistance,

accept, and suggest specific things others can do. Sometimes, people hesitate to offer assistance because they are unsure of the caregiving role. Allow time to help family and friends who offer assistance to feel comfortable.

5 Know their strengths and limitations and become more knowledgeable about caregiving and HIV as a chronic illness.

6 Encourage independence of their loved ones. Realize there is a difference between caring and doing. Be open to strategies that promote autonomy of the care recipient, promoting their self-confidence, sense of control, and self-perceived independence.

7 Recognize that caregiving is not a perfect process and caregivers should allow themselves to celebrate successes as well as what they learn when they make mistakes.

CONCLUSION

In summary, caregivers, including health care workers, family members, and significant others, face many challenging issues in caring for PLWH. This chapter provides an overview of these ongoing concerns and suggests strategies for dealing with them. Caregivers of PLWH will continue to face many challenges as they manage the challenges of providing care. Research into the concerns and issues of formal and informal caregivers holds promise for the identification of best practices in caregiving for this demanding disease.

REFERENCES

Akintola, O. (2008). Defying all odds: Coping with the challenges of volunteer caregiving for patients with AIDS in South Africa. *Journal of Advanced Nursing, 63*, 357–365.

Bakas, T., Austin, J. K., Okonkwo, K. F., Lewis, R. R., & Chadwick, L. (2002). Needs, concerns, strategies, and advice of stroke caregiver the first 6 months after discharge. *Journal of Neuroscience Nursing, 34*, 242–251.

Cadell, S., & Marshall, S. (2007). The (re)construction of self after the death of a partner to HIV/AIDS. *Death Studies, 31*, 537–548.

Centers for Disease Control (CDC). (2008). HIV/AIDS statistics and surveillance. Retrieved November 1, 2008, from www.cdc.gov/Hiv/topics/surveillance/basic.htm#aidscases.

Delgado, J., Heath, K. V., Yip, B., Marion, S., Alfonso, V., & Montaner, J. S. (2003). Highly active antiretroviral therapy: Physician experience and enhanced adherence to prescription refill. *Antiviral Therapy, 8,* 471–478.

Durham, J. D. (1994). The changing HIV/AIDS epidemic: Emerging psychosocial challenges for nurses. *Nursing Clinics of North America, 29*(1), 9–18.

Edward, K. (2005). The phenomenon of resilience in crisis care mental health clinicians. *International Journal of Mental Health Nursing, 14,* 142–148.

Engler, P., Anderson, B., Herman, D., Bishop, D., Miller, I., Pirraglia, P., et al. (2006). Coping and burden among informal HIV caregivers. *Psychosomatic Medicine, 68,* 985–992.

Fife, B. L., Scott, L. L., Fineberg, N. S., & Zwickl, B. E. (2008). Promoting adaptive coping by persons with HIV disease: Evaluation of a patient/partner intervention model. *Journal of the Association of Nurses in AIDS Care, 19,* 75–78.

Garmezy, N. (1993). Resiliency and vulnerability to adverse development al outcomes associated with poverty. *American Behavioral Scientist, 34,* 416–430.

Gilman, B. H., & Green, J. C. (2008). Understanding the varia-tion in costs among HIV primary care providers. *AIDS Care, 20,* 1050–1056.

Goffman, E. (1963) *Stigma: Notes on the management of spoiled iden-tity.* Englewood Cliffs, NJ: Prentice-Hall.

Grant, J. S., Elliott, T. R., Weaver, M., Bartolucci, A. A., & Giger, J. N. (2002). A telephone intervention with family caregivers of stroke survivors after rehabilitation. *Stroke, 33,* 2060–2065.

UNAIDS (Joint United Nations Programme in HIV/AIDS). (2008). *Caregiving in the context of HIV/AIDS.* Retrieved February 7, 2009 from http://www.un.org/womenwatch/daw/egm/equalsharing/EGM-ESOR-2008-BP.4%20UNAIDS_Expert%20Panel_Paper_%20Final.pdf

Joseph, E. B., & Bhatti, R. S. (2004). Psychosocial problems and coping patterns of HIV seropositive wives of men with HIV/AIDS. *Social Work in Health Care, 39,* 29–47.

Kipp, W., & Nkosi, T. (2008). Factors associated with the self-reported health status of female caregivers of AIDS patients. *Western Journal of Nursing Research, 30*(1), 20–33.

London, A. S., Fleishman, J. A., Goldman, D. P., McCaffrey, D. F., Bozzette, S. A., & Leibowitz, A. A. (2001). Use of unpaid and paid home care services among people with HIV infection in the USA. *AIDS Care, 13,* 99–121.

Maneesriwongul, W., Panutat, S., Putwatana, P., Srirapo-ngam, Y., Ounprasertong, L., & Williams, A. (2004). Educational needs of family caregivers of persons living with HIV/AIDS in Thailand. *Journal of the Association of Nurses in AIDS Care, 15*(3), 27–36.

Martin, S. C., Wolters, P. L., Klaas, P. A., Perez, L., & Wood, L. V. (2004). Coping styles among families of children with HIV infection. *AIDS Care, 16,* 283–92.

McCausland, J., & Pakenham, K. I. (2003). Investigation of the benefits of HIV/AIDS caregiving and relations among caregiving adjustment, benefit finding, and stress and coping variables. *AIDS Care, 15,* 853–869.

Meadows, J., Le Maréchal, K., & Catalán, J. (1999). The burden of care: The impact of HIV-associated dementia on caregivers. *AIDS Patient Care and STDS, 13,* 47–56.

Miller, I. W., Bishop, D. S., Herman, D. S., & Stein, M. D. (2007). Relationship quality among HIV patients and their caregivers. *AIDS Care, 19,* 203–211.

Moody, A. L., Morgello, S., Gerits, P., & Byrd, D. (2007, September 18; Epub ahead of print). Vulnerabilities and caregiving in an ethnically diverse HIV-infected population. *AIDS and Behavior.* Retrieved September 9, 2008, from www.springerlink.com/content/5254001j172072l5/fulltext.pdf.

Moroney, R. M., Dokecki, P. R., Gates, J. J., & Haynes, K. N. (Eds.). (1998). *Caring and competent caregivers.* Athens: University of Georgia Press.

Munro, I., & Edward, K. L. (2008). The lived experience of gay men caring for others with HIV/AIDS: Resilient coping skills. *International Journal of Nursing Practice, 14,* 122–128.

National Family Caregivers Association. (2008a). Believe in yourself—and take charge of your life. Retrieved September 28, 2008, from www.nfcacares.orgimproving_caregiving/believe_in_your_family.cfm.

National Family Caregivers Association. (2008b). Caregiving resources. Retrieved September 28, 2008, from www.nfcacares.org/caregiving_resources.

Ogden, J., & Nyblade, L. (2005). HIV related stigma across contexts. Retrieved November 1, 2008, from www.icrw.org/docs/2005_report_stigma_synthesis.pdf.

Pakenham, K. I., & Dadds, M. R. (1995). Carers' burden and adjustment to HIV. *AIDS Care, 7,* 189–203.

Pakenham, K. I., Dadds, M. R., & Lennon, H. V. (2002). The efficacy of a psychosocial intervention for HIV/AIDS caregiving dyads and individual caregivers: A controlled treatment outcome study. *AIDS Care, 14,* 731–750.

Palattiyil, G., & Chakrabarti, M. (2008). Coping strategies of families in HIV/AIDS care: Some exploratory data from two developmental contexts. *AIDS Care, 20,* 881–885.

Pirraglia, P. A., Bishop, D., Herman, D., Trisvan, E., Lopez, R. A., Torgersen, C. S., et al. (2005). Caregiver burden and depression among informal caregivers of HIV-infected individuals. *Journal of General Internal Medicine, 20,* 510–514.

Ploeg, J., Biehler, L., Willison, K., Hutchison, B., & Blythe, J. (2001). Perceived support needs of family caregivers and implications for a telephone support service. *Canadian Journal of Nursing Research, 33,* 43–61.

Poindexter, C., & Shippy, R. A. (2008) Networks of older New Yorkers with HIV: Fragility, resilience, and transformation. *AIDS Patient Care and STDs, 22,* 723–733.

Prachakul, W., & Grant, J. S. (2003). Informal caregivers of persons with HIV/AIDS: A review and analysis. *Journal of the Association of Nurses in AIDS Care, 14,* 55–71.

Prachakul, W., Grant, J. S., Pryor, E., Keltner, N. L., & Raper, J. L. (2009). Family relationships in people living with HIV in a city in the U.S.A. *AIDS Care, 21,* 384–388.

Sheriff, L. (2009) Caring for the caregivers in the face of HIV and TB: A clinical review (part one). Retrieved February 7, 2009, from www.aidsmap.com/cms1283957.aspx.

Snyder, M., Omoto, A. M., & Crain, A. L. (1999). Punished for their good deeds: Stigmatization for AIDS volunteers. *American Behavioral Scientist, 42,* 1175–1192.

Stetz, K., & Brown, M. (2004). Physical and psychosocial health in family caregiving: A comparison of AIDS and cancer patients. *Public Health Nursing, 21,* 533–540.

Stewart, M. J., Doble, S., Hart, G., Langille, L., & MacPherson, K. (1998). Peer visitor support for family caregivers of seniors with stroke. *Canadian Journal of Nursing Research, 30*, 87–117.

Thampanichawat, W. (2008). Maintaining love and hope: Caregiving for Thai children with HIV infection. *Journal of the Association of Nurses in AIDS Care, 19*, 200–210.

Thommessen, B., Wyller, T. B, Bautz-Holter, E., & Laake, K. (2001). Acute phase predictors of subsequent psychosocial burden in carers of elderly stroke patients. *Cerebrovascular Disease, 11*, 201–206.

Toseland, R. (2004). Caregiver education and support programs: Best practice models. San Francisco: Author. Retrieved on February 9, 2009, from www.aoa.gov/alz/prof/ADDGS/docs/Caregiver_Education_Support_Programs.pdf.

UNAIDS (Joint United Nations Programme in HIV/AIDS). (2008). *Caregiving in the context of HIV/AIDS.* Retrieved February 7, 2009, from www.un.org/womenwatch/daw/egm/equalsharing/EGM-ESOR-2008-BP.4%20UNAIDS_Expert%20Panel_Paper_%20Final.pdf.

van den Heuvel, E. T., de Witte, L. P., Schure, L. M., Sanderman, R., & Meyboom-de Jong, B. (2001). Risk factors for burn-out in caregivers of stroke patients, and possibilities for intervention. *Clinical Rehabilitation, 15*, 669–677.

Wacharasin, C., & Homchampa, P. (2008). Uncovering a family caregiving model: Insights from research to benefit HIV-infected patients, their caregivers, and health professionals. *Journal of the Association of Nurses in AIDS Care, 19*, 385–396.

Werner, E. (1993). Risk, resilience, and recovery: Perspectives from the Kauai longitudinal study. *Development and Psychopathology, 5*, 503–515.

Wight, R. G., Aneshensel, C. S., Murphy, D. A., Miller-Martinez, D., & Beals, K. P. (2006). Perceived HIV stigma in AIDS caregiving dyads. *Social Science & Medicine, 62*, 444–456.

Wight, R. G., Beals, K. P., Miller-Martinez, D., Murphy, D. A., & Aneshensel, C. S. (2007). HIV-related traumatic stress symptoms in AIDS caregiving family dyads. *AIDS Care, 19*, 901–909.

Wrubel, J., & Folkman, S. (1997). What informal caregivers actually do: The caregiving skills of partners of men with AIDS. *AIDS Care, 9*, 691–706.

11

HIV Disease and Gay, Lesbian, Bisexual, and Transgender Persons

J. CRAIG PHILLIPS
ELIZABETH M. SAEWYC

Over the course of the HIV epidemic the disease has disproportionately affected members of vulnerable (minority) populations, including racial, ethnic, gender, and sexual minorities. Persons from ethnic and gender minority groups face multiple challenges when seeking health care. Challenges faced by minorities are often contextually based and require nurses and other health care providers to examine complex interrelationships between person and environment. The specific care needs of gender or sexual minorities may be overlooked by health care providers because of limited scientific evidence and preconceived notions about health care needs of gay, lesbian, bisexual, and transgender (GLBT) individuals. Beliefs may be based on stereotypical portrayals from the media or other sources. Although the evidence base to guide nurses' clinical practice with GLBT persons living with HIV is expanding, considerable knowledge gaps still exist. For many individuals, the experience of living with HIV disease is further complicated by the experience of being a member of multiple minorities, for example, being a gay black man. Challenges for GLBT persons may arise from their social environment, including geographic location and isolation from other GLBT persons, the social acceptability of their sexuality in their local community, their socioeconomic status, the legal framework of their region, the potential lack of recognition for their supportive relationships, and a limited availability of a social support network.

This chapter provides an overview of issues faced by GLBT persons globally. In many regions the information available is limited because

365

of the underlying sociopolitical context. Sociopolitical constraints limit discussion about same-gender sexual interactions, and GLBT individuals may face severe criminal and civil penalties. For example, same-gender sex is a capital offense in Iran (Canadian Broadcasting Corporation, 2007). Penalties may have ramifications for nurses and other health care providers. In contexts where same-gender sexual behavior is censured, the emphasis of nurses and other health care providers is to provide factual information about HIV and other health issues of concern to GLBT persons.

SEXUALITY: WHAT IS SEXUAL IDENTITY AND SEXUAL ORIENTATION?

Sexuality is not a dichotomous variable but rather a continuum (Norman et al., 1996). Sexual identity and sexual orientation do not equate directly with sexual practices (Arend, 2003; Kennedy et al., 1995). Human sexuality can be defined as the way in which people experience and express themselves as sexual beings. It is a complex and dynamic expression of human nature that includes cognitive, emotional, and behavioral aspects. Sexuality is often discussed in terms of an individual's sexual identity or his or her sexual orientation. Sexual identity (how an individual self-labels) and sexual orientation (manifestation of sexual attraction) are often used interchangeably in scientific literature and popular media. Using these terms interchangeably may be problematic and reinforce stereotypes about sexuality and beliefs that a person's expression of sexuality is based solely on personal choice or a biological predisposition--an oversimplification of the complex influences that model sexuality and reinforce an individual's expression of his or her sexuality.

Aspects of Sexuality

Wolitski, Stall, and Valdiserri (2007) describe three distinct aspects of sexuality: sexual desire or attraction, sexual behavior, and sexual identity. *Sexual desire* or *attraction* is the degree to which an individual is sexually attracted to members of his or her own or opposite gender, or both, or neither gender. *Sexual behavior* is the actions one takes with regards to sexual contact with others. Sexual behavior may not be consistent with an individual's sexual desire or attraction. For example, some persons may report having a sexual desire for persons of the opposite sex, but engage in sexual acts only with members of the same sex. *Sexual identity* is the label an individual uses to characterize his or her sexual orientation. Sexual identity is culture bound and dynamic. Labels change meanings and popularity, so labels previously accepted may no longer be appropriate at a given time, age, or developmental stage or within a particular social setting or larger societal context.

The Nurse's Role and Obligations Related to Patients' Sexuality

Nurses should understand sexual identity does not predict sexual behavior and should not make assumptions regarding HIV risk based on self-reported or presumed sexual identity (Arend, 2003; Kennedy et al., 1995). Obtaining accurate information from a patient during the health history and assessment is critical. In fact, nurses are obligated to their patients and the profession by nursing's ethical principles and laws established to protect persons in their care. Nurses must make themselves aware of these ethical and legal constraints and determine what influence these will have on their practice when caring for GLBT persons living with HIV/AIDS. Nurses need to be aware of potential social or legal risks they face by working with all patients in their practice area.

Factors Influencing Sexuality

Many factors have been identified that influence an individual's expression of sexuality (Wolitski et al., 2007). Beyond physiological factors that help determine sexuality, there are also environmental and social factors that shape how an individual expresses sexual identity and sexual orientation. Table 11.1 separates these factors into internal and external spheres of influence.

Internal Factors Influencing Sexuality

Internal factors influencing sexuality are those individuals bring to a given context or setting and include personal beliefs and attitudes, internalized stigma, and age and/or developmental stage. Beliefs and attitudes that individuals have about what are acceptable or desirable sexual behaviors to them affect how they express sexuality. For example, if a person believes same-gender sexual activities are immoral and he or she experiences physical attraction to a member of the same gender, this

Table 11.1

FACTORS INFLUENCING SEXUALITY	
Internal Factors	Personal beliefs and attitudes
	Internalized stigma
	Age and/or developmental stage
External Factors	Cultural norms regarding sexual relationships
	Familial expectations
	Availability of partners (incarceration, military service, same-gender boarding school, sociopolitical demographic factors [e.g., one-child birth policy in China])
	Drug dependency and substance misuse
	Economic need (survival sex)
	History of sexual abuse or sexual assault

Based on Phillips (2008) and Wolitski, Stall, & Valdiserri (2007).

attraction may create internal conflict. Internalized stigma occurs when persons accept the negative valuation society has about them (Simbayi et al., 2007) and may influence how they express themselves sexually. During adolescence many individuals contemplate gender identity issues and may experiment with same-gender sexual behaviors. At other times during the life course individuals may contemplate or engage in same-gender sexual behaviors. Contemplation and experimentation about sexuality may be a normal part of development.

External Factors Influencing Sexuality

External factors influencing sexuality are factors imposed on an individual by their social context, setting, or environment. These factors include cultural norms regarding sexual relationships, familial expectations, and availability of partners (incarceration, military service, and same-gender boarding school). Additional external factors include drug dependency, economic need, and/or history of sexual abuse or sexual assault. Internal and external factors are interrelated and influence each other.

STIGMA AND DISCRIMINATION IN HEALTH CARE AND SOCIAL SERVICES SETTINGS

Stigma is a process of devaluing a person based on a characteristic, trait, or attribute of that individual. Sources of stigma can be both internal and external. The complexity with which stigma is experienced by GLBT individuals is determined by context and mediated by coping strategies and mechanisms the individual uses to adapt to or remove themselves from the environment.

HIV/AIDS-Related Stigma

HIV/AIDS-related stigma is "a 'process of devaluation' of people either living with or associated with HIV and AIDS" (UNAIDS, 2003). Stigma is a form of social control, in which socially dominant groups determine who is devalued and use a variety of strategies to target the rejected group, in this case, people with HIV/AIDS (Nyblade, 2006). These strategies include direct actions toward people who are HIV positive, or who are suspected to have HIV/AIDS, from negative comments, refusals to touch someone or to interact with them, to threats of violence, even actual physical assault. Other strategies are directed toward the community, to shape responses to people with HIV disease. For example, this can take the form of gossip or negative jokes and threats of exclusion if people express support for or associate with the stigmatized group. People may even advocate for laws and policies that discriminate against people with HIV or may encourage others to engage in violence toward the outcast group. These activities are all considered forms of *enacted stigma*.

When either a large portion of the general population, or an influential smaller group within the community, accepts this devaluing of a stigmatized group, this acceptance is *perceived* stigma. The nonstigmatized majority recognizes that there may be social risks to identifying with the stigmatized group or associating too closely with someone who has the stigma. For those with HIV disease, perceived stigma affects individuals who are aware that others could devalue or reject them because of their disease status. As a result, they may take steps to try to deflect that potential social hostility or to cope with the stigma they face (Miller & Kaiser, 2001). They may avoid being tested for HIV, try to hide their HIV-positive status, or resist negative perceptions by trying to find other HIV-positive people and sympathetic allies to create a separate support network.

Internalized Stigma

Internalized stigma happens when stigmatized people accept the negative valuation society has about them (Simbayi et al., 2007). They often feel worthless and may accept hostility and discrimination aimed at them as what they deserve. People with internalized stigma related to HIV/AIDS may be less motivated to seek health care or maintain treatment regimens. They may isolate themselves or avoid opportunities for social support.

Orientation Stigma, Multiple Stigmas, and Issues of Racial/Ethnic Stigma

GLBT persons living with HIV/AIDS may experience stigmas related to sexuality, sexual identity, and sexual orientation. They may face multiple stigmas related to race or ethnicity, substance use, homelessness, and possible engagement in sex work. Multiple stigmas have been documented as factors that reduce access to health care and therapeutic interventions provided through the health care system (Krawczyk et al., 2006). Lichtenstein (2003) identified four dimensions of stigma salient to health-seeking behaviors. First, religious convictions affected health care workers' perceptions of the sexual behaviors of patients (especially females). Second, privacy fears of male patients discouraged them from seeking treatment. Third, mistrust in the health care system in general affected willingness to seek treatment. Finally, stigma transference and perception of being the target of local gossip decreased the likelihood of an individual's willingness to seek treatment.

HIV-Related Discrimination

HIV-related discrimination is the unfair and unjust treatment of an individual based on his or her real or perceived HIV status and refers to actions that are based on stigma (UNAIDS, 2003). It is critical for nurses and other health care providers who work with GLBT persons living with HIV/AIDS to become aware of the laws and policies, both codified and unwritten, in their area relating to discrimination and, when possible, to advocate for eliminating discriminatory practices and policies:

> Discrimination against people living with HIV and those perceived to be living with HIV occurs within families and other social networks, and is

often institutionalized. Examples of institutionalized discrimination include government laws, policies, and procedures that negatively target people living with HIV or groups perceived to be living with HIV, and discrimination in workplace settings or health-care settings. Omission can also be a form of discrimination where, for example, the needs and interests of people living with HIV or stigmatized populations are ignored or minimized (UNAIDS, 2008b).

Additionally, nurses must be aware that discrimination is a human rights violation, prohibited by international human rights law (UNAIDS, 2008b). Although not all nations abide by these international laws, nurses and other health care professionals are held to account for their actions

Table 11.2

NURSE-APPROPRIATE STIGMA REDUCTION STRATEGIES

LEVEL	NURSING STRATEGIES
Intrapersonal	Facilitate development of and engagement in self-help, advocacy, and support groups
	Empowerment
	Individual and group counseling*
	Cognitive-behavioral therapy*
Interpersonal	Nursing care and support in all clinical settings, including acute care, primary care, and community-based settings
Organizational/ Institutional	Involvement in training programs
	Advocate for and institute policies that use an integrative approach to patient care
Community	Education
	Contact
	Advocacy
	Protest
Governmental/ Structural	Advocate and lobby for legal and policy changes
	Provide information to governmental and structural level stakeholders regarding human rights-based approaches to HIV

*Requires the nurse to have post-basic training and preparation.
Based on Heijnders & van der Meij (2006).

with regards to human rights laws by professional codes of ethics. (See for example, the International Council of Nurses' Code of Ethics (2006) and the World Medical Association's International Code of Medical Ethics (2006).)

Providing Competent Care to GLBT Persons Living with HIV/AIDS

Table 11.2 provides nurse-appropriate stigma reduction strategies for multilevel intervention consistent with a human rights-based approach to HIV.

EPIDEMIOLOGY OF HIV

Categories to describe HIV risk behaviors (e.g., the use of the CDC's HIV transmission risk categories of men who have sex with men [MSM], women who have sex with women [WSW], heterosexual transmission, and intravenous drug users [IVDU]) simplifies the mathematical models used for comparison of epidemiological profiles of HIV disease and allows for a clearer understanding of broad categories of risk behavior. However, some persons may engage in high-risk behaviors but not realize they are at risk for HIV because they do not identify as an MSM because, for example, they engage in sexual relations only with transgender women (Operario et al, 2008). Individuals who use drugs may not believe they are at increased risk for HIV because they do not inject drugs. Further, the use of categories to articulate exposure risks are often inadequate to identify all persons at risk; hence, high numbers of persons are identified as having "no identifiable risk." Additionally, persons may not report all potential risk factors if potential censure or discrimination is associated with a specific risk behavior. Race and ethnicity categories may be problematic if these persons represent a small percentage of large populations, complicating interpretation of epidemiological data reported and extrapolation of results to other members of that racial/ethnic category within a population.

Discussions throughout this chapter are based on the assumption that risks are similar for persons with anatomically and physiologically similar body structures. Therefore, gay and bisexual men and lesbian and bisexual women are grouped together because their risks for HIV exposure are similar (e.g., anal or vaginal intercourse). The following sections highlight practice, research, and policy issues that are unique to specific GLBT groups.

Gay and Bisexual Men

HIV epidemiology data on gay and bisexual men globally demonstrate that MSM represent an important segment of the HIV-infected population. On a global scale, epidemiology of HIV among MSM remains underestimated and underreported in many areas of the world because some countries deny the existence of the practice and may have harsh penalties for men, including death, who admit to, are suspected of, or are caught engaging in sex with other men (Burris & Cameron, 2008; UNAIDS, 2008a). These laws and policies reinforce the importance of a human rights-based approach to HIV and management of HIV disease as a global population health concern (UNAIDS, 2008b). Viewing epidemiological trends based on WHO geographic regions helps articulate regional differences. In general, the HIV epidemic has stabilized, but there remains considerable variability in the epidemic profile in many regions with some regions having subepidemics in specific at-risk populations (e.g., men of color who have sex with men, men who engage in high-risk sexual behavior with other men). Trends in regions where sex between men was previously considered a less important factor driving the epidemic are disconcerting (UNAIDS, 2008b). Recent studies in sub-Saharan Africa found considerable HIV prevalence rates in Dakar, Senegal (22%), Zambia (33%), and Mombasa, Kenya (43%) among male participants who reported having sex with men (Sanders et al., 2005; UNAIDS, 2008b; Wade et al., 2005; Zulu, Bulawo, & Zulu, 2006). In Asia, unprotected anal sex between men is a potentially significant but underresearched factor in the HIV epidemic. Male sex workers in Asia are at particularly high risk of HIV infection (UNAIDS, 2008b). In Eastern Europe and Central Asia unprotected sex between men is considered to be underestimated with less than 1% of newly registered HIV cases attributed to this mode of transmission (UNAIDS, 2008b). There is limited HIV information available for the Middle East and North Africa, but unprotected sex between men may be a factor in several of the region's epidemics. Sex between men is socially stigmatized and officially censured throughout the region; in some cases, it is a capital crime, and men who have sex with men have been executed (Canadian Broadcasting Corporation, 2007; UNAIDS, 2008b).

Although officially denied in many Caribbean countries, sex between men is a significant factor in several national epidemics. Unprotected sex between men is the main mode of HIV transmission in Cuba and Dominica (UNAIDS, 2008b). In Latin America, MSM is the main mode of HIV transmission. High HIV prevalence has been documented among MSM in several South American countries (Argentina, Bolivia, Colombia, Ecuador, Peru, Uruguay) with research uncovering several hidden epidemics among MSM in several Central American countries (Belize, Costa Rica, El Salvador, Guatemala, Mexico, Nicaragua, and Panama). Many of these men also report having sex with women and having not used condoms with sex partners of both genders (UNAIDS, 2008b).

Most HIV epidemics in Oceania are small, but unprotected sex between men is the primary mode of HIV transmission in Australia and New Zealand (UNAIDS, 2008b). North America and Western and Central Europe also have epidemics, with MSM as the main mode of HIV transmission in these countries (UNAIDS, 2008b). For these countries, the epidemic appears to be in flux, and there are increases in the numbers of HIV cases in specific demographic groups (e.g., black MSM) or among MSM that engage in specific high-risk sexual activities (e.g., bug chasers).

In the United States, decreases in HIV/AIDS diagnoses were observed in all transmission categories except MSM from 2001 through 2006. MSM accounted for more than 50% of the estimated HIV incidence in the United States in 2006 (Hall et al., 2008). The observed number of HIV/AIDS diagnoses among black MSM aged 13 to 24 years of age increased by 93%. Black MSM in this age group had approximately twice as many HIV/AIDS diagnoses as white MSM of the same age (CDC, 2008). According to Sandfort & Dodge (2008):

> Bisexual Black and Latino men are at significantly higher risk for HIV infection and transmission in comparison to both exclusively heterosexual and homosexual men. Since bisexual men have most frequently been categorized with exclusively homosexual men, most previous research on male bisexuality has focused on homosexuality with scant and questionable extrapolations made to bisexuality. Serious shortcomings and inadequate knowledge exist in regards to bisexual men's individual, social, and sexual lives, as well as subjective experiences of their sexualities. (p. 678)

Lesbian and Bisexual Women

Epidemiologically, the incidence and prevalence of HIV among lesbian and bisexual women are deceptively low. Although lesbians were erroneously defined as a "high-risk group" in the early years of the epidemic (Richardson, 2000), myths of lesbian "immunity" or "invulnerability" with respect to HIV/AIDS have subsequently become widespread among both WSW and providers (Arend, 2003; Bull, 2003; Dolan & Davis, 2003; Goldstein, 1995; Stevens & Hall, 2001). These myths have served to (a) negatively influence lesbians' risk perceptions and behaviors, (b) limit education and prevention efforts for lesbians and bisexual women, (c) delay early diagnosis and treatment for lesbians, and (d) restrict resources for research on HIV transmission in WSW (Arend, 2003; Bull, 2003; Saunders, 1999; Stevens, 1993).

Through December 2004, the number of women in the United States who were reported as HIV infected reached 246,461, of whom 7,381 were WSW. It is important to note, however, that information on whether a woman had sex with women was missing in 60% of reported cases because either physicians did not elicit the information or women did not volunteer it. A vast majority of the 7,381 WSW had other risks (e.g., intravenous drug use [IVDU], sex with high-risk men, receipt of blood or blood products). Of the 534 WSW (of 7,381) who reported sex with only women, 91% also had another risk, usually injection drug use (CDC, 2006). Thus, female-to-female sexual transmission of HIV has been considered rare (Bull, 2003; CDC, 2006). This is not the only risk, however. Diamant and colleagues (1999) found three in four self-identified lesbians reported sex with one or more male partners in their lifetime (77.3%) and 5.7% within the past year; nearly two-thirds of those reported unprotected vaginal or anal intercourse. More than half (53.2%) reported having had an HIV test at some point in their lifetime, with a low rate of HIV infection (0.1%). Similarly, in a study of more than 1,400 WSW versus controls in Australia, Fethers and colleagues (2000) found WSW were much more likely to report sexual intercourse with gay or bisexual men, reported more lifetime male sexual partners, had equal rates of HIV (0.3%), and seven times higher rates of hepatitis C, primarily due to higher rates of injection drug use. While most risks for HIV may be due to factors other than female-to-female transmission, other STIs are transmitted among women who exclusively have sex with women. A study of women in Minnesota found 13% of exclusive WSW reported a lifetime history of STIs; and, when all other known risk factors were controlled for, the lifetime number of female sexual encounters independently predicted STI history (Bauer & Welles, 2001). The true risk of female-to-female HIV transmission has not been adequately identified.

Internationally scant information has documented the epidemiology of HIV among WSW. Few studies in developed nations explore

WSW's risk for HIV, and even fewer studies in developing nations do. In the United States, considerable variability in seroprevalence rates for WSW has been reported. In a sample of 498 lesbian and bisexual women, Lemp and colleagues (1995) documented a seroprevalence rate of zero for women who had sex only with women since 1978 and 1.2% for WSW who had other risk factors. However, among 27,370 women who accessed counseling and testing services in New York over one year, Shotsky (1996) found a seroprevalence rate of 3.0% among women who reported sex exclusively with women and 4.8% among women who reported sex with both women and men. Norman and colleagues (1996) noted that of the 1,057 lesbian and bisexual women in their sample, 44% were tested for HIV at least once with a seroprevalence rate of 1.4%.

Transgender Persons

HIV epidemiology trends among transgender persons are difficult to quantify at the international level, due in part to categories of data collection. The CDC, for example, reports incidence data only by male and female, and transgender people do not fit categories of WSW or MSM. Countries may have widely different definitions of transgender populations. In Canada and the United States, the term *Two-Spirit* can sometimes denote a transgender identity, and it is sometimes used as a sexual orientation with clear gender identity (Evans-Campbell et al., 2007; Jacobs, Thomas, & Lang, 1997; Simoni et al., 2006). Similarly, transgender people may not self-identify as transgender in research but indicate the preferred gender identity (Garofalo et al., 2006). Internationally, available empirical evidence about transgender persons is often limited to subsets of study samples that may not provide adequate information about numbers of persons affected (Girault et al., 2004; Pisani et al., 2004). Herbst and colleagues (2008) conducted a systematic review of 29 research studies and found that 27.7% of male-to-female transgender persons tested positive for HIV and African Americans were at highest risk. A study of transgender persons in the United States highlights the need for further research with this group, as more than three-quarters of participants reported current or future intent to engage in high-risk sexual behaviors (Kenagy, 2002).

HIV RISK FACTORS AND VULNERABILITY

Risk factors associated with HIV among GLBT include biological and behavioral factors that put an individual at risk for HIV transmission, such as unprotected intercourse. Risk is "the probability or likelihood that a person may become infected with HIV" (UNAIDS, 2008b). In addition to risk, there are social and environmental contexts (beyond the individual's control) that increase the likelihood of an individual transmitting HIV to another person, which is referred to as *vulnerability* (UNAIDS, 2008b).

HIV Risk Factors Common to All GLBT Persons

Most of the factors common to increased risk of HIV for GLBT persons more precisely meet the definition of vulnerabilities than risk factors. These factors in and of themselves may not predispose an individual to becoming HIV infected; however, they may create the environmental context whereby an individual may perceive a need to engage in HIV risk behaviors. Social and environmental contexts associated with HIV transmission include homelessness, poverty, sex work, sexual abuse and violence, substance misuse, and age and/or developmental stage.

Homelessness

The risk of becoming homeless knows no ethnic, racial, sexual orientation, or gender bounds. There is little information about the prevalence of homeless GLBT persons globally; however, research in North America has found a disproportionate level of GLBT youth among homeless and street-involved populations of adolescents (Ensign & Santelli, 1997, 1998; Smith et al., 2007). Characterizing a person as a gender or sexual minority in many jurisdictions limits his or her ability to find adequate housing and contributes to his or her remaining homeless. The percent of transgender persons who are homeless is unknown. The number of homeless persons living with HIV globally is similarly difficult to discern. However, existing data that describe the numbers of persons living with HIV who are homeless suggest the number is high. Catastrophic illness such as HIV often contributes to a person's becoming homeless. In the United States it is estimated that the homeless population has a median rate of HIV prevalence more than three times (3.4% versus 1%) the general population with a range between 3% and 20% (National Coalition for the Homeless, 2007).

Unstable housing creates challenges that complicate HIV disease management and antiretroviral therapy (ART) adherence. Lack of a safe and secure location to store medications is one problem for persons who are homeless or marginally housed (Phillips, 2008). Some ART medications (e.g., Saquinavir) can be rendered useless if they are not stored properly. Access to adequate amounts and quality of food also may be problematic (Campa et al., 2005). Inconsistent structure in the environment or continually moving from place to place, including transitions between the street, shelters, jails, and health care or drug treatment facilities, complicate HIV treatment (Phillips, 2008).

In the United States, an innovative approach to address the challenge of being homeless for persons living with HIV/AIDS is the "Housing and Health Study" conducted by the CDC and the Department of Housing and Urban Development (Kidder et al., 2007). Although the study is not specific to gender or sexual minorities, it explored five primary health-related outcomes, including treatment adherence, medical care access and use, mental and physical health, HIV disease progression, and risks of transmitting HIV in a sample (n = 630) of mostly black (79%) males (68%). Final analysis of the study data is pending (Kidder et al., 2007); however, the focus of this innovative study draws attention to the possible influence of homelessness on HIV treatment and prevention, factors that are critical to GLBT persons living with HIV.

Poverty

Poverty as an HIV vulnerability is insidious, creating challenges for persons who are in at-risk groups for HIV, especially GLBT persons living with HIV. Poverty has the potential to create the socioeconomic context in which a person may perceive the only means for economic survival is engaging in survival sex or commercial sex work or being involved in dealing in illegal substances, both of which increase the risk of injection drug use. Poverty also creates a downward spiral for persons who are HIV-infected by limiting their ability, in many parts of the world, to gain access to health care and social services required for effective HIV disease management. Although the effects of poverty are not the sole purview of GLBT persons worldwide, in many nations GLBT persons are disproportionately affected by poverty, often the result of oppression and criminalization of sexual behavior for gender minorities. Even in developed nations, GLBT persons living with HIV are at high risk for poverty because of social structures. For example, the structure of the health care system in the United States, with most health insurance coverage financed by employers, creates the potential for financial hardship for GLBT persons if they disclose their sexuality. Many jurisdictions do not have antidiscrimination laws in place to prevent the loss of employment for GLBT persons identified as gender or sexual minorities, which amplifies the risk of losing health insurance coverage (Mayer et al., 2008).

Sex Work and Sex for Money, Drugs, or Other Survival Needs

Survival sex and commercial sex work increase vulnerability of persons to HIV. When minors exchange sex for money or other consideration, this exchange is considered sexual exploitation, not sex work, in a number of legal jurisdictions. The exchange of sex for needed commodities like shelter occurs among vulnerable populations of all ethnicities, races, sexual orientations, and genders. In a recent study of street-involved, sexually exploited youth in western Canada, GLBT youth were disproportionately more likely to report exchanging sex for money, drugs, or basic necessities than were heterosexual youth (Saewyc et al., 2008). Exchanging sex for commodities increases a person's vulnerability to HIV in many ways, including sexual contact with multiple partners, potential for engaging in high-risk sexual behavior (e.g., sex without condoms for higher pay), and exposure to violence. Nurses and other health care providers must explore issues of sexual exploitation or sex work with all patients to determine potential risk. Open-ended questions about sexual behavior during a history and physical may offer insight into this behavior. For example, the nurse may ask, "What concerns/questions do you have about sexual health?" Nurses must be nonjudgmental and aware that persons engaging in sex work may be coping with issues of stigma related to exchanging sex for commodities.

Sexual Abuse and Sexual Violence

Persons who are in sexually abusive and sexually violent situations are more vulnerable to HIV disease and may not be able to protect themselves from the spread of HIV. In the case of sexual abuse, a person who is being abused may not be able to request the use of barriers as a means of protection against HIV without increasing the likelihood of further abuse. In the case of sexual violence, it is often not possible for a person being raped to request that a condom be used. Nurses working with persons who have experienced sexual abuse or sexual violence must be sensitive to the needs of the individual person. It is critical that the nurse include questions about sexual abuse and sexual violence when conducting a history and physical exam. WHO (2003) has published guidelines to help health care providers who are responsible for obtaining history and physical information from victims of sexual violence.

Drug and Alcohol Use—Substance Misuse

Early GLBT research efforts may have resulted in selection bias that overrepresents substance-using GLBT persons because subjects were recruited from bars (Mayer et al., 2008). This recruitment strategy may have been justified as part of early attempts to gain access to hard-to-reach populations. However, these research efforts represent a challenge because interpretation of the results of this early research may lead nurses and other health care providers to stereotype all GLBT as substance users or at risk for substance misuse. Nurses and other health care providers must be aware of this potential bias and be sensitive to the fact that not all GLBT persons have problematic substance use. Nonetheless, nurses and other health care providers must inquire about substance use with GLBT persons to obtain accurate assessment information to guide appropriate and effective interventions.

Age and/or Developmental Stage Risk Factors

Youth. Adolescent lesbian and bisexual girls may be at higher risk for acquiring HIV than heterosexual teens their same age, but they may also have higher risk than older lesbian and bisexual women. This higher risk may be due in part to the greater likelihood of certain HIV-related risks during adolescence, such as increased rates of sexual abuse (Saewyc et al., 2006) and for teen pregnancy involvement among lesbian and bisexual girls (Saewyc, 2005). Adolescent girls may also have higher physiological vulnerability. Younger women and teens tend to have a higher percentage of cervical ectopy, i.e., larger zones of the thinner and more friable columnar epithelium in the cervix, rather than the more mature stratified squamous epithelium. Cervical ectopy has been associated with increased risk for HIV infection, both among older women (Meyer et al., 2006) and among adolescent girls (Moscicki et al., 2001).

Donenberg and Pao (2005) conducted a research literature review and identified HIV risk factors among youths. Although these are not specific to GLBT youths, they highlight important risk factors that must be considered by nurses working with GLBT persons. The nurse caring for a GLBT person may need to determine whether the individual experienced any of these factors during their youth. Individual attributes of youths at risk for HIV disease include HIV-related cognitions (knowledge, attitudes and beliefs, and impaired decision making), affect regulation and the ability of the youth to cope with distress, external-ized mental health problems (e.g., aggression, delinquency), internal-ized mental health problems (e.g., depression, anxiety), personality traits (e.g., sensation seeking, value on health, achievement motivation), and a history of sexual abuse (Donenberg & Pao, 2005). History of childhood sexual abuse has been associated with HIV risk among female samples and gay and bisexual male samples alike (Brennan et al., 2007).

Family context and dynamics of relationships among teens, parents, and siblings are important to youth development. The following areas of family functioning have also been associated with sexual risk-taking behaviors and may contribute to HIV risk behavior:

- The affective characteristics of the family, including levels of warmth, support, and hostility influence behavior of teens.
- Monitoring, supervision, and parental involvement and whether a parent is strict or permissive also influence youth behavior.
- The quality and quantity of communication between teens and parents affect the youth's sexual behavior.
- The parental behaviors and attitudes that are role modeled influ-ence sexual and other risk behaviors (e.g., if a child's first exposure to heroin is when father helps him or her inject, he or she may be inclined to engage in other high-risk behaviors) (Donenberg & Pao, 2005).

As teens mature, their friends and romantic partners become increas-ingly more important in influencing behavior. For example, romantic relationships can be anxiety provoking because of doubts and fear about rejection and abandonment. The importance of maintaining friendships and a sense of belonging may also lead adolescents to engage in HIV risk behaviors (Donenberg & Pao, 2005).

Older persons. The number of persons 50 years of age and older living with HIV disease is increasing (Bhavan, Kampalath, & Overton, 2008). Two primary reasons account for this: Persons diagnosed in their middle adult years (ages 30 to 49) are living longer, and older persons engage in HIV-risk behaviors. The number of older GLBT persons living with HIV is also increasing, posing unique challenges for health care systems. For example, there is an increased demand for GLBT-friendly senior housing facilities. In addition to the psychosocial needs of these individuals, other health-related changes occur in persons living with HIV as they age. These health-related changes include potential age-related changes to the immune response to ART (although the scientific evidence is contentious), bone disease and low bone mineral density, cardiovascular disease and the metabolic syndrome, increased risk for malignancy with aging, additive effects of age related neurocognitive dysfunction (age-related dementia and HIV dementia), and the potential that HIV disease may speed the aging process (Bhavan et al., 2008). Erectile dysfunction medications have contributed to older persons engaging in sexual activities. HIV prevention messages must include content geared to older persons, who may not perceive themselves to be at risk for HIV disease. HIV counseling that routinely offers HIV testing to older adults is important for their health and that of their sexual partners (Bhavan et al., 2008).

Internet Dating

The Internet increases the likelihood of meeting persons with similar interests and desires in a nonthreatening venue. People are able to share information with others on the Internet that they would not normally divulge in other contexts. It creates a perception of safety for some, contributing to its popularity among GLBT persons. The Internet provides opportunities for persons who may not have been able to gain access to others with similar interests and desires in the past. Use of the Internet has been reported in studies of MSM and WSW persons. HIV-negative MSM were more likely to have unprotected anal intercourse (UAI) with potentially serodiscordant partners met on the Internet compared with those met at bars and dance clubs (Berry et al., 2008). In studies that compare risk behaviors of MSM who meet sexual partners on the Internet versus settings in the community, those who met sexual partners on the Internet engage in higher-risk behaviors, such as UAI, club drug use, or having sex with multiple partners (Berg, 2008; Fernandez et al., 2005; Golden et al., 2007). These findings highlight the erroneous belief among some GLBT persons that the Internet may be a safer place to meet others.

Bisexual Persons

Risk factors for bisexuals are specific to sexual behaviors in which the person engages and may include any of the risk behaviors identified for heterosexuals as well as gays, lesbians, and transgender persons. Bisexual persons are at risk for HIV/AIDS from all types of HIV risk behavior. In addition to being at risk for acquiring HIV from any of the HIV risk behaviors in which they engage, they are also at risk for transmitting the virus to others.

Gay and Bisexual Men

The natural history of HIV has been well documented to significantly influence the lives of gay men. Since the identification in the United States of a previously unknown disease entity that would later become HIV in the early 1980s, the lives of gay men have been intimately connected to the science and politics of HIV/AIDS (Rowe & Dowsett, 2008). In North America, Western and Central Europe, and Oceania, the HIV epidemic is primarily centered in the subpopulations of MSM. This connectedness with gay men and their lives for the duration of the HIV epidemic has posed unique challenges for them and their nurses and other health care providers. Davis (2008) and Rowe and Dowsett (2008) theorize that changes in HIV risk behaviors among MSM, primarily gay men, can be best understood as changes in the perception of "gay community." Davis argues that the interrelationships among sexual altruism (the norm prescribed by society that it is the individual's responsibility and obligation to prevent HIV transmission to others), sexual transgression (the individual engaging in HIV risk behavior in light of an awareness of transmission risk), hyper-individualization (the adoption of a "buyer beware" approach to condom use [Adam, 2005] and other HIV risk behavior), and loss of community contribute to the collective thinking of gay men that may contribute to them engaging in HIV risk behaviors. Davis further argues that "sexual citizenship provides a method for addressing how social expectations, such as HIV prevention responsibilities and obligations, are brought into the sexual practice of individuals" (Davis, 2008, p. 184). Sexual citizenship offers a method for determining connections between sexual relating and citizenship duties associated with HIV prevention (Davis, 2008). Understanding the complex dynamics involved with HIV risk behaviors of gay and bisexual men enhances behavioral risk assessment by nurses and other health care providers.

Unprotected Anal Intercourse and "Barebacking"

UAI is one of the highest risk behaviors for transmission of HIV. The popular media and research literature have articulated various other terms that reconceptualize UAI to understand why MSM continue to engage in high-risk sexual behavior (Barker et al., 2007; Crossley, 2004). One such term, *barebacking* emerged in the mid-1990s in the gay community, and early research reported the practice to be understood by gay men as intentional unprotected anal sex (Berg, 2008; Halkitis & Parsons, 2003; Halkitis, Parsons, & Wilton, 2003). In research literature, differentiation between UAI and barebacking was based on intentionality or premeditation on the part of one or both sexual partners (Berg, 2008). However, this conceptualization has lost meaning over time, with MSM increasingly defining barebacking as anal sex without a condom (Berg, 2008; Halkitis, Wilton & Galatowitsch, 2005; Huebner, Proescholdbell, & Nemeroff, 2006; Wilton et al., 2005). The extent to which MSM engage in this HIV risk behavior, the sociodemographic characteristics of MSM who engage in bareback sex, and risk factors associated with barebacking are currently unknown (Berg, 2008). There is some evidence that most MSM who engage in this practice live in urban areas with large gay and bisexual populations (Halkitis et al., 2003; Halkitis et al., 2005; Mansergh et al., 2002), although HIV-negative men also report barebacking (Berg, 2008). HIV-positive men are more likely to engage in bareback sex with serodiscordant men or men of unknown HIV status than are HIV-negative men (Bimbi & Parsons, 2005; Elford et al., 2007; Halkitis & Parsons, 2003; Halkitis et al., 2003, 2005; Mansergh et al., 2002; Wilton et al., 2005). Barebacking among MSM is of concern to nursing and other health care providers because it can lead to sexually transmitted infections, HIV transmission among serodiscordant partners, and HIV reinfection among HIV-positive partners (Chin-Hong et al., 2005).

Another conceptualization of HIV risk behavior among MSM is a subculture of "bug chasers" and "gift givers" at "bug parties" (Freeman, 2003; Moskowitz & Roloff, 2007). "Bug chasers" are HIV-negative MSM who actively seek to become infected with HIV. "Gift givers" are HIV-positive MSM who are willing to engage in UAI with "bug chasers" with the intent of transmitting HIV. Many "bug chasers" misperceive that living with HIV is like living with diabetes or any other chronic illness that can be managed by medications, and some believe they are destined to become infected and would rather not delay the inevitable (Freeman, 2003). Nurses and other health care providers must provide factual information about HIV disease and transmission risk to MSM. Health care providers need to be aware of the psychological state of MSM patients and investigate HIV risk behaviors. They need to be prepared to discuss alternative sexual behaviors and refer MSM for counseling when issues of self-esteem and loss of self-worth emerge during patient encounters.

Club Drugs and the Circuit

Gay and bisexual men are also at risk for HIV through nonsexual behaviors commonly attributed to "gay culture," including use of "club drugs." The club drugs most commonly used by MSM are cocaine, methylenedioxymethamphetamine (MDMA/ecstasy), methamphetamines (crystal, meth, speed), ketamine (special K, kit kat), gamma hydroxybutyrate (GHB), amyl nitrites (poppers), and more recently Viagra and other substances for the treatment of erectile dysfunction (Fernandez et al., 2005; Parsons, Halkitis, & Bimbi, 2006). Because these drugs are perceived to have direct aphrodisiac effects or to enhance sexual pleasure, they are often used in social contexts where sexual activity (frequently UAI) is a primary outcome (Fernandez et al., 2005). These social contexts, often referred to as "the circuit" or "circuit parties," are multiday events where gay and bisexual men have the opportunity to engage in risky sex and club drug use (Fernandez et al., 2005). Club drugs have been associated with HIV risk behavior among MSM in the research literature (Fernandez et al., 2005; McCready & Halkitis, 2008; Mimiaga et al., 2008; Wohl, Frye, & Johnson, 2008). McCready and Halkitis (2008) describe how HIV-positive participants in a qualitative study exploring serostatus disclosure among MSM report that their most recent sexual encounter under the influence occurred in a public environment and/or included multiple partners. Crystal methamphetamine use among MSM in the United States has been reported to be 20 times that of the general population (Mimiaga et al., 2008). For example, in a Los Angeles County sample ($n = 683$) of sociodemographically diverse men, lifetime methamphetamine use was 35% for MSM and 14% for non-MSM (Wohl et al., 2008).

Lesbian and Bisexual Women

Lesbian and bisexual women are not a homogenous group but represent a diverse mosaic of cultural and social backgrounds (Arend, 2003). Major paradoxes with respect to lesbians and HIV risk have been identified including (a) discrepancy between lesbians' perceived personal HIV risk and their perceptions of risk for WSW in general, (b) disconnect between lesbians' perceived personal HIV risk and testing history, and (c) disparities between lesbians' perceived personal HIV risk and reported risk factors and behaviors (Patsdaughter, O'Connor, Grindel, Roberts, & Tarmina, 2003).

Lesbian and bisexual women are at risk for HIV through unprotected sexual activity with men, including a higher likelihood of male sexual partners being gay or bisexual men (Fethers et al., 2000; Marrazzo, Koutsky, & Hunter Hansfield, 2001). Nurses and other health care providers should assess this potential risk factor with patients who identify as lesbian or bisexual. It is important to ask about sexual encounters with a male partner and determine whether they were mutually consensual or if they were rapes or forced sexual encounters. Although there have not been documented cases of WSW HIV transmission through engaging in unprotected sex or sharing of sex toys among women, these behaviors potentially pose risk, and there have been anecdotal reports of HIV transmission. HIV safer sex education for WSW has focused heavily on oral sex and has ignored the fact that penetration with fingers, hands, and shared sex toys provides more contact with a partner's bodily fluids (Kennedy et al., 1995; Patsdaughter et al., 2003).

In addition to injection drug use and sex with men, including IVDUs and gay or bisexual men, risk factors for lesbians identified in the literature include (a) sex under the influence of drugs or alcohol (Perry, 1995; Stevens & Hall, 2001); (b) donor insemination for pregnancy (Kennedy et al., 1995; Norman et al., 1996; White, 1997); (c) receipt of blood or blood products (Norman et al., 1996; White, 1997); and (d) piercing, cutting, or whipping to the point of bleeding (Lemp et al., 1995). Risk of HIV infection through artificial insemination stems primarily from the use of semen from sources other than sperm banks (Kennedy et al., 1995; Patsdaughter et al., 2003). Research is needed to explore effects of cofactors such as HPV, herpes, yeast infections, and other STDs on the mechanics of possible HIV transmission between WSW.

Transgender Persons

Transgender persons (sometimes referred to as "transgendered" persons) are often at heightened risk for HIV because they may engage in high-risk sexual behavior (e.g., unprotected insertive anal intercourse, unprotected receptive anal intercourse) (Garofalo et al., 2006; Girault et al., 2004; Herbst et al., 2008; Kenagy, 2005; Pisani et al., 2004). Nearly one-third of transgender persons in the United States report multiple sex partners, and nearly half report sex with casual partners. These persons may not perceive themselves to be at risk for HIV or may underestimate their risk. Prevalence data on other sexually transmitted infections in transgender populations vary widely (Herbst et al., 2008). Transgender persons may be at increased risk of HIV from engaging in sex work to support high costs associated with the gender reassignment process or for shelter and basic necessities (Garofalo et al., 2006). The proportion of transgender persons who reported engaging in sex work vary widely and ranges between 24% and 75% across the studies reviewed by Herbst and colleagues (2008). Transgender persons are at increased risk for violence in sex work because they are low in the social order of the sex trade. More than half of study respondents reported being forced to have sex, experiencing violence in their home, and being physically abused (Garofalo et al., 2006; Kenagy, 2005).

In addition to high-risk sexual behaviors and potential for violence exposure, transgender persons are at risk for nonsexual transmission of HIV. Injecting hormones and silicone were reported by approximately one-fourth of transgender persons in the United States, but injection of street drugs was much lower at 12% (Herbst et al., 2008). Slightly higher rates of injecting hormones (44%) and silicone (29%) were reported in a study of ethnic minority transgender youth, with needle sharing reported by 17% of those using needles (Garofalo et al., 2006). Transgender persons are also at risk for suicide. Nearly one-third of respondents in United States studies report that they have attempted suicide (Clements-Nolle et al., 2001; Herbst et al., 2008; Kenagy, 2005), and more than half report suicidal thoughts (Herbst et al., 2008). Social isolation, economic marginalization, homelessness, and unmet transgender-specific health care needs may also increase HIV risk for transgender persons (Herbst et al., 2008).

PREVENTION, COUNSELING, AND TESTING

HIV prevention interventions for GLBT persons should be based on the risk profile of the specific group and whenever possible tailored to the individual's HIV risk behavior. Interventions should address the complex behavioral and contextual issues that place members of GLBT populations at risk for HIV. Prevention messages should encourage routine HIV testing for gay men, bisexual men, and transgender persons. Prevention interventions for lesbian and bisexual women should include assessment of HIV risk behaviors, counseling, and, when indicated, HIV testing.

Gay and Bisexual Men

Based on global epidemiologic trends, gay and bisexual men remain at high risk for HIV disease. HIV prevention interventions must continue to focus on these men. Nurses can be effective liaisons for gay and bisexual men who are at risk for HIV and can provide HIV prevention interventions and advocate for legal and policy change. There are currently many different types of HIV prevention interventions for gay and bisexual men, including serosorting, strategic positioning, and negotiation around viral load (Jin et al., 2007).

Serosorting (limiting unprotected anal sexual partners to those who are of the same HIV status [Eaton et al., 2007]) as a risk-reduction strategy may seem sound in theory. Little empirical evidence exists to support its efficacy, with conflicting evidence about the environmental contexts that are most appropriate for its use. There is evidence that the practice results in increased incidence of HIV and the possibility of reinfection for persons living with HIV (Butler & Smith, 2007). They conclude that "serosorting on the basis of mutual disclosure of perceived HIV status is a flawed strategy for reducing sexual transmissions of HIV when it does not consider the prevalence of recent HIV infections in specific populations" (Butler & Smith, 2007, p. 1220). Van der Bij and colleagues (2007) observed that a higher level of unprotected anal intercourse with anonymous or nonconcordant traceable partners more likely explained increased HIV incidence among STI outpatient clinic attendees than a difference in serosorting behavior (Van der Bij et al., 2007). In other words, condom use is a more effective HIV prevention strategy than serosorting. As with all HIV risk-reduction efforts, serosorting involves complex risk–benefit analysis to determine its efficacy across all at-risk populations. The ease with which serosorting can occur in the virtual environment of the Internet is one potential benefit to the practice.

Strategic positioning is "the practice of taking the sexual position believed to be less likely to result in HIV transmission, that is, the HIV-negative man in the insertive role and the HIV-positive man in the receptive role" (Van de Ven et al., 2002). Negotiation around the viral load is based on the principle that an HIV-positive partner who has a lower viral load is less likely to transmit the HIV virus to a seronegative partner (Jin et al., 2007; Van de Ven et al., 2005). It is critical for nurses and other health care providers to inform patients about risks involved in engaging in these practices, namely that they do little to protect against transmission of HIV when a partner is unaware he is HIV infected. Further, these practices offer little protection against other sexually transmitted infections. More research is needed to determine the efficacy of serosorting, strategic positioning, and negotiation around viral load as HIV prevention strategies.

Lesbian and Bisexual Women

HIV education and prevention interventions for WSW need to be gender appropriate as well as targeted toward specific risk factors and behaviors and tailored to specific subgroups (e.g., age cohorts, cultural/ethnic groups, socioeconomic groups, geographic regions) (Arend, 2003; Shotsky, 1996). HIV education for WSW should enable them to make a realistic choice about the level of risk they are willing to take in the context of their everyday life (Munson, 1999). It is important to acknowledge that lesbian and bisexual-identified WSW may also have sex with men, especially gay or bisexual peers, and HIV prevention education and counseling should incorporate discussion of potential risks.

Transgender Persons

Because of high rates of HIV infection and involvement of transgender persons in HIV risk behaviors, prevention interventions and counseling and testing are critical issues. HIV prevention interventions need to be transgender specific and address the risk factors and social environmental contexts of HIV risk (Herbst et al., 2008; Kenagy, 2005). Nurses and other health care providers working with transgender persons should encourage routine HIV testing.

HIV TREATMENT AND OTHER HEALTH-RELATED ISSUES

Treatment of HIV disease has seen major improvements since the epidemic began. Medications have been formulated or developed to optimize efficacy and reduce adverse effects, but many challenges remain. Treatment of HIV disease among GLBT persons internationally may pose additional challenges related to treatment access. Where same-gender sexual behavior and HIV disease transmission are criminalized, the likelihood of GLBT persons seeking medical care may be severely diminished. In all health care settings where persons at risk for or who are living with HIV disease seek services, the importance of a "safe and secure" environment with supportive and nonjudgmental health care providers who are competent and willing to work with GLBT persons is paramount (Dawson-Rose et al., 2005; Kenagy, 2005; Phillips, 2008).

Antiretroviral Therapy Initiation

Initiation of ART for GLBT persons should be guided by an individual's clinical presentation (Gallant, 2008) in the context of a collaborative patient–provider relationship (Dawson-Rose et al., 2005). The complex nature of ART and the interrelationship between ART agents and HIV requires near-perfect adherence to achieve optimal benefit. Treatment should be consistent with treatment guidelines as for other persons with similar disease state markers and age and gender constraints.

Psychosocial Considerations Influencing Treatment

Comprehensive HIV disease management entails not only prescribing ART but also includes assessment of the psychosocial environment in which the GLBT person with HIV/AIDS lives. Nurses and other health care providers need to be aware of facilitators and barriers to HIV treatment and must intervene when appropriate to facilitate optimal therapeutic benefit (Reeves & Piefer, 2005; Sanders et al., 2005; Yasuda et al., 2004). While many treatment barriers have been identified in the literature, those specific to GLBT persons are summarized as follows (Mayer et al., 2008):

- Reluctance by some GLBT patients to disclose sexual or gender identity when receiving medical care.
- Insufficient numbers of providers competent in dealing with GLBT issues as part of the provision of medical care.
- Structural barriers that impede access to health insurance and limit visiting and medical decision-making rights for GLBT persons and their partners.
- Lack of culturally appropriate prevention services.
- Criminalization of sexual behaviors (e.g., sodomy laws) and HIV transmission in some nations and jurisdictions may limit access

to medical care for GLBT persons and create an ethical–legal conundrum for health care providers.

"Family" and Supportive Others

Significant relationships in an individual's life are important for optimal functioning and provide interpersonal social support (Phillips, 2008; Wolitski et al., 2007). Supportive significant others often provide a reason to continue fighting HIV disease (Gaskins, 2006). Bodenlos et al. (2007) found that the presence of social support was associated with appointment attendance, a proxy measure for adherence, but satisfaction with social support was not. The degree (e.g., parent, sibling, intimate partner) may not be as important as the presence of a supportive other in a person's life as he or she faces the challenges of ART adherence and a chronic illness such as HIV disease (Phillips, 2008). Nurses need to be sensitive to how GLBT persons define "family" and explore this issue to determine relationship dynamics within the context of HIV disease.

Socioeconomic, Ethical, and Legal Considerations

Insurance and the Financing of HIV Care and Treatment. How to finance HIV treatment is a major concern for GLBT persons living with HIV disease. Throughout much of the world, governments and nongovernmental organizations have developed strategies to provide ART to all persons for whom ART is clinically indicated. There are many gaps in these strategies, and not all eligible persons have been able to gain access to HIV treatment. Beyond these governmental and quasi-governmental programs, many GLBT persons living with HIV rely on health insurance to cover HIV-related treatment costs. This reliance becomes challenging in communities and national contexts where domestic partnerships, civil unions, or same-gender marriages are not recognized legally. Insurance benefits and coverage for the GLBT person living with HIV may not be honored. Similarly, survivor benefits for same-gender partners may not be honored under life insurance policies in many jurisdictions internationally (Mayer et al., 2008; Wolitski et al., 2007).

Medico-Legal and Ethical Issues. The right to die and who will make decisions about health care and end-of-life care are of concern to GLBT persons living with HIV disease. Living wills and health care surrogacy must be considered in collaboration with nurses, other health care providers, attorneys, and most importantly GLBT persons living with HIV and their "family." In many legal jurisdictions, the individual whom the GLBT person living with HIV disease may choose to have make decisions on his or her behalf may not have the legal authority, thus necessitating dialogue among multiple "family" members. Intervention from legal and medical ethics teams may be needed to facilitate the health care decision-making process. Existence of living wills and health care surrogacy documentation may reduce complex legal issues, but nurses and health care providers need to be aware that these may be challenged in courts of law (Mayer et al., 2008; Stein & Bonuck, 2001; Wolitski et al., 2007; Williams & Freeman, 2007). Nurses must make themselves aware of the legal, ethical, and policy standards regarding living wills and health care surrogacy in their community and work environments.

Anticipatory Guidance Regarding Parenthood. Procreation and the desire to be a parent are important to many GLBT persons. Gay and lesbian couples who chose to act on their desire to become parents are unique in that they require a facilitator to do so. Whether the facilitator is a donor, surrogate, or birth parents (if the child is adopted), an additional layer of complexity is added to the family dynamics (Mitchell & Green, 2007). This complexity may contribute to psychological distress for GLBT persons. The manner in which a donor or surrogate is obtained may contribute to increased HIV risk. GLBT persons considering parenthood should consult health care providers and seek medical advice whenever possible and feasible if they plan to use a donor or surrogate to become parents. Nurses and health care providers working with GLBT persons must be aware of legal ramifications and provide accurate information about parenting options and work with GLBT patients to explore all possible parenthood alternatives (Hare & Skinner, 2008; Stacey, 2006; Tasker & Patterson, 2007).

Aging with Dignity and End of Life Care. Life expectancy has risen over the last century in many parts of the world, including among GLBT persons. Older persons represent the fastest-growing segment of populations in North America and Western Europe (Jackson, Johnson, & Roberts, 2008). ART has extended life for many GLBT persons living with HIV disease, creating a growing urgency to consider how and where these persons will grow old and what services they will require (Jackson et al., 2008; Smolinski & Colon, 2006; Stein & Bonuck, 2001). As

GLBT persons age, many are confronted with the likelihood of entering long-term care facilities and may have concerns about the potential for discrimination based on sexual orientation. This fear of discrimination may lead GLBT persons to choose to live out their lives in isolation or to forego long-term care options that may offer needed health care and social services (Jackson et al., 2008; Williams & Freeman, 2007). GLBT persons may require guidance about end-of-life care. Unlike heterosexual persons, GLBT persons and their partners often face significant legal challenges and societal attitudes that can hinder their ability to die in dignity (Smolinski & Colon, 2006).

Comorbid Health Conditions

GLBT health issues have historically been insufficiently understood, and research has been sporadic and often dependent on the political will of global leaders. Nurses and health care providers of GLBT persons living with HIV need to be aware of other health issues among GLBT patients. Table 11.3 provides examples of health-related topics that should be assessed when working with GLBT persons.

Recommended Routine Nursing Assessment for GLBT persons

Nurses providing care for GLBT persons, regardless of HIV serostatus, should conduct a thorough health history and physical examination as appropriate at the first patient encounter and routinely thereafter. Nurses should regularly assess for signs and symptoms of: (1) substance abuse or misuse (including prescription and over-the-counter medications, herbal and traditional medicines, illegal and illicit substances, and alcohol), (2) depression and other mental health and psychological distress issues, (3) stigma and the individual's adaptation and coping strategies, and (4) potential for and presence of discrimination and how the individual adapts and copes.

For GLBT persons living with HIV disease who are prescribed ART, nurses and health care providers must assess levels of adherence to these and other therapeutic interventions. Nurses are uniquely positioned to facilitate ART adherence and advocate on behalf of GLBT persons living with HIV. For example, nurses can be involved in ART adherence intervention programs and provide patient education and adherence counseling. Nurses may be involved in case management activities and

Table 11.3

HEALTH ISSUES AND PROBLEMS COMMONLY OCCURRING IN GLBT PERSONS

GAY AND BISEXUAL MEN	LESBIAN AND BISEXUAL WOMEN	TRANSGENDER PERSONS
HIV/AIDS, safer sex	Breast cancer	Access to health care
Substance use	Depression/anxiety	Health history
Depression/anxiety	Heart health	Hormones
Hepatitis immunization	Gynecological cancer	Cardiovascular health
Sexually transmitted infections	Fitness	Cancer
Prostate, testicular, and colon cancer	Tobacco use	Sexually transmitted infections, safer sex
Alcohol use	Alcohol use	Alcohol and tobacco
Tobacco use	Substance use	Depression/anxiety
Fitness (diet, exercise)	Domestic violence	Injectable silicone
Anal papilloma	Osteoporosis	Fitness (diet, exercise)

Adapted from Gay and Lesbian Medical Association (GLMA) (2006) and GLMA (nd).

advocate for structural changes such as adequate housing and employment. These interventions require an effective nurse–patient relationship based on trust and mutual respect (Dawson-Rose et al., 2005; Phillips, 2008).

CONCLUSION

GLBT persons living with HIV disease encounter many challenges for which nurses are uniquely positioned within the health care system and society to advocate for change in how care is delivered. This chapter offers nurses an understanding of the complex issues surrounding sexuality and how they influence health behaviors of GLBT persons. Stigma is conceptually defined, and specific types of stigma are discussed in relation to GLBT persons living with HIV disease. The epidemiological profile of HIV disease among GLBT persons highlights the economic, legal, and political realities for them globally. HIV risk factors and vulnerabilities specific to GLBT persons are highlighted. Issues of prevention, counseling, testing, and treatment were discussed in the context of GLBT persons. Legal and ethical foundations for the nurses' role with GLBT persons living with HIV is described, including a call for advocacy to change social policy where possible. Recommendations for routine nurses assessment of health and psychosocial needs of GLBT persons have been articulated.

REFERENCES

Adam, B. (2005). Constructing the neoliberal sexual actor: Responsibility and care of the self in the discourse of barebackers. *Culture, Health and Sexuality, 7*(4), 333–346.

Arend, E. D. (2003). The politics of invisibility: HIV-positive women who have sex with women and their struggle for support. *Journal of the Association of Nurses in AIDS Care, 14*(6), 37–47.

Barker, M., Hagger-Johnson, G., Hegarty, P., Hutchison, C., & Riggs, D. (2007). Responses from the lesbian and gay psychology section to Crossley's "making sense of 'barebacking.'" *British Journal of Social Psychology, 46,* 667–677.

Bauer, G., & Welles, S. L. (2001). Beyond assumptions of negligible risk: Sexually transmitted diseases and women who have sex with women. *American Journal of Public Health, 91,* 1282–1286.

Berg, R. C. (2008). Barebacking among MSM Internet users. *AIDS and Behavior, 12,* 822–833.

Berry, M., Raymond, H. F., Kellogg, T., & McFarland, W. (2008). The Internet, HIV serosorting and transmission risk among men who have sex with men, San Francisco. *AIDS, 22*(6), 787–789.

Bhavan, K. P., Kampalath, V. N., & Overton, E. T. (2008). The aging of the HIV epidemic. *Current HIV/AIDS Reports, 5,* 150–158.

Bimbi, D. S., & Parsons, J. T. (2005). Barebacking among Internet based male sex workers. *Journal of Gay & Lesbian Psychotherapy,* 9(3/4), 85–105.

Bodenlos, J. S., Grothe, K. B., Whitehead, D., Konkle-Parker, D. J., Jones, G. N., & Brantley, P. J. (2007). Attitudes toward health care providers and appointment attendance in HIV/AIDS patients. *Journal of the Association of Nurses in AIDS Care, 18*(3), 65–73.

Brennan, D. J., Hellerstedt, W. L., Ross, M. W., & Welles, S. L. (2007). History of childhood sexual abuse and HIV risk behaviors in homosexual and bisexual men. *American Journal of Public Health,* 97(6), 1107–1112.

Bull, C. (2003). An AIDS wake-up call. *The Advocate, 885,* 35–36.

Burris, S., & Cameron, E. (2008). The case against criminalization of HIV transmission. *Journal of the American Medical Association, 300*(5), 578–581.

Butler, D. M., & Smith, D. M. (2007). Serosorting can potentially increase HIV transmissions. *AIDS, 21*(9), 1218–1220.

Canadian Broadcasting Corporation. (2007, March). Out in Iran: Inside Iran's secret gay world. *CBC News: Sunday.* Retrieved on September 19, 2008, from www.cbc.ca/sunday/2007/03/030407_1.html.

Campa, A., Yang, Z., Lai, S., Xue, L., Phillips, J. C., Sales, S., et al. (2005). HIV- related wasting in HIV-infected drug users in the era of highly active antiretroviral therapy. *Clinical Infectious Diseases, 41*(8), 1179–1185.

Centers for Disease Control. (2006, June). *HIV/AIDS and U.S. women who have sex with women (WSW).* Retrieved October 10, 2008, from www.cdc.gov/hiv/topics/women/resources/factsheets/wsw.htm.

Centers for Disease Control. (2008). Trends in HIV/AIDS diagnoses among men who have sex with men—33 States, 2001–2006. *Morbidity Mortality Weekly Report, 57*(25), 681–686.

Chin-Hong, P. V., Deeks, S. G., Liegler, T., Hagos, E., Krone, M. R., Gant, R. M., et al. (2005). HIV-risk sexual behavior in adults with genotypically proven antiretroviral-resistant HIV infection. *Journal of Acquired Immune Deficiency Syndrome, 40,* 79–83.

Clements-Nolle, K., Marx, R., Guzman, R., & Katz, M. (2001). HIV prevalence, risk behaviors, health care use, and mental health status of transgender persons: Implications for public health intervention. *American Journal of Public Health, 91*(6), 915–921.

Crossley, M. (2004). Making sense of 'barebacking': Gay men's narratives, unsafe sex and the 'resistance habitus.' *British Journal of Social Psychology, 43,* 225–244.

Dawson-Rose, C., Shade, S. B., Lum, P. J., Knight, K. R., Parsons, J. T., & Purcell, D. W. (2005). Health care experiences of HIV positive injection drug users. *The Journal of Multicultural Nursing and Health, 11*(1), 23–30.

Davis, M. (2008). The "loss of community" and other problems for sexual citizenship in recent HIV prevention. *Sociology of Health and Illness, 30*(2), 182–196.

Diamant, A. L., Schuster, M. A., McGuigan, K., & Lever, J. (1999). Lesbians' sexual history with men. *Archives of Internal Medicine, 159,* 2730–2736.

Dolan, K. A., & Davis, P. W. (2003). Nuances and shifts in lesbian women's constructions of STI and HIV vulnerability. *Social Science and Medicine, 57*(1), 25–38.

Donenberg, G. R., & Pao, M. (2005). Youth's and HIV/AIDS: Psychiatry's role in a changing epidemic. *Journal of the American Academy of Child and Adolescent Psychiatry, 44*(8), 728–747.

Eaton, L. A., Kalichman, S. C., Cain, D. N., Cherry, C., Stearns, H. L., Amaral, C., M., et al. (2007). Serosorting sexual partners and risk for HIV among men who have sex with men. *American Journal of Preventive Medicine, 33*(6), 479–485.

Elford, J., Bolding, G., Davis, M., Sherr, L., & Hart, G. (2007). Barebacking among HIV-positive gay men in London. *Sexually Transmitted Diseases, 34,* 93–98.

Ensign, J., & Santelli, J. (1997). Shelter-based homeless youth. Health and access to care. *Archives of Pediatric and Adolescent Medicine, 151,* 817–823.

Ensign, J., & Santelli, J. (1998). Health status and service use: Comparison of adolescents at a school-based health clinic with homeless adolescents. *Archives of Pediatric & Adolescent Medicine, 152*(1), 20–24.

Evans-Campbell, T., Fredriksen-Goldsen, K. I., Walters, K. L., & Stately, A. (2007). Caregiving experiences among American Indian Two-Spirit men and women: Contemporary and historical roles. *Journal of Gay & Lesbian Social Services, 18*(3/4), 75–92.

Fernandez, M. I., Perrino, T., Bowen, G. S., Hernandez, N., Cardenas, S. A., Marsh, D., et al. (2005). Club drug use, sexual behavior, and HIV risk among community and Internet samples of Hispanic MSM: Implications for clinicians. *Journal of Social Work Practice in the Addictions, 5*(4), 81–100.

Fethers, K., Marks, C., Mindel, A., & Estcourt, C.S. (2000). Sexually transmitted infections and risk behaviours among women who have sex with women. *Sexually Transmitted Infections, 76*, 345–349.

Freeman, G. A. (2003). Bug chasers: The men who long to be HIV+. *Rolling Stone.com.* Retrieved on June 19, 2008, from www.rolling stone.com/news/story/ 5939950/bug_chasers.

Gallant, J. E. (2008). When to start antiretroviral therapy: A swinging pendulum? *Topics in HIV Medicine, 16*(2), 82–88.

Garofalo, R., Deleon J., Osmer, E., Doll, M., & Harper G.W. (2006). Overlooked, misunderstood and at-risk: Exploring the lives and HIV risk of ethnic minority male-to-female transgender youth. *Journal of Adolescent Health, 38*, 230–236.

Gaskins, S. W. (2006). Disclosure decisions of rural African American men living with HIV disease. *Journal of the Association of Nurses in AIDS Care, 17*(6), 38–46.

Gay and Lesbian Medical Association (GLMA). (2006). *Guidelines for care of lesbian, gay, bisexual, and transgender patients.* San Francisco, GLMA. Retrieved on August 12, 2008, from http://ce54.citysoft. com/_data/n_0001/resources/live/ GLMA%20guidelines%202006%2 0FINAL.pdf.

Gay and Lesbian Medical Association (GLMA). (nd). *Top ten issues to discuss with your healthcare provider.* San Francisco, GLMA. Retrieved on August 12, 2008, from www.glma.org/index.cfm?fuseaction=Page. viewPage&pageId=586& parentID=533&nodeID=1.

Girault, P., Saidel, T., Song, N., de Lind Van Wijngaarden, J. W., Dallabette, G., Stuer, F., et al. (2004). HIV, STIs, and sexual behaviors among men who have sex with men in Phnom Penh, Cambodia. *AIDS Education and Training, 16*(1), 31–44.

Golden, M. R., Wood, R. W., Buskin, S. E., Fleming, M., & Harrington, R. D. (2007). Ongoing risk behavior among persons with HIV in medical care. *AIDS and Behavior, 11*, 726–735.

Goldstein, N. (1995). Lesbians and the medical profession: HIV/AIDS and the pursuit of visibility. *Women's Studies, 24*, 531–552.

Halkitis, P. N., & Parsons, J. T. (2003). Intentional unsafe sex (barebacking) among HIV-positive gay men who seek sexual partners on the internet. *AIDS Care, 15*, 367–378.

Halkitis, P. N., Parsons, J. T., & Wilton, L. (2003). Barebacking among gay and bisexual men in New York City: Explanations for the emergence of intentional unsafe behaviors. *Archives of Sexual Behavior, 32*, 351–358.

Halkitis, P. N., Wilton, L., & Galatowitsch, P. (2005). What's in a term? How gay and bisexual men understand barebacking. *Journal of Gay and Lesbian Psychotherapy, 9*(3/4), 35–48.

Hall, H. I., Song, R., Rhodes, P., Prejean, J., An, Q., Lee, L. M., et al. (2008). Estimation of HIV incidence in the United States. *Journal of the American Medical Association, 300*(5), 520–529.

Hare, J., & Skinner, D. (2008). "Whose child is this?": Determining legal status for lesbian parents who used assisted reproductive technologies. *Family Relations, 57,* 365–375.

Heijnders, M., & van der Meij, S. (2006). The fight against stigma: An overview of stigma-reduction strategies and interventions. *Psychology, Health and Medicine, 11,* 353–363.

Herbst, J. H., Jacobs, E. D., Finlayson, T. J., McKleroy, V. S., Neuman, M. S., Crepaz, N., et al. (2008). Estimating HIV prevalence and risk behaviors of transgender persons in the United States: A systematic review. *AIDS and Behavior, 12,* 1–17.

Huebner, D. M., Proescholdbell, R. J., & Nemeroff, C. J. (2006). Do gay and bisexual men share researchers' definition of barebacking? *Journal of Psychology and Human Sexuality, 18,* 67–77.

International Council of Nurses. (2006). *Code of Ethics.* Geneva: Author. Retrieved on May 28, 2009, from http://icn.ch/ethics.htm.

Jackson, N. C., Johnson, M. J., & Roberts, R. (2008). The potential impact of discrimination fears of older gays, lesbians, bisexuals, and transgender individuals living in small- to moderate-sized cities on long-term health care. *Journal of Homosexuality, 54*(3), 325–339.

Jacobs, S. E., Thomas, W., & Lang, S. (1997). Introduction. In S. E. Jacobs, W. Thomas, & S. Lang (eds.), *Two-Spirit people: Native American gender identity, sexuality, and spirituality.* Urbana & Chicago: University of Illinois Press, pp. 1–18.

Jin, F., Prestage, G. P., Ellard, J., Kippax, S. C., Kaldor, J. M., & Grulich, A. E. (2007). How homosexual men believe they became infected with HIV: The role of risk-reduction behaviors. *Journal of Acquired Immune Deficiency Syndromes, 46*(2), 245–247.

Kenagy, G. P. (2002). HIV among transgendered people. *AIDS Care, 14*(1), 127–134.

Kenagy, G. P (2005). Transgender health: Findings from two needs assessment studies in Philadelphia. *Health & Social Work, 30*(1), 19–26.

Kennedy, M. B., Scarlett, M. I., Duerr, A. C., & Chu, S. Y. (1995). Assessing HIV risk among women who have sex with women: Scientific and communication issues. *Journal of the American Medical Women's Association, 50*(3/4), 103–107.

Kidder, D. P., Wolitski, R. J., Royal, S., Aidala, A., Courtney-Quirk, C., Holtgrave, D. R., et al. (2007). Access to housing as a structural intervention for homeless and unstably housed people living with HIV: Rationale, methods, and implementation of the housing and health study. *AIDS and Behavior,* ePub date: June 2, 2007, (DOI 10.1007/s10461-007-9249-0).

Krawczyk, C. S., Funkhouser, E., Kilby, J. M., & Vermund, S. H. (2006). Delayed access to HIV diagnosis and care: Special concerns for the Southern United States. *AIDS Care, 18* (Suppl. 1), S35–S44.

Lemp, G. F., Jones, M., Kellogg, T. A., Nieri, G. N., Anderson, L., Withum, D., et al. (1995). HIV seroprevalence and risk behaviors among lesbians and bisexual women in San Francisco and Berkley, California. *American Journal of Public Health, 85,* 1549–1552.

Lichtenstein, B. (2003). Stigma as a barrier to treatment of sexually transmitted infection in the American Deep South: Issues of race, gender and poverty. *Social Science & Medicine, 57*(12), 2435–2445.

Mansergh, G., Marks, G., Colfax, G. N., Guzman, R., Rader, M., & Buchbinder, S. (2002). "Barebacking" in a diverse sample of men who have sex with men. *AIDS, 16,* 653–659.

Marrazzo, J. M., Koutsky, L. A. & Hunter Handsfield, H. (2001). Characteristics of female sexually transmitted disease clinic clients who report same-sex behaviour. *International Journal of STD & AIDS, 12,* 41–46.

Mayer, K. H., Bradford, J. B., Makadon, H. J., Stall, R., Goldhammer, H., & Landers, S. (2008). Sexual and gender minority health: What we know and what needs to be done. *American Journal of Public Health, 98*(6), 989–995.

McCready, K. C., & Halkitis, P. N. (2008). HIV serostatus disclosure to sexual partners among HIV-positive methamphetamine-using gay, bisexual, and other men who have sex with men. *AIDS Education and Prevention, 20*(1), 15–29.

Meyer, L., Wright, T. C., Denny, L., & Kuhn, L. (2006). Nested case–control study of cervical mucosal lesions, ectopy, and incident HIV infection among women in Cape Town, South Africa. *Sexually Transmitted Diseases, 33,* 683–687.

Miller, C. T., & Kaiser, C. R. (2001). A theoretical perspective on coping with stigma. *Journal of Social Issues, 57,* 73–92.

Mimiaga, M. J., Fair, A. D., Mayer, K. H., Koenan, K., Gortmaker, S., Tetu, A. M., et al. (2008). Experiences and sexual behaviors of HIV-infected MSM who acquired HIV in the context of crystal metham-phetamine use. *AIDS Education and Prevention, 20*(1), 30–41.

Mitchell, V., & Green, R. (2007). Different storks for different folks: Gay and lesbian parents' experiences with alternative insemination and surrogacy. *Journal of GLBT Family Studies, 3*(2/3), 81–104.

Moscicki, A. B., Ma, Y., Holland, C., & Vermund, S. H. (2001). Cervical ectopy in adolescent girls with and without human immunodeficiency virus infection. *Journal of Infectious Disease, 183,* 865–870.

Moskowitz, D. A., & Roloff, M. E. (2007). The existence of a bug chasing subculture. *Culture, Health and Sexuality, 9*(4), 347–357.

Munson, M. (1999). Safer sex and the polyamorous lesbian. *Journal of Lesbian Studies, 3*(1/2), 209–216.

National Coalition for the Homeless. (2007). *HIV/AIDS and homeless-ness.* Retrieved on August 8, 2008, from www.nationalhomeless.org/pulications/facts/HIV.pdf.

Norman, A. D., Perry, M. J., Stevenson, L. Y., Kelley, J. A., & Roffman, R. A. (1996). Lesbian and bisexual women in small cities—at risk for HIV? *Public Health Reports, 111,* 347–352.

Nyblade, L. C. (2006). Measuring HIV stigma: Existing knowledge and gaps. *Psychology, Health & Medicine, 11,* 335–345.

Operario, D., Burton, J., Underhill, K., & Sevelius, J. (2008). Men who have sex with transgender women: Challenges to category-based HIV prevention. *AIDS and Behavior, 12,* 18–26.

Parsons, J. T., Halkitis, P. N., & Bimbi, D. S. (2006). Club drug use among young adults frequenting dance clubs and other social venues in New York City. *Journal of Child & Adolescent Substance Abuse, 15*(3), 1–14.

Patsdaughter, C. A., O'Connor, C. A., Grindel, C. G., Roberts, S. J., & Tarmina, M. S. (2003). *The lesbian paradox in HIV risk* [Abstract]. Conference Program of the 16th Annual Association of Nurses in AIDS Care Conference (Spotlight on HIV/AIDS Nursing), 70, New York City, NY.

Perry, S. M. (1995). Lesbian alcohol and marijuana use: Correlated of HIV risk behaviors and abusive relationships. *Journal of Psychoactive Drugs, 27,* 413–419.

Phillips, J. C. (2008). Social factors influencing antiretroviral therapy (ART) adherence among black men living with HIV who use illicit drugs. *Dissertation Abstracts International, 69* (06). (UMI No. 3319008)

Pisani, E., Girault, P., Gultom, M., Sukartini, N., Kumalawati, J., Jazan, S., et al. (2004). HIV, syphilis infection, and sexual practices among transgenders, male sex workers, and other men who have sex with men in Jakarta, Indonesia. *Sexually Transmitted Infections, 80,* 536–540.

Reeves, J. D., & Piefer, A. J. (2005). Emerging drug targets for antiretroviral therapy. *Drugs, 65*(13), 1747–66.

Richardson, D. (2000). The social construction of immunity: HIV risk perception and prevention among lesbians and bisexual women. *Culture, Health, and Sexuality, 2*(1), 33–49.

Rowe, M. S., & Dowsett, G. W. (2008). Sex, love, friendship, belonging and place: Is there a role for "gay community" in HIV prevention today? *Culture, Health & Sexuality, 10*(4), 329–344.

Saewyc, E. M. (2005). Teen pregnancy among gay, lesbian, and bisexual youths: Influences of stigma, sexual abuse, and sexual orientation. Chapter 5 in A. Omoto & H. Kurtzman, (eds.), *Sexual orientation and mental health: Examining identity and development in lesbian, gay, and bisexual people,* pp 95–116. Washington DC: APA Press.

Saewyc, E., M., MacKay, L. J., Anderson, J., & Drozda, C. (2008). *It's not what you think: Sexually exploited youth in British Columbia.* Vancouver: University of British Columbia School of Nursing. Retrieved on October 10, 2008, from www.nursing.ubc.ca/PDFs/ItsNotWhatYouThink.pdf.

Saewyc, E. M., Richens, K., Skay, C. L., Reis, E., Poon, C., & Murphy, A. (2006). Sexual orientation, sexual abuse, and HIV-risk behaviors among adolescents in the Pacific Northwest. *American Journal of Public Health, 96*(6), 1104–1110.

Sanders, G. D., Bayoumi, A. M., Sundaram, V., Bilir, S. P., Neukermans, C. P., Rydzak, C. E., et al. (2005). Cost-effectiveness of screening for HIV in the era of highly active antiretroviral therapy. *New England Journal of Medicine, 352*(6), 570–585.

Sandfort, T. G. M., & Dodge, B. (2008). "...And then there was the down low": Introduction to black and Latino male bisexualities. *Archives of Sexual Behavior, 37*(5), 675–682.

Saunders, J. M. (1999). Health problems of lesbian women. *Nursing Clinics of North America, 34,* 381–391.

Shotsky, W. J. (1996). Women who have sex with other women: HIV seroprevalence in New York State counseling and testing programs. *Women and Health, 24*(2), 1–15.

Simbayi, L. C., Kalichman, S., Strebel, A., Cloete, A., Henda, N., & Mqeketo, A. (2007). Internalized stigma, discrimination, and depression among men and women living with HIV/AIDS in Cape Town, South Africa. *Social Science & Medicine, 64,* 1823–1831.

Simoni, J. M., Walters, K. L., Balsam, K. F., & Meyers, S. B. (2006). Victimization, substance use, and HIV risk behaviors among gay/bisexual/Two-Spirit and heterosexual American Indian men in New York City. *American Journal of Public Health, 96*(12), 2240–2245.

Smith, A., Saewyc, E. M., Albert, M., Mackay, L., Northcott, M., & the McCreary Centre Society. (2007). *Against the odds: A profile of marginalized and street-involved youth in BC.* Vancouver, BC: McCreary Centre Society.

Smolinski, K. M., & Colon, Y. (2006). Silent voices and invisible walls: Exploring end of life care with lesbians and gay men. *Journal of Psychosocial Oncology, 24*(1), 51–64.

Stacey, J. (2006). Gay parenthood and the decline of paternity as we knew it. *Sexualities, 9*(1), 27–55.

Stein, G. L., & Bonuck, K. A. (2001). Attitudes on end-of-life care and advanced care planning in the lesbian and gay community. *Journal of Palliative Medicine, 4*(2), 173–190.

Stevens, P. E. (1993). Lesbians and HIV: Clinical, research, and policy issues. *American Journal of Orthopsychiatry, 63,* 289–294.

Stevens, P. E., & Hall, J. M. (2001). Sexuality and safer sex: The issues for lesbians and bisexual women. *Journal of Obstetric, Gynecologic, and Neonatal Nursing, 30,* 439–447.

Tasker, F., & Patterson, C. J. (2007). Research on gay and lesbian parenting: Retrospect and prospect. *Journal of GLBT Family Studies, 3*(2/3). 9-34.

UNAIDS. (2003). *Fact sheet on stigma and discrimination.* Geneva: Author.

UNAIDS. (2008a). *Policy Brief: Criminalization of HIV transmission.* Geneva: Author.

UNAIDS. (2008b). *Report on the global HIV/AIDS epidemic 2008.* Geneva: Author.

Van der Bij, A. K. Kolader, M. E., de Vries, H. J. C., Prins, M., Coutinho, R. A., & Dukers, N. H. T. M. (2007). Condom use rather than serosorting explains differences in HIV incidence among men who have sex with men. *Journal of Acquired Immune Deficiency Syndrome, 45*(5), 574–580.

Van de Ven, P., Kippax, S., Crawford, J., Rawstorne, P, Prestage, G., Grulich, A., et al. (2002). In a minority of gay men, sexual risk practice indicates strategic positioning for perceived risk reduction rather than unbridled sex. *AIDS Care, 14*(4), 471–480.

Van de Ven, P., Mao, L. Fogarty, A., Rawstorne, P., Crawford, J., Prestage, G., et al. (2005). Undetectable vial load is associated with sexual risk taking in HIV serodiscordant gay couples in Sydney. *AIDS, 19*(2), 179–184.

Wade, A. S., Kane, C. T., Diallo, P. A., Diop, A., K., Gueye, K., Mboup, S., et al. (2005). HIV infection and sexually transmitted infections among men who have sex with men in Senegal. *AIDS, 19*(18), 2133–2140.

White, J. C. (1997). HIV risk assessment and prevention in lesbians and women who have sex with women: Practical information for clinicians. *Health Care for Women International, 18*, 127–138.

Williams, M. E., & Freeman, P. A. (2007). Transgender health: Implications for aging and caregiving. *Journal of Gay & Lesbian Social Services, 18*(3/4), 93–108.

Wilton, L., Halkitis, P. N., English, G., & Roberson, M. (2005). An exploratory study of barebacking, club drug use, and meanings of sex in black and Latino gay and bisexual men in the age of AIDS. *Journal of Gay & Lesbian Psychotherapy, 9*(3/4), 49–72.

Wohl, A. R., Frye, D. M., & Johnson, D. F. (2008). Demographic characteristics and sexual behaviors associated with methamphetamine use among MSM and non-MSM diagnosed with AIDS in Los Angeles County. *AIDS and Behavior, 12*, 705–712.

Wolitski, R. J., Stall, R., & Valdiserri, R. O., Eds. (2007). *Unequal opportunity: Health disparities affecting gay and bisexual men in the United States.* New York: Oxford University Press.

World Health Organization (WHO). (2003). *Guidelines for medico-legal care for victims of sexual violence.* Geneva: Author. Retrieved on September 21, 2008, from whqlibdoc.who.int/publications/2004/924154628X.pdf.

World Medical Association. (2006). *International Code of Medical Ethics.* Ferney-Voltaire, France: Author. Retrieved on May 28, 2009, from http://www.wma.net/e/policy/c8.htm.

Yasuda, J. M., Miller, C., Currier, J. S., Forthal, D. N., Kemper, C. A., Beall, G. N., et al. (2004). The correlation between plasma concentrations of protease inhibitors, medication adherence and virological outcome in HIV-infected patients. *Antiviral Therapy, 9*(5), 753–761.

Zulu, K. P., Bulawo, N. D., & Zulu, W. (2006). *Understanding HIV risk behavior among men who have sex with men in Zambia* [Abstract]. XVI International AIDS Conference, WEPE0719. Toronto, Ontario.

12

HIV Disease in Minority Communities: Current Progress and Future Directions

JUDITH B. CORNELIUS
ANN C. WHITE

According to the White House's Office of National AIDS Policy, President Clinton in 1998 declared HIV/AIDS to be a "severe and ongoing health crisis in racial and ethnic minority communities" and announced an initiative to improve the nation's effectiveness in preventing and treating HIV/AIDS in the African American, Hispanic, and other minority communities (Office of the Press Secretary, 1998). Shortly thereafter, the Minority AIDS Initiative was established to address the disproportionate rates of HIV infection among racial and ethnic minorities in the United States (U.S.).

A decade after President Clinton's announcement, HIV infection continues to exact a disproportionate toll on U.S. minority communities, with ongoing disparities in HIV infection rates in racial, ethnic, and sexual minority communities. HIV prevention and treatment efforts in minority communities have been hindered by mistrust of the biomedical community, stigma, complacency and denial in affected minority communities, inadequate funding, discrimination, and cultural barriers to care. This chapter covers HIV risk factors that affect ethnic and minority communities; HIV federal, state, and local funding for ethnic and minority communities; and HIV service agencies and programs targeted to minority communities. The chapter concludes with a discussion of future directions for HIV research in minority communities.

405

DISPROPORTIONATE IMPACT OF HIV/AIDS
ON MINORITY COMMUNITIES

Of the estimated new rates of HIV infections in the United States, 46% are occurring among African Americans, 36% among whites, and 18% among Hispanics (CDC, 2008b, 2008e). Although African Americans represent 12.9% of the U.S. population (U.S. Census Bureau, 2000), they have been affected by HIV more than any other racial or ethnic group. HIV infection among African Americans peaked in the late 1980s and has been at a high level ever since (CDC, 2008a, 2008c). In 2006, the rate of HIV infection in African Americans was seven times the rate for whites. In a CDC study of late versus early testing of HIV, African Americans represented 56% of those who were diagnosed with AIDS within one year of their HIV diagnosis (CDC, 2003).

In 2005, Hispanics represented 14% of the nation's population (CDC, 2008e) yet accounted for 17% of new HIV infections. According to recent CDC (2008b) surveillance data, the rate of new HIV infections among Hispanics is three times that for whites.

While Asians, Pacific Islanders (APIs), American Indians and Alaska Natives (AI/ANs) total 4.2% of the population, they represent approximately 2% of new HIV infections (CDC, 2004a, 2004b, 2008a, 2008c). Over a recent four-year period, however, APIs had a significantly greater increase in HIV infection rates than other racial and ethnic groups (CDC 2004a, 2006a; Chin et al., 2007). The estimated AIDS diagnosis rate for AI/AN adults and adolescents is the third highest after African Americans and Hispanics (CDC, 2006a, 2006b).

In 2006, the rate of new HIV infections for African American males was seven times that for whites and more than twice the rate for Hispanic males (CDC, 2008c). Among API and AI/AN males the rates of new HIV infections were 17.7% and 13.5%, respectively (CDC, 2008c). Most importantly, 81% of API males acquired the virus by having sex with men, compared to 61% of all racial and ethnic groups combined (CDC, 2008b). When HIV diagnosis and disease progression rates were examined among men who have sex with men (MSM), researchers found that the three-year survival rate was lower for African American than for white or Hispanic MSM (Hall et al., 2007). Predictors of unprotected sex varied among young MSM based on race, ethnicity, and culture. For young African American MSM, predictors of unprotected sex were being in an established relationship and being kicked out of the home for initiating sexual acts with men at a young age. For young Hispanic MSM, strong ethnic identification and initiation of sexual acts with men at an older age were predictors of unprotected sex. For young white MSM, there were no predictors of unprotected sex (Warren et al., 2008).

In 2006, the rate of new HIV infections for African American females was 19 times the rate for white females and three times the rate for Hispanic females. The HIV infection rate for Hispanic females was twice the rate for white females (CDC 2006b, 2008d). In 2004, HIV/AIDS was the leading cause of death among African American women 25 to 34 years of age and the fifth leading cause of death for all women 35 to 44 years of age. Additionally, HIV was the fourth leading cause of death for Hispanic women 35 to 44 years of age (CDC, 2008d). While HIV has been considered a disease of younger women, older women are emerging as a high-risk group. In 2006, women 50 years of age and older represented 10% of HIV-infected individuals. In a study with older (50 years of age and older) African American women, Cornelius, Moneyham, and LeGrand (2008) found that over half of the sample lacked knowledge about HIV risk factors and the great majority wanted an HIV prevention program that targeted their unique needs. (See Chapter 1 for a discussion of the epidemiology of HIV/AIDS.)

Sexual minorities have also been affected by HIV. (See Chapter 11.) African American transgender individuals have higher rates of HIV infection than other racial and ethnic groups (Kellogg et al., 2001; Simon, Reback, & Bemis, 2000). Further, infection rates continue to rise, with reported increases of 3 to 8% per year (Kellogg et al., 2001; Simon et al., 2000). Because there is a latency period between HIV infection and the appearance of clinical symptoms sufficient to warrant an AIDS diagnosis, many African American transgender adults appear to have been infected with the virus that causes AIDS when they were adolescents. While the overall incidence of AIDS is declining, there has not been a comparable decline in the incidence of new HIV cases among transgender women (18 to 35 years of age).

MISTRUST OF THE BIOMEDICAL COMMUNITY: CONSPIRACY THEORY BELIEFS

Since the infamous "Tuskegee Study of Untreated Syphilis in the Negro Male," conducted from 1932 to 1972, racial and ethnic minorities have mistrusted the biomedical community. This mistrust has been referred to by one writer (Fullilove, 2004) as "the elephant in our living room":

The elephant in our living room is the failure of HIV policy makers, researchers, and providers to admit that we are not speaking directly to the doubts, beliefs, and fears of many, and that our failure to talk about those doubts only fuels the oft-expressed belief that "They don't want us to talk about it because their domination and eventual extinction of us is possible only if we are ignorant." (p. 3)

A number of studies have examined the extent to which HIV conspiracy theories exist within minority communities. A large community-based anonymous survey ($n = 1,494$) conducted by Ross, Essien, and Torres (2006) with four racial or ethnic groups of men and women (African American, Latino, non-Hispanic white, and Asian subjects), found that 50% African Americans, 41% Latino, and 33% API men believed the genocidal conspiracy theory of HIV origin. The findings from this study suggest that an understanding of these beliefs is essential to HIV prevention efforts and recruitment of racial minorities into clinical trials. In their 2005 cross-sectional survey at four public facilities of 113 HIV-infected subjects diagnosed with HIV for three years or less, Clark and colleagues (2008) found that 63% endorsed one or more conspiracy beliefs. More African Americans held conspiracy beliefs than other ethnic and racial groups, yet these beliefs did not have a negative impact on access or adherence to HIV treatment care. The researchers concluded that efforts to improve adherence to HIV care may not need to focus on eliminating conspiracy beliefs.

In a telephone survey of 500 African Americans aged 15 to 44 years, Bogart and Thorburn (2005) found that a significant number supported HIV conspiracy theory beliefs. In their national cross-sectional exploratory telephone survey examining the relationship of HIV/AIDS conspiracy beliefs to sexual attitudes and behaviors ($n = 71$ African American adults), Bogart and Bird (2003) found that men's attitudes about condom use and greater number of sexual partners were partially mediated by the effects of conspiracy theories. Hutchinson and colleagues (2007) reported similar findings in their study with minority men who have sex with men (MSM). Of the 696 MSM subjects in their study, 86% agreed at least somewhat with one or more conspiracy beliefs. Bird and Bogart (2005) concluded from their review of conspiracy theory research that African Americans believed that the government was trying to reduce the number of African American births by encouraging condom use. Bogart and Thorburn (2005, 2006), in a digitally dialed sample of 500 African Americans (15 to 44 years old), found that stronger HIV conspiracy theories were associated with male gender, lower income, and lower education. Conversely, Klonoff and Landrine (1999), in a door-to-door sample of 520 African American adults, found that the HIV conspiracy theory was endorsed by traditional college-educated men who had a history of considerable racial discrimination.

Finally, a study by Gilley and Keesee (2007) that addressed HIV conspiracy beliefs of American Indian men who have sex with men found that one-third believed that HIV was developed by whites, white Christians, or the federal government. No published study, other than that of Ross and colleagues (2006), has examined Asian Pacific Islanders' beliefs about HIV conspiracy theories.

THE ROLE OF ORGANIZED RELIGION

In minority communities, many of the places of worship attended by persons at risk for HIV infection condemn behaviors that place persons at risk of infection, including injection drug use, promiscuity, sex work, and homosexuality (Baker, 1999). Early in the AIDS epidemic (and to a lesser extent today) some, and perhaps most, of organized religions serving minority communities were not actively involved in HIV/AIDS prevention, education, and support. This reluctance on the part of many churches to become involved stemmed from myriad causes, but certainly some churches were concerned that active involvement might give the appearance that they were contributing to and condoning the spread of HIV and increasing its impact on the communities they served (Kelly, 2003). Also, some churches failed to become involved as a result of their denial that members of their congregation and community engaged in behaviors placing them at risk of infection. Not talking about HIV/AIDS in these churches was a reflection of the denial that their communities had a problem. A turning point in the African American community came in 1991 when Magic Johnson announced that he had HIV, followed by Arthur Ashe's death from AIDS in 1993. Other issues that churches have struggled with and continue to confront with varying degrees of difficulty include the use of condoms, the moral condemnation of HIV/AIDS because of its association with stigmatized behaviors, the "AIDS-Silence" stance of some organized religions, patriarchal approaches that negate the equality of women, and a wide range of cultural beliefs that may not be consistent with religion. For religion to assume a leadership role in efforts to control HIV/AIDS, Kelly (2003) offers the following suggestions for the global community:

- Cease "putting down," discrediting, or sidelining the importance of religion or religious organizations in the struggle against both the disease and the epidemic.
- Secure the full participation of religious bodies in programs and projects.
- Ensure that religious leaders are involved in the development of AIDS-related policies, plans, and strategies.
- Establish a strong desk for religious issues at UNAIDS.
- Enable religious bodies to have access to funding for their anti-AIDS and orphans programs.
- Facilitate religious organizations in developing a common internationally supported approach to reducing HIV transmission and mitigating the impacts of the epidemic. (p. 7)

Kelly (2003) offers several suggestions for religious bodies as well:

- Come out loud and clear in every possible way about HIV/AIDS, overcoming silence or denial, in their own personnel, in their members, and in their teaching.
- Adamantly reject every utterance, pronouncement, or practice that carries any connotation of stigma or discrimination.
- Pour their human resources into the major tasks of eliminating poverty and ending the subjugation of women.
- Recognize the dimensions of the orphans challenge and mobilize their communities for a massive response to it in humane and practical ways.
- Galvanize their members into action for the reduction of HIV transmission, provision of care and support for those infected or affected, and mitigation of the impact of the disease and epidemic.
- Work in cooperation and harmony with one another, the representatives of local cultures, civic personnel, and local, national, and international leaders.
- Maintain a multidimensional response to HIV/AIDS at the top of their agenda and as an integral element in their seminary and other training programs.
- Put the condom debate to rest. (p. 7)

Organized religion can play a pivotal role in combating HIV/AIDS at local, regional, national, and international levels. However, to do so, religious leaders may need to set aside the dogma that has reduced their influence in the HIV/AIDS epidemic. Ansari (2008), writing about the role of religious leaders in the epidemic, has concluded that these leaders "need to communicate that after one becomes infected with HIV, the only relevant responsibility is that of the community to unconditionally take care of those who are ill" (¶10).

PARTICIPATION IN CLINICAL TRIALS

In 1993 Congress passed a law (PL 103-43) aimed at including greater numbers of women and racial and ethnic minorities in clinical research. The law was further strengthened in 2001 to mandate the inclusion of women and racial and ethnic minorities in federally funded research. Yet, despite these efforts, members of minority communities have been slow to participate in HIV clinical trials, for a range of reasons, including: (1) conspiracy beliefs about vaccines, (2) bleak views of the future, (3) misinformation and confusion about the effectiveness of HIV vaccines, (4) failure to be asked to participate, and (5) desire not to be "guinea pigs" (Roberts et al.., 2005; Sullivan et al., 2007). There is some evidence that HIV-infected minority women are more likely to participate in clinical trials, while racial or ethnic minority men are less likely (Sullivan et al., 2007). Researchers have suggested several actions to increase the participation of racial and ethnic minorities in clinical research, including HIV/AIDS research. These include taking steps to gain the trust of minority communities and negate the effects of conspiracy beliefs while disseminating HIV prevention information. Other actions to increase minority participation in clinical research include: (1) making efforts to reach potential subjects by providing more multipronged community-based education about clinical trials; (2) providing more information and education about available clinical research to nurses and physicians, especially those who themselves are from racial or ethnic minority groups, to encourage them to increase their efforts to interest more minority participants in clinical research; (3) including more racial and ethnic minorities in research teams; (4) including minority community members on research advisory boards; and (5) gaining the input and support of community leaders. Because minority populations are disproportionately affected by the HIV/AIDS epidemic, greater efforts to encourage participation of minority subjects in clinical research are critical to ensure that results from such research are applicable to diverse populations.

COUPLE INTERVENTIONS WITH MINORITY POPULATIONS

HIV prevention and treatment present a public health problem that is exacerbated by multiple environmental, sociocultural, and systematic health system problems. Because of some minorities' beliefs in HIV conspiracy theories, condom use remains low in established relationships between African American and Latino men and women (Sly et al., 2001). Prevention efforts targeting heterosexual couples have been minimal in settings that serve urban, low-income clients. Prevention efforts have primarily targeted MSM. Women have been targeted to be the change agents in negotiating condom use with their partners, and condom negotiation has often resulted in isolation, intimate partner violence, infidelity, and mistrust for many women of color. Yet few programs have been funded to examine condom use in established couple relationships.

One program that has met success with couple relationships and safer sex practices is Project Connect, funded by the National Institute of Mental Health (NIMH). This relationship-based HIV and other sexually transmitted disease prevention intervention for heterosexual couples living in a low-income neighborhood in New York included 217 couples, 55% African American and 39% Latino (El-Bassel et al., 2001; El-Bassel et al., 2003). The intervention consisted of an orientation session and multiple relationship-based sessions, six conjointly to couples and seven to women without their partners. The interventions focused on couple relationships, communication, and choices for risk reduction behaviors. The researchers concluded that: (1) behavioral change relative to HIV can be maintained over time (12 months) and (2) HIV prevention interventions can be delivered to women alone, if the partner is aware of and willing to participate in the intervention through the female partner. However, although this project was effective with many of the program participants, some couples indicated that they did not intend to adopt safer sex practices in their relationships because they insisted that they were not at risk for sexually transmitted infections, including HIV.

The Eban Project, also funded by the NIMH (2008), is a multisite study being conducted in Philadelphia, Atlanta, Los Angeles, and New York. Five hundred and thirty-five HIV serodiscordant heterosexual African American couples will be examined to see if protected vaginal and anal intercourse occurs within the couple index and if a proportion of participants become infected with an STI over the 12-month postintervention period.

Women in established relationships with an incarcerated partner are at particularly high risk for HIV infection (Auerswald et al., 2006; CDC, 2004b; Comfort et al., 2005; Grinstead et al., 2008; Johnson & Raphael, 2006). Approximately 80% of HIV infections in women have been associated with having a partner who was incarcerated (CDC, 2004b). These high infection rates probably stem from the fact that HIV seroprevalence rates are significantly higher among men who are incarcerated because of behaviors prior to incarceration that placed them at higher risk of HIV infection. Second, the emotional strain of having an incarcerated partner may place some female partners at a higher risk of HIV infection. Grinstead and her research team at the University of California at San Francisco (2008) implemented HIV interventions tailored to meet the needs of African American women with incarcerated partners. The Health Options Mean Empowerment (HOME) project included a 17-minute video presenting stories of women whose partners had been incarcerated and men who have served time and explored the challenges faced by women after their partners are released from prison. The project also included training for peer educators and provided support for participants in regard to incarceration issues. Being in the project reinforced information that participants had learned about safer sex practices. The women who participated found that maintaining partner intimacy was feasible.

St. Lawrence and colleagues (2001) found that minority women in established relationships were less likely than others to negotiate condom use and exhibited low condom use with their main sexual partner (Saul et al., 2000). Minority women have been found to place the value of their relationship with a man over their own well-being. One study of 362 low-income African American women in established relationships found that women who had recently used condoms were more likely to use them than women who had not used condoms with their main partners (Perrino et al., 2006). Women who experienced abuse (emotional, physical, or sexual) were less likely to negotiate safer sex behaviors with their main partners than women who had not. Women who feared that condom negotiations would result in accusations of infidelity from their main partner did not discuss condom use (Witte et al., 2007). Financial dependence in a relationship has also resulted in less condom use. Further, a lack of marriageable men in some minority communities has made women panic and avoid discussions of safer sex practices for fear of "losing their man."

In a mixed-ethnicity study involving 393 low-income non-Hispanic black, Hispanic, and non-Hispanic white women, the non-Hispanic black and Hispanic women were more likely to insist on condom use with their sexual partners than were white women (Soler et al., 2000). One of the few studies that targeted couple interventions with Latinos showed promise with Latino adolescent mothers and their partners. A sample of 49 couples completed a six-session culturally appropriate intervention. Findings at six-month follow-up showed that unprotected sex was significantly reduced and condom use intentions were increased (Koniak-Griffin et al., 2008). Another study of 39 couples of Mexican origin (Harvey et al., 2002) found that simply providing a single education session for couples was cheap and effective in the adaptation of safer sex behaviors, especially when women had the power to make unilateral decisions.

The female condom is the only female-initiated safer sex method. However, research on the use of this safer sex method is limited. In one study by Witte and colleagues (2006b) with 217 women in established relationships, the researchers found that a relationship-based intervention was efficacious in promoting the use of the female condom among long-term heterosexual couples. A women-only intervention was also effective in promoting female condom use. One educational session was effective in increasing female condom use among heterosexual couples. Subjects reported a relatively high intent to use the female condom within the next 90 days of the research intervention. In their study with 108 minority women comparing satisfaction with female and male condoms, Kulczycki and associates (2004) concluded that satisfaction with the female condom was significantly lower than that for the male condom, but neither condom scored high on user satisfaction measures. According to the U.N. Population Fund (2006), in 2005 only 14 million female condoms were available for distribution worldwide, costing $1.15 to $2.75 in the United States and 80 cents in other parts of the world, while 6 to 9 *billion* male condoms (costing much less than female condoms) were provided worldwide. A second-generation female condom ("FC2") is now under consideration for possible approval by the FDA in 2009. The FC2 is reported to be 30% less expensive than its first-generation predecessor.

The importance of women in committed monogamous relationships being able to reduce their risk of HV infection has been underscored over the past decade in articles in the popular press and in professional literature on the lives of "straight" African American men who engage in extra relationship sexual activity with other men, referred to as "down low" (DL) sex. Men who "live on the DL" (King, 2004) come from all socioeconomic, racial, and ethnic backgrounds, although much of the literature has focused on this sexual behavior by African American men. King (2004) has identified five categories of DL behaviors: (1) the mature brother; (2) the thug brother; (3) the professional brother; (4) "I have a wife/girlfriend"; and (5) "I'm just curious." King suggests that these categories illustrate the difficulty of recognizing a man on the DL. King also believes that more African American men are living on the DL because gay white men are less stigmatized and have better support systems. Denizet-Lewis (2003) concurs, saying, "It seems that the majority of those having sex with men still lead secret lives, products of a black culture that deems masculinity and fatherhood as a black man's responsibility—and homosexuality as a white man's perversion" (p. 1).

O'Leary and associates (2007) have reported that African American men are less likely than white men to view themselves as gay and are more likely to engage concurrently in sexual behavior with women; thus, a woman may unknowingly engage in sex with a man who is "living on the DL," greatly increasing her risk of HIV infection. Whyte, Whyte, and Cormier (2008) interviewed 11 women with an average age of 59.6 years and living in monogamous relationships. These 11 women, who became HIV positive as a result of sex with their partner, reported feeling betrayed by their partners, and this sense of betrayal was magnified by their own HIV-positive status; most stayed in their relationship after reflecting on the nature of that relationship. Many felt ashamed before God, their community, and their family; and most felt a need to care for their infected partners. The researchers noted that the findings suggest a need to provide educational approaches "that alert and assist African-American women to accurately determine the trustworthiness of their husbands or partners" (p. 430).

While HIV-related research to date with racial and ethnic heterosexual couples is relatively limited, findings from some studies are encouraging. A benefit to couple intervention is the presentation of choices for safer-sex behaviors that are presented to both a woman and her sexual partner. However, there are challenges that must be addressed before undertaking couple intervention research (Pappas-Deluca et al., 2006). For example, getting couples together who work and have children may be a challenge, or one partner may be willing and the other not willing to participate in the research. Witte and colleagues (2006a) identify recruitment and retention strategies that have worked effectively in couple intervention research, including:

- Using project recruiters of the same race/ethnicity as the study participants.
- Using recruiters who are familiar with the community.
- Emphasizing the importance of language, body language, and dress .
- Demonstrating respect for each participant.
- Engaging site staff as partners in the recruitment process.
- Stressing the benefits of couple research such as social conscience, financial compensation, and an opportunity to improve relationships.
- Inviting the woman's main partner into the study using brokering strategies.
- Using corecruitment strategies of mail, phone, or face-to-face approaches.
- Using role-play strategies to help women troubleshoot recruiting their main partner into the study.

HOMELESSNESS, POVERTY, AND HIV INFECTION IN MINORITY COMMUNITIES

Homelessness, poverty, and HIV infection intersect in minority communities. Minorities experience adverse social determinants and are disproportionately represented among the uninsured and marginalized (Betancourt & Maina, 2004). The rate of HIV infection among homeless individuals is 20 to 40 times higher than that for nonhomeless individuals (CDC, 2007). According to a U.S. Conference of Mayors study of 25 major U.S. cities in 2004, the urban homeless population is estimated to be 42% African American, 39% white, 13% Latino, 4% Native American, and 2% Asian. The impoverished, including the homeless, are at high risk for HIV because of the social circumstances in which they live. For example, in one study individuals who were uninsured recipients of Medicaid, homeless, and living in low-income zip code areas were four times as likely to be HIV-positive as those who were insured and lived in high-income zip code areas (Murrain & Barker, 1997). Older residents living in a low-income senior housing complex reported engaging in high-risk sexual practices but perceived themselves to be at risk if someone who was HIV-infected coughed on them (Schensul, Levy, & Disch, 2003).

In a longitudinal study conducted at Columbia University in New York (CHAIN study), stable housing was identified as a primary need of HIV-positive individuals. Homeless individuals are especially vulnerable to HIV by engaging in risky sexual behaviors (Forney, Lombardo, & Toro, 2007). Homelessness or imminent risk of homelessness, especially among those with a history of incarceration and/or substance abuse, has been identified as a marker for HIV risk behaviors (Courtenay-Quirk et al., 2008; Forney et al., 2007). HIV-infected individuals who are homeless report higher levels of stigma and drug and alcohol use (Wolitski et al., 2008). Situational homelessness with poor-quality housing results in increased HIV-risk behaviors. Stein, Dixon, and Nyamathi (2008) found that sexual risk behaviors were more common among homeless men who lived on the streets or in abandoned buildings than among those who lived in stable housing. Yet Rotheram-Borus and others (2008) found that a Healthy Living Program administered to marginally housed HIV-infected individuals was effective in decreasing the number of sexual partners, drug and alcohol use, and risky sexual behaviors. In another study, 20% of homeless people living with HIV/AIDS had intentionally abstained from sexual encounters in the past three months because of lack of interest, fear of transmission, and/or lack of a sexual partner (Courtenay-Quirk, Zhang, & Wolitski, 2008).

American Indians and Alaska Natives (AI/ANs) are disproportionately affected by economic factors that contribute to HIV risk behaviors. Thirty-two percent of AI/ANs live below the poverty level, compared to 13% of the general population (Baldwin et al., 2000). In addition, the AI/AN poverty rate is higher among families on reservations than among AI/AN families in other areas. High levels of substance abuse contribute to unprotected sex, high rates of STIs, and intimate partner violence. Alaska Native (AN) women are more likely to use drugs, have more sexual partners who abuse drugs, and have higher rates of STIs than women of other racial and ethnic groups (Advocates for Youth, 2007; Baldwin et al., 1996, 2000; CDC, 2008c; Fisher et al., 2000; Hamill & Dickey, 2005). Hamill and Dickey (2005) believe that working with AI/ANs to prevent HIV infection requires gaining their trust because "history depicts how U.S. government policy has affected Native-American communities by depriving AI/AN people of their rich culture, traditions, language, spirituality, and extended family and social systems" (p. 66). These authors note that health care providers must become culturally competent if they are to be effective. Cultural competence requires that health care providers understand the importance of AI/AN history, be respectful of traditional healing approaches, allow clients to decide how much to share about their traditional approaches, communicate support and acknowledge traditional approaches and teachings, become familiar with AI/AN communication styles, engage a community leader to serve as a cultural consultant, and provide cultural training for staff.

Many transgender persons lack employment and live below the poverty level. The psychosocial consequences of stigma include depression, low self-esteem, substance abuse, and indiscriminant sex in some transgender persons (Nemoto et al., 2004). When transgender sex workers of color experience homelessness, they often engage in "survival sex" (i.e., the exchange of sex for money, gifts, drugs, shelter, health care, or other needs). Limited social networks, fear of deportation, and experiences of racism, sexism, and transphobia (i.e., fear of or actual discrimination against transsexuality and transsexual or transgender people) are factors that influence transgender sex workers' decisions to engage in sex work. (Nemoto et al., 2004; Sausa, Keathley, & Operario, 2007).

Homelessness is related to persons' well-being and HIV risk behaviors in minority communities. Health care providers and nurses need to target individuals who are homeless, are marginally homeless, or have a history of incarceration for HIV prevention and treatment services. A social intervention strategy that addresses socioeconomic influences on HIV transmission should be the basis for HIV services for racial and ethnic minorities (Fournier & Carmichael, 1998; Lyles et al., 2007). Works by Woods (2007) and Osemene, Essien, and Egbunike (2001) address the need for culturally sensitive curricula and interventions.

EFFECTS OF PATIENT–PROVIDER INTERACTIONS ON MINORITIES

Disparities in access to care are evident at minority-serving HIV clinics. African Americans and Hispanics reported longer travel and wait times to see health care providers than did whites (Korthuis et al., 2008). As a result of perceived stigma and discrimination by health care providers, some high-risk individuals do not disclose their sexual orientation and other behaviors that might be perceived negatively by health care providers. For example, in one study, 39% of MSM respondents did not disclose their sexual orientation to their health care providers, missing opportunities for HIV testing (Bernstein et al., 2008). Minorities are more likely to report discrimination and distrust of health care providers and to have poorer adherence to medication treatment (Thrasher et al., 2008). HIV-positive individuals frequently report deterioration in formerly trustful patient–provider relationships.

A physician's gender and race or ethnicity may influence the frequency with which HIV risk reduction information is discussed with patients (Gardner et al., 2008). In one study, fewer than half of physicians used opportunities to discuss reducing HIV transmission risk with HIV-positive patients (Korthius et al., 2008). While 65% of physicians agreed that they had sufficient time and knowledge to discuss safer-sex behaviors with HIV-positive patients, they did not use these opportunities to reinforce disease prevention information. Hispanic, Asian Pacific Islander, and female physicians and physicians with fewer patients discussed HIV transmission risk-reduction behaviors more often with their infected patients. In their study of 308 HIV-infected New York City subjects, Sohler and associates (2007) concluded that patient–physician race and ethnicity concordance was associated with lower mistrust in the health care system but was not associated with trust in the provider. These researchers expressed surprise that patient–provider racial and ethnic concordance was not associated with trust in the provider because this finding was inconsistent with previous research findings. They speculated that the lack of association between trust in provider and race and ethnicity concordance may indicate improvement in cross cultural patient–provider relationships. However, a number of other studies and papers that considered the influence of gender and/or race on patient–physician trust and health care outcomes have, in general, found that provider–patient concordance may benefit patients (Cooper-Patrick et al., 1999; King et al., 2004; LaVeist & Nuru-Jeter, 2002; Malat & van Ryn, 2005; Saha et al., 2000).

The competence and attitudes of nurses who provide HIV patient care are important factors in patient satisfaction of racial or ethnic minority patients. A study by Jones and colleagues (2002) found that, while nurses and physicians were deficient in pain management, did not always discuss side effects of HIV medications, and spoke to fewer than half of their minority patients about HIV clinical trials, minority infected patients were satisfied with the care they received. Because minority HIV-infected patients were not informed of experimental drugs, however, they were potentially denied equal access to clinical drug trials. These findings underscore the need for health care providers, regardless of race, to inform all patients, and particularly racial and ethnic minorities, of opportunities to participate in clinical trials.

One study compared the quality of patient care delivered by HIV nursing consultants to the quality of care delivered by general-practice nurses and HIV nurse specialists (Hekkink et al., 2005). The quality of care delivered by the HIV nursing consultants was rated "good with room for improvement," yet their professional performance and attitudes scores were below that of the general practitioners and HIV specialists.

Nursing students' attitudes and care intentions toward HIV-positive patients are influenced by their personal contacts with HIV-infected individuals (Cornelius, 2004). Cornelius (2004) found that an HIV-experiential teaching method entitled "To be touched by AIDS" increased nursing students' knowledge about HIV by 60%, improved attitudes toward HIV-positive individuals, and increased behavioral intents to provide HIV patient care. Male nursing students expressed higher levels of homophobia than female nursing students. Penny (2008) found that a role-playing experiential teaching-learning experience with nursing students increased their empathy for HIV-infected patients. When HIV-experiential teaching-learning strategies are used, however, they should include discussions of social and personal factors such as religion, morality, homophobia, transphobia, and fear of contagion.

CULTURAL ISSUES AND HIV RISKS IN MINORITY COMMUNITIES

Culture plays a dominant role in racial and ethnic minorities' perceived susceptibility to HIV infection and the way they disclose their HIV serostatus to family and friends. In a study involving 249 women sampled from nine Asian and Pacific Islander communities in 1993 through 1995, Cooper, Loue, and Lloyd (2001) found that acculturation (measured by years in the United States) and ethnicity appeared to modify risk behaviors and perceived susceptibility to HIV. Education, age (30 years or older), personally knowing someone HIV positive, and personal risk behaviors were strongly associated with perceived HIV susceptibility among these API women.

API gay, bisexual, and MSM experience significant conflicts between family loyalty and sexual identity. Cultural expressions of giving to others, love and intimacy, and reluctance to suspend unsafe sexual practices, stigma, discrimination, and power dynamics in relationships with white men may compromise HIV risk reduction in this population (Kanuha, 2000; Nemoto et al., 2003). Han (2008) has speculated that the increasing unsafe sex found among gay API men may be related to sexual norms in Asian cultures, a lack of culturally relevant and/or linguistically appropriate intervention material, lack of integration into the mainstream gay community, and internalized homophobia.

Asian men find that self-disclosure of HIV status is emotionally draining. Cultural ties to the home country and its prevailing cultural norms significantly influence the migration experience and acculturation to life in the United States (Ching et al., 2003). The values of harmony and avoidance of conflict, which are rooted in cultural norms, pose additional barriers to disclosure. Yoshioka and Schustack (2001) conducted in-depth interviews with 16 HIV-positive Asian men and found that protection of family from shame, protection of family from an obligation to help, and avoidance of highly personal communication were the main barriers to self-disclosure to family members. Asian MSM find support with gay friends and disclose to their families only when necessary for health care reasons. APIs living with HIV/AIDS are susceptible to HIV-related stigma due to social cultural norms and their sexual activities (Kang et al., 2005). Psychological distress has been found to be high among this ethnic minority group because of a diminished sense of self-worth and fear of social rejection.

American Indian (AI) and Alaska Natives (AN) also experience cultural barriers to HIV risk-reduction practices. Subgroups and individual differences are evident among this population. AI/AN women report more sexual risk behaviors than men (Stevens, Estrada, & Estrada, 2000). In response to cultural barriers, substance abuse and mental health services have been integrated into a cultural context in San Francisco's Holistic Native Network program. Culture and community are included at every stage of service provision, from outreach to case management to substance abuse and mental health services, in an effort to meet clients' spiritual, medical, and psychosocial needs (Nebelkopf & Penagos, 2005). This program includes: (1) monthly interdisciplinary meetings and bimonthly interagency clinical case conferences, (2) strategic community outreach through phone calls and home or hotel visits by outreach workers to increase treatment adherence and follow-ups, and (3) peer advocacy to increase rapport and trust with patients or clients and provide assistance with social support and transportation. These interventions have led to positive treatment outcomes. Other activities of the project include those to increase adherence to holistic HIV/AIDS treatments, confidential HIV testing and counseling, HIV prevention services for high-risk AI/ANs, and use of cultural and traditional wellness approaches. Project leaders have concluded that: (1) effective holistic HIV/AIDS services should include interdisciplinary treatment approaches to improve treatment adherence, coordinate care and referrals, and support each component of treatment; (2) ongoing sensitivity and community awareness trainings and in-services on homophobia, stigma, community building, and culturally relevant and appropriate treatment strategies must be implemented; (3) the integration of cultural wellness practices, practitioners, and principles can enhance HIV/AIDS services and care and support community awareness of HIV/AIDS and community development; and (4) effective and comprehensive HIV/AIDS services and care must encompass co-occurring disorders and complex trauma issues.

Other researchers have stressed the importance of cultural factors in conducting HIV research involving Latinos. Cultural values of familialism (family obligation), simpatias (respectful interaction), confianzia (support and trust) ,respeto (respect), and machismo (sense of masculinity) have been found to be essential in involving Latinos in HIV treatment and research (Villarruel et al., 2006).

The impact of HIV/AIDS on minority individuals underscores the need to implement and sustain effective HIV treatment and prevention efforts. Barriers to recognition of HIV susceptibility and HIV risk reduction have been associated with conspiracy theories, homelessness, poverty, lack of provider–patient interactions and cultural beliefs. HIV prevention efforts with racial and ethnic minorities must include culturally appropriate individual, group, and couple interventions. Funding for HIV services must focus on the unique needs of each of these cultural groups. Current progress in these efforts can be seen in the services provided by HIV/AIDS service organizations. One program that has met success in providing culturally competent HIV services is the Metrolina AIDS Project (MAP) in North Carolina. Their efforts have been funded by national, state, and regional funds. MAP offers a broad range of services, including case management and service coordination, individual counseling, multiple support groups, primary care services, a food pantry, an adolescent speakers' bureau for advocacy benefits, and counseling and testing.

PROGRESS IN HIV SERVICES: FUNDING SOURCES

HIV treatment services in minority communities are managed by health care agencies and funded by federal, state, and regional funds. In 2007, the requested federal budget for HIV/AIDS treatment services was $22.8 billion (Henry J. Kaiser Family Foundation, 2007), an 8.3% increase over the 2006 fiscal year budget. HIV/AIDS federal programs are organized into general categories of care, education, housing assistance, prevention and treatment research, and global or international activities. Some key agencies include the following:

- AIDS Education and Training Centers (www.aidsetc.org/)
- The AIDS Drug Assistance Program (ADAP) (http://hab.hrsa.gov/programs/adap/)
- The Centers for Disease Control and Prevention (www.cdc.gov)
- The Centers for Medicare and Medicaid Services (CMS) (www.cms.hhs.gov/home/medicaid.asp)
- The Health Resources and Services Administration (HRSA) (www.hrsa.gov)
- The Housing Opportunities for Persons with AIDS (HOPWA) Program (www.hud.gov/offices/cpd/aidshousing/programs)
- The Office of Minority Health (www.omhrc.gov)
- The Office of Health Disparities (CDC) (www.cdc.gov/NCHSTP/OD/OHD/default.htm)
- The Pediatric AIDS Clinical Trials Group (http://pactg.s-3.com/sites.htm)
- The Ryan White AIDS Program (http://hab.hrsa.gov)
- National HIV and STD Testing Resources (CDC) (www.hivtest.org)
- The National Institute of Allergy and Infectious Diseases (www3.niaid.nih.gov)
- The Substance Abuse and Mental Health Services Administration (SAMHSA) (www.samhsa.gov)
- Vaccine and Treatment Evaluation Units (NIAID) (www3.niaid.nih.gov/research/resources/vteu)

While not a federal agency, the National Minority AIDS Coalition (www.nmac.org/home) seeks to develop leadership around HIV/AIDS in communities of color. It accomplishes its mission through a variety of public policy education programs, national conferences, treatment and research programs and training, electronic and printed resource materials, and a website.

These resources and others are described more fully in the appendices accompanying this book.

HIV RESEARCH IN MINORITIES COMMUNITIES

Because minority communities are bearing the burden of HIV/AIDS, research on prevention and care is urgently needed (see the Office of AIDS Research's [OAR] fiscal year 2009 Trans-NIH Plan for HIV-related Research [2007] and the OAR's NIH Strategic Plan for AIDS Research Related to Racial and Ethnic Minorities [2002]) . The goal of two federally funded programs is to increase minority HIV researchers. The Collaborative HIV Prevention Research in Minority Communities program (www.caps.ucsf.edu/CAPS/about/fellows/minorityindex.php), prepares university researchers to work with community-based organizations to reach individuals in need of HIV services and treatment. This program was developed to address the scourge of HIV in communities of color. Housed in the Center for AIDS Prevention Studies (CAPS) at the University of California at San Francisco, the 27-month program provides visiting professors with small grant funding, summer seminars, long-term research collaboration, access to behavioral and methodological expertise, and internal peer review (Marín & Diaz, 2002). One benefit of this program is collaboration with other researchers, reducing the isolation that many scientists of color experience. The program has created a network of community-based researchers who provide support and encouragement for each other. Visiting professors include a multidisciplinary team of psychologists, social workers, anthropologists, sociologists, and nurses. To date, three nurses have participated in the program: Drs. Emma J. Brown, Sheldon Fields, and Judith B. Cornelius.

The second program, Cyber Mentors, is funded by the National Institute of Mental Health (NIMH). The Cyber Mentors program uses cyber mentoring to sustain a model for developing minority HIV researchers. The principal investigators, Drs. John Anderson and Maria Fernandez of the American Psychological Association, work with a group of senior scientists to mentor junior faculty to develop successful independent research careers in HIV/AIDS prevention in communities of color. The program uses technology such as distance learning to prepare mentees to develop their programs of research. Seminars include topics on methodology, research, grant writing, and budget management. The first cohort of 15 mentee/mentor pairs has been selected.

CONCLUSION

While much has been done to address the impact of the HIV/AIDS on minority communities in the United States, much still needs to be accomplished. With new HIV infections still increasing in minority communities, prevention and early diagnosis and treatment efforts need to be increased. Major barriers such as conspiracy beliefs, substance abuse, mental illness, lack of faith-based support, homelessness, cultural beliefs, and patient–provider interactions continue to hinder progress. Innovative and appealing interventions need to be developed to address cultural, social, and contextual factors that affect this disease in minority communities. Effective model programs targeted to the needs of minority communities at individual, family, and community levels need to receive funds from federal, state, and regional sources. Research programs such as CAPS and Cyber Mentors must continue to prepare HIV scientists to address HIV issues in minority communities. Research training for new investigators should include collaborations with community and health agencies, religious institutions, and historically black colleges and universities. Finally, research relevant to cultural beliefs about sexuality will facilitate the development of interventions that address health, substance abuse, mental illness, poverty, homelessness, conspiracy theories, and HIV health risk-reduction behaviors in the context of minority communities.

REFERENCES

Advocates for Youth. (2007). *HIV and young American Indian/Alaska Native women.* Retrieved February 31, 2009, from www.advocates foryouth.org/PUBLICATIONS/factsheet/fsnative.pdf.

Ansari, D. (2008, February 26). HIV in Senegal: Religion and Responsibility. *The Lancet Student.* Retrieved February 2, 2009, from www.thelancetstudent.com/2008/02/28/hiv-in-senegal-religion-and-responsibility.

Auerswald, C., Muth, S., Brown, B., Padian N., & Ellen, J. (2006). Does partner selection contribute to sex differences in sexually transmitted infection rates among African American adolescents in San Francisco? *Sexually Transmitted Disease, 33*(8), 480–484.

Baker, S. (1999). HIV/AIDS, nurses, and the black church: A case study. *Journal of the Association of Nurses in AIDS Care, 10*(5), 71–79.

Baldwin, J., Maxwell, C., Fenaughty, A., Trotter, R., & Stevens, S. (2000). Alcohol as a risk factor for HIV transmission among American Indian and Alaska Native drug users. *American Indian Alaska Native Mental Health Research, 9*(1), 1–16.

Baldwin, J., Rolfe, J., Johnson, J., Bowers, J., Benally, C., & Trotter, R. (1996). Developing culturally sensitive HIV/AIDS and substance abuse prevention curricula for Native American youth. *Journal of School Health, 66*(9), 322–327.

Bernstein, K., Liu, K., Begier, E., Koblin, B., Karpati, A., & Murrill, C. (2008). Same-sex attraction disclosure to health care providers among New York City men who have sex with men: Implications for HIV testing approaches. *Archives of Internal Medicine, 13*(168), 1458–1464.

Betancourt, J., & Maina, A. (2004). The Institute of Medicine report "Unequal Treatment": Implications for academic health centers. *Mt. Sinai Journal of Medicine 71*(5), 314–321.

Bird, S., & Bogart, L. (2005). Conspiracy beliefs and HIV/AIDS and birth control among African Americans: Implications for the prevention of HIV and other STIs, and unintended pregnancy. *Journal of Social Issues, 61*(1), 109–126.

Bogart, L., & Bird, S. (2003). Exploring the relationship of conspiracy beliefs about HIV/AIDS to sexual behaviors and attitudes among African-American adults. *Journal of the National Medical Association, 95*(11), 1057–1065.

Bogart, L., & Thorburn, S. (2005). Are HIV/AIDS conspiracy beliefs a barrier to HIV prevention among African Americans? *Journal of Acquired Immune Deficiency Syndrome, 38*(2), 213–218.

Bogart, L., & Thorburn, S. (2006). Relationship of African Americans' sociodemographic characteristics to belief in conspiracies about HIV/AIDS and birth control. *Journal of the National Medical Association, 98*(7), 1144–1150.

Centers for Disease Control and Prevention (CDC). (2003). Late versus early testing of HIV-16 sites, United States, 2002–2003. *Morbidity and Mortality Weekly Report, 52*(25), 581–586.

Centers for Disease Control and Prevention (CDC). (2004a). *HIV/AIDS among Asians and Pacific Islanders.* Rockville, MD: Author.

Centers for Disease Control and Prevention (CDC). (2004b). *HIV/AIDS surveillance report, 15.* Retrieved January 29, 2009, from www.cdc.gov/hiv/topics/surveillance/resources/reports/2003report/pdf/2003SurveillanceReport.pdf.

Centers for Disease Control and Prevention (CDC). (2006a). *HIV/AIDS among American Indians and Alaska Natives.* Rockville, MD: Author.

Centers for Disease Control and Prevention (CDC). (2006b). *HIV/AIDS among Hispanics.* Rockville, MD: Author.

Centers for Disease Control and Prevention (CDC). (2007). *Communities at risk.* Rockville, MD: Author.

Centers for Disease Control and Prevention. (2008a). *Estimates of new HIV infections in the United States.* Retrieved September 28, 2008, from www.cdc.gov/hiv/topics/surveillance/resources/factssheets/incidence.htm

Centers for Disease Control and Prevention (CDC). (2008b). *HIV and AIDS in the United States: A picture of today's epidemic.* Retrieved September 28, 2008, from www.cdc.gov/hiv/topic/surveillance/united_states.htm.

Centers for Disease Control and Prevention (CDC). (2008c). *HIV/AIDS among American Indians and Alaska Natives.* Retrieved February 1, 2009, from www.cdc.gov/hiv/resources/factsheets/aian.htm.

Centers for Disease Control and Prevention (CDC). (2008d). *HIV/AIDS among women.* Retrieved September 28, 2008, from www.cdc.gov/hiv/topics/women/resources/factsheets/women.htm.

Centers for Disease Control and Prevention (CDC). (2008e). Subpopulation estimates from the H IV incidence surveillance system—United States, 2006. *Morbidity and Mortality Weekly Report, 57*(36), 985–989. Retrieved September 8, 2008, from www.cdc.gov/mmwrrhtml/mm576al.htm.

Chin, J., Leung, M., Sheth, L., & Rodriguez, T. (2007). Let's not ignore a growing HIV problem for Asians and Pacific Islanders in the U.S. *Journal of Urban Health, 84*(5), 642–647.

Ching, C., Wong, F., Park, R., Edberg, M., & Lai, D. (2003). A conceptual model for understanding sexual health among Asian American/ Pacific Islander (AAPI) men who have sex with men (MSM) in the United States. *AIDS Education and Prevention, 15.A,* 21–28.

Clark, A., Mayben, J., Hartman, C., Kallen, M., & Giordano, T. (2008). Conspiracy beliefs about HIV infection are common but not associated with delayed diagnosis or adherence to care. *AIDS Patient Care STDs, 22*(9), 753–759.

Comfort, M., Grinstead, O., McCartney, K., Bourgois, P., & Knight, K. (2005). "You can't do anything in this damn place": Sex and intimacy among couples with an incarcerated male partner. *The Journal of Sex Research, 42*(1), 3–12.

Cooper, M., Loue, S., & Lloyd, L. (2001). Perceived susceptibility to HIV infection among Asian and Pacific Islander women in San

Diego. *Journal of Health Care for the Poor and Underserved, 12*(2), 208–223.

Cooper-Patrick, L., Gallo, J., Gonzales, J. , Vu, H., Powe, N., & Nelson, C., et al. (1999). Race, gender, and partnership in the patient-physician relationship. *Journal of the American Medical Association, 282,* 583–589.

Cornelius, J. B. (2004). Senior nursing students respond to an HIV experiential-teaching method with an African-American female. *Journal of National Black Nurses Association, 15*(2), 11–15.

Cornelius, J., Moneyham, L., & LeGrand, S. (2008). Adaptation of an HIV prevention curriculum for use with older African American women. *Journal of the Association of Nurses in AIDS Care, 19*(1), 16–27.

Courtenay-Quirk, C., Pals, S., Kidder, D., Henny, K., & Emshoff, J. (2008). Factors associated with incarceration history among HIV-positive persons experiencing homelessness or imminent risk of homelessness. *Journal of Community Health, 33*(6), 434–443.

Courtenay-Quirk, C., Zhang, J., & Wolitski, R. (2008, September 26). Intentional abstinence among homeless and unstably housed persons living with HIV/AIDS. *AIDS and Behavior,* Epub ahead of print: PMID: 18818997.

Denizet-Lewis, B. (2003, August 3). Double lives on the down low. *New York Times.* Retrieved February 2, 2009, from http://query.nytimes.com/gst/fullpage.html?sec=health&res=9F0CE0D61E3FF930A357 5BC0A9659C8B63.

El-Bassel, N., Witte, S., Gilbert, L., Sormanti, M., Moreno, C., Pereira, L., et al. (2001). HIV prevention for intimate couples: A relationship-based model. *Families, Systems and Health, 19*(4), 379–395.

El-Bassel, N., Witte, S., Gilbert, L., Wu, E., Chang, M., Hill, J., et al. (2003). The efficacy of a relationship-based HIV/STD prevention program for heterosexual couples. *American Journal of Public Health, 93*(6), 963–969.

Fisher, D., Fenaughty, A., Paschane, D., & Cagle, H. (2000) Alaska Native drug users and sexually transmitted disease: results of a five-year study. *American Indian Alaskan Native Mental Health Research, 9*(1), 37–57.

Forney, J., Lombardo, S., & Toro, P. (2007). Diagnostic and other correlates of HIV risk behaviors in a probability sample of homeless adults. *Psychiatric Services, 58*(1), 92–99.

Fournier, A., & Carmichael, C. (1998). Socioeconomic influences on the transmission of human immunodeficiency virus infection: The hidden risk. *Archives of Family Medicine, 7*(3), 214–217.

Fullilove, R. (2004). The elephant in the room: AIDS conspiracies in the black community. *Focus: A guide to AIDS Research and Counseling,* *19*(2), 1–4.

Gardner, L., Marks, G., O'Daniels, C., Wilson, T., Golin, C., Wright, J., et al. (2008). Implementation and evaluation of a clinic-based behavioral intervention: Positive steps for patients with HIV. *AIDS Patient Care, 22*(8), 627–635.

Gilley, B., & Keesee, M. (2007). Linking "white oppression" and HIV/ AIDS in American Indian etiology: Conspiracy beliefs among MSMs and their peers. *American Indian Alaska Native Mental Health Research, 14*(1), 44–62.

Grinstead, O., Comfort, M., McCartney, K., Koester, K., & Neilands, T. (2008). Bringing it home: Design and implementation of an HIV/ STD intervention for women visiting incarcerated men. *AIDS Education and Prevention, 20*(4), 283–300.

Hall, H., Byers, R., Ling, Q., & Espinoza, L. (2007). Racial/ethnic and age disparities in HIV prevalence and disease progression among men who have sex with men in the United States. *American Journal of Public Health,* 97(6), 1060–1066.

Hamill, S., & Dickey, M. (2005). Cultural competence: What is needed in working with Native Americans with HIV/AIDS. *Journal of the Association of Nurses in AIDS Care, 16*(4), 64–69.

Han, C. (2008) A qualitative exploration of the relationship between racism and unsafe sex among Asian Pacific Islander gay men. *Archives of Sexual Behavior,* 37(5), 827–837.

Harvey, S., Beckman, L., Browner, C., & Sherman, C. (2002). Relationship power, decision making, and sexual relations: An exploratory study with couples of Mexican origin. *Journal of Sex Research, 39*(4), 284–291.

Hekkink, C., Wiggersma, L., Yzermans, C., & Bindels, P. (2005). HIV nursing consultants: Patients preferences and experiences about the quality of care. *Journal of Clinical Nursing, 14*(3), 327–333.

Henry J. Kaiser Family Foundation. (2007). *Trends in U.S. government funding for HIV/AIDS fiscal years 1981–2004.* Menlo Park, CA: Author. Retrieved February 2, 2009, from www.kff.org/hivaids/loader. cfm?url=/commonspot/security/getfile.cfm&PageID=33622.

Hutchinson, A., Begley, E., Sullivan, P., Clark, H., Boyett, B., & Kellerman, S. (2007). Conspiracy beliefs and trust in information about HV/AIDS among minority men who have sex with men. *Journal of Acquired Immune Deficiency Syndrome, 45*(5), 603–605.

Johnson, R., & Raphael, C. (2006). The effects of male incarceration dynamics on AIDS infection rates among African American women and men (National Poverty Center Worker Paper No. 06-22). Retrieved on February 2, 2009, from http://paa2006.princeton.edu/download.aspx?submissionId=61207.

Jones, S., Messmer, P., Charron, S., & Parns, M. (2002). HIV-positive women and minority patients' satisfaction with inpatient hospital care. *AIDS Patient Care, 16*(3), 127–134.

Kang, E., Rapkin, B., Remien, R., Mellins, C. A., & Oh, A. (2005). Multiple dimensions of HIV stigma and psychological distress among Asians and Pacific Islanders living with HIV illness. *AIDS and Behavior, 9*(2), 145–154.

Kanuha, V. (2000). The impact of sexuality and race/ethnicity on HIV/AIDS risk among Asian and Pacific Island American (AI/P/IA) gay and bisexual men in Hawaii. *AIDS Education and Prevention, 12*(6), 505–518.

Kellogg, T., Clements-Nolle, K., Dilley, J., Katz, M., & McFarland, W. (2001). Incidence of HIV among male to female transgendered persons in San Francisco. *Journal of Acquired Immune Deficiency Syndrome, 28*(4), 380–384.

Kelly, M. (2003). *The role of religion in the HIV/AIDS epidemic.* Retrieved February 2, 2009, from www.missioncouncil.se/download/18.51ddd3b10fa0c64b24800024901/religion_hiv_aids_michael_kelly.pdf.

King, J. (2004). *On the down low.* New York: Broadway Books.

King, W., Wong, M., Shapiro, M., Landon, B., & Cunningham, W. (2004). Does racial concordance between HIV-positive patients and their physicians affect the time to receipt of protease inhibitors? *Journal of General Internal Medicine, 19*(11), 1146–1153.

Klonoff, E., & Landrine, H. (1999). Do blacks believe that HIV/AIDS is a government conspiracy against them? *Preventive Medicine, 28*(5), 451–457.

Koniak-Griffin, D., Lesser, J., Henneman, T., Huang, R., Huang, X., Tello, J., et al. (2008). HIV prevention for Latino adolescent mothers and their partners. *Western Journal of Nursing Research, 30*(6), 724–742.

Korthius, P., Saha, S., Fleishman, J., McGrath, M., Josephs, J., Moore, R., et al. (2008). Impact of patient race on patient experiences of access and communication in HIV care. *Journal of General Internal Medicine, 23,* 2046–2052.

Kulczycki, A., Kim, D., Duerr, A., Jamieson, D., & Macaluso, M. (2004). The acceptability of the female and male condom: A randomized crossover trial. *Perspectives on Sexual and Reproductive Health, 36*(3), 114–119.

LaVeist, T., & Nuru-Jeter, A. (2002). Is doctor–patient race concordance associated with greater satisfaction with care? *Journal of Health and Social Behavior, 43,* 296–306.

Lyles, C., Kay, L., Crepaz, N., Herbst, J., Passin, W., Kim, A., et al. (2007). Best-evidence interventions: Findings from a systematic review of HIV behavioral interventions for US populations at high risk, 2000–2004. *American Journal of Public Health, 97,* 133–143.

Malat, J., & van Ryn, M. (2005). African-American preference for same-race health care providers: The role of health care discrimination. *Ethnicity and Disease, 15,* 740–747.

Marín, B., & Díaz, R. (2002). Collaborative HIV Prevention Research in Minority Communities Program: A model for developing investigators of color. *Public Health Reports, 117*(3), 218–230.

Murrain, B., & Barker, T. (1997). Investigating the relationship between economic status and HIV risk. *Journal of Health Care for the Poor & Underserved, 8,* 416–423.

National Institute of Mental Health Multisite HIV/STD Prevention Trial for African American Couples Group. (2008). Measure of HIV/STD risk-reduction: Strategies for enhancing the utility of behavioral and biological outcome measures for African American couples. *Journal of Acquire Immune Deficiency Syndrome, 1*(49), S35–41.

Nebelkopf, E., & Penagos, M. (2005). Holistic Native network: Integrated HIV/AIDS, substance abuse, and mental health services for Native Americans in San Francisco. *Journal of Psychoactive Drugs, 37*(3), 257–264.

Nemoto, T., Operario, D., Soma, T., Bao, D., Vajrabukka, A., & Crisostomo, V. (2003). HIV risk and prevention among Asian/Pacific Islander men who have sex with men: Listen to our stories. *AIDS Education Prevention, 15*(1 Suppl. A), 7–20.

Nemoto, T., Operario, D., Keatley, J., Han, L., & Soma, T. (2004). HIV risk behaviors male-to-female transgender persons of color in San Francisco. *American Journal of Public Health, 94,* (7), 1193–1199.

Office of AIDS Research. (2002). *NIH strategic plan for AIDS research related to racial and ethnic minorities.* Retrieved February 2, 2009, from http://minority-health.pitt.edu/archive/00000088/01/OAR.pdf.

Office of AIDS Research. (2007). *FY 2009 trans-NIH plan for HIV-related research.* Retrieved February 2, 2009, from www.drugabuse.gov/whatsnew/meetings/hiv_aids_specialrep/powerpoint/Whitescarver.ppt#257,1, NIH AIDS Research Priorities.

Office of the Press Secretary. (1998). President Clinton declares HIV/AIDS in racial and ethnic minority communities to be a "severe and ongoing health care crisis" and unveils a new initiative to address this problem (Press Release). Retrieved January 31, 2009, from www.hhs.gov/news/press/1998pres/19981028.html.

O'Leary, A., Fisher, H., Purcell, D., Spikes, P., & Gomez, C. (2007). Correlates of risk patterns and race/ethnicity among HIV positive men who have sex with men. *AIDS and Behavior, 11,* 706–715.

Osemene, N., Essien. E., & Egbunike, I. (2001). HIV/AIDS behind bars: An avenue for culturally sensitive interventions. *Journal of the National Medical Association, 93,* 481–486.

Pappas-Deluca, K., Kraft, J., Edwards, S., Casillas, A., Harvey, S., & Huszti, H. (2006). Recruiting and retaining couples for an HIV prevention intervention: Lessons learned from the PARTNERS project. *Health Education Research, 21*(5), 611–620.

Penny, K. (2008). HIV/AIDS role-play activity. *Journal of Nursing Education, 47*(9), 435–436.

Perrino, T., Fernandez. I., Bowen, S., & Arheart, K. (2006). Low-income African American women's attempts to convince their main partner to use condoms. *Cultural Diversity and Ethnic Minority Psychology, 12*(1), 70–83.

Roberts, K., Newman, P., Duan, N., & Rudy, E. (2005). HIV vaccine knowledge and beliefs among communities at elevated risk: Conspiracies, questions, and confusion. *Journal of National Medical Association, 97*(12), 1662–1671.

Ross, M., Essien, E., & Torres, I. (2006). Conspiracy beliefs about the origin of HIV/AIDS in four racial/ethnic groups. *Journal of Acquired Immune Deficiency Syndrome, 41*(3), 342–344.

Rotheram-Borus, M., Desmond, K., Comulada, S., Arnold, E., Johnson, M., & the Healthy Living Trial Group. (2008). Reducing risky sexual behavior and substance use among currently and formerly homeless adults living with HIV. *American Journal of Public Health, 98*(11), 1–11.

Saha, S., Taggart, S., Komaromy, M., & Bindman, A. (2000). Do patients choose physicians of their own race? *Health Affairs, 159,* 997–1004.

St. Lawrence, J., Wilson, T., Eldridge, G., Brasfield, T., & O'Bannon, R. (2001). Community-base interventions to reduce low income, African American women's risk of sexually. *Journal of Community Psychology, 29*(6), 937–964.

Saul, J., Erwin, J., Bruce, J., & Peters B. (2000). Ethnic and demographic variations in HIV/AIDS presentation at two London referral centres 1995–9. *Sexually Transmitted Infections, 76*(3), 215.

Sausa, L., Keathley, J., & Operario, D. (2007). Perceived risks and benefits of sex work among transgender women of color in San Francisco. *Archives of Sex Behavior, 36*(6), 768–777.

Schensul, J., Levy, J., & Disch, W. (2003). Individual, contextual, and social network factors affecting exposure to HIV/AIDS risk among older residents living in low-income senior housing complexes. *Journal of Acquired Immune Deficiency Syndrome, 1*(33, Suppl. 2), S138–152.

Sly, D., Harrison, D., Moore, T., & Soler, H. (2001). HIV transmission risks of females and males in paired partner relationships. *Journal of Health and Human Service Administration, 24*(2), 144–170.

Simon, P. A., Reback, C. J., & Bemis, C. C. (2000). HIV prevalence and incidence among male-to-female transsexuals receiving HIV prevention services in Los Angeles County. *AIDS, 14*, 2953–2955.

Sohler, N., Fitzpatrick, L., Lindsay, R., Anastos, K., & Cunningham, C. (2007). Does patient–provider racial/ethnic concordance influence ratings of trust in people with HIV infection? *AIDS and Behavior, 11*, 884–896.

Soler, H., Quadagno, D., Sly, D., Richman, K., Eberstein, I., & Harrison, D. (2000). Relationship dynamics, ethnicity and condom use among low-income women. *Family Planning Perspectives, 32*(2), 82–88.

Stein, J., Dixon, E., & Nyamathi, A. (2008). Effects of psychosocial and situational variables on substance abuse among homeless adults. *Psychology Addict Behavior, 22*(3), 410–416.

Stevens, S. J., Estrada, A. L., & Estrada, B. D. (2000). HIV drug and sex risk behaviors among American Indian and Alaska Native drug users: Gender and site differences. *American Indian Alaska Native Mental Health Research, 9*(1), 33–46.

Sullivan, P., McNaghten, A., Begley, E., Hutchinson, A., & Cargill, V. (2007). Enrollment of racial/ethnic minorities and women with HIV in clinical research studies of HIV medicines. *Journal of the National Medical Association, 99*(3), 242–250.

Thrasher, A., Earp, J., Golin, C., & Zimmer, C. (2008). Discrimination, distrust, and racial/ethnic disparities in antiretroviral therapy adherence among a national sample of HIV-infected patients. *Journal of Acquired Immune Deficiency Syndrome, 49*(1), 84–93.

U.N. Population Fund. (2006). *Female condom: A powerful tool for protection.* New York: Author. Retrieved January 31, 2009, from http://67.205.89.177/webdav/site/global/shared/documents/publications/2006/female condom.pdf.

U.S. Census Bureau 2000. (2000). *The black population 2000.* Retrieved September 25, 2007, from www.census.gov/prod/2001pubs/c2kbr01-5.pdf.

U.S. Conference of Mayors. (2004, December). *Hunger and homelessness survey.* Retrieved February 1, 2009, from www.usmayors.org/hungersurvey/2004/onlinereport/HungerAndHomelessnessReport2004.pdf.

Villarruel, A., Jemmott, L., Jemmott, J., & Eakin, B. (2006). Recruitment and retention of Latin Adolescents to a research study: Lessons learned from a randomized clinical trial. *Journal of Specialists in Pediatric Nursing, 11*(6), 244–250.

Warren, J., Fernandez, M., Harper, G., Hidalgo, M., Jamil, O., & Torress, R. (2008). Predicators of unprotected sex among young sexually active African American, Hispanic, and white MSM: The importance of ethnicity and culture. *AIDS and Behavior, 12*(3), 459–468.

Whyte, J., Whyte, M., & Cormier, E. (2008). Down low sex, older African American women, and HIV infection. *Journal of the Association of Nurses in AIDS Care, 19*(6), 423–431.

Witte, S., El-Bassel, N., Gilbert, L., Wu, E., & Chang, M. (2007). Predicators of discordant reports of sexual and HIV/sexually transmitted infection risk behaviors among heterosexual couples. *Sexually Transmitted Diseases, 34*(5), 302–308.

Witte, S., El-Bassel, N., Gilbert, L., Wu, E., Chang, M., & Hill, J. (2006a). Promoting female condom use to heterosexual couples: Findings from a randomized clinical trial. *Perspectives on Sexual Reproductive Health, 38*(3), 148–154.

Witte, S., El-Bassel, N., Gilbert, L., Wu, E., Chang, M., & Steinglass, P. (2006b). Recruitment of minority women and their main sexual partners in an HIV/STI prevention trial. *Journal of Women's Health, 13*(10), 1137–1147.

Wolitski, R., Pals, S., Kidder, D., Courtenay-Quirk, C., & Holtgrave, D. (2008, September 4). The effects of HIV stigma on health, disclosure of HIV status, and risk behavior of homeless and unstably housed persons living with HIV. Epub ahead of print: PMID: 18770023.

Woods, C. (2007). Towards a culturally sensitive HIV/AIDS education curriculum: Kenyan Literacy Project. *The International Journal of Learning, 14*(10), 69–74.

Yoshioka, M., & Schustack, A. (2001). Disclosure of HIV status: Cultural issues of Asian patients. *AIDS Patient Care STDs, 15*(2), 77–82.

13 HIV Infection in Women

SUSAN W. GASKINS

Women face unique challenges, issues, and considerations with respect to HIV/AIDS, and it is important that health care providers are aware of their special needs. As the number of women infected with HIV has increased steadily since the beginning of the pandemic in the early 1980s, we have learned about differences and similarities in the impact the disease has on women versus men. Sadly, women are often at risk for HIV infection because of behaviors of their sexual partners rather than their own risk behaviors. Many women with HIV infection live in poverty, and most have important family responsibilities. This chapter will address women's clinical manifestations and issues relative to women, contraception and pregnancy, transmission and prevention, and psychosocial issues relevant to women. The epidemiology of HIV/AIDS in women is discussed in Chapter 1. Nurses, who play a key role in the care, education, research, and policy development related to women and HIV/AIDS, must be aware of the special HIV/AIDS issues for women to ensure that transmission is decreased, the best care is provided, and the quality of life is enhanced for HIV-infected women.

437

STATISTICS

Around the world, women account for half of all people infected with HIV (UNAIDS, 2008). Early in the HIV/AIDS pandemic, there were few cases diagnosed in women and female adolescents the United States. However, today in the United States, women represent almost 19% of the estimated cumulative number of AIDS cases reported through 2006 (189,566 cases out of 1,014,797) and 27% of adults and adolescents living with HIV/AIDS (CDC, 2008, 2009). Racial minorities are dispro-portionately represented in cases of HIV/AIDS. In 2006 black women (12% of the U.S. female population) accounted for 65% of the estimated number of cases of HIV/AIDS in women 13 years of age and older; Hispanics (13% of the U.S. female population) accounted for 15%; and whites (68% of the U.S. female population) accounted for 18% of cases (CDC, 2008, 2009). The rate of diagnosis of AIDS for black women is approximately 23 times the rate for white women (45.5/100,000 for black women and 2/100,000 for white women) and four times higher than the rate for Hispanic women (11.2/100,000) (CDC, 2008). While African American and Hispanic women represented 24% of all U.S. women, they accounted for 82% of women diagnosed with AIDS in 2005 (CDC, 2008). In 2004, HIV infection was the leading cause of death among African American women aged 25 to 44 years; the third leading cause of death for black women aged 35 to 44 years; the fourth leading cause of death for black women aged 45 to 55 years; and the fourth leading cause of death for Hispanic women aged 35 to 44 (CDC, 2008). Also in 2004, HIV infection was the fifth leading cause of death among all U.S. women 35 to 44 years of age and the sixth leading cause of death in all women 25 to 34 years of age (CDC, 2008). For adolescent females, HIV infection rates are three to six times higher than for adolescent males (Simon, Ho, & Karim, 2006).

CLINICAL ISSUES AND MANIFESTATIONS

In the beginning of the epidemic, injection drug use (IDU) was the mostly likely mode of HIV transmission to women, but today IDU is the second most common mode of transmission in women. Currently, the most likely route of transmission in women is high-risk heterosexual contact, which accounted for almost 75% of the new cases of AIDS in women in 2006 (CDC, 2008). Several biological factors influence women's susceptibility to heterosexual transmission of HIV. Once infected, however, there is little evidence of differences between men and women in HIV disease progression or response to antiretroviral therapy (ART) (Perez-Hoyos et al., 2007; Prins, Meyer, & Hessol, 2005). Women do have gynecological manifestations related to HIV infection. A major concern for women is human papillomavirus (HPV) infection.

Transmission

Biologically, women are more susceptible to heterosexual transmission of HIV than men. This increased risk is related to female anatomy and physiology, as well as individual sexual practices. Women's risk for infection is increased by aspects of the female genital tract including the vagina and cervical epithelium, pH, vaginal fluid, microbial flora, and cervical mucus. Additionally, a woman's risk of infection is influenced by changes that occur with aging, sexual excitement, effects of systemic steroids on the genital tract, menstruation, and contraceptive practices, including barrier methods and sexual and hygienic practices (Cotton & Watts, 1997). The presence of sexually transmitted infections (STIs) also accentuates the risk of transmission and acquisition of HIV among women for a variety of reasons, including the presence of inflammatory cells that act as targets for the virus and disruption of the integrity of the epithelial or mucus membrane. Both ulcerative STIs, such as syphilis, genital herpes, and chancroid, and inflammatory STIs, such as gonorrhea, chlamydia, and HPV, have been associated with HIV transmission (Kojic & Cu-Uvin, 2007). The rates of gonorrhea and syphilis are higher in women of color than in white women, contributing to their increased vulnerability to HIV. These higher rates are significantly higher for 15- to 24-year-old females of color (CDC, 2008). In many women, STIs are asymptomatic, making diagnosis and treatment difficult (Turmen, 2003).

Clinical Manifestations

There is little difference in opportunistic processes or disease progression in women and men with HIV/AIDS. HIV-infected women often present with gynecological manifestations that are influenced by their disease (Cotton & Watts, 1997). Mucosal candidiasis has been reported to be more common in women than men, and persistent Candida vulvovaginitis is often a presenting symptom of HIV infection, indicating severely compromised immunity. In 1993, the expanded AIDS surveillance case definition of AIDS included invasive cervical cancer, recognizing women as a high-risk subpopulation with an increased incidence of AIDS. While cervical neoplasia is not the most common gynecological manifestation of HIV infection, it is the most serious. The inclusion of this preventable cancer in the list of AIDS-defining conditions increases attention to the importance of gynecological care for women with HIV/AIDS.

HIV, Human Papilloma Virus, and Cervical Cancer

HPV is an STI that is of particular concern to women with HIV infection. While most HPV infections are transient, the persistent high-risk types lead to cervical dysplasia and cancer. HPV infection is common among all women, but it is are more prevalent and persistent in HIV-infected women, especially in those with a low CD4 count. Also, HIV-infected women with HPV (especially types 16, 18, and several others) have been reported to develop cervical dysplasia and progress to cervical intraepithelial neoplasm, to be more likely to develop cervical or other genital cancers, and to be more likely to relapse after treatment compared to HIV-negative women (Harris et al., 2005). Research on the impact of antiretroviral therapy (ART) on cervical HPV infection in HIV-infected women has been inconclusive. However, evidence suggests that a strong immune system helps keep HPV infection in check. Women with higher CD4 counts are less likely to become infected with HPV and to have a lower risk of precancerous cervical changes if infected (Harris et al., 2005). Anal HPV has been reported in both men and women. Anal HPV infection, which can progress to anal cancer, is reported to be more common than cervical HPV infection in women who practice anal sex. High-risk HPV types are more prevalent in anal infections than in cervical infections (Kojic & Cu-Uvin, 2007). A quadrivalent human papillomavirus recombinant vaccine (Gardasil and Cervarix) is available and recommended for use in girls and women 9 through 26 years old. (It may also prevent genital warts in boys and men.) This vaccine protects against four strains of HPV (6, 11, 16, and 18) which cause 70% of cervical cancers and 90% of genital warts in women (Vetter & Geller, 2007). It is effective only before a person becomes infected with HPV and has not been studied in HIV-infected adults.

Medical experts recommend that women have a Papanicolaou test (also called Pap smear, Pap test, cervical smear, or smear test) when diagnosed with HIV or when care for HIV is sought and again six months later. For women with negative tests who are asymptomatic and have a CD4 count of >200 cells/mm3, annual screening is then recommended.

For women with previous abnormal Pap tests, other signs of cervical abnormalities, or advanced disease, screening should be continued every six months (Highleyman, 2007).

MENSTRUATION, MENOPAUSE, CONTRACEPTION, AND PREGNANCY

Because the majority of HIV-infected women are of reproductive age, there are concerns about the effects of HIV and its treatment on their menstrual cycles, contraception decisions, and pregnancies. Issues and concerns related to HIV and pregnancy are important because of the possibility of perinatal transmission to the baby as well as potential effects on the mother's and the baby's health. As women live longer on ART, the effects of HIV on menopause have also become a concern.

Menstruation

The interaction between HIV and menstruation remains unclear. A report from the Women's Interagency HIV Study (WIHS) reports that while many women with HIV/AIDS report abnormalities with their menstrual cycles, findings from studies have been conflicting (Highleyman, 2007). Studies have been complicated by other variables such as weight loss, substance abuse, and stress, all of which are associated with menstrual abnormalities in women. More problems have been reported in women with CD4 counts below 50 cells/mm3. Women on ART with a well-preserved immune system are less likely to experience serious menstrual problems (Harlow et al., 2000; Massad et al, 2006). HIV is present in menstrual blood, and intercourse during menses has been reported to increase the risk of transmission to the male partner (European Study Group on Heterosexual Transmission of HIV, 1992). The vaginal pH during menses is raised to the neutral range, improving the viability of HIV shed in menstrual blood and in semen deposited vaginally. Therefore, menstruation may serve to enhance a woman's infectiousness or her susceptibility to infection (Cotton & Watts, 1997).

Contraception

Because the majority of HIV-infected women are of reproductive age, contraceptive counseling is an essential component of their health care. Barrier methods (male and female condoms) of contraception are recommended because they prevent pregnancy and the transmission of sexually transmitted diseases, including HIV. (In March 2009 the FDA approved a second-generation female condom known as FC2 Female Condom.) Combination hormonal contraceptives widely used by women are more effective in preventing pregnancy but offer no protection against STIs. Oral hormonal birth control pills can interact with antiretroviral medications, reducing the efficacy of the contraceptives. Nevirapine, lopinavir-ritonavir, ritonavir, and nelfinavir have been reported to decrease the levels of estradiol and norethindrone, leading to an increased risk of pregnancy. Side effects and toxicity of estradiol and norethindrone are accentuated with atazanavir, indinavir, and efavirenz because the levels are increased. For these reasons, coadministration of oral contraceptives and ART is not recommended (Kojic & Cu-Uvin, 2007). Other forms of hormonal contraceptives, such as patches and injections (Depo-Provera) do not interact with ART (Richardson et al., 2007). None of the hormonal contraceptives have been found to have an effect on HIV disease progression (Richardson et al., 2007). Intrauterine devices (IUDs) initially were not recommended for women with HIV/AIDS because of the risk of complications, such as pelvic inflammatory disease. Studies in Kenya have reported that the copper T intrauterine device is equally safe in HIV-infected or uninfected women (Morrison et al., 2001) and have also concluded that HIV-infected women can safely use IUDS if they are on ART and their HIV disease is well controlled. Complications for HIV-infected women, including infection, are no more common than for women who are not infected with HIV.

Pregnancy Decisions

It is important for clinicians to be aware of the myriad of issues related to pregnancy decisions for HIV-infected women. Accurate information and guidance are crucial to help women make the best decisions for themselves and their babies. While there is a risk of perinatal HIV transmission, today that risk can minimized. Pregnancy decisions include considerations about becoming pregnant, treatment during pregnancy and delivery, and whether to continue an existing pregnancy. Many HIV-infected women wish to have children. Indeed, the intensity of the desire for children has been reported to be no different in HIV-infected women and uninfected women (Wesley, 2003). Craft and colleagues (2007) found that a decision to become pregnant is more highly influenced by the desire for children than by family members, friends, partners, or a woman's concern for her own health. That desire correlates with increased self-esteem and self-efficacy; however, women with a negative self-image and a high level of personalized HIV stigma may also choose to become pregnant. If the stigma is from external sources, HIV-infected women have reportedly been less likely to choose to become pregnant (Craft et al., 2007).

There are many factors that influence HIV-infected women's pregnancy decisions. Older, more religious black women have been reported to be more likely to become pregnant than younger, less religious white women. However, younger women with HIV infection, in general, are more likely to become pregnant than older HIV-infected women. Women who have had previous abortions are less likely to desire having children or to carry a pregnancy to term than those who have not had abortions or who have had fewer abortions (Kline, Strickler, & Kempf, 1995). Women who receive their diagnosis of HIV infection during pregnancy have been reported to be more likely to terminate the pregnancy than women who were diagnosed prior to becoming pregnant (Craft et al., 2007).

HIV Testing and Counseling

In 2003, in an effort to reduce perinatal HIV transmission, the CDC recommended the universal HIV testing of all pregnant women and the use of rapid tests during intrapartum or postpartum if the mother had not been screened prenatally. The revised testing recommendations in 2006 reiterated these recommendations but simplified the process by not requiring a separate written consent form for HIV testing. HIV testing should be a routine component of preconception care. Testing early in pregnancy makes it possible for HIV-infected women to benefit from care that minimizes the risk of perinatal HIV transmission (CDC, 2006). The new recommendations are for diagnostic HIV testing and opt-out screening for all adults and adolescents as part of routine clinical care in all health care settings. (See Chapter 2 for a fuller discussion of opt-out and other issues related to screening and testing.) These recommendations foster earlier detection of HIV infection, thereby making it possible to identify and counsel people with unrecognized HIV infection and link them to care and services. The effectiveness in detecting unsuspected maternal HIV infection by screening all pregnant women is one rationale for the 2006 recommendations.

Pregnancy

ART has improved the health and extended the lives of HIV-infected women, many of whom are of childbearing age. Research has not found that pregnancy leads to worse HIV disease progression and has even reported that pregnant women infected with HIV had a lower risk of developing AIDS-defining conditions or dying than nonpregnant HIV-infected women (Tia et al., 2007). While HIV infection confers a risk of perinatal transmission, with appropriate care and treatment the transmission rate is less than 2% (Cooper et al., 2002). It is important that the viral load be suppressed to an undetectable level during pregnancy to decrease the likelihood of transmission (Warszawski et al, 2008). Kojic and Cu-Uvin (2007) discuss other maternal factors that are associated with higher rates of perinatal transmission, including advanced HIV disease, a low CD4 count, poor nutrition, drug use, and concomitant STIs. Obstetrical factors that increase the likelihood of perinatal transmission of HIV include a vaginal delivery, prolonged rupture of membranes, invasive fetal monitoring, and chorioamnionitis. Pregnant women with HIV infection should be monitored during pregnancy and should follow the same recommendations as those for other pregnant women for a healthy pregnancy, including: (1) good nutrition; (2) avoidance of smoking, recreational drugs, and alcohol; and (3) prenatal vitamins.

The AIDS Clinical Trial Group (ACTG) Protocol 076 in 1994 demonstrated that the use of zidovudine (ZDV) in HIV-infected pregnant women during antepartum, intrapartum, and, for six weeks prophylaxis treatment of the infant, reduced perinatal transmission from 25.5% to 8.3% (Connor et al., 1994). Both ZDV (Retrovir) and nevirapine (Viramune) monotherapy have been found to reduce the risk of vertical transmission dramatically, but today ART is recommended for pregnant women with HIV/AIDS to prevent perinatal HIV transmission regardless of CD4 count or viral load (Public Health Service Task Force, 2008). Antepartal antiretroviral prophylaxis should be started by 28 weeks gestation for maximum effectiveness. For women who do not require antiretroviral treatment for their own health, postponing initiation of prophylaxis treatment can be a consideration (Public Health Service Task Force, 2008). If antepartal antiretroviral drugs are not received, combined intrapartal and postpartal drug administration has demonstrated the capacity to reduce HIV transmission. However, intrapartal drug administration alone is not effective without postexposure prophylaxis in the infant (Petra Study Team, 2002). Regardless of the use of antiretrovirals during antepartum, intrapartum intravenous ZDV and six weeks of infant ZDV are recommended to reduce perinatal HIV transmission (Public Health Service Task Force, 2008).

Research has also demonstrated the low rate of perinatal transmission (1.2%) in mothers during pregnancy who receive combination therapy that includes a protease inhibitor (Cooper et al, 2002). While there are limited data on drug resistance among pregnant women, resistance testing is recommended for all treatment-naïve pregnant women and for those with suboptimal viral suppression to ensure the efficacy of the drugs in preventing transmission of the virus (Public Health Service Task Force, 2008). Unless there is severe toxicity or resistance, zidovudine is the preferred nucleoside analog reverse transcriptase inhibitor (NRTI) for use in ART and is recommended in all antepartal regimens based on documented efficacy. There are certain antiretrovirals that are contraindicated in pregnant women because of the possibility of birth defects or serious side effects for pregnant women (Highleyman, 2007). Efavirenz (Sustiva) is contraindicated because it can cause birth defects such as anencephaly, anophthalmia (absence of an eye[s]), and cleft palate (Public Health Service Task force, 2008.) Nelfinavir (Viracept) contained an impurity, ethyl methanesulfonate (EMS), that was potentially harmful to pregnant women or young children and was not recommended for pregnant women or infants. By March 2008 the Food and Drug Administration and Pfizer, the U.S. manufacturer of nelfinavir, had agreed on a limit for EMS in nelfinavir, leading to the lifting of the recommendation against its use by children and pregnant women (Public Health Service Task Force, 2008). Nevirapine (Viramune) is associated with liver toxicity and deaths from hepatic failure in pregnant women and should only be used as a component of ART if a women's CD4 count is greater than 250 and the benefits outweigh the risks. Maternal deaths from lactic acidosis have also been reported in HIV-infected pregnant women taking d4T (stravudine, Zerit) and ddI (didanosine, Videx). There is a need to continue to study and monitor the effects of ART on pregnant women and infants.

For HIV-infected women whose viral loads are fully suppressed, a cesarean section is not warranted. Complications, especially postpartal infections related to the surgery, are more likely to be experienced by HIV-infected women. An elective cesarean section in women with plasma viral load greater than 1,000 copies/ml close to the time of delivery is recommended (Public Health Service Task Force, 2008).

During pregnancy, HIV-infected women should have their CD4 count assessed at the first visit and then every three months. To monitor antiretroviral therapy, plasma HIV RNA should be assessed at the first visit, two to six weeks after initiating or changing therapy, and monthly until RNA levels are undetectable. Then HIV levels should be monitored every two months and at 34 to 36 weeks gestation for decisions about the need for a cesarean section delivery (Public Health Service Task Force, 2008).

HIV is also transmitted through breast-feeding, and there are no safe methods to treat breast milk to prevent the risk of transmission. Additionally, little is known about the level of penetration of antiviral drugs into breast milk, which causes concerns about toxicity in the infant or possible development of drug-resistant virus. Therefore, breast-feeding is not recommended in the United States and in other countries where safe formula feeding is available, affordable, acceptable, and sustainable (Public Health Service Task Force, 2008). A fuller discussion of breast-feeding is provided in Chapter 14.

Menopause

There is a growing population of HIV-infected women who are living longer on HAART and will experience menopause. There is a dearth of data on HIV infection and menopause, and extant research has produced conflicting results. Thinning of the vaginal epithelial thickness that occurs because of decreased estrogen increases a woman's risk of HIV infection during menopause. The thinner epithelium is a less effective barrier and may be injured during coitus (Cotton & Watts, 1997). The common symptoms associated with menopause, including hot flashes, night sweats, mood swings, vaginal dryness, memory loss, and depression are often associated with HIV infection and have not been found to differ in intensity or frequency in women with HIV/AIDS (Kojic & Cu-Uvin, 2007). Factors that accentuate these symptoms, like smoking, stress, drug use, and low body mass, are prevalent in women with HIV/AIDS. A major concern for postmenopausal women is bone loss and increased heart disease risk related to falling estrogen levels. For women with HIV/AIDS, the concern is greater because ART is also associated with bone loss and increased heart disease (Anastos et al., 2007). It is important to monitor bone health with periodic dual energy X-ray absorptiometry (DEXA) scans in women with HIV/AIDS and to treat them with medications for the prevention and treatment of osteoporosis.

PREVENTION

The steady increase in the number of women infected with HIV, plus the heavy burden of HIV experienced by women in resource-limited countries, underscore the need for prevention strategies targeted at women. The ABC (abstinence, be faithful, and condoms) approach is not sufficient, practical, or even possible for many women. Abstinence is not an option for married women or victims of sexual violence. Being faithful is effective in preventing HIV transmission only if both people in a relationship are monogamous. While male and female condoms are effective in reducing the transmission of HIV when properly used, they are not always acceptable to both parties. Women's rights are elusive in many cultures, and thousands of females are infected with HIV daily because saying no to sex or insisting on condom use is not an option in view of cultural factors, financial dependence, or the threat of violence. HIV prevention programs for women need to be gender specific and culturally appropriate. Effective, safe, and acceptable prevention strategies that are female initiated and controlled are urgently needed. Vaginal microbicides offer hope to make a dramatic decrease in HIV transmission in women, but effective and safe microbicides are not yet available.

Female Condoms

The female condom is the only female-controlled method of pregnancy and STI prevention available at this time and has been available in theUnited States since 1994. Female condoms were heralded for their disease and contraceptive prevention capability as well as their potential to address power differences in heterosexual relationships. Much of the research on female condoms has focused on acceptability rather than effectiveness in disease prevention (Vijayakumar et al., 2006). Studies on the use of female condoms have reported increased protected sex acts when female condoms are introduced to a population as an option for protection from STIs (Vijayakumar et al., 2006). Greater protection would result from the use of the female condom, male condoms or, more often, a combination of the two. The purpose of the female condom is to augment existing prevention strategies, not to replace the ones that are known to be effective.

Research on the effectiveness of female condoms in preventing transmission of STIs has provided inconsistent results. Two randomized intervention studies reported decreased STI incidence in the groups that included female condoms (Fontanet et al., 1998; French et al., 2003). One study by Feldblum and colleagues (2001) addressing STI prevalence and the use of female condoms did not find a difference in the intervention and control groups. Female condoms are slightly less effective than male condoms as contraceptives, and their use in the United States is low (Status Report of the Female Condom, 2008). The ability of the female condom to prevent HIV infection has not been studied directly (Padian et al., 2008).

Studies on patterns of use of female condoms have also yielded mixed and inconsistent results (Vijayakumar et al., 2006). For example, studies in the United States and Zimbabwe have found younger women more likely to use them, while older women were more likely to use them in Uganda. In the United States. black and Hispanic women have been reported as more likely to try and use female condoms consistently than white women (Vijayakumar, et al. 2006). Greater acceptance of the female condom has been reported in women with indicators of risk for HIV, such as being tested for HIV, having had an STI, having been pregnant, or trading sex for drugs. Studies on female condom use and type of sexual partners have found that women in the United States and Brazil are more likely to use them with steady partners than casual or new ones. Commercial sex workers in Zimbabwe were less likely to use the female condom with steady partners than with their clients (Napierala et al., 2008).

Issues related to female condom use include acceptability, convenience, and cost. Cost is particularly a barrier to use in developing countries. A new generation female condom, the FC2, is reported to have a more acceptable design, be easier to use, and be less expensive, which may lead to increased use. Studies on the cost effectiveness of the female condom are lacking and needed.

Female condoms are most needed and have the potential to make the biggest impact on HIV transmission in the countries with the highest rates of HIV infection. Their use and acceptance in such areas are reportedly inconsistent. Future research on female condom use needs to focus on assessing its effectiveness in prevention of HIV transmission and on best practices to target and promote its use in specific populations.

Microbicides

Microbicides are prophylactic agents that are used vaginally to prevent the transmission of HIV and other STIs. There are a number of different delivery formulations including gels or creams, films, foaming pills, suppositories, sponges or vaginal rings, and preloaded diaphragms. The vaginal ring has many advantages such as ease of use and a lower compliance burden because of the 30-day duration of drug delivery (Cates & Rosenberg, 2008). Microbicides have several mechanisms of action that reduce transmission of HIV: (a) vaginal defense enhancers, (b) membrane disruption, (c) entry or fusion inhibitors, (d) replication inhibitors, and (e) combination of actions (Alliance for Microbicide Development, 2008).

Early microbicide candidates were entry inhibitors that work by blocking attachment of the virus or creating conditions in the vagina that inhibited infection. Two of these candidates are in efficacy trials. The latest microbicide candidates use ARVs that specifically target HIV or its target cells and are referred to as reverse transcriptase inhibitors (International Partnership for Microbicides, 2008). They are expected to be more effective in preventing HIV Infection. Prior to approval and availability for use, each microbicide must pass a series of rigorous tests and meet a number of criteria (Global Campaign for Microbicides, 2006). After testing in the laboratory, then in animals, a compound must undergo three levels of clinical (human) trials. Currently the microbicide pipeline includes more than 50 candidates in preclinical development and 12 candidates in clinical trials (Alliance for Microbicide Development, 2008). All of the candidates in Phase III efficacy trials are coitally dependent and must be used right before sexual intercourse. The goal is to develop microbicides that can be used independent of sex to facilitate use and compliance. A challenge in microbicide development is determining the optimal dose level. Absorption of microbicides must be minimal to reduce the possibility of toxicity, as well as the possibility of the development of drug-resistant HIV when ARVs are used as microbicides.

Safety studies are critical for microbicides because of their potential for chronic use. Researchers recognize the importance of extreme diligence in studying safety after nonoxynol-9 was found to enhance the transmission of HIV in comparison to the placebo being used in the study (Van Damme et al., 2002). Local toxicity or irritation is a concern for all topically applied microbicides. Not only do breaches to the mucosal epithelium provide a passage to the systemic circulation for HIV, but cells involved in inflammatory reactions are target cells for the virus. To be effective, microbicides must be used correctly, so they must be easy to use, be acceptable to users, and not interfere with sexual intercourse.

Additionally it is important that they be stable at high temperatures like those found in developing countries, where the need is most critical (Mantell et al., 2005).

Social and behavioral studies are an integral part of microbicide research. It is important to understand people's motivation to use them and the types of sexual relationships in which they are involved (Voelker, 2006). This research must be part of the development phase of microbicides as well as the implementation phase. This research will be crucial in determining: (a) user preferences and concerns, (b) partners' knowledge preference and attitudes toward use, and (c) strategies for introducing the products. Research related to developing educational and training materials for users and health care providers is needed to ensure the appropriate use of microbicides.

Once a microbicide is licensed, its success will depend on its introduction into HIV-prevention programs and its use by women and their partners. The majority of HIV-infected women live in low-income countries and sub-Saharan Africa, and this is where microbicides have the greatest potential to have an impact in preventing the transmission of HIV. A major concern with introducing microbicides in these countries is that the majority of the people lack access to existing HIV-prevention services. Early planning and timely mobilization of resources are critical to ensure that microbicides reach and can be used by women who need them when they become available. It will be important that microbicides can be produced in sufficient supply and at a cost that is affordable if they are to be successful in decreasing HIV transmission.

The Alliance for Microbicide Development (2008) emphasizes the need for increased funding for research in microbicide development. Government and philanthropic donors must step forward to fund the work and research that must be done rather than depending on pharmaceutical companies. Once licensed, the support of policy makers and global leaders will be critical to ensure that the women who most need microbicides receive them. While the development of a successful microbicide is complex and expensive, it has the potential to be one of the greatest public health accomplishments of our generation, with the ability to change and save the lives of women around the world.

Prevention Programs

There are different individual, interpersonal, sociocultural, and temporal factors related to HIV transmission for women in comparison to men that underscore the need for gender-relevant and culturally sensitive prevention programs. The most effective programs have been found to: (a) use social psychological models that emphasize gender-related influences, (b) be peer led, (c) use multiple intervention sessions of low intensity (one to four sessions) versus high intensity (over five sessions), (d) be focused on specific populations, (e) include only women, and (f) move beyond education to empowerment of individuals (Ickovics & Yoshikaw, 1998; Wingood & DiClemente, 1996). Empowerment can come from increased education and information, but services, policies, and programs are necessary to ensure that women have the resources and support needed to enact what they learn. Goals of prevention programs include reducing the number of unprotected sexual encounters, reducing sexual partners, reducing or eliminating high-risk sexual behaviors, and increasing consistent condom use.

PSYCHOSOCIAL ISSUES

Multiple psychosocial issues influence women's risk for and response to HIV infection. Two specific ones are stigma and violence. HIV-positive women experience and fear stigmatization by others, and this is a central part of their lives. Stigma is a major influence in disclosure decisions for women. High rates of violence have been reported in women with HIV infection, both prior to and after infection (Liebschutz et al., 2000).

Stigma

HIV-related stigma is recognized as a stressor for people with HIV/AIDS that negatively affects their lives and is associated with low self-esteem, depression, anxiety, loneliness, suicidal ideation, and poor treatment adherence. Stigma can be perceived or felt from an internal source, or it can be the effect of overt actions or behaviors of others.

From a metasynthesis of the findings of qualitative studies on stigma in HIV-positive women, Sandelowski, Lambe, and Barroso (2004) found perceived or felt and enacted stigma to be pervasive in the lives of the women. While only 16 of the 93 reports reviewed were specifically focused on stigma, the majority of the other reports included stigma findings from the descriptions of living with HIV/AIDS. Study participants described how they lived with the fear and negative effects of being stigmatized, including social rejection, discrimination, and violence. Their fear of stigma was related to internalizing negative cultural views of people with HIV and how they had contracted the infection. The fact that women have the ability to bear and infect children added to their stigmatization. Mode of HIV transmission was also an issue. Many women become infected in a heterosexual monogamous relationship but are assumed to have become infected by drug use, promiscuity, or prostitution.

Fear of stigma has been identified as a critical issue in disclosure decisions regardless of how the disease is contracted (Greene et al., 2003; Sayles et al., 2007). Perceptions of HIV-related stigma shape individuals' concerns about the consequences of disclosure. Consequently, higher levels of perceived stigma have been reported to decrease the likelihood of disclosure (Clark et al., 2003; Yang et al., 2006). Disclosure decisions are difficult and complex for all people infected with HIV (Holt et al., 1998; Levy et al., 1999). In contrast to men, women have been found to worry more about disclosing their infection to their children and disclose to others sooner after their diagnosis (Levy et al., 1999). HIV-infected women want to protect their children from possible negative effects of disclosure, such as having to cope with their mother's disease and being stigmatized because of their mother's infection. The timing of disclosure to children is difficult as women worry about the possibility of the children telling others or of other people informing children who do not know about their mother's infection (Sandelowski et al., 2004). Strategies used by women to manage disclosure of their HIV infection to others include lying about signs and symptoms of HIV infection, avoiding social interactions, and ensuring safer sex with condom use.

Violence

The prevalence of violence, both physical and sexual abuse, has been reported to be high among HIV-infected women (Liebschutz et al., 2000). Disclosure violence is feared and has been experienced by many HIV-infected women, especially from their sexual partners. However, violence has a much broader context in the lives of women with HIV/AIDS. Prior to infection, many HIV-infected women report having a history of physical abuse as an adult (Gielen et al., 2000; Vlahov et al., 1998). Abuse is a factor to be considered in HIV transmission if women are the victims of rape or as a consequence of their refusal to practice unsafe sexual behaviors. After disclosure, violence continues to be a fear and issue for many women, particularly for those women with a history of abuse. Liebschutz and colleagues (2000) reported episodic and chronic disease, injuries, emergency room visits, and hospitalizations to be more likely in abused HIV-infected women than in women not abused. This increased disease and health care use can serve as a warning sign to clinicians to assess HIV-infected women for abuse and to make appropriate referrals to address inherent psychosocial issues of the women.

NURSING IMPLICATIONS

To ensure that all women receive the appropriate information and care necessary to prevent transmission, promote their health, and enhance their quality of life, nurses must recognize the special and unique challenges of HIV/AIDS for women. HIV primary prevention messages and programs need to reach all women, including adolescents, to equip them with the knowledge, skills, and strategies necessary to protect themselves from high-risk sexual behaviors or encounters.

Services and resources for HIV-infected women need to be available and easily accessed. Examples of the services and resources needed include family planning, drug treatment, legal services, and case management (Dole, 2003). Coordination of these services with clinical care is important. When scheduling appointments for women, health care providers need to consider the child care responsibilities of women and either provide child care or work around children's schedules.

Thorough sexual and drug use histories in women are critical in assessing risk for HIV, prevention counseling, and making appropriate referrals. These histories provide nurses with opportunities to identify behaviors associated with HIV transmission, give patient-centered education that will help women protect themselves from all STIs, and determine the need for further counseling.

As HIV testing is expanded it is critical for health care systems to develop diagnosis protocols that include personnel trained in counseling and specific strategies to assist infected individuals' response to a diagnosis of HIV infection. These protocols need to include linkages to needed care, treatment, and support services (Stevens & Hildebrandt, 2006). Nurses are in key positions to ensure that the staffs of health care facilities understand the new recommendations and that they receive the skills, education, and resources necessary to address the patient's concerns and appropriate care (Burrage et al., 2008).

Contraceptive counseling is essential for all HIV-infected women of reproductive age. Nurses play a key role in guiding women to select the effective and appropriate contraception to prevent unintended pregnancy. They also need to be cognizant of the specialized treatment necessary for HIV-infected women during pregnancy. At this time, clinicians must consider ART for maternal infection and ART chemoprophylaxis to reduce the risk of perinatal HIV transmission.

CONCLUSION

Today women with HIV/AIDS are benefiting from ART and living healthier, longer lives. Prevention of HIV transmission in women continues to be a challenge as new programs and methods are developed. It is important for nurses to have current information and skills to be able to provide appropriate care to women with or at risk for HIV infection. Nurses also need to be aware of the unique needs of HIV-infected women. Research is still needed on women and HIV/AIDS. It is important that women be represented in clinical trial studies to ensure that findings address gender differences as well as similarities.

REFERENCES

Alliance for Microbicide Development. (2008). *Microbicide Pipeline.* Retrieved August 20, 2008, from www.microbicide.org/cs/microbicide-pipeline.

Anastos, K., Lu, D., Shi, O., Mulligan, K., Tien, P. C., Freeman, R., et al. (2007). The association of bone mineral density with HIV infection and antiretroviral treatment for women. *Antiviral Therapy, 12*(7), 1049–1058.

Burrage, J. W., Zimet, G. D., Cox, D. S., Cox, A. D., Mays, R. M., Fife, R. S., et al. (2008). The Center for Disease Control and Prevention Revised Recommendations for HIV testing: Reactions of women attending community health clinics. *Journal of the Association of Nurses in AIDS Care, 19*(1), 66–74.

Cates, W., & Rosenberg, Z. (2008). Vaginal microbicides: What does the future hold? *Contemporary OB/GYN, 22-4, 26, 22-28.* Available online at http://www.research4development.info/PDF/Outputs/Microbicides/Vaginal_Microbicides_What_does_the_future_hold_ZRosenberg_and_WCates_Apr2008.pdf

Centers for Disease Control and Prevention (CDC). (2006). Revised Recommendation for HIV testing of adults, adolescents and pregnant women in health-care settings. *Morbidity and Mortality Weekly Report, 15*(RR14:1–17).

Centers for Disease Control and Prevention (CDC). (2008). *HIV/AIDS among women.* Retrieved March 1, 2009, from www.cdc.gov/hiv/topics/women/resources/factsheets/pdf/women.pdf.

Centers for Disease Control and Prevention (CDC). (2009). *HIV/AIDS Surveillance Report: Cases of HIV infection and AIDS in the United States and dependent areas, 2007.* Retrieved March 12, 2009, from www.cdc.gov/HIV/topics/surveillance/resources/reports/2007report/pdf/2007SurveillanceReport.pdf.

Clark, H. J., Lindner, G., Armistead, L., & Austin, B. (2003). Stigma, disclosure and psychological functioning among HIV-infected and non-infected African American women. *Women & Health, 38*(40), 57–71.

Connor, E., Sperling, R., Gelber, R., Kiselev, P., Scott, G., O'Sullivan, M., et al. (1994). Reduction of maternal infant transmission of human immunodeficiency virus Type 1 with zidovudine treatment. *New England Journal of Medicine, 331,* 1173–1187.

Cooper, E. R., Charurat, M., Mofenson, L. M., Hanson, I. C., Pitt, J., Diaz, C., et al. (2002). Combination antiretroviral strategies for the treatment of pregnant HIV 1-infected women and prevention of perinatal HIV 1-transmission. *Journal of Acquired Immune Deficiency Syndromes (1999), 29*(5), 484–95.

Cotton, D., & Watts, D. H. (1997). *The medical mammogram of AIDS in women.* New York: Wiley-Liss.

Craft, S. M., Delaney, R. O., Bautista, D. T., & Serovich, J. M. (2007). Pregnancy decisions among women with HIV. *AIDS Behavior, 11,* 927–935.

Dole, P. (2003). Concerns of special populations: Women. In C. Kirton (Ed.), *ANAC's care curriculum for HIV/AIDS nursing* (2nd ed.) (pp. 229–233). Thousand Oaks, CA: Sage.

European Study Group on Heterosexual Transmission of HIV. (1992). Comparison of female-to-male and male-to-female transmission of HIV in 563 stable couples. *British Medical Journal, 304,* 809–813.

Feldblum, P. J., Kuyoh, M. A., Bwayo, J. J., Omari, M., Wong, E. L., Tweedy, K. G., et al. (2001). Female condom introduction and sexually transmitted prevalence results of a community intervention trial in Kenya. *AIDS, 15*(8), 1037–1044.

Fontanet, A.L., Saba, J. Chadelying, V., Sakondhavat, C., Bhiraleus, P., Rugpao, S., et al. (1998). Protection against sexually transmitted disease by granting sex workers in Thailand the choice of using the male or female condom: results from a randomized controlled trial. *AIDS, 12,* 1851–1859.

French, P., Latka, M., Gollub, E., Rogers, C., Hoover, D., & Stein, Z. (2003). Use-effectiveness of the female versus male condom in preventing sexually transmitted disease in women. *Sexually Transmitted Disease, 30,* 433–439.

Gielen, A. C., McDonnell, K. A., Burke, J. G., & O'Campo, P. O. (2000). Women's lives often an HIV-positive diagnosis: Disclosure and Violence. *Maternal and Child Health Journal, 4*(2). 111–120.

Global Campaign for Microbicides. (2006). *Clinical testing.* Retrieved September 20, 2006, from www.globalcampaign.org/clinical-testing. htm. Greene, K., Derlega, V. J., Yep, G. A., & Petronio, S. (2003). Privacy and disclosure in interpersonal relationships. Mahwah, NJ: Lawrence Erlbaum Associates.

Harlow, S. D., Schuman, P., Cohen, M., Ohmit, S. E., Cu-Uvin, S., Lin, X., et al. (2000). Effect of HIV infection on menstrual cycle length. *Journal of Acquired Immune Deficiency Syndromes, 24,* 68–75.

Harris, T. G., Burk, R. D., Palefsky, J. M., Massad, L. S., Bank, J. Y., Anastos, K., et al. (2005). Incidence of cervical lesions associated with HIV serostatus, CD cell counts, and human papilloma virus results. *Journal of the American Medical Association, 293* (T2), 1471–1476.

Highleyman, L. (2007). *Women and HIV.* Retrieved August 16, 2008, from www.nichd.nih.gov/research/supported/WIHS.CFM.

Holt, R., Court, P., Vedhara, L., Note, K. H., Holme, J., & Snow, M. H. (1998). The role of disclosure in coping with HIV infection. *AIDS Care, 10*(11), 49–61.

Ickovics, J. R., & Yoshikaw, H. (1998). Prevention intervention to reduce heterosexual risk for women. Current perspectives, future directions. *AIDS, 12,* 197–208.

International Partnership for Microbicides. (2008). *Microbicide Research and Development* (3rd ed.). Silver Spring, Maryland: Author. Available online at http://ipm-microbicides.org/pdfs/english/ipm_publications/2008/ipm_ib_rd_feb2008_20080328v4.pdf

Kline, A., Strickler, J., & Kempf, J. (1995). Factors associated with pregnancy and pregnancy resolution in HIV seropositive women. *Social Science Medicine, 40,* 1539–1547.

Kojic, E. M., & Cu-Uvin, S. (2007). Special care issues of women living with HIV/AIDS. In Naya, K. (Ed.) *Infectious disease clinics of North America, HIV AIDS.* Philadelphia: Saunders.

Levy, A., Laska, F., Abelhauser, A., Delfraissy, J. F., Gouiard, C., & Dormont, J. (1999). Disclosure of HIV seropositivity. *Journal of Clinical Psychology, 66,*(9), 1041–1049.

Liebschutz, J. M., Feinman, G., Sullivan, L., Stein, M., & Samet, J. (2000). Physical and sexual abuse in women infected with Human Immunodeficiency Virus: Increased illness and health care utilization. *Archives of Internal Medicine, 160,* 1659–1664.

Mantell, J. E., Myer, L., Carballo-Dièqiez, A., Stein, A., Ramjee, G., Morar, N. S., et al. (2005). Microbicide acceptability research: Current approaches and future directions. *Social Science and Medicine, 60*(20), 319–330.

Massad, L. S., Evans, C. T. Minkoff, H., Watts, D. H., Greenblatt, R. M., Levine, A. M., et al. (2006). Effects of HIV infection and its treatment on self-reported menstrual abnormalities in women. *Journal of Women's Health, 15*(5), 591–8.

Morrison, C. S., Sekadde-Kigondu, C. Sinei, S. K., Weiner, D. H., Kwok, C., & Kokonya, D. (2001). Is the intrauterine device appropriate contraception for HIV 1-infected women? BJOG: An International *Journal of Obstetrics and Gynaecology, 108*(8), 784–790.

Napierala, S., Kang, M., Chipato, T., Padian, N., & van der Straten, A. (2008). Female condom uptake and acceptability in Zimbabwe. *AIDS Education and Prevention, 20*(2), 121–134.

Padian, A. Buve, A., Balkus, J. Serwadda, D., & Cates, W. (2008). Biomedical intervention to prevent HIV infection: Evidence, challenges, and forward. *The Lancet, HIV Prevention,* 21–35.

Perez-Hoyos, S., Rodriguez-Arenas, A., De La Hara, M. G., Iribarren, J. A., Moreno, S., ViCiana, P., et al. (2007). Progression to AIDS and death and response to HAART in men and women from a multicenter hospital-based cohort. *Journal of Women's Health, 16*(7), 1052–1061.

Petra Study Team. (2002). Efficacy of three short-course regimens of zidovudine, lamivudine, in preventing early and late transmission of HIV-1 from mother to child in Tanzinia, South Africa, and Uganda (Petra study): A randomized, double-blind, placebo-controlled trial. *Lancet, 359,* 1178–1186.

Prins, M., Meyer., L., & Hessol, N. A. (2005). Sex and the course of HIV infection in the pre- and highly active antiretroviral therapy eras. *AIDS, 19*(4), 357–370.

Public Health Service Task Force. (2008). *Recommendations for use of antiretroviral drugs in pregnant HIV-infected women for material health and interventions to reduce perinatal HIV transmission in the*

United States. Retrieved August 18, 2008, from http://AIDSinfo.nih. gov.

Richardson, B. A., Otieno, P. A., Mbori-Ngacha, D., Overbaugh, J., Farquhar, C., & John-Stewart, G. C. (2007). Hormonal contraception and HIV-1 disease progression among postpartum Kenyan women. *AIDS, 21*(6), 749–753.

Sandelowski, M., Lambe, C., & Barroso, J. (2004). Stigma in HIV-positive women. *Journal of Nursing Scholarship, 36*(2), 122–128.

Sayles, J. N., Ryan, G. R., Silia, J. S. Sarkisian, C. A., & Cunningham, W. E. (2007). Experience of social stigma and implications for healthcare among a diverse population of HIV positive adults. *Journal of Urban Health: Bulletin of the New York Academy of Medicine,* (84), 814–828.

Simon, V., Ho, D. D., & Karim, Q. A. (2006). HIV/AIDS epidemiology, pathogensis, prevention, and treatment. *Lancet, 368,* 489–504.

Status report of the female condom: What will increase use in the U.S.? (2008, February). *Contraceptive Technology Update, 29*(2), 13–24.

Stevens, P. E., & Hildebrandt, E. (2006). Life changing words: Women's responses to being diagnosed with HIV infection. *Advance in Nursing Science, 29*(3), 207–221.

Tia, J. H., Udoji, M. A., Barkanic, G., Byrne, D. W., Rebiero, P. F., Byram, B. R., et al. (2007). Pregnancy and HIV progression during the era of highly active anti retrovial therapy. *Journal of Infectious Diseases, 196,* 1044–1052.

Turmen, T. (2003). Gender and HIV/AIDS. *International Journal of Gynecology and Obstetrics, 82,* 411–418.

UNAIDS. (2008). *Report on the global AIDS epidemic.* Geneva: Author.

Van Damme, L., Ramjee, G., Alary, M., Vuylsteke, B., Chandeying, V., Rees, H., et al. (2002). Effectiveness of COL-1492. A nonoxynol-9 vaginal gel, on HIV-1 transmission in female sex workers: a randomized, controlled trial. *Lancet, 300,* 962–964.

Vetter, K. M., & Geller, S. E. (2007). Moving forward: Human papillomavirus vaccination and the prevention of cervical cancer. *Journal of Women's Health, 16*(9), 1258–1268.

Vijayakumar, G., Mabude, Z. Smit, J., Beksinska, M., & Lurie, M. (2006). A review of female condom effectiveness: Patterns of use and impact on protected sex acts and STI incidence. *International Journal of STD and AIDS, 17:* 652–659. (2001).

Vlahov, D., Wientge, D. Moore, J., Flynn, C. Shuman, P. Schoenbaum, F., et al. (1998). Violence among women with or at risk of HIV infection. *AIDS Behavior, 2,* 53.

Voelker, R. (2006). Anti-HIV microbicide efforts press on. *Medical News and Perspectives, 296,* 735, 755.

Warszawski, J., Tubiana, R., Chenadec, J., Blanche, S., Teglas, J. P., Dollfus, C., et al. (2008). Mother to child transmission despite antiretroviral therapy in the ANRS French perinatal cohort. *AIDS, 22*(2) 289–299.

Wesley, Y. (2003). Desire for children among black women with and without HIV infection. Journal of Nursing Scholarship, 35(1), 37–43.

Wingood, G. M., & DiClemente, R. J. (1996). HIV sexual risk reduction for women. A Review. *American Journal of Preventive Medicine, 12,* 209–217.

Yang, H., Li, X., Stanton, B., Fang, X., Lin, D., & Naar-King, S. (2006). HIV-related knowledge, stigma, and willingness to disclose: A mediation analysis. *AIDS Care, 18*(7), 717–724.

14 Children and HIV Prevention and Management

MARY G. BOLAND
DEBORAH S. STORM

CHILDREN AND HIV PREVENTION AND MANAGEMENT

HIV infection affects children throughout the world and is a chronic, treatable, but not curable condition. Prevention of mother-to-child transmission (PMTCT) interventions and use of highly active antiretroviral therapy (HAART) are effective in reducing transmission and mortality among children and adolescents infected with HIV. With improved survival, follow-up care is necessary to monitor adverse events associated with the prolonged use of HAART and to address the long-term effects of therapy on immune function, growth, sexual maturation, and quality-of-life parameters. In low-resource settings, the growing numbers of infected children add to the cumulative burden of family disease across multiple generations. This chapter will focus on the nursing care of children living with HIV infection, recognizing that nurses play a significant role both in providing individual patient care and in creating health care delivery systems. Regardless of context and resources available, the goal remains the same—providing competent, evidence-based care to the child within a family-focused and community-centered model. This chapter will provide an overview of current knowledge and understanding related to the comprehensive management of HIV disease in children. We review the history of three decades of HIV disease in children; address prevention, care, and treatment in high- and low-resource settings; present principles and guidelines for antiretroviral therapy; and provide evidence-based recommendations to guide the nurse caring for the child and family.

THREE DECADES OF HIV DISEASE IN CHILDREN

The recognition of the global transmission of HIV infection focused attention on both women and children. The initial reports of AIDS in children in the United States were followed closely by the understanding that transmission from mother to child accounted for the majority (92%) of cases (CDC, 2004). To prevent new infections, it was critical to prevent or interrupt transmission from mother to child. For infants and children infected perinatally, the goal was to develop therapeutic strategies that suppress viral replication, preserve immune function, and reduce development of viral resistance. Over the past 25 years, there have been dramatic advances in the scientific understanding of disease transmission, virus behavior, and use of antiretroviral drug therapy. While combination antiretroviral therapy is effective in reducing viral load and in maintaining and improving immune function, HIV/AIDS is still incurable, and drug treatment confers a range of risks. Nevertheless, the significant reduction in mortality has made antiretroviral therapy an essential part of the treatment for all HIV-infected individuals world-wide, including children (Working Group on Antiretroviral Therapy and Medical Management of HIV-Infected Children, 2008).

Even though antiretroviral therapy prolongs and improves the lives of HIV-infected children, the number of new infections in children around the world continues to increase (UNAIDS, 2008). HIV-infected infants and children currently face the prospect of lifelong treatment with combination antiretroviral drug regimens, medications for prevention of opportunistic infections, and therapies to manage symptoms of HIV infection and complications of its treatment. Long-term follow-up of HIV-infected infants, children, and youth who have received antiretroviral therapy remains a critical priority and challenge to the worldwide effort to control HIV infection and prolong progression to AIDS. Access to such treatment and long-term monitoring also remain major challenges in many parts of the world.

With the detection of HIV, followed quickly with the ability to test and screen blood by the late 1980s, the majority of subsequent cases of HIV infection in children reflected maternal-to-child transmission. Such transmission occurring during pregnancy, labor and delivery, or breast feeding is referred to as perinatal or "mother-to-child" transmission. In 1987, the U.S. Surgeon General convened a cross-disciplinary group of clinicians and scientists to discuss the rapidly emerging numbers of infected children. This group addressed the call for action and set the national agenda that guided efforts relative to HIV-infected children for the next decade (U.S. Public Health Service, 1987). Federal funding for research and care soon followed this meeting. At a time when national advocacy efforts increased for the U.S. government to assist stigmatized populations affected by HIV, women and children represented a small number of infections. However, the pediatric medical and nursing communities came together to provide the voice and advocacy necessary to obtain the resources needed to address the rapidly increasing numbers of new infections in women and children. In 1987, the Health Resources Services Administration (HRSA) provided funding for pediatric AIDS demonstration projects. This effort created a national network of programs that evolved into a model for comprehensive interdisciplinary care that was both family focused and community based. Up to this time, the health care delivery model, including that of nursing, was symptom driven and individual focused. While children's hospitals were moving to a family-friendly model, providing access to services across a continuum of care that included case management was not commonplace. Following passage of the 1990 Ryan White Comprehensive AIDS Resources Emergency Act, continuing funding for pediatric care was supported. Concurrently, researchers were working intensely to understand transmission of the virus with the hope of finding a drug or regimen that could prevent transmission and treat the infection. Throughout this first decade of the HIV epidemic, nursing care focused on preventing and treating complications, assuring continuity of care across acute and community settings, and providing palliative care.

The National Institute of Allergy and Infectious Disease (NIAID) at the National Institutes of Health (NIH) created the AIDS Clinical Trials Group to address the emergence of HIV/AIDS. This national network of units was charged to develop and conduct clinical trials to determine medical treatment for HIV/AIDS. The pediatric arm, the Pediatric AIDS Clinical Trials Group (PACTG), focused initial efforts on use of zidovudine as a vehicle to interrupt transmission. Without antiretroviral intervention, 25% of pregnant infected women will transmit HIV to their infant (Lindegren et al., 1999). The Pediatric AIDS Clinical Trial Group Protocol 076 (ACTG 076) is a complex protocol that required administration of zidovudine to the mother during late pregnancy and intravenously during childbirth, along with oral treatment of the neonate at birth and for 6 weeks. This study demonstrated that zidovudine significantly reduced the risk of HIV transmission to the neonate (Connor et al., 1994). The CDC launched a national effort to provide access to HIV counseling and testing to all pregnant women. Within a few years, the U.S. perinatal transmission rate decreased significantly (CDC, 2006). Subsequent protocols with newer agents and the widespread use of antiretroviral treatment for women have decreased the U.S. perinatal transmission rate to 2% (Public Health Service Task Force [PHS], 2008). By October 2007, the CDC noted that approximately 100 to 200 infants in the United States are infected annually (CDC, 2007a). Lack of awareness of HIV serostatus and uneven HIV testing rates (in large part due to lack of prenatal care) account for the small but continuing number of new infant infections (CDC, 2007a).

The Working Group on Antiretroviral Therapy and Medical Management of HIV-Infected Children (2008) created an evidence-based process to develop guidelines for the use of HAART in pediatric HIV infection. The continuously updated guidelines, along with resources for HIV/AIDS treatment and clinical trials, are available through AIDSinfo at www.aidsinfo.nih.gov. In the United States and Western Europe, the rapid translation of research findings from bench to bedside and community has resulted in dramatic decreases in the perinatal transmission rate, effectively preventing disease in children born to infected women (McKenna & Hu, 2007). National efforts focusing on translation of findings into treatment and care guidelines have transformed patient management. In the United States, HIV mortality in children has decreased 80 to 90% since the introduction of HAART regimens that include protease inhibitors. This improvement in the treatment of HIV infection in children has created the opportunity to transform HIV infection into a chronic and manageable infection with prolonged survival and improved quality of life.

The CDC (2007b) reports an estimated 6,051 persons infected perinatally were living with HIV/AIDS in the United States at the end of 2005. An estimated 115 new HIV/AIDS cases were attributable to perinatal transmission in 2006 (CDC, 2008a). Today, increased survival of children is associated with access to treatment, adherence to medical regimens, and management of the toxicity and complications of antiretroviral therapy. The nursing competencies needed in the first decade, when much care was provided in the acute setting, required skills to manage the opportunistic infections, multiorgan system failure, and palliation of chronic infection. Today the nurse's ability to succeed in supporting adherence, sustaining access to HAART, and providing social support are critical to maintaining the gains of the second decade.

The underlying social and economic disparities that create the vulnerability to HIV infection in women and young teens still exist. Creating and delivering effective interventions to families struggling with multiple stresses continues to challenge nursing. The present Ryan White HIV/AIDS Treatment Modernization Act of 2006 provides funds for the care of women, infants, children, and youth though Part D (formerly Title IV). The act requires grantees "to provide care, treatment, and support services or create a network of medical and social service providers, who collaborate to supply services. In addition, grantees are to educate clients about research and research opportunities and inform all clients about the benefits of participation, and how to enroll in research" (HRSA, 2008, p. 1). These grantees, in cooperation with the restructured NIAID HIV/AIDS research networks, are the focal points for HIV prevention and treatment within the United States. Pregnant women and children can participate in studies within the International Maternal-Pediatric-Adolescent AIDS Clinical Trials (IMPAACT) network (http://pactg.s-3.com/), which resulted from the merger of the PACTG with the Perinatal Scientific Working Group of the HIV Prevention Trials Network (HPTN).

The aging of the population of children living with HIV/AIDS in the United States presents continuing and new challenges for nursing care. Both individual care delivery and care models were originally designed to support families with life-threatening illness. Child-rearing families and their health care providers were focused on addressing day-to-day concerns. The rapid and effective scale up of HAART has resulted in an unanticipated plunge in mortality. Families and children who once faced a grim prognosis now have to plan for a future. In this respect, they have much in common with survivors of other chronic childhood conditions. Areas of self-management of treatment, sexuality, reproduction, education, and employment must be addressed.

Low-Resource Settings

The success of PMTCT efforts in the United States has yet to be realized in the developing world (Little, Bland, & Newell, 2008). Of the nearly 33.2 million people estimated to be living with HIV infection worldwide at the end of 2007, UNAIDS estimates that children compose 2.5 million of this population (U.N. Children's Fund [UNICEF] & WHO, 2008). Of these, 2 million live in sub-Saharan Africa and acquired HIV from their mothers during pregnancy, birth, or breastfeeding. The proven PMTCT interventions that demonstrated success in the United States are not easily implemented in countries lacking the system, human, and fiscal resources required for scale-up of prevention and treatment efforts. In recognition of the need for a global response, several public and private efforts are underway. WHO, the Global Fund, and the President's Emergency Plan for AIDS Relief (PEPFAR) are all committed to decreasing new infection and increasing access to life-saving treatment. Private efforts by the Elizabeth Glaser Pediatric AIDS Foundation, the Clinton Foundation, the Gates Foundation, and others are focusing on specific areas of need. The UNAIDS Report on the Global AIDS Epidemic (UNAIDS, 2008, p. 3) documents:

> . . . considerable progress in many countries in addressing their national epidemics. A six fold increase in financing for HIV programmes in low- and middle-income countries from 2001–2007 is beginning to bear fruit, as gains in lowering the number of AIDS deaths and preventing new infections are apparent in many countries. Progress remains uneven, however, and the epidemic's future is still uncertain, underscoring the need for intensified action to move towards universal access to HIV prevention, treatment, care and support.

Ginsburg and colleagues (2007) reported that the Glaser Foundation efforts had reached 1 million pregnant women with counseling and testing. Of the 10% of women who tested seropositive for HIV, 81,000 received antiretroviral prophylaxis. In this group, 52,000 of the HIV-exposed infants received antiretroviral prophylaxis, and 9,000 infants received opportunistic infection prophylaxis at 6 weeks of age. Early PMTCT programs focused on finding effective strategies to deliver interventions to pregnant women. In many countries, these programs evolved as separate efforts from maternal child health and adult HIV programs. Funders are now seeking to integrate these efforts and ensure that women and children receive access to the full package of care, treatment, and support services. Preexisting resource constraints will continue to impact scaling up of efforts. In particular, the lack of nurses and other health care workers limits delivery of services (Holzemer, 2008).

While progress is occurring, the number of new pediatric infections in 2007 was estimated at 420,000. WHO has noted, however, that low- and middle-income countries are making progress in building capacity to provide care, support, and treatment for children. At the close of 2006, more than 125,000 children were receiving treatment in contrast to 75,000 in 2005. Participants at the 2008 International AIDS Conference in Mexico City complained that the global response has "shortchanged children" (International AIDS Society, 2008). Speakers noted that both infected and affected children require physiological and nutritional support—and that need is critical in those communities severely impacted by HIV.

PREVENTION OF MOTHER-TO-CHILD TRANSMISSION OF HIV INFECTION (PMTCT)

New cases of pediatric HIV infection in the United States are often the result of missed opportunities and barriers to prevention, such as lack of prenatal care or mothers becoming infected during pregnancy. The elimination of pediatric HIV infection requires understanding of the chain of events leading to an infected child in conjunction with the implementation of a continuum of prevention interventions. These range from provider-initiated HIV testing as part of the health care for women of reproductive age to the specialized care of pregnant women, women with HIV infection, and HIV-exposed infants. Nurses play a key role in these interventions, including taking roles to champion changes in their institutions that are needed to translate emerging research and updated guidelines into practice, e.g., implementation of rapid testing in labor and delivery (Burr et al., 2007).

Maternal Diagnosis

Maternal HIV diagnosis is the focal point of perinatal HIV prevention. The CDC recommends universal prenatal testing using the opt-out approach, whereby women are informed that HIV testing is part of routine prenatal care and given the opportunity to decline (i.e., "opt out") (CDC, 2006). Specific testing requirements, including requirements for pretest counseling, written informed consent, and mandatory newborn testing if the mother's HIV status is unknown, vary by state. Some states are modifying testing legislation in response to evidence supporting the opt-out approach to prenatal testing and other advances, including rapid testing in labor and delivery and third trimester retesting. Information about legislation or regulations governing practices related to HIV testing is available through state departments of health, and summary information about all states is available on-line through the National HIV/AIDS Clinicians' Consultation Center (www.nccc.ucsf.edu/StateLaws/Index.html) (State HIV Testing Laws Compendium, 2008).

Antiretroviral Prophylaxis and Treatment for PMTCT

PMTCT interventions include antiretroviral prophylaxis or treatment of women during pregnancy (i.e., intrapartum zidovudine and zidovudine chemoprophylaxis for the newborn) (PHS Task Force, 2008). Three-drug, highly active antiretroviral treatment (HAART) regimens are recommended for pregnant women with HIV infection who meet standard criteria for initiating HIV treatment and for antiretroviral prophylaxis in women who have not met indicators for ongoing HIV treatment. Issues regarding a drug's use in pregnancy, risk of teratogenicity, and future treatment needs (for women receiving antiretroviral prophylaxis regimens) are considerations when caring for pregnant women and their infants. Based on substantial evidence of effectiveness for PMTCT and safety, zidovudine is included whenever possible. Use of efavirenz, a drug with known teratogenic effects, is avoided, particularly in the first trimester. For detailed discussion and information about antiretroviral therapy for women, refer to Chapter 13.

National guidelines (Working Group on Antiretroviral Therapy and Medical Management of HIV-Infected Children, 2008) recommend that all HIV-exposed infants receive a six-week course of zidovudine chemoprophylaxis, beginning within 6 to 12 hours of birth. The standard zidovudine dose of 2 mg/kg every 6 hours is appropriate for infants with a gestational age of at least 35 weeks. Although data are limited and there is no definitive evidence related to equivalent efficacy for PMTCT, national guidelines suggest that it may be appropriate to double the dose and give zidovudine at 12-hour intervals when adherence is a significant concern. Zidovudine dosing should be adjusted for premature infants of less than 35 weeks gestation. These infants should receive 2 mg/kg orally every 12 hours or 1.5 mg/kg intravenously every 12 hours. Experts may recommend additional antiretroviral drugs as part of the infant prophylactic regimen based on maternal history and receipt of antiretroviral drugs, but additional drugs are not recommended for premature infants.

HIV Diagnosis in Infants and Children

A positive HIV immunoglobulin G (IgG) antibody test, with confirmatory Western blot, is used to diagnose HIV infection in children 18 months of age and older. Due to the presence of maternal HIV antibodies, virologic testing is required to definitively diagnose HIV infection in infants and young children less than 18 months of age. Polymerase chain reaction (PCR) HIV, DNA, and RNA assays are the preferred virologic tests. National guidelines recommend diagnostic testing of HIV-exposed infants at ages 14 to 21 days, 1 to 2 months and 4 to 6 months, with positive test results confirmed by repeat testing as soon as possible (Working Group on Antiretroviral Therapy and Medical Management of HIV-Infected Children, 2008). For non–breastfed infants, HIV infection can be diagnosed in most infants by age 1 month and virtually all infants by age 4 months. To definitively exclude HIV infection, children with negative tests at 14 to 21 days and 1 to 2 months require repeat testing and a negative virologic test at age 4 to 6 months. The 2008 revised surveillance case definitions for HIV infection and AIDS now require laboratory-confirmed evidence of HIV infection for children 18 months and older and have made changes in the case definition for presumptively uninfected in children less than 18 months (CDC, 2008b). Due to the complexity of HIV diagnosis in children less than 18 months of age, children with AIDS-defining conditions born to mothers with laboratory-confirmed HIV infection may be classified as presumptively HIV infected. Details of surveillance case definitions diagnosis or exclusion of HIV infection in children are available at www.cdc.gov/mmwr/PDF/rr/rr5710.pdf.

HIV DNA and RNA assays are highly sensitive for HIV subtype B, which is the predominant HIV subtype in the United States, but are less sensitive to non–subtype B viruses that predominate in other parts of the world, i.e., subtype C in parts of Africa and India and subtype E in much of Southeast Asia (Working Group on Antiretroviral Therapy and Medical Management of HIV-Infected Children, 2008). It is important to be alert to the potential for a false-negative HIV DNA PCR test in children whose mothers may be infected with a non–subtype B virus.

Levels of maternal HIV antibodies acquired by transplacental transfer decrease over time; many HIV-exposed, uninfected infants will test HIV antibody negative by age 6 months. By age 12 months, most children will have cleared maternal antibodies, although it may take until 15 to 18 months of age for some children. HIV antibody testing can be used to exclude HIV infection in HIV-exposed, non-breastfeeding children 6 months of age and older. Two negative antibody tests in the absence of any clinical, virologic, or laboratory indicators of HIV provide clear evidence the child is not HIV infected. At age 12 to18 months, HIV antibody testing is used to document seroconversion of HIV-exposed infants with negative virologic tests.

Supporting the Family

Successful referral and linkages to specialized care for HIV-exposed infants are essential for effective HIV screening and early diagnosis with appropriate care and follow-up. Clinical programs with Ryan White Part D funding focus on the care of women, children, and families and serve as information resources for pediatric providers in the general community. Established linkages between pediatric and obstetric care providers help to support outreach to women with HIV infection during pregnancy or immediately after delivery, assuring continued access to services and reducing loss to follow-up.

The HIV-infected childbearing woman and her family require support as they cope during the infant diagnostic period. The prolonged period of time after birth before an HIV diagnosis can be ruled out contributes to maternal and family stress. The expected concerns related to parenting, increased financial responsibilities, and physical fatigue are present. At the same time, the woman is responsible for administering prophylactic medication to her infant, adhering to her own treatment regimen, and making and keeping medical appointments for herself and the infant. Shannon, Kennedy and Humphreys (2008) reported that maternal concerns showed a temporal pattern in association with infant testing and obtaining results. Infant infection was a continuous concern expressed by mothers, and only when an HIV diagnosis was excluded did mothers' concern shift to nonhealth areas. In addition to maintaining family stability and financial insecurity, women worried about inadvertent disclosure of diagnosis. In spite of the normalization of HIV in media and through advocacy efforts, concern about stigma continues to shadow those living with infection. (See Chapter 11.)

Early follow-up care for HIV-exposed infants includes management and adherence support for antiretroviral prophylaxis, screening for clinical or laboratory indicators of HIV infection, and initiating trimethoprim sulfamethoxazole (TMP/SMX) for prophylaxis of *Pneumocystis jiroveci* (formerly *carinii*) pneumonia after antiretroviral prophylaxis is complete until HIV infection is definitely excluded. Because zidovudine may cause anemia, hematologic monitoring is often performed. In cases of severe anemia, infants may be monitored as frequently as twice a week to continue zidovudine as long as possible. Anemia must be profound for zidovudine to be discontinued prematurely.

Low-Resource Settings

As discussed earlier, the widespread recognition of the impacts of the disease on global health are bringing about mobilization efforts funded by public donor agencies and private foundations. At the core of such low-resource setting effort is the ability to provide simple, effective interventions in an organized package of services. Testing and intervention schedules will differ from those of high-resource settings. With consultation, each country develops its national program guidelines based on its burden of disease, access to resources, and ability to deliver the interventions. Chapter 13 covers primary prevention of HIV infection in women. WHO-recommended PMTCT interventions are found in Table 14.1 (WHO, Department of HIV/AIDS, 2007).

Breastfeeding is the most common and supported infant feeding practice regardless of resource setting. However, HIV is present in human milk and can be transmitted with rates varying from 10 to 20% depending on duration and other risk factors (De Cock et al., 2000). While formula feeding avoids the risks associated with breastfeeding transmission, the risk of HIV infection needs to be balanced with the risk of replacement feeding, such as increased infant morbidity and mortality (Coutsoudis, Coovadia, & Wilfert, 2008). In resource-limited settings, U.N. guidance currently recommends exclusive breastfeeding for six months for children born to HIV-infected mothers unless replacement feeding is acceptable, feasible, affordable, sustainable, and safe before that time (WHO, 2007a). Mothers need support to practice exclusive breastfeeding effectively. Mixed breastfeeding is common and has been associated with higher rates of transmission. A recent study in KwaZulu Natal, South Africa, estimated a transmission rate of about 4% by age 6 months in exclusively breastfed infants who were HIV negative at 6 weeks of age. The rate of transmission was doubled in infants who received both formula and breast milk and was elevenfold higher in those who also received solids (Coovadia et al., 2007). Clinical trials are ongoing to evaluate interventions to make breastfeeding safer by preventing transmission including

Table 14.1

PMTCT INTERVENTIONS WITHIN THE CONTEXT OF A COMPREHENSIVE APPROACH
CORE

ELEMENT	KEY ACTIVITIES TO BE CONSIDERED	
Primary prevention of HIV infection among women, especially young women	• Health information and education • HIV testing and counseling—regular retesting for those with exposure • Couple counseling and partner testing • Safer-sex practices, including dual protection (condom promotion) • Delay of onset of sexual activity • Behavioral change communications to avoid high-risk behavior	
Prevention of unintended pregnancies among HIV-infected women	• Family planning (FP) counseling and services to ensure women can make informed decisions about their reproductive health • HIV testing and counseling in Reproductive health/FP services • Safer-sex practices, including dual protection (condom promotion)	
Provision of appropriate treatment, care, and support to HIV-infected mothers, their infants, and family	Package of services for mothers • Antiretroviral treatment for eligible women • Co-trimoxazole prophylaxis • Continued infant feeding counseling and support • Nutritional counseling and support • Sexual and reproductive health services, including FP • Psychosocial support	Package of services for HIV-exposed children • Antiretroviral prophylaxis • Routine immunization and growth monitoring and support • Co-trimoxazole prophylaxis starting at 6 weeks • Early diagnosis testing for HIV infection at 6 weeks where virological tests are available • Continued infant feeding counseling and support • Screening and management of tuberculosis • Prevention and treatment of malaria • Nutrition care and support • Psychosocial care and support • Antiretroviral therapy for eligible HIV-infected children • Symptom management and palliative care if needed

Source: World Health Organization (WHO). (2007). Prevention of mother-to-child transmission (PMTCT) briefing note [Electronic Version]. Retrieved October 8, 2008, from www.who.int/hiv/pub/toolkits/PMTCT%20HIV%20Dept%20brief%20Oct%2007.pdf.

use of vaccines, combining immune prophylaxis with short duration anti-retroviral prophylaxis. Researchers have called for review of the present UNICEF, WHO, and UNAIDS feeding guidelines based on documented increased morbidity and mortality with mixed feeding and emerging data about exclusive breastfeeding (Coovadia et al., 2007).

To address the complexities of PMTCT in settings with varying resource capacities, WHO and CDC partnered with the François-Xavier Bagnoud Center, School of Nursing, University of Medicine and Dentistry of New Jersey, to develop the PMTCT Generic Training Package (GTP), first completed in 2004 and updated in 2008. The GTP is a comprehensive, evidence-based course developed for PMTCT program implementation in resource-limited settings. It is designed to be adapted at the country or regional level to meet participant learning needs and to reflect national policy and local context. The process of adapting the curriculum for country use facilitates stakeholder input and provides a context for reviewing existing materials (policies, procedures, and curricula) in light of current science and evidence-based practice. The GTP also provides a framework for updating existing policy, developing materials where needed and considering the implications of implementing PMTCT services in a range of clinical settings. The package is available at www.womenchildrenhiv.org.

CDC REVISED SURVEILLANCE AND CLASSIFICATION SYSTEM FOR HIV IN CHILDREN LESS THAN 13 YEARS OF AGE

The 1994 revised classification system for HIV in children less than 13 years of age (see Tables 14.2 and 14.3) shows the similarities and differences in immunologic and clinical manifestations of the disease compared to adults (CDC, 1994). Infants have high levels of CD4 T-lymphocytes. Normal, age-related declines in CD4 number occur most rapidly during the first year of life, with levels comparable to adults achieved after age 5 years (see Table 14.2). For this reason, CD4 percentage is most often used for monitoring HIV disease progression in children. The clinical categories of the pediatric classification of HIV infection in children reflect the problems commonly seen in children, such as recurrent bacterial infections, failure to thrive, and encephalopathy. Problems such as Kaposi's sarcoma or lymphoma, seen commonly in adults, are rare in children. HAART slows the expected disease progression to category

Table 14.2

1994 REVISED HIV PEDIATRIC CLASSIFICATION SYSTEM: IMMUNOLOGIC CATEGORIES BASED ON AGE-SPECIFIC CD4+ T-LYMPHOCYTE COUNTS AND PERCENTAGE OF TOTAL LYMPHOCYTES

	AGE OF CHILD					
	<12 MOS		1–5 YRS		6–12 YRS	
IMMUNOLOGIC CATEGORY	NO./µL	(%)	NO./µL	(%)	NO./µL	(%)
Category 1: No evidence of suppression	≥ 1,500	(≥ 25%)	≥ 1,000	(≥ 25%)	≥ 500	(≥ 25%)
Category 2: Evidence of moderate suppression	750–1,499	(15–24)	500–999	(15–24)	200–499	(15–24)
Category 3: Severe suppression	< 750	(< 15%)	< 500	(< 15%)	< 200	(< 15%)

Source: Centers for Disease Control and Prevention (CDC) (1994). Revised classification system for human immunodeficiency virus infection in children less than 13 years of age. *MMWR*, 1994. 43 (No. RR-12): p. 1–10. Available at www.cdc.gov/mmwr/preview/mmwrhtml/00032890.htm.

Table 14.3

1994 REVISED HIV PEDIATRIC CLASSIFICATION SYSTEM: CLINICAL CATEGORIES

Category N: Not Symptomatic
Children who have no signs or symptoms considered to be the result of HIV infection or who have only one of the conditions listed in category A.

Category A: Mildly Symptomatic
Children with two or more of the following conditions but none of the conditions listed in category C:
• Lymphadenopathy (≥0.5 cm at more than two sites; bilateral = one site)
• Hepatomegaly
• Splenomegaly
• Dermatitis
• Parotitis
• Recurrent or persistent upper respiratory infection, sinusitis, or otitis media

Table 14.3

1994 REVISED HIV PEDIATRIC CLASSIFICATION SYSTEM: CLINICAL CATEGORIES *continued*

Category B: Moderately Symptomatic

Children who have symptomatic conditions, other than those listed for category A or category C, that are attributed to HIV infection. Examples of conditions in clinical category B include, but are not limited to, the following:

- Anemia (<8 gm/dL), neutropenia (<1,000 cells/mm³), or thrombocytopenia (<100,000 cells/mm³) persisting ≥30 days
- Bacterial meningitis, pneumonia, or sepsis (single episode)
- Candidiasis, oropharyngeal (i.e., thrush) persisting for >2 months in children aged >6 months
- Cardiomyopathy
- Cytomegalovirus infection with onset before age 1 month
- Diarrhea, recurrent or chronic
- Hepatitis
- Herpes simplex virus (HSV) stomatitis, recurrent (i.e., more than two episodes within 1 year)
- HSV bronchitis, pneumonitis, or esophagitis with onset before age 1 month
- Herpes zoster (i.e., shingles) involving at least two distinct episodes or more than one dermatome
- Leiomyosarcoma
- Lymphoid interstitial pneumonia (LIP) or pulmonary lymphoid hyperplasia complex
- Nephropathy
- Nocardiosis
- Fever lasting >1 month
- Toxoplasmosis with onset before age 1 month
- Varicella, disseminated (i.e., complicated chickenpox)

Category C: Severely Symptomatic

Children who have any condition listed in the 1987 surveillance case definition for acquired immunodeficiency syndrome, with the exception of LIP (which is a category B condition):

- Serious bacterial infections, multiple or recurrent (i.e., any combination of at least two culture-confirmed infections within a 2-year period), of the following types: septicemia, pneumonia, meningitis, bone or joint infection, or abscess of an internal organ or body cavity (excluding otitis media, superficial skin or mucosal abscesses, and indwelling catheter-related infections)
- Candidiasis, esophageal or pulmonary (bronchi, trachea, lungs)
- Coccidioidomycosis, disseminated (at site other than or in addition to lungs or cervical or hilar lymph nodes)
- Cryptococcosis, extrapulmonary
- Cryptosporidiosis or isosporiasis with diarrhea persisting >1 month
- Cytomegalovirus disease with onset of symptoms at age >1 month (at a site other than liver, spleen, or lymph nodes)

(continued)

Table 14.3

**1994 REVISED HIV PEDIATRIC CLASSIFICATION SYSTEM:
CLINICAL CATEGORIES** *continued*

- Encephalopathy (at least one of the following progressive findings present for at least 2 months in the absence of a concurrent illness other than HIV infection that could explain the findings): (a) failure to attain or loss of developmental milestones or loss of intellectual ability, verified by standard developmental scale or neuropsychological tests; (b) impaired brain growth or acquired microcephaly demonstrated by head circumference measurements or brain atrophy demonstrated by computerized tomography or magnetic resonance imaging (serial imaging is required for children <2 years of age); (c) acquired symmetric motor deficit manifested by two or more of the following: paresis, pathologic reflexes, ataxia, or gait disturbance
- Herpes simplex virus infection causing a mucocutaneous ulcer that persists for >1 month; or bronchitis, pneumonitis, or esophagitis for any duration affecting a child >1 month of age
- Histoplasmosis, disseminated (at a site other than or in addition to lungs or cervical or hilar lymph nodes)
- Kaposi's sarcoma
- Lymphoma, primary, in brain
- Lymphoma, small, noncleaved cell (Burkitt), or immunoblastic or large-cell lymphoma of B-cell or unknown immunologic phenotype
- Mycobacterium tuberculosis, disseminated or extrapulmonary
- Mycobacterium, other species or unidentified species, disseminated (at a site other than or in addition to lungs, skin, or cervical or hilar lymph nodes)
- Mycobacterium avium complex or Mycobacterium kansasii, disseminated (at site other than or in addition to lungs, skin, or cervical or hilar lymph nodes)
- Pneumocystis jiroveci pneumonia
- Progressive multifocal leukoencephalopathy
- Salmonella (nontyphoid) septicemia, recurrent
- Toxoplasmosis of the brain with onset at >1 month of age
- Wasting syndrome in the absence of a concurrent illness other than HIV infection that could explain the following findings: (a) persistent weight loss >10% of baseline; *or* (b) downward crossing of at least two of the following percentile lines on the weight-for-age chart (e.g., 95th, 75th, 50th, 25th, 5th) in a child ≥1 year of age; *or* (c) <5th percentile on weight-for-height chart on two consecutive measurements, ≥30 days apart *plus* (1) chronic diarrhea (i.e., ≥ two loose stools per day for >30 days), *or* (2) documented fever (for ≥30 days, intermittent or constant)

Source: Centers for Disease Control and Prevention. (1994). 1994 Revised classification system for human immunodeficiency virus infection in children less than 13 years of age. *MMWR*, 1994. 43 (No. RR-12): p . 55-56 from Working Group on Antiretroviral Therapy and Medical Management of HIV-Infected Children. (2008a). Guidelines for the Use of Antiretroviral Agents in Pediatric HIV Infection July 29, 2008 [Electronic Version]. Retrieved July 7, 2008, from http://aidsinfo.nih.gov.

C or AIDS. Young children may have long periods of asymptomatic or mildly symptomatic illness, and even children who have had more severe clinical conditions (category B or C) have fewer acute illnesses and dramatically improved survival. The revised surveillance case definitions for HIV infection and AIDS released in 2008 did not alter the 1994 clinical and immunologic classifications for HIV infection in children under 13 years of age. However, children 18 months and older now require laboratory-confirmed evidence of HIV infection to meet criteria for AIDS (CDC, 2008b). The immature and developing immune system in infants and young children influences the initial presentation, clinical manifestations, and trajectory of illness in perinatally acquired HIV infection. Infants experience a higher peak HIV RNA level and a slower decline in HIV RNA levels after infection with HIV when compared to adults. The clinical categories of the 1994 Revised HIV Pediatric Classification Systems (see Table 14.3) highlight the nonspecific nature of frequent early symptoms of HIV infection in infants, such as fever, failure to thrive, hepatomegaly and splenomegaly, generalized lymphadenopathy, parotitis, and diarrhea. Prior to the advent of early, aggressive treatment with HAART, most infants (90%) would show one or more symptoms during the first year of life, and about 20% experienced a rapid, severe disease course with deterioration of immune function and/or development of an AIDS-defining condition (Brady, 2005). In contrast to adults, immunologic and virologic parameters are less predictive of clinical course in infants and children. There have been reports of infants under 1 year of age who developed *Pneumocystis* pneumonia (PCP) with a normal CD4 count (Brady, 2005). A recent study from South Africa documented a 75% reduction in mortality during the 6 months after enrollment when HAART was initiated prior to 12 weeks of age in perinatally infected infants who were asymptomatic with a normal CD4 percentage (>25%) rather than delaying treatment until specific clinical or immunological indicators of disease progression become evident (Violari et al., 2007).

ANTIRETROVIRAL THERAPY

In pediatric populations, antiretroviral therapy increases survival and reduces complications of HIV, including opportunistic infections; improves growth and neurocognitive function; and leads to better quality of life (Working Group on Antiretroviral Therapy and Medical Management of HIV-Infected Children, 2008). Guidelines for the use of antiretroviral agents in pediatric HIV infection are continuously updated based on new information and data. The U.S. Working Group on Antiretroviral Therapy and Medical Management of HIV-Infected Children is composed of clinicians, researchers, consumers, and government agencies. Their national guidelines are available on the AIDSinfo web site. Through this continuous review process, clinicians can have access to the most current findings and recommendations for initiation and management of antiretroviral therapy. Because these guidelines are targeted to high-resource settings, the WHO convenes a parallel process to make recommendations for mid- and low-resource settings. WHO uses a similar evidence-based process to guide deliberations, and the WHO Paediatric Antiretroviral Working Group reports are posted on its website. Both groups are challenged by the lack of available palatable drug formulations and pharmacokinetic information to guide drug dosing in the various age groups. Drug resistance can develop in both multidrug-experienced and older children whose initial treatment with one or two drug regimens led to incomplete virus suppression on initiation of HAART. Decisions about when to start therapy and what drugs to choose are complicated. Treatment is best directed and/or managed in consultation with a multidisciplinary team in an experienced pediatric HIV treatment program.

The U.S. Working Group recognizes that infants, children, and adolescents present particular issues related to therapy. The principles guiding their deliberations are found in Table 14.4. Highly active treatment regimens (HAART), including at least three drugs, are recommended. Antiretroviral drug resistance testing should be done before starting therapy in those children who are drug naïve.

Goals of treatment are similar to those for adults, including reduction of mortality and morbidity; restoring and preserving immune function; maximally and durably suppressing viral replication; minimizing drug related toxicity; and improving quality of life. In addition, treatment of infants and children must address maintaining normal physical growth and neurocognitive development. Choice of regimens must consider that treatment will be lifelong, requiring sequencing to preserve options due to failure to suppress virus, side effects, and toxicity.

Current recommendations call for initial therapy with two classes of drugs—nonnucleoside reverse transcriptase inhibitor (NNRTI) or protease inhibitor (PI)-based regimens consisting of one NNTRI in combination with a two-drug backbone of nucleoside or nucleotide reverse transcriptase inhibitors (NRTIs) or one or two PIs in combination with 2 NRTIs.

Table 14.4

UNIQUE CONSIDERATIONS FOR ANTIRETROVIRAL THERAPY FOR HIV-INFECTED INFANTS, CHILDREN, AND ADOLESCENTS

- Acquisition of infection through perinatal exposure for many infected children
- In utero, intrapartum, and/or postpartum neonatal exposure to zidovudine and other antiretroviral medications in most perinatally infected children
- Requirement for use of HIV virologic tests to diagnose perinatal HIV infection in infants under age 18 months
- Age-specific differences in CD4 cell counts
- Changes in pharmacokinetic parameters with age caused by the continuing development and maturation of organ systems involved in drug metabolism and clearance
- Differences in the clinical and virologic manifestations of perinatal HIV infection secondary to the occurrence of primary infection in growing, immunologically immature persons
- Special considerations associated with adherence to antiretroviral treatment for infants, children, and adolescents.

Source: Working Group on Antiretroviral Therapy and Medical Management of HIV-Infected Children. (2008). *Guidelines for the use of antiretroviral agents in pediatric HIV infection* February 28, 2008 (p. 1) [Electronic Version]. Retrieved July 7, 2009 from http://aidsinfo.nih.gov.

This approach spares three classes of drugs for second-line treatment. As of November 2008, efavirenz is the preferred NNTRI for children age 3 years and older, with nevirapine recommended for children under age 3 due to the availability of a liquid formulation. Nevirapine is considered an alternative NNRTI for children age 3 and older due to potential toxicity. Skin and hypersensitivity reactions have been reported in children, although hepatic toxicities associated with nevirapine use in adults have not been reported in prepubertal children. Lopinavir/ritonavir is the preferred PI for initial treatment. It is essential that clinicians refer to the web-based guidelines to remain up-to-date with changing recommendations based on emerging data, new drugs, and new formulations.

For treatment purposes, children are placed into three categories: children less than 12 months regardless of clinical status; children age 1 to less than 5 years; and children and adolescents greater than or equal to 5 years (Table 14.5). Using age, along with clinical (symptom) immune status (CD4 percentage or count) and virologic status (plasma HIV RNA) as criteria, treatment may be recommended, considered, or deferred. The

Table 14.5

INDICATIONS FOR INITIATION OF ANTIRETROVIRAL THERAPY IN CHILDREN INFECTED WITH HUMAN IMMUNODEFICIENCY VIRUS (HIV)*

AGE	CRITERIA	RECOMMENDATION
<12 Months	• Regardless of clinical symptoms, immune status, or viral load	*Treat*
1–<5 Years	• AIDS or significant HIV-related symptoms[1]	*Treat*
	• CD4 <25%, regardless of symptoms or HIV RNA level[2]	*Treat*
	• Asymptomatic or mild symptoms[3] *and* ■ CD4 ≥25% and ■ HIV RNA ≥ 100,000 copies/mL	*Consider*
	• Asymptomatic or mild symptoms[3] *and* ■ CD4 ≥25% *and* ■ HIV RNA <100,000 copies/mL	*Defer[4]*
≥5 Years	• AIDS or significant HIV-related symptoms[1]	*Treat*
	• CD4 <350 cells/mm³ [5]	*Treat*
	• Asymptomatic or mild symptoms[3] *and* ■ CD4≥ 350 cells/mm³ and ■ HIV RNA ≥ 100,00 copies/mL	*Consider*
	• Asymptomatic or mild symptoms[3] *and* ■ CD4 ≥ 350 cells/mm³ *and* ■ HIV RNA <100,00 copies/mL	*Defer[4]*

*This table provides general guidance rather than absolute recommendations for an individual patient. Factors to be considered in decisions about initiation of therapy include the risk of disease progression as determined by CD4 percentage or count and plasma HIV RNA copy number, the potential benefits and risks of therapy, and the ability of the caregiver to adhere to administration of the therapeutic regimen. Issues associated with adherence should be fully assessed, discussed, and addressed with the child, if age appropriate, and caregiver before the decision to initiate therapy is made.

[1]CDC Clinical Category C and B (except for the following Category B conditions: single episode of serious bacterial infection or lymphoid interstitial pneumonitis).

[2]The data supporting this recommendation are stronger for those with CD4 percentage <20% than for those with CD4 percentage between 20% and 24%.

[3]CDC Clinical Category A or N or the following Category B conditions: single episode of serious bacterial or interstitial pneumonitis.

[4]Clinical and laboratory data should be reevaluated every 3 to 4 months.

[5]The data supporting this recommendation are stronger for those with CD4 counts between 200 and 350 cells/mm³.

Source: Working Group on Antiretroviral Therapy and Medical Management of HIV-Infected Children (2008). *Guidelines for the Use of Antiretroviral Agents in Pediatric HIV Infection February 28, 2008* (p. 62) [Electronic Version], Retrieved July 7, 2008, from http://AIDSinfo.nih.gov.

guidelines provide evidence-based criteria to guide decision making, but each child and family requires an individualized approach. Adherence assessment is critical when considering treatment initiation.

Controversy is ongoing regarding when to initiate therapy in asymptomatic patients. Proponents of early therapy believe that it provides the best opportunity to control viral replication before mutation occurs, thereby preserving immune function and slowing clinical progression. Others believe that using clinical progression or immune suppression to begin therapy decreases the risk of drug-resistant viral evolution. The burden of treatment and ability to manage adherence is specific to each family and its circumstances. Keeping the therapy goals in mind can serve as common ground for provider–parent collaborative decision making on therapy. Once therapy begins, management consists of ongoing monitoring as described in Table 14.6.

HIV disease is more rapidly progressive in infants, and laboratory testing does not predict progression in infants less than 12 months of age (Dunn et al., 2008). CD4 percentage and HIV RNA are both independently predictive of progression with CD4 percentage a stronger predictor. Therapy is recommended for all infants under 12 months of age regardless of clinical status, CD4 percentage, or viral load. Clinicians need to recognize the hazards when using HAART in young infants. Potential problems include incomplete viral suppression, leading to development of resistance and compromise of future treatment options. Other potential problems include possible toxicities associated with HAART, including lipodystrophy, dyslipidemia, glucose intolerance, osteopenia, and mitochondrial dysfunction. Children with significant clinical AIDS or significant symptoms will benefit from treatment regardless of immunologic or virologic status. Guidelines are available to identify the most appropriate initial regimen for this group based on age and immune status.

Adherence to Antiretroviral Therapy

Drug therapy is the mainstay of management of HIV disease and treatment will be lifelong. Several studies have linked adherence with virologic outcomes of therapy in children and youth. In a long-term, observational follow-up study of 2,088 children and adolescents using three-day recall of missed doses, the median HIV RNA level was tenfold higher in those who had missed one or more doses compared to those with 100% adherence (Williams et al., 2006); most children (84%) had no missed doses. In an open-label trial of lopinavir/ritonavir-based therapy in 21 infants

Table 14.6

EXAMPLE OF MINIMUM SCHEDULE FOR MONITORING OF CHILDREN ON ANTIRETROVIRAL THERAPY

TIME AFTER STARTING THERAPY	TOXICITY MONITORING[1]	ADHERENCE AND EFFICACY MONITORING
Baseline (prior to initiation of therapy)	Clinical history, complete blood count and differential, chemistries[3]	CD4+ cell count/ percentage, IIIV RNA
1–2 weeks[2]	Clinical history	Adherence screen
4–8 weeks	Clinical history, complete blood count and differential, chemistries[3]	Adherence screen, CD4+ cell count/percentage. HIV RNA
Every 3–4 months	Clinical history, complete blood count and differential, chemistries[3]	Adherence screen, CD4+ cell count/percentage, HIV RNA
Every 6–12 months	Lipid Panel	

[1] For children receiving nevirapine, serum transaminase levels should be measured every 2 weeks for the first 4 weeks of therapy, then monthly for 3 months, followed by every 3 to 4 months.

[2] Children starting a new antiretroviral regimen should be evaluated in person or by a phone call within 1 to 2 weeks of starting medication to screen for clinical side effects and to assure that they are taking medication properly; many clinicians will plan additional contacts (in person or by telephone) with the child and caregivers to support adherence during the first few weeks of therapy.

[3] Chemistries may include electrolyses, glucose, liver function tests (hepatic transaminases and bilirubin), renal function tests (BUN, creatinine), calcium, and phosphate). Additional evaluations should be tailored to the particular drugs the child is receiving; for example, pancreatic enzymes (amylase and lipase) may be considered if the child is starting drugs with potential pancreatic toxicity, such as ddl.

Source: Working Group on Antiretroviral Therapy and Medical Management of HIV-Infected Children. (2008). *Guidelines for the Use of Antiretroviral Agents in Pediatric HIV Infection February 29, 2008* (p. 72) [Electronic Version]. Retrieved July 7, 2008, from http:// AIDSinfo.nih.gov.

6 weeks to 6 months of age, Chadwick and colleagues (2008) reported that suboptimal adherence was associated with delayed viral suppression in five infants. Intensive adherence training and support or change in caregiver resulted in achievement of viral suppression in all five infants. These findings point out the potential family impact of poor adherence and underscore the importance of effective adherence support and in-

tervention, particularly for families adjusting to a new diagnosis of HIV infection in their child.

Family assessment for ability to adhere to treatment begins when treatment is under consideration. Careful assessment and family education before initiating or changing antiretroviral therapy should be coupled with frequent contacts and monitoring immediately after starting therapy, decreasing in frequency over time. Effective adherence support requires obtaining a comprehensive baseline assessment, providing anticipatory guidance regarding daily medication administration, managing side effects or toxicities, and engaging parents or caregivers—and children when indicated—to track progress toward treatment goals, such as preserving or restoring CD4 count and achieving target HIV RNA levels. Anticipatory and ongoing guidance tailored for the developmental stage of the child and family context should address difficulties giving medication to children, developing a schedule with reminders, and side effects specific to the planned regimen because these issues are commonly reported causes of missed doses and interruptions in treatment. In addition, assessing strengths and difficulties experienced by mothers living with HIV infection related to their own adherence to therapy provides an opportunity for a family-centered approach with individualized adherence intervention prior to initiation of therapy in the child. Approaches to support adherence must be comprehensive and address issues related to the family, child, regimen, and relationships with health care providers, as described in the summary of strategies to improve adherence shown in Table 14.7.

Once treatment begins, ongoing assessment with monitoring is required to ensure that full benefit is achieved and viral suppression is maintained. Regular adherence assessment, integrated with monitoring for toxicities and treatment efficacy, facilitates early detection and management of problems. Regular adherence assessment is a central element of ongoing monitoring for all children. Even in families who have successfully managed antiretroviral medications, the potential for some nonadherence should be anticipated as the child grows and the family faces inevitable stresses. Negative life events in families have been associated with poor adherence (Mellins et al., 2004).

Although pediatric studies often show high rates of adherence, many have a limited time frame of assessment, do not assess issues such as timing of doses, or were done in the context of a clinical trial. In care settings, it can be helpful to begin with a standard assessment, such as recall of missed doses in the past three days or in the past month and to use an interactive approach to assess how and when medications are taken and supervised and to identify actual or potential barriers to adherence. Both the parent

Table 14.7

STRATEGIES TO IMPROVE ADHERENCE WITH ANTIRETROVIRAL MEDICATIONS (UPDATED OCTOBER 26, 2006)

INITIAL INTERVENTION STRATEGIES

- Establish trust and identify mutually acceptable goals for care.
- Obtain explicit agreement on need for treatment and adherence.
- Identify depression, low self-esteem, drug use or other mental health issues for the child/adolescent and/or caregiver that may decrease adherence. Treat prior to starting antiretroviral drugs, if possible.
- Identify family, friends, health team members, or others who can help with adherence support.
- Educate patient and family about the critical role of adherence in therapy outcome.
    - ■ Specify the adherence target: 95% of prescribed doses.
    - ■ Educate patient and family about the relationship between partial adherence and resistance.
    - ■ Educate patient and family about resistance and constraint of later choices of antiretroviral drug; i.e., explain that while a failure of adherence may be temporary, the effects on treatment choice may be permanent.
- Develop a treatment plan that the patient and family understand and to which they feel committed.
- Establish readiness to take medication by practice sessions or other means.
- Consider a brief period of hospitalization at start of therapy in selected circumstances, for patient education and to assess tolerability of medications chosen.

MEDICATION STRATEGIES

- Choose the simplest regimen possible, reducing dosing frequency and number of pills.
- Choose a regimen with dosing requirements that best conform to the daily and weekly routines and variations in patient and family activities.
- Choose the most palatable medicine possible (pharmacists may be able to add syrups or flavoring agents to increase palatability).
- Choose drugs with the fewest side effects; provide anticipatory guidance for management of side effects.
- Simplify food requirements for medication administration.
- Prescribe drugs carefully to avoid adverse drug–drug interactions.

FOLLOW-UP INTERVENTION STRATEGIES

- Monitor adherence at each visit, and in between visits by telephone or letter as needed.
- Provide ongoing support, encouragement, and understanding of the difficulties of the demands of attaining >95% adherence with medication doses.
- Use patient education aids including pictures, calendars, stickers.
- Use pill boxes, reminders, alarms, pagers, timers.
- Provide nurse, social worker, or other practitioner adherence clinic visits or telephone calls.

Table 14.7

STRATEGIES TO IMPROVE ADHERENCE WITH ANTIRETROVIRAL MEDICATIONS (UPDATED OCTOBER 26, 2006) *continued*

FOLLOW-UP INTERVENTION STRATEGIES

- Provide access to support groups, peer groups, or one-on-one counseling for caregivers and patients, especially for those with known depression or drug use issues that are known to decrease adherence.
- Provide pharmacist-based adherence support.
- Consider gastrostomy tube use in selected circumstances.
- Consider a brief period of hospitalization for selected circumstances of apparent virologic failure, to assess adherence and reinforce that medication adherence is fundamental to successful antiretroviral therapy.
- Consider directly observed therapy at home, in the clinic, or during a brief inpatient hospitalization.

Source: Working Group on Antiretroviral Therapy and Medical Management of HIV-Infected Children (2008). *Guidelines for the Use of Antiretroviral Agents in Pediatric HIV Infection February 28, 2008* (p. 61) [Electronic Version]. Retrieved July 7, 2008, from http://AIDSinfo.nih.gov.

or caregiver and the child should be involved in adherence assessment and support. A nonjudgmental, problem-solving attitude is important to establishing honest communication because the "right" answer is that no doses were missed. A key issue is helping parents recognize the need to closely supervise children when they are taking medication to avoid situations where medications are spit out, not taken, or hidden. Large pill or capsule size and unpalatable liquid formulations contribute substantially to nonadherence in children. At times, families may report excellent adherence, but HIV RNA monitoring indicates a lack of response, a suboptimal response to treatment, or treatment failure following initial viral suppression. Viral resistance provides additional information because lack of viral suppression and absence or specific resistance mutations suggest that medication is not being taken. Whenever possible, home visits should be used to fully assess adherence problems and develop a package of interventions and support that are appropriate for the child and family.

COMPREHENSIVE CARE OF THE CHILD

The prevention and treatment of pediatric HIV infection in the United States and Western Europe are often termed a success story. Widespread public health efforts, which have focused on increasing access to HIV counseling and testing, coupled with interventions to interrupt transmission in HIV-infected pregnant women, have dramatically altered the course of the epidemic in the United States. By 2001, 78% of HIV-infected children were receiving antiretroviral therapy (McConnell et al., 2005). Concurrently, access to care and antiretroviral treatment has decreased morbidity and mortality. A review of selected AIDS-defining conditions reported in children from 1992 to 2001 showed that PCP, wasting, lymphocytic interstitial pneumonia (LIP), HIV encephalopathy, and bacterial infections dropped from 13% to just 2% (CDC, 2006). From 1994 to 2006, the mean age of death in children increased from 8.9 years to 18.2 years (CDC, 2006). Multiorgan system failure, sepsis, and renal disease have replaced AIDS-related opportunistic infections as the cause of mortality.

By 2007, the median age of over 3,500 HIV-infected U.S. children was 14.8 years (CDC, 2006). However, this cohort of youth continues to face a chronic life-threatening illness with physical, emotional, and social consequences. With the emergence of this cohort of long-term survivors has come the realization that inadequate evidence-based knowledge exists to guide interventions. Recent published reviews of the literature indicate that, aside from antiretroviral therapy, most evidence consists of papers presented at scientific meetings and descriptive reports of groups of patients. Such clinical evidence can be used to provide background and guide development of interventions for children and families. Nurses may find it convenient to draw parallels from work in other chronic illnesses and disability but must be cautious. Similarities abound, including impacts on growth and development, challenges to self-esteem, long-term treatment, and need to develop self-management skills. Differences are clear as well. The multigenerational nature of the disease in families coping with socioeconomic stressors of poverty, racism, and drug use is significant. Further, stigmatization and disclosure concerns are unlike those faced by any other group of children and families coping with a chronic condition.

Primary Care of the HIV-Exposed Infant

Care may be provided through a comprehensive treatment center or in conjunction with a community-based provider. In the asymptomatic infant, establishing the presence or absence of infection is critical in the first months of life (see previous description). While testing is underway, the infant should receive primary care in accordance with American Academy of Pediatrics guidelines. Because breastfeeding can transmit HIV, the mother should be counseled prenatally regarding her feeding choice. Alternative feeding with formula is safe and accessible in the United States. Table 14.8 discusses key nursing actions for the care of HIV-exposed infants. The CDC provides detailed guidance for administration of recommended vaccinations to HIV-exposed and -infected children. Those determined to be immunocompromised (CD4 age-specific T-lymphocyte percentages <15% or lymphocyte count <200 cells/mm^3 in children or adolescents) should not receive measles, mumps, and rubella (MMR) and varicella vaccines. The immunization schedule for HIV-exposed and -infected children aged 0 to 6 years and 7 to 18 years may be found in the publication *Guidelines for Prevention and Treatment of Opportunistic Infections among HIV-Exposed and HIV-Infected Children* (pp. 195–196), available online at http://aidsinfo.nih.gov/contentfiles/Pediatric_OI.pdf. (Also see Appendix I.) Both sets of recommendations were developed by the Working Group on Guidelines for the Prevention and Treatment of Opportunistic Infections Among HIV-Exposed and HIV-Infected Children (2008).

Table 14.8

NURSING CARE FOR THE HIV-EXPOSED INFANT

AREA	ACTION
Provide support during the HIV testing period	• Explain the diagnostic process to family • Support family to address concerns and answer questions • Stay in touch and schedule appointments or telephone calls during the testing period • Refer family to AIDS support organizations
Nutrition	• Counsel mother about the risk of HIV transmission through breastfeeding • Support feeding choice
Antiretroviral and Opportunistic Infection prophylaxis	• Monitor adherence with infant and maternal regimens • Teach parent or caregiver about administering the drug regimen and the side effects of drugs • Provide method to contact health care provider
Health teaching	• Teach parent or caregiver about early signs and symptoms of HIV infection

Opportunistic Infections

HAART regimens are effective in suppressing viral replication with maintenance or restoration of immune function. In both children and adults, effective ongoing HAART is the most important factor in controlling opportunistic infection (Working Group on Antiretroviral Therapy and Medical Management of HIV-Infected Children, 2008). That said, prevention and management of opportunistic infections require continual vigilance from health care providers.

Children are believed to acquire opportunistic pathogens from an infected mother or household member coinfected with opportunistic pathogens. While OIs in adults represent reactivation of latent infection, the child experiences primary infection after HIV infection is established and may be immunocompromised; thus symptoms and natural history of the infection may differ, particularly in the younger child. OIs include bacterial, mycobacterial, fungal, parasitic, and viral agents. In children receiving HAART, significant decreases in reporting of such infections has occurred (Gona et al., 2006). Detailed Guidelines for Prevention and Treatment of Opportunistic Infections among HIV-Exposed and HIV-Infected Children can be retrieved online at http://Aidsinfo.nih.gov.

Pneumocystis jiroveci (formerly *Pneumocystis carinii*) pneumonia continues as the most commonly reported AIDS-defining condition in children. Typically, life-threatening PCP occurs in the first 3 to 6 months of life and presents with fever, tachypnea, dyspnea, and cough. Primary prophylaxis to prevent PCP is recommended for all infants born to HIV-infected women and is highly effective in the prevention of PCP. Criteria for its use are based on the child's age and CD4 count or percentage. Prophylaxis is recommended for all HIV-infected children aged ≥6 years with CD4 counts <200 cells/mm^3 or CD4 <15%, for children aged 1 to 5 years with CD4 counts of <500 cells/mm^3 or CD4 <15%, and for all HIV-infected infants aged 12 months regardless of CD4 count and percentage (see Table 14.9) (Working Group on Guidelines for the Prevention and Treatment of Opportunistic Infections Among HIV-Exposed and HIV-Infected Children, 2008). Infants born to HIV-infected mothers should be considered for prophylaxis beginning at 4 to 6 weeks of age. Those infants determined to be infected should be given prophylaxis until 1 year of age, at which time treatment is reassessed on the basis of the age-specific CD4 count or percentage thresholds mentioned above. Infants with indeterminate HIV infection status should receive prophylaxis until they are determined to be HIV-uninfected or presumptively uninfected with HIV.

Table 14.9

PROPHYLAXIS TO PREVENT FIRST EPISODE OF OPPORTUNISTIC DISEASE AMONG HIV-EXPOSED AND HIV-INFECTED INFANTS AND CHILDREN

	PREVENTIVE REGIMEN		
PATHOGEN	INDICATION	FIRST CHOICE	ALTERNATIVE
I. STRONGLY RECOMMENDED AS STANDARD OF CARE			
Pneumocystis pneumonia	HIV-infected or HIV-indeterminate infants aged 1 to 12 mo; HIV-infected children aged 1 to 5 yr with CD4 count <500 cells/mm^3 or CD4 percentage <15%; HIV-infected children aged 6 to 12 yr with CD4 count <200 cells/mm^3 or CD4 percentage <15%	• Trimethoprim-sulfa-methoxazole (TMP-SMX), 150/750 mg/m2 body surface area per day daily divided into two doses and given three times weekly on consecutive days (AI); • Acceptable alternative dosage schedules for same dosage (AI): single dose by mouth three times weekly on consecutive days; two divided doses by mouth given daily; or two divided doses by mouth three times weekly on alternate days	• Dapsone (children aged ≥1 mo), 2 mg/kg body weight (max 100 mg) by mouth daily or 4 mg/kg body weight (max 200 mg) by mouth weekly (BI) • Atovaquone (children aged 1 to 3 mo and >24 mo, 30 mg/kg body weight by mouth daily; children aged 4 to 24 mo, 45 mg/kg body weight by mouth daily) (BI) • Aerosolized pentamidine (children aged ≥5 yr), 300 mg every month via Respirgard II™ (manufactured by Marquest, Englewood, Colorado) nebulizer (BI)

Source: Working Group on Guidelines for the Prevention and Treatment of Opportunistic Infections Among HIV-Exposed and HIV-Infected Children. (2008). *Guidelines for Prevention and Treatment of Opportunistic Infections among HIV-Exposed and HIV-Infected Children June 20, 2008* (p. 147) [Electronic Version]. Retrieved October 8, 2008, from http://AIDSinfo.nih.gov.

Care of the HIV-Infected Child

Once an HIV diagnosis is confirmed and the family enters care, nursing involvement is supportive to guide the family in understanding the diagnosis and its implications. Comprehensive management of the infected child requires the skills and expertise of a range of health disciplines working together across settings. Keeping in mind that the family delivers care in a home or community setting, the health care provider role is focused on education, counseling, supporting adherence, and serving as a resource to the family over a period of many years. The range of support services available for a family will vary by community. Nurses can maintain an up-to-date resource list and assist families in getting access to such services and supports. When the child resides with his or her HIV-infected parent, nurses should assess the health of the parent or parents and support them in gaining access to health care. Weglarz and Boland (2005) recommend that the home assessment address the housing, daily routine, family structure, knowledge of HIV, disclosure status, family supports, child behavior, medication administration, and need for additional resources. Because all of these areas are fluid, the home and family should be reassessed at intervals, the frequency determined on the basis of the health status of infected members. At a minimum, the reassessment should be done at least once a year. The infant and child represent a vulnerable population who depend on parents, caretakers, and social institutions. As a child enters adolescence, this dependency decreases over time. Regardless of setting or role responsibilities, the nurse must have specific competencies to deliver effective nursing care in the context of a comprehensive effort (Table 14.10).

Neurodevelopmental Functioning

Recent studies report that, when compared to children from similar socioeconomic situations, children with HIV experience greater impairment of neurologic, cognitive, and psychosocial functioning (Steele, Nelson, & Cole, 2007). Studies show that HIV is carried on monocytes or macrophages and CD4 lymphocytes in the central nervous system (CNS) early in infection. Some evidence suggests that the developing brain may be more susceptible to disruption and development of encephalopathy. Data in adults and observations in children indicate that HIV infection is compartmentalized within the brain as measured by difference in genetic sequencing or drug resistance patterns between plasma and cerebrospinal fluid (CSF). Observations in children seem to indicate the same pattern.

Understanding the evolution of the child's neurodevelopment in the context of active HIV infection is important. Key features of HIV "neuroAIDS," also referred to as progressive HIV encephalopathy (or PHE), in children and adults are described in Table 14.11 (Van Rie et al.,

Table 14.10

NURSING COMPETENCIES	
Basic understanding	• Immune system function • Assessment of immune function with emphasis on cell-mediated system • Virology of HIV including replication, mutation, and drug resistance • Impacts of chronic childhood illness in the context of a family with more than one infected family member
Highly active anti-retroviral treatment (HAART)	• Concepts and goals considered in formulating pediatric HIV treatment regimen • Strategies to support adherence • Management of side effects
Ability to	• Perform pediatric nursing and developmental assessment • Perform family assessment • Provide age-appropriate education to the child and ongoing education to the family • Collaborate with family and other care providers to choose the plan of care • Link with community-based providers including schools • Maintain confidentiality and respect family privacy while advocating for the needs of the child

2006). Factors associated with CNS disease in children with HIV infection include maternal and child immune status, elevated CSF and plasma viral load, and timing and route of infection. Risk is higher in those infants born to mothers with advanced disease (low CD4 count and high viral load) at time of delivery. Also, children with immune suppression and high plasma load have higher rates of encephalopathy. Concurrently, environmental factors including maternal drug use, poverty, low maternal education, and foster care placement also influence adjustment and may contribute to developmental delay. Because several of the published papers in this area include studies conducted prior to the widespread use of HAART, their results must be interpreted cautiously.

HAART, which reduces plasma and CSF viral load, also reduces risk of encephalopathy. While HAART halts PHE progression in children and adults, high rates of residual impairment remain, including behavioral problems as well as neurological, cognitive, and scholastic impairments

Table 14.11

KEY FEATURES OF HIV-1 NEUROAIDS IN CHILDREN AND ADULTS

ADULTS	CHILDREN
CNS HIV-1 invasion during primary infection, often followed by compartmentalization	CNS HIV-1 invasion during primary infection, likely also often followed by compartmentalization
Target cells include macrophages, microglia, and, to a lesser degree, astrocytes	Same target cells, but astrocytes may play a more central role and neurons may also be actively infected
Long latent period between infection and neurological manifestations	Neurological disease more often the first AIDS-defining illness, even before important immunodeficiency
Deterioration of mature CNS with brain atrophy	Impairment of immature CNS and impaired brain growth
Both motor and cognitive functions deteriorate	Motor, cognitive, and language functions are impaired
CNS opportunistic infections and cerebrovascular disease are common	Cerebrovascular disease and CNS opportunistic infections are rare, but the latter may be more frequent in developing countries
Antiretroviral treatment reduces incidence and can reverse neurological manifestations present at start of treatment	Similar preventive and therapeutic effects of antiretroviral treatment on CNS manifestations

Source: Reprinted from page 3 of Van Rie, A., Harrington, P.R., Dow, A., & Robertson, K. (2006). Neurologic and neurodevelopmental manifestations of pediatric HIV/AIDS: a global perspective. *European Journal of Paediatric Neurology, 11,* 1–9. Copyright 2006, with permission from Elsevier.

(Van Rie et al., 2006). Van Rie and colleagues postulate that the cognitive effects are due to ongoing viral replication in the CNS or residual effects of static neuropathy. Because both environmental and neurologic factors increase the vulnerability of the child, behavioral specialists are needed on the treatment team. Regular neurocognitive and developmental testing should be included into the child's ongoing care.

Psychosocial functioning. Because of a paucity of large controlled longitudinal studies, the true effects of HIV on psychosocial functioning are unclear. The small body of literature on psychosocial function of children with HIV infection is mixed. The numerous, continuing, and varied stressors experienced by this group of children do heighten concern related to psychosocial functioning. Regular assessment and communication with the child and family is key to providing timely intervention if or when a problem is noted. Caregiver coping style would be expected to influence the child's experience, and studies note that HIV-infected parents report poorer emotional health compared to noninfected caregivers. Child coping style is believed to serve as a moderator of adjustment for children. Bachanas and colleagues (2001) found children using emotion-focused strategies reported more problems that those using problem-focused efforts. They suggest that building emotion-focused skills could be an effective intervention.

Disclosure of HIV Status

While the American Academy of Pediatrics in 1999 recommended disclosure of HIV status, both clinicians and families have been cautious in embracing this recommendation (American Academy of Pediatrics Committee on Pediatric AIDS, 1999). Concerns include parental discomfort, fear of stigma, worry about the child's ability to cope, and parental distress. Today, the improved survival and transition to adolescence and adulthood provide a stronger imperative for considering a process for disclosure as a component of ongoing care, including how and when to disclose.

A review of the psychology literature related to life-threatening illness in children can inform providers so that they help allay the fears of both providers and parents. The growing body of research shows that the concepts proposed by Piaget related to movement from preoperational to concrete and operational stages of reasoning are valid. Wiener and colleagues (2007) conducted a systematic review and synthesis of the literature to guide development of efficacy-based interventions and to begin creating clinical guidelines. Partial disclosure, i.e., giving some but not all the information about an illness, was used frequently with younger children. They reported mixed findings on the impact of disclosure, with some studies showing benefits, others risks, and others no difference. They concluded that there is no clear evidence that children who have experienced full disclosure fare better or worse than those who do not. Lacking clear evidence and recognizing that clinicians require some guidance, they made five recommendations: (1) consider the child's abilities; (2) assess caregiver abilities to cope with the stress of disclosure, to gain access to support, and to discuss other family secrets; (3) rehearse and prepare for the actual disclosure through role playing;

(4) identify sources of family and community support; and (5) encourage ongoing open communication within the family and support systems. Viewing disclosure as a process that occurs along a continuum may be helpful. The cognitive and behavioral impairments discussed earlier will influence the child's ability to understand and create a context for the information. Creating a safe environment where the child is able to repeatedly ask questions and receive answers appropriate to their level of understanding is critical. The provider can be prepared to correct misinformation, address magical thinking, and provide opportunities for ongoing dialogue between the child and caregiver.

Low-Resource Settings

Untreated HIV infection in infants is an aggressive disease, with 30% of those infected dying by age 1 year and 50% by age 2 (Working Group on Antiretroviral Therapy and Medical Management of HIV-Infected Children, 2008). WHO estimated that HIV accounts for 3% of deaths in all children under 5 years of age (WHO, 2007b). In Africa, HIV disease accounts for 7% of child deaths but may be as much as 50% in the most-affected countries. According to WHO, many of the 290,000 children who died from HIV in 2007 never were diagnosed or entered care for their infection (UNICEF & WHO, 2008). With early diagnosis, infection prophylaxis, and access to HAART, many of these deaths could be prevented.

HIV infection is decreasing gains in child survival in certain parts of the world. Improving child survival requires a comprehensive approach that includes country health systems for immunizations, essential nutritional intervention, care for newborn infants, and care for sick children (Gilks et al., 2006). With this foundation, such programs have a potential to improve life expectancy in HIV-infected infants and children in low-resource settings.

In 2008, UNICEF and WHO created a programming framework to accelerate the scale-up of programs to prevent, diagnose, and treat HIV infection in infants and children. UNICEF and WHO (2008, p. 12) have put forth the following principles to guide program development and scale-up:

- *Urgency.* HIV prevention, diagnosis, care, and treatment must be immediately scaled up to avert hundreds of thousands of deaths among children who are exposed to or have HIV.
- *Universal access.* All children in need should have access to HIV prevention, diagnosis, care and treatment services.

- *Life-long care.* HIV disease is a chronic disease and requires ongoing care and treatment; national governments have a responsibility to ensure uninterrupted care and treatment.
- *Family-centered care.* Family members should receive care in a manner that recognizes and responds to the family as a unit.
- *High-quality care.* Care provided should be of the highest quality possible and should be monitored and improved through a system of improvement.

Recognizing the varying levels of resources across and within countries, UNICEF and WHO recommend that countries use a public health approach, including selecting interventions based on the best available evidence and the burden of disease; optimizing the use of available human resources; implementing standardized treatment protocols and simplified clinical monitoring; simplifying clinical decision making by facilitating the provision of services by more types of health care workers; involving community members; and using strategies such as generic medications and alternative laboratory technologies to minimize costs. The country's Ministry of Health, with expert working groups and advisors, is responsible for determining the national program for HIV prevention, diagnosis, care, and treatment. Because access, capacity, and cost must influence decisions, the program and corresponding clinical algorithms and guidelines will vary with the country's resources.

These recommendations are largely dependent on delivery by the health care workforce, mainly nurses. They come at a time when WHO itself acknowledges a global shortage of over 4 million health care workers that is most acute in regions burdened with HIV infection. Scaling up AIDS programs and building strong country health systems need to be viewed as allied and not competitive goals (International AIDS Society, 2008). Government, donors, and foundations must begin to direct attention and resources to building or retaining their nursing workforce. While developing new cadres of workers may be needed in the most severely affected regions, building capacity for nursing education and increasing numbers of trained and competent nursing professionals is a much more effective and viable long-term solution. Such nurses can contribute to improved outcomes, including overall infant mortality and morbidity. Nursing education across borders can be accomplished, and several partnership models have evolved in recent years. The emergence of global nursing curriculum and competencies can support such efforts. There is an urgent need to move from an approach focused on "training" to one that educates the workforce to meet a range of health needs, including

HIV, across borders. Major nursing schools from high-resource settings are actively engaged and funded in the area of HIV care and research. Using PEPFAR funds, countries could potentially scale up nursing education to build a workforce to deliver direct care, supervise new cadres of workers, and contribute to country health programs. If prevention efforts could halt transmission to women and PMTCT programs were fully implemented, decreases in pediatric HIV infection rates in low-resource settings could mirror the successes described earlier in this chapter. While countries mobilize to address these challenges, nurses will need to care for those infants and children with HIV infection. In low-resource settings, the nurse is expected to perform a variety of functions and may be expected to provide care for all age groups. In some settings, she or he is the only care provider and manages treatment using approved algorithms. For example, a nurse working in a health center will manage all the clinics that occur in a given week and be available as patients drop in with problems. In the hospital, the family may be rooming in with the patient and providing meals and direct care. These settings provide opportunities for case finding and family-centered care and support the family unencumbered by established barriers to service. At the district hospital level in Africa, one report found considerable confusion regarding diagnosis, opportunistic infection prophylaxis, and antiretroviral therapy and noted a lack of health care interventions such as pain relief, palliative care, and emotional support. Services and support are most needed at this level where care is delivered. Those committed to ending suffering have a responsibility to ensure that generous donor resources make their way beyond construction and research to those suffering from HIV (De Baets et al., 2007).

Virologic testing at 4 to 8 weeks of age will identify >95% of infants infected intra- and postpartum and is the recommended standard. WHO suggests that all infants have their HIV status established at their first contact with the health system. The WHO case definition for HIV infection is based on virologic testing for infants under 18 months and includes antibody testing for those older than 18 months. In the absence of virologic testing, clinical or immunologic criteria can be used to make the diagnosis and guide initiation of HAART. Recent advances using heel stick for dried blood spot testing for HIV DNA PCR in central or regional laboratories are being implemented in resource limited settings, allowing early laboratory diagnosis and treatment of infants and young children (Creek et al., 2007).

In most low-resource settings, status will be established by asking the mother, checking the health cards, and requesting the history of maternal HIV testing. Because disease progression occurs so rapidly, over 80% of diagnosed infants are eligible to start therapy before 6 months of age to achieve the reported dramatic reduction in mortality and disease progression. WHO recommends that all infants with confirmed infection should be started on antiretroviral therapy, irrespective of clinical or immunologic stage. Recommendations from the WHO Technical Working Group, Paediatric HIV/ART Care Guideline Group Meeting are found on the WHO website (www.who.int/hiv/pub/paediatric/WHO_Paediatric_ART_guideline_rev_mreport_2008.pdf).

Reports indicate that all infants born to HIV-infected women are at risk for adverse outcomes. Both exposed and infected children require close follow-up and access to ongoing primary care. Laboratory testing is ideal for guiding diagnosis and management of cotrimoxazole prophylaxis and antiretroviral therapy. Immune status, measured by CD4 (either percentage count or absolute number) is believed to be more informative than clinical presentation. When immunologic testing is not available, WHO provides a clinical staging scheme to guide care providers.

AIDS Orphans

AIDS orphans have received considerable attention in professional and lay literature (Guest, 2003; Li et al., 2008; Meier, 2003; Salaam, 2005, Smart, 2003; Williamson, Foster, & Levine, 2006). The AIDS pandemic has orphaned millions of children around the world, primarily in low-resource nations (an estimated about 11.6 million living in sub-Saharan Africa). These children have lost one or both parents to AIDS. UNAIDS (2008) estimates that worldwide more than 15 million children under 18 years of age have been orphaned as a result of AIDS. By some estimates, by 2010 20 million children will be orphaned by AIDS. In some countries (e.g., Zambia and Botswana), an estimated 20% of children under 17 are orphans. About half of the world's orphans are 9 years of age or younger. The loss of one or both parents to AIDS can have a negative impact on these children's lives. The effects of losing one or more parents may result in neglect, developmental delays, psychological distress (depression and anxiety), not having basic necessities (including food, shelter, and health care), educational difficulties, exploitation (labor and sex work), and stigmatization and discrimination. The international AIDS charity AVERT (2008), in discussing AIDS orphans, notes that until adult deaths can be prevented,

AIDS orphans will need the following interventions: (1) support for their caregivers, (2) attention to their emotional needs, (3) resources to stay in school, and (4) protection of their human and legal rights. Numerous national and international governmental and nongovernmental organizations have developed statements and policies regarding AIDS orphans; but, as the number of these children increases over the next several years, the international community will be challenged to provide the assistance these children need to survive into adulthood.

CONCLUSION

Three decades of experience and research provide an evidence-based framework for the diagnosis, care, and treatment of children with pediatric HIV infection. Effective scale-up of PMTCT programs in high-resource settings has decreased the number of new infections; effective HAART for children prolongs both quality and length of life; and nurses participate actively in all aspects of these efforts. Long-term complications of HIV infection and antiretroviral therapy in children require close monitoring and management. Mental health and psychosocial functioning assessment and management will ensure that long-term survivors are prepared to move from adolescence to adulthood in school and community. In low-resource settings, scale-up of PMTCT is slow while the number of new infections continues to increase. The lack of capacity in health systems in the context of a global nursing shortage challenges efforts to diagnose, manage, and treat pediatric infection. The gains discussed in this chapter are not yet within the grasp of many low-resource countries. Long-standing obstacles in the global effort to reduce transmission of HIV to children and provide antiretroviral therapy to infected children are continuing challenges.

The authors acknowledge Marla Acosta who assisted in preparing this manuscript.

REFERENCES

American Academy of Pediatrics Committee on Pediatrics AIDS. (1999). Disclosure of illness status to children and adolescents with HIV infection. *Pediatrics, 103*(1), 164–166.

AVERT. (2008). *AIDS orphans.* Retrieved February 8, 2009, from www.avert.org/aidsorphans.htm.

Bachanas, P. J., Kullgren, K., Schwartz, K. S., Lanier, B., McDaniel, J. S., Smith, J., et al. (2001). Predictors of psychosocial adjustment in school-age children infected with HIV. *Journal of Pediatric Psychology, 26*(6), 343–352.

Brady, M. T. (2005). Pediatric human immunodeficiency virus-1 infection. *Advances in Pediatrics, 52,* 163–193.

Burr, C. K., Lampe, M. A., Gross, E., Clark, J., & Jones, R. (2007, November 4–7). *A strategic planning approach to influencing hospital practice regarding rapid HIV testing in labor and delivery.* Paper presented at the Annual Meeting of the American Public Health Association, Washington, DC. Abstract 161680.

Centers for Disease Control and Prevention (CDC). (1994). 1994 revised classification system for human immunodeficiency virus infection in children less than 13 years of age [Electronic Version]. *Morbidity and Mortality Weekly Report, 43,* 1–10. Retrieved November 18, 2008, from www.cdc.gov/mmwr/previewmmwrhtml/0032890.htm.

Centers for Disease Control and Prevention (CDC). (2004). *HIV/AIDS surveillance report* [Electronic Version]. 16, Retrieved August 8, 2008, from www.cdc.gov/hiv/topics/surveillance/resources/reports/index.htm.

Centers for Disease Control and Prevention (CDC). (2006). *Pediatrics HIV/AIDS surveillance (through 2006).* Atlanta, GA: Author.

Centers for Disease Control and Prevention (CDC). (2007a). *CDC HIV/AIDS fact sheet: Mother-to-child (perinatal) HIV transmission and prevention* [Electronic Version]. Retrieved July 7, 2008, from www.cdc.gov/hiv/topics/perinatal/resources/factsheets/perinatal.htm.

Centers for Disease Control and Prevention (CDC). (2007b). *HIV/AIDS surveillance report, 2005,* Rev. June 2007 [Electronic Version]. Retrieved August 8, 2008, from www.cdc.gov/hiv/topics/surveillance/resources/reports/2005report/table8.htm.

Centers for Disease Control and Prevention (CDC). (2008a). *HIV/AIDS statistics and surveillance* [Electronic Version]. Retrieved February 8, 2009, from www.cdc.gov/hiv/topics/surveillance/basic.htm.

Centers for Disease Control (CDC). (2008b). Revised surveillance case definitions for HIV infection among adults, adolescents, and children aged <18 months and for HIV infection and AIDS among children aged 18 months to <13 years—United States, 2008. [Electronic Version]. *Morbidity and Mortality Weekly Report, 57,* 1–8. Retrieved February 20, 2009, from www.cdc.gov/mmwr/preview/mmwrhtml/rr5710a1.htm.

Chadwick, E. G., Capparelli, E. V., Yogev, R., Pinto, J. A., Robbins, B., Rodman, J. H., et al. (2008). Pharmacokinetics, safety and efficacy of lopinavir/ritonavir in infants less than 6 months of age: 24 week results. *AIDS, 22*(2), 249–255.

Connor, E., Sperling, R. S., Gelber, R., Kiselev, P., Scott, G., O'Sullivan, M. J., et al., and the Pediatric AIDS Clinical Trials Group Protocol 076 Study Group. (1994). Reduction of maternal–infant transmission of human immunodeficiency virus 1 with zidovudine treatment: Results of AIDS Clinical Trials Group Protocol 076. *New England Journal of Medicine, 331*(18), 1173–1180.

Coovadia, H. M., Rollins, N. C., Bland, R. M., Little, K., Coutsoudis, A., Bennish, M. L., et al. (2007). Mother-to-child transmission of HIV-1 infection during exclusive breastfeeding in the first 6 months of life: an intervention cohort study. *Lancet, 369*(9567), 1107–1116.

Coutsoudis, A., Coovadia, H. M., & Wilfert, C. M. (2008). HIV, infant feeding and more perils for poor people: New WHO guidelines encourage review of formula milk policies. *Bulletin of the World Health Organization, 86*(3), 161–240.

Creek, T. L., Sherman, G. G., Nkengasong, J., Lu, L., Finkbeiner, T., Fowler, M. G., et al. (2007). Infant human immunodeficiency virus diagnosis in resource-limited settings: Issues, technologies, and country experiences. *American Journal of Obstetrics and Gynecology, 197*(Suppl. 3), S64–71.

De Baets, A. J., Bulterys, M., Abrams, E. J., Kankassa, C., & Pazvakavambwa, I. E. (2007). Care and treatment of HIV-infected children in Africa: Issues and challenges at the district hospital level. *Pediatric Infectious Disease Journal, 26*(2), 163–173.

De Cock, K. M., Fowler, M. G., Mercier, E., de Vincenzi, I., Saba, J., Hoff, E., et al. (2000). Prevention of mother-to-child HIV transmission in resource-poor countries. *Journal of the American Medical Association, 283*(9), 1175–1182.

Dunn, D., Woodburn, P., Duong, T., Petro, J., Phillips, A., Gibb, D., et al., for the HIV Paediatric Prognostic Markers Collaborative Study Group. (2008). Current CD4 cell count and the short-term risk of AIDS and death before the availability of effective antiretroviral therapy in HIV-infected children and adults. *Journal of Infectious Diseases, 197*(3), 398–404.

Gilks, C. F., Crowley, S., Ekpini, R., Gove, S., Perriens, J., Souteyrand, Y., et al. (2006). The WHO public-health approach to antiretroviral treatment against HIV in resource-limited settings. *Lancet, 368*(9534), 505–510.

Ginsburg, A. S., Hoblitzelle, C. W., Sripipatana, T. L., & Wilfert, C. M. (2007). Provision of care following prevention of mother-to-child HIV transmission services in resource-limited settings. *AIDS, 21*(18), 2529–2532.

Gona, P., Van Dyke, R. B., Williams, P. L., Dankner, W. M., Chernoff, M. C., Nachman, S. A., et al. (2006). Incidence of opportunistic and other infections in HIV-infected children in the HAART era. *Journal of the American Medical Association, 296*(3), 292–300.

Guest, E. (2003). *Children of AIDS: Africa's orphan crisis.* Scottsville, South Africa: University of Natal Press.

Health Resources and Services Administration. (2008). *The HIV/AIDS program: Ryan White parts A-F* [Electronic Version]. Retrieved October 8, 2008, from http://hab.hrsa.gov/treatmentmodernization.partd.htm.

Holzemer, W. L. (2008). Building a qualified global nursing workforce. *International Nursing Review, 55,* 241–242.

International AIDS Society. (2008). *HIV experts underscore natural alliance between the response to AIDS and efforts to expand primary care, strengthen health systems in poor countries* [Electronic Version]. Retrieved July 7, 2008, from www.aids2008.org/admin/images/upload/813.pdf.

Li, X., Naar-King, S., Barnett, D., Stanton, B., Fang, X., & Thurston, C. (2008). A developmental psychopathology framework of the psychosocial needs of children orphaned by HIV. *Journal of the Association of Nurses in AIDS Care 19,* 147–157.

Lindegren, M. L., Byers, R. H., Thomas, P., Davis, S. F., Caldwell, B., Rogers, M., et al. (1999). Trends in perinatal transmission of HIV/AIDS in the United States. *Journal of the American Medical Association, 282*(6), 531–538.

Little, K. E., Bland, R. M., & Newell, M. L. (2008). Vertically acquired paediatric HIV infection: The challenges of providing comprehensive packages of care in resource-limited settings. *Tropical Medicine and International Health, 13*(9), 1098–1110.

McConnell, M. S., Byers, R. H., Frederick, T., Peters, V. B., Dominguez, K. L., Sukalac, T., et al. (2005). Trends in antiretroviral therapy use and survival rates for a large cohort of HIV-infected children and adolescents in the United States, 1989–2001. *Journal of Acquired Immune Deficiency Syndromes, 38*(4), 488–494.

McKenna, M. T., & Hu, X. (2007). Recent trends in the incidence and morbidity associated with perinatal human immunodeficiency virus infection in the United States. *American Journal of Obstetrics and Gynecology, 197*(3, Suppl. 1), S10–S16.

Meier, E. (2003). Growth of AIDS orphans and policy solutions. *Pediatric Nursing, 29*(1), 75–76.

Mellins, C. A., Brackis-Cott, E., Dolezal, C., & Abrams, E. J. (2004). The role of psychosocial and family factors in adherence to antiretroviral treatment in human immunodeficiency virus-infected children. *Pediatric Infectious Disease Journal, 23*(11), 1035–1041.

National HIV/AIDS Clinicians' Consultation Center.)2009). *State HIV testing laws compendium.* Retrieved June 2, 2009, from http://www.nccc.ucsf.edu/StateLaws/Index.html

Public Health Service Task Force (PHS). (2008). *Recommendations for Use of Antiretroviral Drugs in Pregnant HIV-Infected Women for Maternal Health and Interventions to Reduce Perinatal HIV Transmission in the United States* [Electronic Version]. Retrieved February 8, 2009, from http://aidsinfo.nih.gov/contentfiles/PerinatalGL.pdf.

Salaam, T. (2005, February 11). *AIDS orphans and vulnerable children: Problems, responses, and issues for Congress.* Retrieved February 7, 2009, from www.law.umaryland.edu/marshall/crsreports/crsdocuments/RL3225202112005.pdf.

Shannon, M., Kennedy, H. P., & Humphreys, J. C. (2008). HIV-infected mothers' foci of concern during the viral testing of their infants. *Journal of the Association of Nurses in AIDS Care, 19*(2), 114–126.

Smart, R. (2003). Policies for orphans and vulnerable children: A framework for moving ahead. Retrieved February 8, 2009, from www.policyproject.com/pubs/generalreport/OVC_Policies.pdf.

State HIV testing laws compendium—2008 . Retrieved November 19, 2008, from www.nccc.ucsf.edu/StateLaws/Index.html.

Steele, R. G., Nelson, T. D., & Cole, B. P. (2007). Psychosocial functioning of children with AIDS and HIV infection: Review of the literature from a socioecological framework. *Journal of Developmental & Biobehavioral Pediatrics, 28*(1), 58–69.

UNAIDS. (2008). *Report on the global HIV/AIDS epidemic 2008.* Geneva: Joint United Nations Programme on HIV/AIDS.

United Nations Children's Fund (UNICEF) & World Health Organization (WHO). (2008). *Scale up of HIV-related prevention, diagnosis, care and treatment for infants and children: A programming framework* [Electronic Version]. Retrieved July 7, 2008, from www.unicef.org/aids/files/UNICEF_WHO_Programming_Framework_June_2008.pdf.

U.S. Public Health Service. (1987). *Report of the Surgeon General's workshop on children with HIV infection and their families.* DHHS Publication No. HRS-D-MC 87-1. Washington, DC: U.S. Government Printing Office .

Van Rie, A., Harrington, P. R., Dow, A., & Robertson, K. (2006). Neurologic and neurodevelopmental manifestations of pediatric HIV/AIDS: A global perspective. *European Journal of Paediatric Neurology, 11,* 1–9.

Violari, A., Cotton, M., Gibb, D., Babiker, A., Steyn, J., & Jean-Phillip, P., et al. (2007, July 22–25). *Antiretroviral therapy initiated before 12 weeks of age reduces early mortality in young HIV-infected infants: Evidence from the Children with HIV Early Antiretroviral Therapy (CHER) study.* Paper presented at the 4th International AIDS Conference on HIV Pathogenesis, Treatment and Prevention, Sydney, Australia.

Weglarz, M., & Boland, M. (2005). Family-centered nursing care of the perinatally infected mother and child living with HIV infection. *Journal for Specialists in Pediatric Nursing, 10*(4), 161–170.

Wiener, L., Mellins, C. A., Marhefka, S., & Battles, H. B. (2007). Disclosure of an HIV diagnosis to children: history, current research, and future directions. *Journal of Developmental and Behavioral Pediatrics, 28*(2), 155–166.

Williams, P. L., Storm, D., Montepiedra, G., Nichols, S., Kammerer, B., Sirois, P. A., et al. (2006). Predictors of adherence to antiretroviral medications in children and adolescents with HIV infection. *Pediatrics, 118*(6), e1745–1757.

Williamson, J., Foster, G., & Levine, C. (Eds.). (2006). *A Generation at risk: The global impact of HIV/AIDS on orphans and vulnerable children.* Cambridge, U.K.: Cambridge University Press.

Working Group on Antiretroviral Therapy and Medical Management of HIV-Infected Children. (2008). *Guidelines for the use of antiretroviral agents in pediatric HIV infection February 28 2008* [Electronic Version]. Retrieved July 7, 2008, from http://AIDSinfo.nih.gov.

Working Group on Antiretroviral Therapy and Medical Management of HIV-Infected Children. (2008a). *Guidelines for the use of antiretroviral agents in pediatric HIV infection July 29, 2008* [Electronic Version]. Retrieved November 15, 2008, from http://AIDSinfo.nih.gov.

Working Group on Guidelines for the Prevention and Treatment of Opportunistic Infections Among HIV-Exposed and HIV-Infected Children. (2008). *Guidelines for prevention and treatment of opportunistic infections among HIV-exposed and HIV-infected children June 20, 2008* [Electronic Version]. Retrieved October 8, 2008, from http://AIDSinfo.nih.gov.

World Health Organization (WHO). (2007a). *HIV and infant feeding: Update based on the technical consultation held on behalf of the Interagency Team (IATT) on Prevention of HIV Infections in Pregnant Women, Mothers and Their Infants.* Geneva, Switzerland: World Health Organization. [Electronic Version]. Retrieved February 20, 2009, from http://whqlibdoc.who.int/publications/2007/9789241595964_eng.pdf.

World Health Organization (WHO). (2007b). *Preferred antiretroviral medicines for treating and preventing HIV infection in younger children: Report of the WHO paediatric antiretroviral working group.* Geneva: Author.

World Health Organization, Department of HIV/AIDS. (2007). *Prevention of mother-to-child transmission (PMTCT) briefing note* [Electronic Version]. Retrieved October 8, 2008, from www.who.int/hiv/pub/toolkits/PMTCT%20HIV%20Dept%20brief%20Oct%2007.pdf.

15

Aging and the Person Infected with HIV

JOE W. BURRAGE, JR.
DAVID E. VANCE

This chapter was written to provide nurses with the information necessary for evidence-based, best practices by furthering their understanding of the synergistic effects of age and HIV within the context of a model of successful aging with HIV. It is beyond the scope of this chapter to address the developmental process of aging or discuss every possible impact that HIV can have on successful aging. However, we will present the components of a model of successful aging, and, based on this model, our clinical experience, research, and review of the literature, we will address some of the more relevant issues that nurses will face as they provide care to their aging HIV-infected patients.

HISTORICAL PERSPECTIVE OF HIV

Since HIV infection in humans was first identified, remarkable progress has been made in the diagnosis and treatment of HIV disease and AIDS. In the 1980s, the majority of those first identified as being infected with HIV were young gay men ranging in age from 20 to 30 years. Due to the high mortality rates experienced during the first decade of the epidemic, few people survived even to 50 years of age. The introduction of highly active antiretroviral therapy (HAART) in the mid-1990s has heralded a new era in the treatment of HIV (Nichols et al., 2002). At the time, the scientific and health care communities did not fully understand how HAART might affect longevity in HIV-infected adults. Now, more than a decade later, HIV is widely viewed as a chronic condition. People are now aging with HIV disease. In fact, of the estimated 1.1 million adults and adolescents infected with HIV in the United States (CDC, 2008b), adults 50 years of age or older made up 15% of all new HIV diagnoses in 2005. In 2005, persons 50 years of age or older also comprised 24% of those living with HIV, 29% of those diagnosed with AIDS, and 35% of those who died of AIDS (CDC, 2008a). Since 1990 the number of AIDS cases in Americans 50 years of age and older has increased fivefold (Oursler et al., 2006). Older persons progress from HIV to AIDS more rapidly than younger HIV-infected persons (Stark, 2007). Older patients are twice as likely to be diagnosed with AIDS and to receive this diagnosis during hospitalization, the possible result of a misperception by some providers that older persons are not at risk of HIV infection because they are perceived as being sexually inactive (Mugavero et al., 2007; Stark, 2007). Because HIV infection in older adults may not be discovered until the onset of AIDS, older persons, as a group, have a shorter survival than younger persons with HIV infection (Deeks & Phillips, 2009; Stark, 2007). The prevalence of HIV infection in older adults is expected to grow, primarily as a result of HAART but partly due to later-life infections as well as the unprecedented growth in the aging population in general (Vance & Robinson, 2004).

The face of HIV/AIDS continually changes as more knowledge and insight result from research and experience in providing care and preventive services for those with and affected by HIV. This illness, once considered an acute life-threatening illness, is now viewed as a chronic illness associated with the challenges of successful aging. A longer lifespan in this group is relatively new, and as such, the state of the science is in the early stages of examining the impact of HIV on those who have survived to the age of 50 years and beyond. This transformation is evident not only in how the disease appears and responds to pharmacologic and other interventions but also in its transmission to many different populations and groups once considered invulnerable. From the perspective of aging, the health care needs of four groups should be considered in terms of HIV:

- Those who are newly infected or not diagnosed.
- Those who are at risk of being infected.
- Those persons living with HIV/AIDS (PLWH).
- Those PLWH who are now entering old age.

This chapter focuses on those who have survived with HIV. Although longer life in this population is obviously welcome news, new challenges and a myriad of questions are emerging about how the process of aging and HIV will interact to affect patient care and quality of life. For instance:

- What does it mean to age with HIV infection?
- How well will HIV medications be tolerated in older adults with HIV?
- Will cognitive changes due to the synergy of HIV and aging have an impact on medication adherence and everyday functioning?
- What age-related conditions and comorbidities will be exacerbated by HIV or the HIV-related medications?
- Are there unique hormonal changes in this group?
- What are the emotional and social consequences of aging with HIV?

Much of what is known is based on clinical experience as well as gerontological and HIV research and literature. Understanding aging and HIV is difficult because they share certain common conditions. For example, many conditions commonly associated with HIV are also common in aging; thus, as people age with HIV, they may possibly become more susceptible to a variety of comorbidities, including osteopenia, osteoporosis, sarcopenia, memory loss and decreased cognition, hypertension, vascular disease, diabetes, cancer, kidney disease, decreased immunity, increased pain, hypogonadism, and frailty, just to name a few conditions (Figure 15.1). This means that, in addition to treating HIV, these other comorbidites may be common with HIV treatment, and treatments for both HIV and the comorbidities must be considered and balanced.

Synergy of Aging and HIV on Comorbidites

Research findings should influence the design and delivery of interventions for this vulnerable population. The number of research studies being conducted to address this demographic change in the HIV-infected population is constantly increasing. For example, research now shows that among survivors 5–10 years post HIV diagnosis, there is an increased incidence of some non-HIV related cancer (Pragna et al., 2008). Also, the assessment of the impact of HIV on the aging process from the perspective of cognition is ongoing through studies to determine whether there is an additive effect of HIV on age-related dementia and vice versa (Valcour, 2009). Although these questions and issues are yet unanswered, findings suggest that the interaction between aging and HIV does have a profound effect on some individuals (Vance & Burrage, 2006b). These are but a few examples of what must be discovered in terms of HIV and aging. Much is still unknown.

Early in the HIV pandemic, nurses who cared for those with AIDS were leaders in the evidence-based practice arena. Because so little was known about HIV during the early years after its discovery, nurses had little choice but to design and deliver care from an evidence-based perspective. This approach continues to drive HIV care delivery and prevention activities. Diligence continues in finding innovative ways to provide care. For example, the Association of Nurses in AIDS Care (ANAC) has developed and published practice standards and a core curriculum specific to the nursing care of people with HIV that includes aspects of aging with HIV (Association of Nurses in AIDS Care [ANAC], 2007; Kirton, 2003).

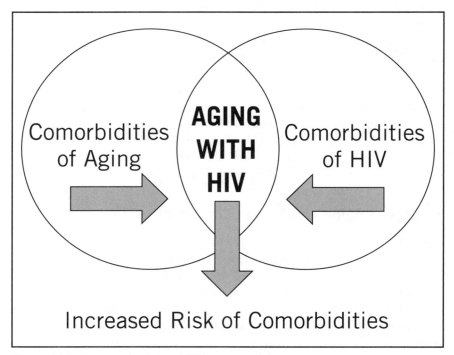

Figure 15.1 Synergy of aging and HIV on comorbidites.

A MODEL FOR SUCCESSFUL AGING WITH HIV

The gerontological literature provides information that helps us to understand what, in general, successful aging means, which in turn provides a context in which to discuss aspects of aging with HIV. Parker and colleagues (2002) hypothesized a parsimonious model of successful aging that consists of four essential components: (1) low levels of disease and disability, (2) high cognitive and physical functioning, (3) active engagement in life, and (4) spirituality within a developmental context. The phrase "low levels of disease and disability" refers to maintaining the optimal health possible in lieu of age-related comorbidities. "High cognitive and physical functioning" involves keeping one's functional abilities intact to perform daily tasks that help to maintain autonomy. "Active engagement in life" means being socially and personally involved in the events of one's life. Such engagement can be a factor in the development of hardiness in older persons with HIV/AIDS (Vance et al., 2008a). Finally, spirituality within a developmental context refers to the personal evolution of one's meaning and purpose in life. Thus, if a person is aging with HIV or any other condition and can maintain some acceptable level of functioning and quality of life in each of these components, then he or she is considered to be aging successfully; however, level of functioning and quality of life are based on personal experience and what one deems acceptable, and are therefore subjective, varying from one person to another. Figure 15.2 is based on the model of Parker and his colleagues.

According to this model of successful aging, one needs to maximize the potential of each of these areas to achieve an acceptable quality of life in lieu of age-related losses and changes. However, aging with HIV presents unique challenges that can compromise each of these components of successful aging. As is emphasized in this model of successful aging, if one component is compromised, other components may be affected and compromised as well. For example, cognitive impairments are common among those aging with HIV, even without dementia (Vance & Burrage, 2006b). These cognitive impairments thus can lead to functional problems in everyday life, such as difficulty adhering to medication schedules or forgetting to go to medical appointments. Compromise of such health-related behaviors by cognitive dysfunction can result in the promotion of disease and disability. Likewise, cognitive functioning is needed to fully engage in activities in life. For example, when socializing with friends and family by playing a card or board game, an individual whose cognitive abilities are so compromised that he or she cannot keep the rules

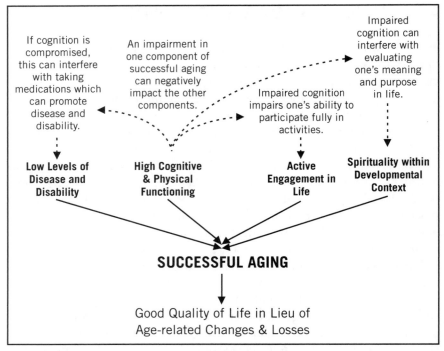

Figure 15.2 Interaction of the components of successful aging.

straight may become frustrated and experience a diminished enjoyment from this activity. Even adults with mild cognitive impairment often experience difficulty paying bills, organizing their money, and dealing with other financial tasks (Griffith et al., 2003). So if one's capacity to manage finances is compromised by a decline in cognitive ability, this decline can result in less money to engage in activities in life. Finally, self- and inner reflection are important for evaluating one's purpose and meaning in life, which is fundamental for spiritual development; however, a decrease in cognitive ability can result in a compromised ability to reflect and sustain attention on personally meaningful activities, thoughts, and events. A decline in cognitive ability thus compromises one's ability to age successfully and can negatively affect the other components of successful aging. In the same manner, a compromise in one or more of the other three components also holds the potential to negatively affect the other components of successful aging, thereby potentially impairing one's quality of life.

Health care professionals sometimes take it on themselves to define what it means to age successfully. While objective criteria for successful aging exist, aging persons, including those with HIV disease, have their own criteria by which to assess their success in aging. So health care professionals must balance these "objective" criteria with the patient's "subjective" criteria of what it means to age well with this disease.

FACTORS AFFECTING SUCCESSFUL AGING

The following information about successful aging of those with HIV is organized according to the impact various factors have on components of the model and an HIV-infected person's ability to age successfully. These factors are not mutually exclusive in their role in successful aging with HIV; an overlapping of factors in the components of the model is indeed possible and logical.

Model Component: Low Level of Disease and Disability

Premise: The lower the level of disease and disability, the better the possibility of achieving or maintaining optimal health and successful aging. Factors that can affect the level of disease and disability include:

- Comorbidities: These are the effect of diseases and other disorders an individual patient might have other than the primary disease of interest. These are conditions that do not cause HIV/AIDS and are not considered to be AIDS-defining illnesses (see Table 15.1).
- Medication issues (see Table 15.2).

Model Component: High Cognitive and Physical Functioning

Premise: The higher the level of cognitive and physical functioning such as performance of daily tasks, the ability to achieve and maintain autonomy is enhanced. Table 15.3 lists factors that can affect the level of cognitive and physical functioning.

Table 15.1

EXAMPLES OF HIV COMORBIDITIES		
Hepatitis	Pancreatitis	Coronary artery disease
Cirrhosis	Diabetes	Peripheral vascular disease
Liver failure		Hyperlipidemia
Hypertension	Stroke/TIA/MI	Renal insufficiency
Congestive heart failure	Bone disease	Renal failure
Pulmonary disease	Neuropsychiatric disorders	Non-HIV related cancer

Based on Casau, 2005; Fine & Atta, 2007; Greenbaum et al., 2008; Manfredi, 2002.

Table 15.2

EXAMPLES OF HIV MEDICATION ISSUES		
Side effects of highly active antiretroviral therapy (HAART)	Side effects of antiretroviral drugs (ART)	Compliance with treatment regimen
	Interactions of drugs and food	
Short- and long-term ART and HAART Toxicity	Interactions with underlying illnesses (examples: cardiovascular disease, liver disease, kidney disease)	Drug–drug interactions Polypharmacy

Model Component: Active Engagement in Life

Premise: As the level of active engagement in life through social and personal involvement in life events rises, the level of quality of life is enhanced. Table 15.4 includes factors that can affect active engagement in life.

Model Component: Spirituality Within a Developmental Context

Premise: As one's personal evolution of meaning and purpose in life becomes more advanced, the level of quality of life is enhanced. Factors

Table 15.3

MODEL COMPONENT: HIGH COGNITIVE AND PHYSICAL FUNCTIONING				
Comorbidities	Stress	Alcohol/sub-stance use	Nutrition	Positive or negative perception of one's own aging
Neurological change: cortical and subcortical vitality	Fatigue	General health status		

Based on Vance, 2004; Vance & Burrage, 2005, 2006a, 2006b; Vance et al., 2008b; Vance & Struzick, 2007.

Table 15.4

MODEL COMPONENT: ACTIVE ENGAGEMENT IN LIFE				
Availability of social support and number of social networks	Perceived level of stigma of HIV	Perceived level of stigma of aging	Depressive symptomatology	Perceived loneliness
Financial status	Physical appearance	Perception of declining health		

Based on Shippy & Karpiak, 2005; Vance et al., 2008b.

that affect the development of one's purpose and meaning in life and spiritual beliefs are included in Table 15.5.

CLINICAL IMPLICATIONS

Use of the model for successful aging as a guide for application of the nursing process to those aging with HIV provides a framework to apply and evaluate interventions specific to this group. Following is a brief discussion of implications for care within the context of aging and HIV infection.

To achieve and maintain a lower level of disease and disability, a careful systematic assessment for HIV comorbidities and medication

Table 15.5

MODEL COMPONENT: SPRITUALITY WITHIN A DEVELOPMENTAL CONTEXT				
Self-perception of a connection to a higher power or supreme being	Degree of internalization of spiritual or religious beliefs	Cultural/ educational background	Value of organized religion or aspects of spirituality	Engagement in institutional or organized religious activities

Based on Vance, 2006; Vance, Struzick & Raper, 2008.

issues should be conducted and appropriate interventions implemented to mitigate problems if present. Likewise, patient education about these issues is always warranted.

High cognitive and physical functioning can be supported by assessing for the presence of model factors such as stress or fatigue, alcohol or other substance use, nutritional status, comorbidities and general health status, perception of aging, and neurologic status. Appropriate interventions can then be applied as needed.

Factors affecting engagement in life should be explored with the patient and family as appropriate. In addition to usual interventions for those factors, referrals to behavioral medicine and/or social services should be considered if indicated. Factors affecting spirituality should also be assessed with careful consideration of how the patient wishes to proceed to support his or her choices and beliefs in this aspect of life.

CONCLUSION

The factors that affect successful aging—level of disease and disability, cognitive and physical functioning, engagement in life, and spirituality—can be both barriers to and facilitators of successful aging with HIV.

Barriers include:
1 Stigma and social isolation
2 Decreased cognitive and physical functioning
3 Synergistic effects with age-related comorbidity
4 Stigma from religious paradigms

Facilitators include:

1 Active engagement with life
2 Maximization of high cognitive and physical functioning
3 Prevention of disease and disability
4 Spirituality in the context of developmental processes
   (Vance, Burrage, Couch et al., 2008)

Nurses play important roles in helping older persons at risk of HIV and those living with HIV. First, nurses need to recall that older persons are sexual beings, and many maintain sexual activity well into their eighth decade and beyond. Like their younger counterparts, some older persons engage in other behaviors that may also place them at risk of HIV infection. Thus, nurses need to assess their older clients' risk of HIV infection and, when appropriate, to recommend screening or testing. Older persons with an HIV diagnosis, especially those diagnosed late in the course of the disease, may need aggressive treatment for both HIV and comorbid conditions. Because the risk of depression and suicide is considerable in older persons, even without an HIV diagnosis, the HIV-infected older adult may need to be referred to sources of support and mental health treatment; many of them may be alone or cannot turn to their families for support. Finally, because older adults with HIV tend to develop AIDS more quickly than their younger counterparts, some will need end-of-life care.

REFERENCES

Association of Nurses in AIDS Care (ANAC). (2007). *HIV/ AIDS nursing: Scope & standards of practice.* Silver Spring, MD: Nursesbooks.

Casau, N. (2005). Perspective on HIV infection and aging: Emerging research on the horizon. *Clinical Infectious Diseases, 41*(6), 855–863.

Centers for Disease Control (CDC). (2008a). *HIV/AIDS among persons aged 50 and older: CDC HIV/AIDS facts.* Retrieved March 11, 2009, from www.cdc.gov/hiv/topics/over50/resources/factsheets/pdf/over50.pdf.

Centers for Disease Control (CDC). (2008b). HIV prevalence estimates—United States, 2006. *Morbidity and Mortality Weekly Review, 57*(39), 1073–1076. Retrieved March 11, 2009, from www.cdc.gov/mmwr/preview/mmwrhtml/mm5739a2.htm.

Deeks, S., & Phillips, A. (2009). HIV infection, antiretroviral treatment, ageing, and non-AIDS related morbidity. *British Medical Journal, 338*, 3172–3181.

Fine, D., & Atta, M. (2007). Review: Kidney disease in the HIV-infected patient. *AIDS Patient Care and STDs, 21*(11), 813.

Greenbaum, A., Wilson, L., Keruly, J., Moore, R., & Gebo, K. (2008). Effect of age and HAART regimen on clinical response in an urban cohort of HIV-infected individuals. *AIDS, 22*(17), 2331–2339.

Griffith, H., Belue, K., Sicola, A., Krzywanski, S., Zamrini, E., Harrell, L., et al. (2003). Impaired financial abilities in mild cognitive impairment: A direct assessment approach. *Neurology, 60,* 449–457.

Kirton, C. (Ed.). (2003). *ANAC's core curriculum for HIV/AIDS nursing* (2nd ed.). Thousand Oaks, CA: Sage.

Manfredi, R. (2002). HIV disease and advanced age: An increasing therapeutic challenge. *Drugs & Aging, 19*(9), 647–669.

Mugavero, M., Castellano, C., Edelman, D., & Hicks, C. (2007). Late diagnosis of HIV infection: The role of age and sex. *American Journal of Medicine, 120,* 370–373.

Nichols, J. E., Speer, D. C., Watson, B. J., Watson, M., Vergon, T. L., Vallee, C. M., et al. (2002). *Aging with HIV: Psychological, social, and health issues.* San Diego, CA: Academic Press.

Oursler, K. Goulet, J., Leaf, D., Akingicil, C., Katzel, L., & Justice, A., et al. (2006) Association of comorbidity with physical disability in older HIV-infected adults. *AIDS Patient Care and STDs, 20,* 782–791.

Parker, M., Bellis, J., Bishop, P., Harper, M., Allman, R., Moore, C., et al. (2002). A multidisciplinary model of health promotion incorporating spirituality into a successful aging intervention with African American and white elderly groups. *Gerontologist, 42*(3), 406–415.

Pragna, P., Hanson, D. Sullivan, P., Novak, R., Moorman, C., Tong, T., et al. for the Adult and Adolescent Spectrum of Disease Project and HIV Outpatient Study Investigators. (2008). Incidence of types of cancer among HIV-infected persons compared with the general population in the United States, 1992–2003. *Annals of Internal Medicine, 148,* 728–736.

Shippy, R., & Karpiak, S. (2005). The aging HIV/AIDS population: Fragile social networks. *Aging & Mental Health, 9*(3), 246–254.

Stark, S. (2007). The aging face of HIV/AIDS. *American Nurse Today, 2*(6), 30–34.

Valcour, V. (2009). Lessons from CROI 2009. 16th Conference on Retroviruses and Opportunistic Infections, Montreal. Retrieved March 17, 2009, from www.natap.org/2009/CROI/croi_112.htm.

Vance, D. (2004). Cortical and subcortical dynamics of aging with HIV infection. *Perceptual and Motor Skills, 98,* 647–655.

Vance, D. (2006). Spirituality of living and aging with HIV: A pilot study. *Journal of Religion, Spirituality & Aging, 19*(1), 57–74.

Vance, D., & Burrage, J. (2005). Cognitive complaints in adults aging wit HIV: A pilot study. *Physical and Occupational Therapy in Geriatrics, 24*(2), 35–51.

Vance, D., & Burrage, J. (2006a). Chemosensory declines in older adults with HIV: Identifying interventions. *Journal of Gerontological Nursing, 32*(7), 42–48.

Vance, D., & Burrage, J. (2006b). Promoting successful cognitive aging in adults with HIV: Strategies for intervention. *Journal of Gerontological Nursing, 32*(11), 34–41.

Vance, D., Burrage, J., Couch, A., & Raper, J. (2008a). Promoting successful aging with HIV through hardiness: Implications for nursing practice and research. *Journal of Gerontological Nursing, 34*(6), 22–31.

Vance, D., Moneyham, L., Fordham, P., & Struzick. T. (2008b). A model of suicidal ideation in adults aging with HIV. *Journal of the Association of Nurses in AIDS Care, 19*(5), 375–384.

Vance, D., & Robinson, F. (2004). Reconciling successful aging with HIV: A biopsychosocial overview. *Journal of HIV/AIDS and Social Services, 3*(1), 59–78.

Vance, D., & Struzick, T. (2007). Addressing risk factors of cognitive impairment in adults aging with HIV: A social work model. *Journal of Gerontological Social Work, 49*(4), 51–77.

Vance, D., Struzick, T., & Raper, J. (2008). Biopsychosocial benefits of spirituality in adults aging with HIV: Implications for nursing practice and research. *Journal of Holistic Nursing, 26*(2), 119–127.

16

Sex Workers and Transmission of HIV

JANE DIMMITT CHAMPION

The phrase *sex work* was conceived as nonstigmatizing and inclusive language that conveys the professionalism of the sex worker rather than a lack of worth as seen by much of society. Sex workers—male, female, and transgender—offer sexually explicit services in return for money or other goods or services. Sex workers are individuals whose reasons for engaging in sex work, and for leaving it, are personally, economically, and socially contextual. Sex workers are not homogenous and include persons of all ages and sexual orientation. Sex work in many parts of the world is illegal. Sex work may be full or part time and freely chosen, coerced, or forced. As a group, persons known to engage in sex work suffer from stigmatization, discrimination, and marginalization. Worldwide, hundreds of millions of persons are believed to be clients of sex workers, although numbers vary greatly across nations and cultures (UNAIDS, 2006). In developing countries, clients of female sex workers are often men living away from home who may become HIV infected and transmit the virus to their wives or partners (Ngugi, Jackson, & Branigan, 1999).

Society has historically blamed sex workers for transmission of sexually transmitted infections (STI), including HIV. The reality, however, may be quite different, although STI and HIV rates are higher than those in the general population in many parts of the world. The inferred association between sex work and HIV is considerable. However, the incidence of HIV infection among sex workers in some parts of the world is unknown. The prevalence of safer-sex practices during commercial sex transactions is also unknown (Cote et al., 2004; Drain et al., 2004;

Epstein, 2004; Ghys, Jenkins, & Pisani, 2001; Harcourt & Donovan, 2005; Vandepitte et al., 2006). Higher rates of STIs and HIV among sex workers have been attributed to numerous factors, including poverty, low educational level, inadequate knowledge about STIs/HIV, poor work environment, limited access to health care and prevention commodities (e.g., condoms), low social status, substance abuse, abusive or violent conditions, sexual exploitation or coercion, and inadequate (or lack of) protective legislation and government polices.

Until recent years sex workers have received little attention from either public health officials or researchers. The stigma and criminality attached to sex work make reliable data hard to come by. Information about male sex workers was nonexistent in past decades. Since the advent of HIV, however, limited numbers of studies have been conducted around the world. These results do not substantiate the premise that sex work *by itself* contributes disproportionately to the spread of HIV; rather, it is the context of the lives of those who participate in sex work that contributes disproportionately to the spread of HIV.

SEX WORK AS A RISK FACTOR FOR HIV

Based on cross-country data from UNAIDS, the number of female sex workers as a percentage of the female adult population is positively correlated with countrywide HIV prevalence levels. Interestingly, confirming other studies, female illiteracy levels, gender illiteracy differences, and income inequality within countries are also significantly positively correlated with HIV/AIDS levels (Talbot, 2007). Generally, writers fail to adequately differentiate among types of sex workers. In relation to issues of health and well-being, differentiation among sex workers on the basis of specific features of their working situation (e.g., contexts, routines, relations, conditions) has hardly been studied (Vanwesenbeeck, 2001).

Sex workers who are injection drug users are more likely to be HIV positive than those who do not inject drugs (Rekart, 2006). Injection risks include sharing needles and injection equipment and being injected by someone else. Injection drug use and other substance use can also affect sexual risks by compromising safe sexual behavior and communication (Alexander, 1998). Persons who use crack cocaine are more likely to enter sex work and have large numbers of partners (Maranda, Han, & Rainone, 2004).

Surveillance within the United States in 1994 for HIV prevalence among female drug injectors found a 12.9% HIV prevalence among those involved in sex work and 14.4% among those who were not involved (Scaccabarrozzi, 2005). Women not involved in sex work were less likely to be in contact with drug treatment or helping agencies and less likely to have been tested for HIV than those engaged in sex work. Study respondents in contact with treatment agencies and those involved in commercial sex work were more likely to be aware of their HIV status. Seventy-two percent of HIV-positive women who were not sex workers were unaware of their status. These results decrease the importance of sex work as a risk factor for HIV. However, drug use among sex workers appears to be high. Sex workers in a Glasgow study were largely IV drug users (89%). Among these women, 98% indicated that they always used condoms during vaginal intercourse with sex work; only 17% always used condoms with their regular sexual partners, who were frequently drug users (Carr et al., 1996).

Transgender women are a key risk group for HIV because sex work may be the only form of employment they can find (Keatley, 2008). Epidemiologic studies have attributed high rates of HIV infection to behaviors associated with sex work in this population. A systematic review compared HIV prevalence among transgender female sex workers with prevalence among transgender women who do not engage in sex work, male sex workers, and biologically female sex workers (Operario, Soma, & Underhill, 2008). Systematic searches were made of six electronic databases, including studies that met preestablished criteria. Searches identified 25 studies with 6,405 participants recruited from 14 countries. Overall crude HIV prevalence was 27.3% in transgender female sex workers, 14.7% in transgender women not engaging in sex work, 15.1% in male sex workers, and 4.5% in female sex workers. Findings indicated that transgender female sex workers experienced higher risk for HIV infection in comparison to all other groups and particularly in comparison to female sex workers. Transgender female sex workers could benefit from targeted HIV prevention interventions, HIV testing, and interventions to help reduce the risk of contracting or transmitting HIV. Structural interventions to reduce reliance on sex work among transgender women may be warranted (Operario et al., 2008).

Rietmeijer and colleagues (1999) conducted a study to explore differences in demographic characteristics, risk practices, and preventive behaviors among subgroups of men who have sex with men (MSM), including gay- and non-gay-identified men who have sex with men, men who have sex with men who inject drugs, and those engaging in sex hustling. Men were interviewed in gay bars, bath houses, adult video arcades, and outdoor cruising areas in Denver and Long Beach. Of 1,290 men who have sex with men, 32% did not identify as gay, 7% were drug injectors, and 9% were hustlers. Of drug-injecting MSM, 55% reported sex hustling, and 40% of hustlers reported injection drug use. Hustling was associated with a higher number of partners, more frequent anal sex with men and women, and less frequent condom use during anal sex with occasional male partners. Hustlers and drug-injecting MSM used condoms less consistently during vaginal intercourse with female partners than did other MSM. Among MSM, subgroups at particularly high risk for HIV can be identified. Although these subgroups may be relatively small, they may be important epidemiologic links to the larger population of men who have sex with men and heterosexual communities and warrant focused behavioral interventions to prevent the further spread of HIV (Rietmeijer et al., 1999).

Sex workers have elevated rates of STIs, including HIV. Female, male, and transgender sex workers in San Francisco, CA, were found to have high rates of gonorrhea (12.4%), chlamydia (6.8%), syphilis (1.8%), and herpes (34.3%) (Cohan et al., 2006). Active STIs increase the likelihood of acquiring HIV. Genital trauma caused by frequent or forced intercourse also increases HIV risk (Rekart, 2006).

African American women have high rates of most STIs, including HIV. A study in central Brooklyn, New York, conducted by Miller and colleagues (2008) found that among 228 black women who used drugs, 17% tested HIV seropositive, and the incidence of other STIs was herpes simplex virus-2 (79%), trichomoniasis (37%), chlamydia (11%), and gonorrhea (2%). Few women knew themselves to be infected with STIs other than HIV. HIV-infected women were more likely than uninfected women to have multiple STIs. Women reported having both lower- and higher-risk sex partners. HIV-infected women were twice as likely as uninfected woman to report current sex work, the only difference in sex risk. Crack cocaine use was uniquely associated with multiple positive STI screens, excluding HIV. These results strongly suggest that individuals with multiple STIs may unknowingly, but efficiently, contribute to high STI and HIV rates (Miller et al., 2008).

Condom use had been posited to reduce the risk of HIV acquisition. A sex worker's decision and ability to use condoms is a complex one that depends on many factors (McMahon et al., 2006; Roxburgh et al., 2005). Negotiating safer sex can be affected by money if business is slow or clients offer more money for unprotected sex. Sex workers may use drugs before or with clients, which affects decision making and ability to use condoms. Sex workers may also be targeted by police if they are carrying condoms (Alexander, 1998). Sex workers, like many people, may choose not to use condoms with their boyfriends, girlfriends, or spouses (Wechsberg et al., 2008).

Violence, and the trauma associated with it, is a concern for many sex workers. Violence can include physical, sexual, and verbal abuse that sex workers experience from their clients and intimate partners. It can also include the violence many street-based sex workers witness daily. Clients may use violence to enforce unsafe sex. A history of violence leaves many sex workers with emotional trauma, and many may turn to drug use to deal with the harsh realities of their daily lives (Romero-Daza, Weeks, & Singer, 2003). Childhood maltreatment has been associated with sex work and HIV in adulthood. A study of physically and sexually abused and neglected children (ages 0 through 11 years) with documented cases from 1967 to 1971 were followed into adulthood. Assessments for sex work were made through in-person interviews and official records of 1,196 participants at the age of approximately 29 years. HIV tests were conducted on 631 participants at the age of approximately 41 years. A history of child maltreatment was associated with sex work. The prevalence of HIV among abused and neglected children was twice that of controls. These findings provide prospective evidence that maltreated children are more likely to engage in sex work by young adulthood and test positive for HIV in middle adulthood (Wilson & Widom, 2008).

INTERNATIONAL RESEARCH ON SEX WORK AND HIV

The incidence of HIV among sex workers is by and large about the same as among the population as a whole, except in Africa. This is true even within developing countries, although the incidence does vary geographically. Among populations or within geographical areas in which HIV has not been specifically studied, researchers often use other STIs as surrogates for HIV to help them gauge the incidence of infection. Evidence exists that high rates of STI incidence are often linked to high HIV incidence rates (Shain et al., 2004). Sex workers typically have high rates of hepatitis C, gonorrhea, Chlamydia, and *Treponema pallidum,* a reminder that there are other STIs besides HIV to which sex workers and their customers may be vulnerable. This increased vulnerability also indicates that concerns should not be focused on stigmatizing the issue of HIV with sex workers but rather on implementing public health programs to provide education and access to care for HIV and STIs for all persons engaging in high-risk behaviors.

Commercial sex plays a critical role in the heterosexual transmission of HIV in China. Existing studies (1990 to 2006) indicate that female sex workers in China are young and mobile, and most have both commercial and noncommercial sex partners; they have low rates of consistent condom use and high rates of STI infection. Some female sex workers are also engaged in drug abuse. Great variation in sexual practices and HIV risks has been found among female sex workers across different work settings (Hong & Li, 2008).

A cross-sectional survey was conducted from October 2000 to January 2001 among female commercial sex workers in Zhengzhou, China, to estimate rates of HIV infection and STIs and to document the workers' sexual behavior patterns. Female sex workers were recruited by the snowball sampling technique and were interviewed anonymously in their working environments. HIV prevalence among the 621 sex workers interviewed was 1.4% for direct and 0.2% indirect contact. A history of STI was reported by 49% of the sex workers. Most sex workers (87%) reported inconsistent condom use. Ten percent of them recognized their clients as drug users. A few sex workers (2.2%) were injection drug users. Inconsistent use of condoms and a high level of STDs underscored the urgent need to implement intervention strategies and condom promotion, particularly among direct sex workers in China (Ding et al., 2005).

Men having sex with men now account for 7% of all HIV cases in China, and there is growing awareness that internal rural-to-urban migration might shift the HIV epidemic within China by broadening social and sexual mixing. About 70% of HIV infections are among rural residents, of whom 80% are males and 60% aged 16 through 29. This young, male, rural-to-urban migrant population has been identified as the "tipping point" for the AIDS epidemic in China. A subgroup of these migrants is the "money boy" population, i.e., those who engage in same-sex transactional sex for economic survival. Wong and associates (2008) conducted a study to elucidate factors for preventing substance abuse and HIV among two types of money boys—"gay-identified" and "non–gay-identified"—living in the Shanghai metropolitan area. The authors found gay and nongay money boys shared similar patterns of substance use and low HIV knowledge. However, sexual orientation differentially predicted HIV testing, with gay money boys more likely to be tested for HIV. Nongay money boys showed fewer sexual risks. HIV prevention targeting money boys within China was recommended, as were outreach strategies most effective for particular subgroups of men who have sex with men.

According to UNAIDS (2006), 4 million people, including 1.2 million children under 18 years of age, may be trafficked within their own countries or across international borders. While few data on HIV seroprevalence are available for these trafficked persons, their risk of STI/HIV infection is high because of their lack of power to negotiate condom use, their multiple partners, and their risk of being victims of violence. Young women and girls in Asia who are trafficked for sex work are emerging as an HIV risk factor, according to a report released by the United Nations at the 8th International Congress on AIDS in Asia and the Pacific (Trafficking of girls, 2007). The report, entitled "Human Trafficking and HIV," focused on the estimated 150,000 to 200,000 people from South Asia trafficked and forced into labor annually, usually as sex workers. The report examined the intersection between HIV and trafficking in Afghanistan, Bangladesh, India, Nepal, Pakistan, and Sri Lanka. According to the AP/PR-Inside.com report, this number represents only 50% of the people who are trafficked in all of Asia. Although there are few reliable statistics about HIV among trafficked people, one study estimated that 25% of trafficked women in Mumbai, India, are HIV positive. Another study found 60% to 70% of 218 trafficked sex workers from Nepal who were later rescued in Mumbai were HIV positive. The increase in the number of infrastructure projects across the region, as well as the sex work that accompanies project workers, had the potential to further spread HIV across the Asia-Pacific region (Trafficking of girls, 2007).

The incidence of HIV in Europe is low among the population as a whole as well as among sex workers. As is typical worldwide, the incidence of HIV rises among populations in which intravenous drug use exists. For example, sex workers in Vienna who were found to be HIV positive reported that they were IV drug users or had sexual partners who were (Stary et al., 1992). Sex workers in Seville, Spain, who used intravenous drugs were eight times as likely to be HIV positive as were those who used nonintravenous drugs (Soriano et al., 1992). Sex work in the Netherlands is legal and regulated, and drug use is largely approached from a public health rather than a criminal perspective. Both non-IV-drug-using female sex workers and their male clients in the Netherlands were found to have an extremely low incidence of HIV. HIV incidence was concentrated among sex workers who were recent immigrants from AIDS-endemic countries.

Other results from the Netherlands include a study of non-IV-drug-using female sex workers in Amsterdam. These sex workers reported no HIV infection and consistent condom use. Contrarily, a group of transgender Dutch sex workers with a fairly high incidence of HIV reported not using condoms during receptive anal sex (van Veen et al., 2008). Findings from a study in Glasgow identified low HIV rates, even among IV drug users (Hart et al., 1999). Almost 75% of female sex workers in Glasgow injected drugs. All of the HIV-positive sex workers studied were found to be IV drug users.

Male sex workers in Sydney were interviewed to assess prevalence of HIV and STI and risk behavior. Estcourt and colleagues (2000) conducted a retrospective review of medical records of patients attending public STI and HIV clinic in Sydney from 1991 until 1998. Although male sex workers used condoms with clients, they were more likely to practice unsafe sex with non–work partners (especially women) and inject drugs than were female sex workers and non–sex worker homosexual men. Men with HIV were working within the commercial sex industry. The authors recommended targeting health education to encourage safer drug use and safer sex outside work.

Information is limited on HIV among sex workers in North and South America. One large-scale study in South America included 960 female Peruvian sex workers over a three-year period. This study was conducted in the early 1990s and showed HIV infection (0.3%). Interestingly, a much higher incidence of hepatitis B and C was found. The hepatitis B antibody was found in 59.8% of sex workers, while 0.7% had hepatitis C antibodies (Hyams et al., 1993). Bautista and colleagues (2006) conducted cross-sectional studies of 13, 600 female commercial sex workers in nine South American countries from 1999 to 2002 and concluded "consistently low HIV seroprevalences were detected among female commercial sex workers in South America, particularly in the Andean region" (p. 311). They also found that predictors of HIV infection across the continent were sexually transmitted diseases and length of commercial sex work. Use of illegal drugs and sexual contacts with foreigners were also found to be associated risk factors in the Southern Cone region. They recommended that interventions for the control of HIV and other STIs be region and country specific.

HIV prevalence is increasing among female sex workers in Tijuana and Ciudad Juarez, two Mexican cities on the U.S. border. Quasi-legal sex work in both cities attracts large numbers of sex tourists. Strathdee et al. (2008) assessed HIV prevalence among 924 female sex workers, 69% of whom had U.S. clients. The prevalences of HIV (6%) and any STI (27%) were high. Female sex workers with U.S. clients were more likely to have HIV (30% versus 20%) or a current STI and to engage in higher-risk behaviors. Findings indicated that intensified binational prevention efforts involving both female sex workers and their clients are urgently needed (Strathdee et al., 2008).

There are relatively limited data on sex workers in the United States, in part because of government refusal and private reluctance to recognize this population. U.S. Sex workers may be at risk for HIV depending on the conditions of their workplace. Male, female, and transgender sex workers who are most vulnerable to HIV are street-based workers, most of whom are poor or homeless and likely to have had a history of sexual or physical abuse (Rekart, 2006). Street-based sex workers are also commonly dependent on drugs or alcohol and at a greater risk for violence from clients and police (Vanwesenbeeck, 2001). Sex work off the street (i.e., in brothels, massage parlors, private homes, or escort services) is less likely to result in HIV infection for the workers because they may exercise greater control over their working conditions and sexual transactions, including condom use.

Few studies have been done on rates of HIV infection among street-based sex workers across the United States. In one study of drug-using female sex workers in Miami, Florida, 22.4% of the women tested HIV positive (Inciardi, Surratt, & Kurtz, 2006). In a study of male sex workers in Houston, TX, 26% reported testing HIV positive (Timpson et al., 2007). Bacon and colleagues (2006) conducted a study in California from January 2000 through November 2001 to learn about the relationship between sex work and HIV infection among young injection drug-using MSM. Sixty-eight percent of participants reported being paid by another man for sex. HIV prevalence was 12%, with 42% of seropositive participants being unaware of their infection. HIV was independently associated with a higher number of paying male partners and history of gonorrhea and inversely associated with the number of female partners, education, and syringe sharing. Consistent condom use overall was 41%, but it varied significantly by type of partner. The researchers concluded that among young injection drug-using men who have sex with men in San Francisco, sex work with men is strongly associated with HIV infection and the prevalence of condom use is low. The recommendation was made to tailor HIV prevention among this group to address the increased risk associated with sex work (Bacon et al., 2006).

Male sex workers and travesti and transgender and transsexual sex workers are among the groups most affected by HIV. They suffer from stigma and discrimination, yet are often absent from the design of educational programs and HIV prevention campaigns. Infante, Sosa-Rubi, and Cuadra (2009) conducted a study in Mexico City to provide an account of the social context in which male sex workers and travesti and transgender and transsexual sex workers function by focusing on their sexual identities, sexual practices, and vulnerability to HIV. Findings revealed a differentiation of vulnerability by subgroup. In general, vulnerability was influenced by the social context and stigma related to homosexuality and sex work, as well as sex workers' access to scarce social capital and the lack of response in terms of social and health programs. The authors suggested that, to diminish the vulnerability of male sex workers and travesti and of transgender and transsexual sex workers and to reduce their risk of HIV infection, preventive measures are needed that take into account their specific health and social needs, that promote meaningful participation, and that encourage respect for human rights (Infante et al., 2009).

Africa is the global center of the HIV epidemic. Epidemiological research in Africa was scarce in the past, particularly with regard to sex workers. Studies conducted early in the 1990s found high and increasing incidence of HIV among female sex workers in Cameroon. Early speculation that HIV might be confined to discrete areas of the continent was rejected in the late 1980s when the infection rate among sex workers in Djibouti escalated. Early on, in 1987, Djibouti sex workers had only a 2% HIV-positive rate, an incidence much lower than that reported in any Eastern African country. Unfortunately, a follow-up study in the early 1990s found HIV infection rates as 6% among street sex workers and 15.3% among sex workers working as bar hostesses.

A recent study by Leclerc and Garenne (2008) compared the association between using the services of sex workers and male HIV seroprevalence in five African countries--Ghana, Kenya, Lesotho, Malawi, and Rwanda. The HIV seroprevalence among men who "ever paid for sex" was compared with men who "never paid for sex." Results were based on 12,929 men, aged 15 to 59 years. The odds ratio of HIV seroprevalence associated with ever-paying for sex was 1.89, with only minor differences by country. These results match previous observations that commercial sex seems to play a minor role in the spread of HIV in mature epidemics (Leclerc & Garenne, 2008).

To identify social and behavioral characteristics associated with sexual risk behaviors among male sex workers who sell sex to men in Mombasa, Kenya, 425 men who had recently sold and were currently willing to sell sex to men were surveyed (Geibel et al., 2008). The researchers identified factors associated with self-reported unprotected anal sex with male clients in the past 30 days. Thirty-five percent of respondents did not know that HIV can be transmitted via anal sex, which was a significant predictor of unprotected anal sex. Other associated factors included drinking alcohol three or more days per week, self-report of burning urination within the past 12 months, and having never been counseled or tested for HIV. Only 21.2% of respondents correctly knew that a water-based lubricant should be used with latex condoms. These results found that male sex workers who sell sex to men in Mombasa are in acute need of targeted prevention information on anal HIV and STI transmission, consistent condom use, and correct lubrication use with latex condoms. Recommendations were made for HIV programs in Africa to consider and develop specific prevention strategies to reach this vulnerable population (Geibel et al., 2008).

Sex work can be contextualized by violence, social and material inequality, and HIV vulnerability. Simić and Rhodes (2008) conducted a qualitative study in Belgrade and Pancevo, Serbia, to explore 31 female and transvestite sex workers' accounts of the HIV risk environment. These researchers identified violence as a key theme and emphasized the ubiquity of multiple forms of everyday violence, including physical, emotional, and social, in street sex work scenes, linked to police as much as clients. Findings emphasized how the risk of violence in street sex work reflects institutionalized social inequalities and injustices. Sex workers were inevitably participants in the cycle of symbolic violence they sought to resist. The challenges for HIV prevention are, therefore, considerable, and require interventions that not only seek to foster safer microenvironments of sex work but structural changes in the welfare, criminal justice, and other social institutions that reproduce the cycle of violence faced by sex workers day to day (Simić & Rhodes, 2008).

SEX WORKER CLIENTS AT RISK OF CONTRACTING HIV

A history of STIs clearly correlates with HIV incidence. Men with STIs have a high risk of acquiring HIV from sex workers. The high rates of

HIV and STI among sex workers have created international concern that male clients may constitute a critical bridge population for HIV and STI transmission. Decker and colleagues (2008) analyzed a U.S. community-based survey of 1,515 men aged 18 to 35 years attending urban health centers to assess the prevalence of engagement in sex purchasing during the past year and to evaluate relations with self-reported HIV and STI diagnosis and symptoms across this same period. They found that more than 1 in 12 (8.7%) men reported exchanging drugs, money, or a place to stay for sex with a female partner in the past year. This behavior was associated with additional sexual risk taking and predicted a self-report diagnosis of HIV, STI, or symptoms. Sex purchasing was a common form of HIV and STI risk among the population sampled. Men engaging in such behavior were more likely to be HIV or STI infected, thereby representing a risk to the sexual health of sex work and non–sex work partners. The authors recommended interventions targeted toward male clients of female sex workers (Decker et al., 2008).

Day, Ward, and Perrotta (1993) conducted a study to describe risk behaviors for infection with HIV in male sexual partners of female sex workers in London, England. Self-identified male sexual partners of female sex workers reported risk behaviors for infection with HIV. The researchers found that, among those who paid for sex, 34% had also had sex with other men, 43% reportedly paid for sex abroad, and 9% said that they had also been paid for sex. The majority (82%) said that they had always used a condom. In contrast, only 18% of nonpaying partners of sex workers reported ever using a condom with their partners. These findings indicated that men who have sex with female sex workers cannot be assumed to be at risk of infection with HIV only by this route—*sexual* contact with men may place them at greater risk. Despite the heterogeneity among male sexual partners of sex workers, patterns of use of condoms were uniform when they were considered as a reflection of the type of relationship a man had with a female sex worker rather than a consequence of an individual's level of risk (Day et al., 1993).

Many behavioral studies of men fail to differentiate between those who have sex exclusively with men and those who have sex with both men and women. Wheeler and colleagues (2008) conducted a study in New York City and Philadelphia among 1,154 black men who have sex exclusively with men and those who have sex with both men and women. The strongest correlate of either insertive or receptive unprotected anal insertive sex among both groups of men was engaging in sex exchange. These findings highlighted the need for specific HIV prevention interventions targeting men who have sex exclusively with men as distinctive from those who have sex with both men and women (Wheeler et al., 2008).

PREVENTION OF HIV IN SEX WORKERS

Because sex workers may be bridge for HIV infection to the larger population in some parts of the world, targeted interventions to reduce HIV infection in sex workers and to prevent transmission of HIV and STIs to their clients are urgently needed. Most prevention interventions reflect a three-tiered effort to prevent HIV infection in sex workers: preventing entry into sex work, protecting those involved in sex work, and helping sex workers leave sex work. However, in many countries where sex work is viewed highly negatively, ideological opposition has prevented the full implementation of prevention programs aimed at sex workers. The UNAIDS Inter-Agency Task Team on Gender and HIVAIDS (2005) has reported that prevention efforts in various parts of the world have "provided evidence that targeted, comprehensive HIV prevention programmes combining STI treatment, condom promotion and provision, and prevention education interventions delivered through outreach, peer education, and sex worker empowerment approaches have made sex work safer" (p. 3). These prevention interventions have included free distribution or promotion of condoms; provision of health services, especially to treat STIs; discussion groups or classroom-based HIV and sexual health education; networking to promote better laws, working conditions, and health services for sex workers; dissemination of information through printed materials and street theater; and economic development programs for sex workers seeking other types of employment (UNAIDS, 2005, 2006). Efforts aimed at preventing HIV in sex workers include the following examples (Ngugi et al., 1999; UNAIDS, 2005, 2006):

- Interventions taking place in a variety of settings, including bars, clubs, brothels, the street, truck stops, and prisons;
- Targeted interventions that also deal with drug addiction;
- Provision of free condoms, including female condoms, to clients and sex workers;
- Provision of free STI/HIV screening, testing, and treatment;
- Contact tracing and contact treatment;
- Mass media campaigns for sex worker clients;

- Interventions directed toward the male clients of female sex workers;
- Emphasis on the power of sex workers to help stop the spread of HIV through the promotion of condom use with clients; and
- Engagement of sex workers in policy and program development and implementation as part of the overall empowerment-building process and for greater program effectiveness.

Other interventions have been developed to prevent violence against sex workers (International HIV/AIDS Alliance, 2008; WHO, 2005), including individual-based, group-based, and community-based strategies.

CONCLUSION

Since the emergence of the HIV epidemic, sex workers have been associated, if not blamed, for the transmission of HIV. While sex workers have higher rates of STIs and HIV in many parts of the world, the true incidence of these infections among sex workers is not fully known in all parts of the world. Efforts to reduce HIV infection, especially in resource-limited nations where "HIV infection has become almost a daily fact of life for almost all CSWs [commercial sex workers]" (Ngugi et al., 1999), are particularly critical. Prevention activities need to be provided at the individual, group, and community levels. Prevention interventions for sex workers must be culturally sensitive and provided by knowledgeable and nonjudgmental peers and experts if they are to be successful. These interventions need to be supported by both national and international organizations and governments and sustained over time. In addition to prevention interventions, STI/HIV-infected sex workers need early medical and other interventions that will not only improve their lives but reduce the risk that they will transmit STIs/HIV to other persons. Finally, leaders in government and nongovernment organizations need to work together to develop policies and laws that seek to balance the human rights of sex workers with larger societal concerns and cultural norms.

REFERENCES

Alexander, P. (1998). Sex work and health: A question of safety in the workplace. *Journal of the American Medical Women's Association, 53,* 77–82.

Bacon, O., Lum, P., Hahn, J., Evans, J., Davidson, P., Moss, A., et al. (2006). Commercial sex work and risk of HIV infection among young drug-injecting men who have sex with men in San Francisco. *Sexually Transmitted Diseases, 33*, 228–34.

Bautista, C., Sanchez, J., Montano, S., Laguna-Torres, A., Suarez, L., Sanchez, J., et al. (2006). Seroprevalence of and risk factors for HIV-1 infection among female commercial sex workers in South America. *Sexually Transmitted Infections, 82*, 311–316.

Carr, S., Goldberg, D. J., Elliott, L., Green, S., Mackie, C., & Gruer, L. (1996). A primary health care service for Glasgow street sex workers—6 years experience of the "drop-in centre," 1989–1994. *AIDS Care, 8*(4), 489–497.

Cohan, D., Lutnick, A., Davidson, P., Cloniger, C., Herlyn, A., Breyer, J., et al. (2006). Sex worker health: San Francisco style. *Sexually Transmitted Infections, 82*, 418–422.

Cote, A., Sobela, F., Dzokoto, A., Nzambi, K., Asamoah-Adu, C., Labbe, A., et al. (2004). Transactional sex is the driving force in the dynamics of HIV in Accra, Ghana. *AIDS, 18*, 917–925.

Day, S., Ward, H., & Perrotta, L. (1993). Prostitution and risk of HIV: Male partners of female prostitutes. *British Medical Journal, 307*, 359–361.

Decker, M. R., Raj, A., Gupta, J., & Silverman, J. G. (2008). Sex purchasing and associations with HIV/STI among a clinic-based sample of US men. *Journal of Acquired Immune Deficiency Syndrome, 4*(3), 355–359.

Ding, Y., Detels, R., Zhao, Z., Zhu, Y., Zhu, G., Zhang, B., et al. (2005). HIV infection and sexually transmitted diseases in female commercial sex workers in China. *Journal of Acquired Immune Deficiency Syndrome, 38*(3), 314–319.

Drain, P. K., Smith, J. S., Hughes, J. P., Halperin, D. T., & Holmes, K. K. (2004). Correlates of national HIV seroprevalence. An ecologic analysis of 122 developing countries. *Journal of Acquired Immune Deficiency Syndrome, 35*(4), 407–420.

Epstein, H. (2004, June 13). The fidelity fix. *New York Times Magazine*, 54–59.

Estcourt, C. S., Marks, C., Rohrsheim, R., Johnson, A. M., Donovan, B., & Mindel, A. (2000). HIV, sexually transmitted infections, and risk behaviours in male commercial sex workers in Sydney. *Sexually Transmitted Infections, 76*, 294–298.

Geibel, S., Luchters, S., King'Ola, N., Esu-Williams, E., Rinyiru, A., & Tun, W. (2008). Factors associated with self-reported unprotected anal sex among male sex workers in Mombasa, Kenya. *Sexually Transmitted Diseases, 35,* 746–752.

Ghys, P., Jenkins, C., & Pisani, E. (2001). HIV surveillance among female sex workers. *AIDS, 15* (Suppl. 3), S33–S40.

Harcourt, C., & Donovan, B. (2005). The many faces of sex work. *Sexually Transmitted Infections, 81,* 201–206.

Hart, G. J., Flowers, P., Der, G. J., & Frankis, J. S. (1999). Homosexual men's HIV related sexual risk behaviour in Scotland. *Sexually Transmitted Infections, 75,* 242–246.

Hong, Y., & Li, X. (2008). Behavioral studies of female sex workers in China: A literature review and recommendation for future research. *AIDS Behavior, 12,* 623–636.

Hyams, K. C., Phillips, I. A., Tejada, A., Wignall, F. S., Roberts, C. R., & Escamilla, J. (1993). Three-year incidence study of retroviral and viral hepatitis transmission in a Peruvian prostitute population. *Journal of Acquired Immune Deficiency Syndrome, 6,* 1353–1357.

Inciardi, J. A., Surratt, H. L., & Kurtz, S. P. (2006). HIV, HBV, and HCV infections among drug-involved, inner-city, street sex workers in Miami, Florida. *AIDS and Behavior, 10,* 139–147.

Infante, C., Sosa-Rubi, S. G., & Cuadra, S. M. (2009). Sex work in Mexico: Vulnerability of male, travesti, transgender and transsexual sex workers. *Culture Health and Sexuality, 12,* 1–12.

International HIV/AIDS Alliance. (2008). *Sex work, violence, and HIV.* Hove, U.K.: Author. Retrieved on February 3, 2009, from www.aidsalliance.org/graphics/secretariat/publications/Sex_%20work_violence_and_HIV.pdf.

Keatley, J. (2008, August 3–8). *Transgender global HIV/AIDS epidemiology.* Paper presented at the XVII International AIDS Conference, Mexico City. PowerPoint slides retrieved February 4, 2009, from http://74.125.95.132/search?q=cache:_mWNo7PU1Y4J:www.caps.ucsf.edu/pubs/presentations/pdf/KeatleyIAC2008.pdf+van+Veen+HIV+and+sexual+risk+behavior+among+commercial+sex+workers+in+the+Netherlands.+Archives+of+Sexual+Behavior&hl=en&ct=clnk&cd=3&gl=us.

Leclerc, P. M., & Garenne, M. (2008). Commercial sex and HIV transmission in mature epidemics: A study of five African countries. *International Journal of STD & AIDS, 19,* 660–664.

Maranda, M. J., Han, C., & Rainone, G. A. (2004). Crack cocaine and sex. *Journal of Psychoactive Drugs, 36*(3), 315–322.

McMahon, J. M., Tortu, S., Pouget, E. R., Hamid, R., & Neaigus, A. (2006). Contextual determinants of condom use among female sex exchangers in East Harlem, NYC: An event analysis. *AIDS and Behavior, 10*(6), 731–741.

Miller, M., Liao, Y., Wagner, M., & Korves, C. (2008). HIV, the clustering of sexually transmitted infections, and sex risk among African American women who use drugs. *Sexually Transmitted Diseases, 35*(7), 696–702.

Ngugi, E., Jackson, E., & Branigan, D. (1999). Interventions for commercial sex workers and their clients. In L. Gibney, R. DiClemente, & Sten H. Vermund (eds.). *Preventing HIV in developing countries: Biomedical and behavioral approaches* (pp. 205–228). New York: Springer.

Operario, D., Soma, T., & Underhill, K. (2008). Sex work and HIV status among transgender women: Systematic review and meta-analysis. *Journal of Acquired Immune Deficiency Syndrome, 48*(1), 97–103.

Rekart, M. L. (2006). Sex-work harm reduction. *The Lancet, 366,* 2123–2134.

Rietmeijer, C. A., Wolitski, R. J., Fishbein, M., Corby, N. H., & Cohn, D. L. (1999). Sex hustling, injection drug use, and non-gay identification by men who have sex with men. Associations with high-risk sexual behaviors and condom use. *Sexually Transmitted Diseases, 26*(2), 93–94.

Romero-Daza, N., Weeks, M., & Singer, M. (2003). "Nobody gives a damn if I live or die": Violence, drugs, and street-level prostitution in inner-city Hartford, Connecticut. *Medical Anthropology, 22,* 233–259.

Roxburgh, A., Degenhardt, L., Larance, B., & Copeland, J. (2005). *Mental health, drug use and risk among street-based sex workers in greater Sydney* (NDARC Technical Report No. 237). Sydney: National Drug and Alcohol Research Centre, University of New South Wales.

Scaccabarrozzi L. (2005). Sex workers and HIV: What is the real story. *AIDS Community Research Initiative of America 15,* 1–5.

Shain, R. N., Piper, J. M., Holden, A. E. C., Champion, J. D., Perdue, S. T., Korte, J. E., et al. (2004). Prevention of gonorrhea and Chlamydia through behavioral intervention: Results of a two-year controlled randomized trial in minority women. *STD, 31,* 401–408.

Simić, M., & Rhodes, T. (2008). Violence, dignity and HIV vulnerability: Street sex work in Serbia. *Sociology of Health and Illness, 31,* 1–16.

Soriano, V., Aguado, I., Fernández, J. L., Granada, I., Pineda, J. A., Valls, F., et al. (1992). Multicenter study of the prevalence of type 2 human immunodeficiency virus infection in Spain (1990). Medicina Clinica (Barcelona), 98, 771–774. (In Spanish)

Stary, A., Kopp, W., Hofmann, H., Heller-Vitouch, C., & Kunz, C. (1992). Seroepidemiologic study of hepatitis C virus in sexually transmitted disease risk groups. *Sexually Transmitted Diseases, 19,* 252–258.

Strathdee, S. A., Lozada, R, Semple, S. J., Orozovich, P., Pu, M., Staines-Orozco, H., et al. (2008). Characteristics of female sex workers with US clients in two Mexico-US border cities. *Sexually Transmitted Diseases, 35,* 263–268.

Talbott, J. R. (2007). Size matters: The number of prostitutes and the global HIV/AIDS pandemic. *PLoS ONE, 2*(6), e543. Retrieved February 4, 2009, from www.plosone.org/article/info:doi/10.1371/journal. pone.0000543.

Timpson, S. C., Ross, M. W., Williams, M. L., & Atkinson, J. (2007). Characteristics, drug use, and sex partners of a sample of male sex workers. *The American Journal of Drug and Alcohol Abuse, 33,* 63–69.

Trafficking of girls, women in Asia for commercial sex work emerging as HIV/AIDS risk factor, report says. (2007, August 24). *Kaiser Daily HIV/AIDS Report.* Retrieved February 2, 2009, from www.kaiser network.org/Daily_Reports/print_report.cfm?DR_ID=47086&dr_cat=1.

UNAIDS Inter-Agency Task Team on Gender and HIV/AIDS. (2005). *Operational guide on gender: HIV/AIDS: A rights-based approach. Amsterdam: KIT Publishers.* Retrieved June 2009 from http://www. genderandaids.org/downloads/events/Operational%20Guide.pdf.

UNAIDS (Joint United Nation Programme on HIV/AIDS). (2006). *At risk and neglected: Sex workers: Report on the global AIDS epidemic.* Geneva: Author. Retrieved February 3, 2009, from http://data.unaids. org/pub/GlobalReport/2006/2006_GR_CH05_en.pdf.

van Veen, M. G., Götz, H. M., van Leeuwen, P. A., Prins, M., & van de Laar, M. J. (2008, September 25). HIV and sexual risk behavior among commercial sex workers in the Netherlands. *Archives of Sexual Behavior* [Epub ahead of print]. Retrieved March 9, 2009, from www.rivm.nl/cib/binaries/van%20Veen_2008_ArchSexBehav_tcm92-56921.pdf.

Vandepitte, J., Lyerla, R., Dallabetta, G., Crabbé, F., Alary, M., & Buvé, A. (2006). Estimates of the number of female sex workers in different regions of the world. *Sexually Transmitted Infections, 82*(Suppl. III), iii18–iii25.

Vanwesenbeeck, I. (2001). Another decade of social scientific work on sex work: A review of research 1990–2000. *Annual Review of Sexuality Research, 12,* 242–289.

Wechsberg, W. M., Luseno, W., Riehman, K., Karg, R., Browne, F., & Parry, C. (2008). Substance use and sexual risk within the context of gender inequality in South Africa. *Substance Use & Misuse, 43,* 1186–1201.

Wheeler, D. P., Lauby, J. L., Liu, K. L., Van Sluytman, L. G., & Murrill, C. (2008). A comparative analysis of sexual risk characteristics of black men who have sex with men or with men and women. *Archives of Sexual Behavior, 37,* 697–707.

Wilson, H. W., & Widom, C. S. (2008). An examination of risky sexual behavior and HIV in victims of child abuse and neglect: A 30-year follow-up. *Health Psychology, 27,* 149–158.

Wong, F. Y., Huang, Z. J., He, N., Smith, B. D., Ding, Y., Fu, C., et al. (2008). HIV risks among gay- and non-gay-identified migrant money boys in Shanghai, China. *AIDS Care, 20,* 170–180.

World Health Organization (WHO). (2005). *Violence against women and HIV/AIDS: Critical intersections.* Geneva: Author. Retrieved February 3, 2009, from   www.who.int/gender/documents/sexworkers.pdf.

17

HIV in Corrections: Care of Incarcerated and Formerly Incarcerated Persons

JACQUELINE C. ZALUMAS

Engaging and retaining incarcerated and formerly incarcerated HIV-positive individuals in care presents special barriers and challenges. This chapter will review the care of HIV positive incarcerated or formerly incarcerated individuals in the United States. The chapter will provide an overview of HIV in corrections facilities, present characteristics of inmate populations, and discuss health care issues relative to incarcerated and formerly incarcerated populations. The role of nurses in corrections and community settings will be emphasized.

At the end of 2004, 9.2 million people were living under the jurisdiction of this country's justice system (Harrison & Beck, 2005; Kantor, 2006). Nearly 2.3 million inmates (including one in every 100 adults) were held in U.S. prisons and jails at midyear 2007, the highest rate of incarceration in the world (Pew Center on the States, 2008; Sabol & Couture, 2008; Sabol & Minton, 2008). Over the course of a year, 13.5 million persons will spend some time in of this nation's 5,000 adult prisons or jails (Vera Institute of Justice, 2006).

Individuals who are incarcerated in U.S. prisons and jails, and those formerly incarcerated and living back in the community, generally have higher rates of HIV and other infectious diseases (e.g., tuberculosis and hepatitis C), substance abuse and mental health issues, and chronic health problems than those in the general population. Rates of hepatitis C virus (HCV) are nine to ten times higher among inmates than in the general population, while estimated prevalence of HIV infection is nearly five times higher for incarcerated populations (2%) than for the

539

general U.S. population (0.43%) (Maruschak, 2005; Weinbaum, Lyerla, & Margolis, 2003). According to a study of 2003 data released in 2005 by the Department of Justice Statistics, 1.8% of men and 2.6% of women in federal and state prisons are HIV positive (Maruschak, 2005). States with the highest percentage of inmates in state and federal prisons who are HIV positive include New York (6.3%), Florida (4.1%), and Maryland (2.7%) (Maruschak, 2008). Female inmates, who account for less than 10% of the prison population, have a higher HIV antibody seroprevalence than male prisoners (Maruschak, 2005). Prisoners who are seronegative for HIV at the point of their entry into the prison system may become infected while incarcerated because of consensual or nonconsensual male–male sexual activity, intravenous drug use, and tattooing (CDC, 2006; Horsburgh et al., 1990; Kantor, 2006).

Policies regarding voluntary and mandatory testing in prisons vary widely across the nation. According to Beckwith and Poshkus (2007), "Correctional testing policies include (1) mandatory upon entrance or exit; (2) routinely offered, but not mandatory; (3) voluntary, upon request by an inmate; (4) performed when clinically indicated, as deemed by the correctional medical staff; and (5) ordered by the court." In 1999, 19 states had laws requiring that all prison inmates to receive an HIV test on entry into jail (CDC, 2001). Some states and the Federal Bureau of Prisons test inmates if they have HIV-related symptoms; some states test inmates after they've been in a fight; fewer then 20 states test inmates who are members of high-risk groups (e.g., injection drug users, those with a sexually transmitted disease or hepatitis); a few states test inmates at the time of release from prison; and a small number of states test inmates randomly. Various organizations, including the American Public Health Association and WHO, have opposed mandatory HIV testing of prisoners because of difficulty in maintaining the confidentiality of test results and the potential segregation and stigmatization of those testing HIV positive, among other concerns. Instead, many of these organizations support offering prisoners routine screening for HIV infection, with the opportunity to opt out of such screening.

Providing competent health care for incarcerated persons presents many challenges rooted in the characteristics of corrections settings and inmate populations, the complexity of treatment regimens for HIV and AIDS, uneven distribution of resources, and the movement of inmate populations within corrections systems. Further, prevention education, testing, and resources to protect immunosuppressed individuals from contracting other infectious diseases (e.g., tuberculosis or hepatitis) while incarcerated are challenges in corrections settings. Most U.S. prisons, for example, do not provide inmates with condoms (a common practice in prisons in other parts of the world), even though the WHO (2007) concluded that condom distribution "is feasible in a wide range of prison settings" (p. 14). The health status of inmates presents both a significant public health risk and an opportunity because most incarcerated individuals will return to the community. Many releasees will be reincarcerated several times, especially in jail settings, which have rapid turnover of "unknown" individuals. Almost one-fourth of people living with HIV/AIDS in the United States have spent time in the correctional system (Hammett, Harmon, & Rhodes, 2002; Kantor, 2006).

PRISONS, JAILS, AND JUVENILE FACILITIES

Caring for inmates at risk for or diagnosed with HIV infection requires an understanding of the correctional system in American society, the challenges of the correctional setting as a health care site, and the requirements of implementing a recommended standard of practice for patients at risk for or diagnosed with HIV/AIDS in that setting. Terminology is an important factor in clarifying the purpose of different types of corrections facilities and understanding who is housed there and for how long.

The concepts of incarceration and punishment are complex. Even defining corrections populations is elusive. About 30% of sentenced individuals are sent to jails or prisons. Although this 30% represents very high numbers of adults incarcerated in the United States, most of those individuals will at some time return to the community. About 70% of individuals sentenced by the courts are not held in prisons but are sentenced to probation, electronic monitoring with home confinement, substance abuse treatment, or drug court supervision. These alternatives to incarceration impose limitations on movement, behavior, employment, and child custody and require periodic reporting to the court. For individuals who encounter the legal and judicial system while residing in the community, effective programming for health care and rehabilitative programs must extend into the community. Most importantly, health care initiatives begun in jail or prison must be continued as inmates are released into the community.

Prisons are maintained and operated by state Departments of Corrections or by the Federal Bureau of Prisons. They house individuals who were accused and arrested, tried, and sentenced to specific terms.

Medical care in prison settings is provided by the state, by contract with university medical departments, or by a private medical and staffing contractor or company. Prison populations are longer term than those in jails, with inmate populations more stable and well known to the medical and nursing staff. Inmates are processed in intake facilities and receive a comprehensive medical workup. Although inmates may be transferred among various prisons because of security designations, their medical record will follow them. Maintaining medications and current orders for ongoing care is of particular importance for effective chronic care management of inmates with HIV or other long-term medical problems that require frequent monitoring of treatment regimens and medication adherence. Inmates with HIV disease and certain other conditions, many from impoverished backgrounds, may experience their best and most continuous health care in corrections settings.

Severe sentencing laws in the past two decades have increased the number of inmates with life sentences. One of the consequences of this trend is an increasing number of aging inmates with chronic illnesses in prisons. As individuals with HIV and AIDS live longer and survive to manage HIV disease as a chronic illness, those incarcerated with HIV or AIDS may be among this aging prison population.

Health care and medical unit organization within jails and prisons are increasingly set by accreditation standards of professional correctional health care organizations. The National Commission on Correctional Health Care (www.ncchc.org) and the American Correctional Health Services Association (www.achsa.org) provide standards for health services, an accreditation process, and national meetings that promote networking and professional excellence and certification. Accreditation of the health care services in jails, prisons, and juvenile facilities is voluntary.

Many prison facilities are located in rural areas and play a major role in the economies of those locales. Rural areas may have fewer resources for health care and education for the general community than are available in the correctional institution, leading some prison workers to resent the care provided to prisoners. Particular vigilance and skill in management and training are essential in these settings. Nurses and physicians in the medical unit may encounter this resentment and require support and procedures to deal with it effectively.

Jails are operated by city or county municipalities and sheriff's departments and hold inmates who are accused of crimes and are awaiting trial and sentencing. Many of the accused qualify for bail and may not be incarcerated while awaiting trial. Jails generally hold accused persons for relatively short periods of time in comparison to prisons. The jail population is recently arrested from the "street" and may be unknown to jail custody and health care staff. The burden of disease is also quite high in jail populations. Newly arrested jail inmates, many with histories of mental illness and/or substance abuse, may have engaged in various high risk behaviors prior to arrest (Harrison & Beck, 2002). Once in jail, they may demonstrate violence, withdrawal from alcohol and drugs, mental health crises, and suicide attempts. This very unstable and unpredictable population may turn over very quickly, within hours or days. This rapid turnover presents particular challenges to planning cost-effective and efficient health care screenings, assessments, and interventions. Nursing and medical staff experience challenges in performing required initial health assessments of newly admitted inmates, as well as challenges to initiating care for current medical conditions. Collaboration with health departments, community-based organizations, and AIDS service organizations can assist in continuity of care and program effectiveness. Nurses and other health care providers who work with incarcerated clients have responsibility for assessment, education, and potential referral of inmates to community services for health care.

Case management strategies for incarcerated or formerly incarcerated persons have been shown to be effective (Healey, 1999). Jails and prisons are sites of recent federally funded transitional case management programs for HIV positive inmates (e.g., Spaulding et al. [2007] and Opening Doors, the HRSA/CDC Corrections Demonstration Projects for Persons Living with AIDS, 1999–2004 [2007]). Both of these multisite projects tested models of transitional care from corrections settings to the community. Strategies that were shown to be effective included transitional case management and care planning; HIV and STD testing and follow-up; HIV, medical, and mental health and substance abuse referrals, appointments, and medications; and housing (U.S. Department of Health and Human Services, Health Resources and Services Administration, 2007).

COMMUNITY STANDARD OF CARE

Jails, prisons, and juvenile facilities are required to provide a community standard of health care to inmates and to avoid "deliberate indifference" to health care needs (Rold, 2006). The Supreme Court developed the standard of "deliberate indifference to serious medical needs" to define the Eighth Amendment obligation to provide health care under the Constitution, in *Estelle v. Gamble* in 1976. It remained unchanged for 30 years. Three basic rights emerged from *Estelle v. Gamble*: the right to access to health care, the right to care that is ordered, and the right to a professional medical judgment (*Estelle v. Gamble*, 429 U.S. 97, 1976; Rold, 2006).

Larger corrections facilities most often maintain medical facilities on-site. These medical units may be operated by the state, the local municipality, or by a health care company or contractor. In the latter case, employees in the medical unit are employees of the contract company rather than the state or local government. If an individual is in a jail or prison, the primary purpose is confinement or custody. While inmates have a mandated right to health care, the dual purposes of care and custody may conflict in day-to-day operations. Inmates are housed in facilities and housing units within facilities according to security designation. Generally, inmates require an escort through the correctional facility to the medical unit by corrections officers or deputy sheriffs. Security disruptions in the facility (e.g., fights between inmates, deliberately set fires, or an inmate head count that does not tally), will interrupt the normal flow of activities of daily living, including operation of the medical unit, inmate work units, movement in the facility for meal time, recreation, and the like.

A "lockdown" situation resulting from a security breach may interfere with health care delivery in other ways. Not only can inmates be delayed in getting to the medical unit for sick call, chronic care clinic appointments, or for medications, but nurses may be prohibited or delayed in going to units where "directly observed therapy" medications are given for TB, HIV, hepatitis C, mental health issues, or seizure disorders. Nurses may also be interrupted in scheduled visits and checks on inmates on suicide watch or on mental health precautions. Security precautions in place to protect inmates and staff can interfere with the established procedures to implement best practices and standards of care. These disruptions usually do not last very long but are a reminder that the primary purpose of corrections facilities is custody.

HIV-positive inmates are increasingly housed in general populations based on security level. In some facilities, however, inmates with HIV/AIDS were the target of stigma, exploitation, and violence. Special nutritional supplements and food rations for inmates with HIV disease may be stolen or bribed, and the inmate may experience intimidation. In addition, self-administered medication (SAM) packets that inmates kept in the housing unit are at risk of theft. Some facilities have been forced to create designated housing units for HIV-positive inmates. This effort makes confidentiality of an HIV-positive diagnosis difficult to maintain.

Even when HIV-positive inmates are housed in the general population housing units, strategies to prevent abuse by other inmates may be required. If medical units attempt to prevent theft of medications, supplemental meal portions, and nutritional supplements by having HIV-positive inmates come to the medical unit for pill call, confidentiality is at risk. This was especially true in earlier days when HIV medications were administered three and four times a day. HIV-positive inmates were visible as a group arriving at "pill call" for medications, not unlike insulin-dependent diabetics who need blood glucose checks and insulin.

Defining a community standard of care generated controversy when inmates were placed on the transplant lists for liver, kidney, and heart transplants. And inmates have received transplanted organs in the past. In January 2002, for example, an inmate received a heart transplant at Stanford Medical Center. The estimated cost of surgery and follow up care exceeded $1 million dollars. Although criticized for the decision to place the inmate on the transplant list, the California Department of Corrections cited the obligation to avoid "deliberate indifference" that can occur when a professional knows of and disregards an excessive risk to an inmate's health or safety. It is common for inmates to receive renal dialysis and elective surgery for non–life-threatening conditions, but the ethical issues surrounding extraordinary interventions remain controversial. These decisions have budgetary implications for state departments of corrections whose budgets are stressed. Similar discussions arise periodically when cost issues related to purchase of HIV or HCV medications strain state budgets. The persistent issues in defining a community standard of care for inmate populations are likely to spark debate in the future in light of constrained resources and expanding options for treatment of medical conditions (Perry, 2002).

CHARACTERISTICS OF THE INMATE POPULATION

Individuals incarcerated in prisons, jails, and juvenile facilities have often had poor access to health care services prior to incarceration. Many have a history of poverty, poor education, inadequate health care, racial discrimination, emotional trauma, physical abuse, and violence. Lack of access to health care for inmates prior to incarceration contributes to high rates of chronic illnesses such as hypertension, seizure disorders, and diabetes. Addictive behaviors are prevalent in the histories of incarcerated persons. Smoking, alcohol, and drug use are common. Pregnant women often arrive in prison or jail with little or no preventive health care during their pregnancy. Mental health disorders among incarcerated persons often received little attention in the community unless they have reached crisis proportions.

Rates of infectious diseases such as HIV/AIDS, TB, hepatitis, and STDs are much higher in corrections settings than in the general population. Inmates participate in behaviors that put them at high risk for HIV and hepatitis B and C while in prison and jail. Unprotected sex, needle sharing for IV drug use, tattooing with shared needles or instruments, and accidental exposure through fights, bites, or exposure to items contaminated with blood or body fluids can result in transmission of HIV and hepatitis B and C (Zalumas & Dawson Rose, 2003). In some facilities, TB infection rates far exceed those in the general population. The issue of multidrug-resistant TB is of particular concern among the incarcerated due to the close environment and unknown populations and the high rates of HIV-positive inmates who may be immunosuppressed. STD rates in some facilities range between 5 and 35% (Maruschak, 2004).

Corrections facilities are critical settings for identification and treatment of HIV and other associated infectious diseases. Brown and Herbert (2002) emphasize that corrections providers are in a key position to provide three essential components of HIV and AIDS prevention: education, testing, and treatment. Effective interventions can have a significant impact on the public health because corrections is a part of the community.

Inmates in correctional facilities have a shared "risk" for disease and incarceration. Behaviors and patterns such as prostitution or sex work, legal and illegal alcohol and drug use, unprotected sex, driving while intoxicated, and IV drug use and sale place individuals at risk for arrest and for disease and injury. Women who are or who have been incarcerated have a disproportionately high prevalence of HIV infection, compared both to incarcerated men and to nonincarcerated women (Arriola, Braithwaite, & Newkirk, 2006). The reasons for this high prevalence are complicated, but many of the factors that increase risk of HIV infections--poverty, exposure to violence and abuse, substance abuse, unemployment, and unstable living conditions--also increase the likelihood of criminal behavior (i.e., sex work and drug use) with resulting incarceration. Increasing numbers of minority women and youth are being incarcerated in the United States, many with HIV/AIDS, hepatitis, and substance abuse issues. The high rates of physical and sexual abuse and assault in the histories of women who are incarcerated are well known. For many women, these issues continue to be a problem after incarceration. Although the Fourth Amendment of the U.S. Constitution prohibits sexual abuse of prisoners, several states do not have laws prohibiting sexual abuse of prisoners. Public attention to the plight of women in prison has been reported widely in the media. These media efforts made visible the complexities surrounding issues of "consensual sex" or trading favors by women prisoners with guards. Such consent is not legally possible because of the woman's powerlessness and fear of retaliation if she does not participate. Indeed, reports of retribution by guards against female prisoners who did not agree to sex have included putting feces in food, withholding medical care, urinating on prisoners, and hanging (Allender & Spradley, 2005). Changes in custody regulations for women evolved in positive ways after these issues became public. Specific regulations about privacy, the ratio of female corrections officers supervising female prisoners, details about access to medical and mental health services, and legal counsel are now in place in many state systems.

HIV AND HEALTH CARE ISSUES IN CORRECTIONS SETTINGS

Medical units in larger jails, prisons, and juvenile facilities resemble clinics in a health department or Ryan White Clinic. Most operate scheduled out-patient appointments in chronic care clinics and also maintain an emergency, symptom-based provider schedule--referred to as "sick call" in corrections settings. Inmates gain access to this clinic by completing a request form that is usually available in the housing units and depositing the form in a closed box in a central location (e.g., the cafeteria or recreation area). Medical staff members collect these forms daily and contact inmates for appointments. If inmates are on a secure or closed housing unit, the custody officers collect forms and take them to the medical unit. Communication can break down and prevent inmates from being seen for sick call. For example, forms may not be available to inmates. Other inmates or corrections staff may exercise coercion to prevent inmates from requesting assistance. Interruptions in collecting requests or scheduling sick call may delay the inmate from receiving care in a timely manner.

Nurses, who are involved in initial and ongoing medical care, are likely to be a consistent factor in the life of an inmate. This is especially true since HIV has been viewed as more of a chronic illness. Nurses can be pivotal in planning and implementing procedures that ensure that sick call is carried out carefully and predictably. When unavoidable delays in scheduling do occur, the nurse manager, clinic nurse, or nurse practitioner can set priorities for inmates at risk, including HIV-positive inmates, with evolving and potentially dangerous symptoms such as drug side effects or fluid and electrolyte imbalances from fever or diarrhea. Procedures can be in place so that these at-risk inmates are seen as quickly as possible.

Risks of exposure to blood and body fluids in corrections settings for staff and inmates are higher than in the general community because of the higher rates of HIV and hepatitis among inmates, the nature of work in the setting, and inmate behaviors. Occupational exposure guidelines require the use of standard precautions and annual staff training (Panlilio et al., 2005). Nurses and other health care providers in the corrections health care setting may be involved in assessing and treating exposures to blood and body fluids among officers, medical staff, and inmates. They may also be involved in training activities. Corrections-specific educational materials and resources are available for these educational purposes at the National Resource Center of the AIDS Education and Training Centers (www.aidsetc.org) (Zalumas, 2005). Nurses are in a position to observe exposure issues in the setting and take steps to ensure that staff and inmates are knowledgeable, that personal protective equipment is available and used properly, that supplies for cleanup of spills are available, and that postexposure assessment and interventions are implemented correctly.

Incarceration places a burden on the relationship between parents and children. Incarcerated parents lose normal contact with their children, have infrequent visits with them, tolerate terrible circumstances of visitation when visits do occur, and generally lose the ability to contribute to their children's development. Relationships between the person incarcerated and his or her parents and children are often complicated by chronic health problems, HIV disease, hepatitis, or other STDs, and by histories of drug use or dealing. The disruption of the arrest and conviction of a parent means that children have to learn to cope with the loss of a parent, stigma of parental imprisonment, and a different support system that may include grandparents, foster care, or new caregivers in their home (Travis & Waul, 2003; Travis, Solomon, & Waul, 2001). Travis describes a ripple effect of incarceration on families and communities. Issues related to incarceration of a parent on children are complex, with far-reaching social and economic effects. Removal of a parent from the home may reduce violence in the setting but may also reduce family income and resources. Reentry of a parent into the home can disrupt patterns that provided stability during incarceration. The nature of the crime may have an impact on family resources. Individuals convicted of a drug felony are not eligible for TANF (Temporary Assistance for Needy Families) or food stamps. Housing, a significant factor for successful transition of individuals with HIV disease and/or mental illness, can be complicated by incarceration status. Housing is often more readily available for women and children than for adult men (U.S. Department of Health and Human Services, Health Resources and Services Administration, 2007).

Some facilities have programs for incarcerated parents and their children. San Quentin operates a summer camp for children so that participation and visitation can occur. Some facilities maintain inviting and pleasant visiting areas so that children can touch, hug, eat, and play with the parent during visits. This is different from many facilities where children must visit the parent behind glass partitions. Some prison programs offer parenting classes and allow pregnant inmates to complete the pregnancy with pre- and postpartum care, with periodic visitation with the infant to promote bonding.

The "Children of Incarcerated Parents Bill of Rights" was published by the San Francisco Partnership for Incarcerated Parents (2003). It articulated rights of children, such as: to be kept safe and informed during the time of arrest of my parent; to have a voice in decisions made about me; to be considered in decisions made about my parent; to be well cared for in my parent's absence; to speak with, see, and touch my parent; to have support as I struggle with my parent's incarceration; to be blameless for my parent's incarceration; and to have a right to a lifelong relationship with my parent. These rights placed the needs of children on the agenda of judicial process and have had impact in many jurisdictions as decisions are made about parents with children. Nurses may encounter children who have been affected by incarceration in many settings. Sensitivity to the issues they face and the impact of their life events may enable the nurse to guide factors that can make a difference in outcomes for child health.

THE ROLE OF THE HEALTH CARE PROVIDER

Corrections settings emerged in the last two decades as an environment for expert HIV care. Because of the mandate to provide a community standard of care and the high rates of HIV disease in jails and prisons, a number of strategies to provide competent care for HIV-positive inmates were developed and implemented across the country. Corrections facilities developed and implemented procedures for HIV testing, pre- and posttest counseling, diagnostic workup, collaborations with infectious disease experts about initiating treatment, beginning antiretroviral medications, and providing essential ongoing laboratory treatment surveillance.

Implementation of standards of care for HIV-positive inmates required substantial commitment of financial resources for the medical budgets for corrections facilities. Corrections settings increasingly focus on obtaining providers with experience in infectious diseases, maintaining training programs for medical and nursing staff, developing infectious disease protocols, and implementing quality improvement programs. As care of HIV patients became more complex, with multiple medications, and issues of resistance patterns and adherence requirements, management by expert providers in HIV care became the standard practice. HIV infectious disease experts are often available as a statewide resource for providers in a system. Local providers can refer an inmate to the prison hospital--usually one or two in a state system--for care there. If the HIV-positive inmate comes back to the local prison, a plan of care must be in place or a complication resolved. Some prisons and jails use telemedicine for consultation, whereby the HIV expert observes the history and physical examination at the local prison, interacts with the inmate and provider, and makes recommendations for care. Other referral and consultation processes are not so formal but involve the local provider using standards of practice and consulting as needed with the infectious disease expert located at a distance from the point of care.

Jurgens (2006), summarizing prisoner-related presentations given at the 2006 International AIDS Conference, reached several conclusions regarding the care, treatment, and support of prisoners:

> When provided with care and access to medications, prisoners respond well to antiretroviral treatment. Adherence rates in prisons can be as high as or higher than that among patients in the community. This is also true for injecting drug users, particularly when they can access methadone main-

tenance treatment; and the gains in health status made during the term of incarceration may be lost unless careful discharge planning and linkage to community care are undertaken. (p. 4)

Jurgens concluded that "Ensuring continuity of care from the community to the prison and back to the community, as well as continuity of care within the jail/prison system, is a fundamental component of successful treatment scale-up efforts" (p. 4).

The current nursing shortage is a major barrier to providing a competent level of care of HIV-positive inmates in corrections settings. Because many corrections facilities are located in rural areas, shortages of qualified nurses may be even more of a challenge than in urban areas. Nursing and other corrections administrators attempt a range of strategies to meet this challenge. Use of incentives, staffing agencies, creative scheduling, bonuses, and educational benefits are common strategies to recruit and retain nursing staff. Contract services and agencies, such as travel nurse groups and corrections health care contractors, are also used to provide nursing staff. Continuing education, such as that provided by the Association of Nurses in AIDS Care (www.anacnet.org) and the AETC National Resource Center (www.aidsetc.org/aidsetc?page=etres-display&resource=etres-92), can expand the knowledge base of nurses employed in corrections settings and serve as a retention strategy. Still another useful source of education for nurses caring for HIV-infected prisoners is the "HIV /AIDS Resources and References for California Correctional Health Care Providers" (available at www.sfaetc.ucsf.edu/CORRECTIONS/index.html). The resources available at this Internet-based resource include a virtual HIV/AIDS reference manual for care providers covering all key aspects of care.

CHRONIC CARE AND TRANSITION TO THE COMMUNITY

In 2006, the Vera Institute of Justice released its Report of the Commission on Safety and Abuse in America's Prisons. The report, entitled *Confronting Confinement,* noted that "What happens inside jails and prisons does not stay inside jails and prisons" (p. 10). The report emphasized that what happens in prisons follows prisoners after their release. This report attributed many of the current problems in U.S. prisons to the shift over 30 years ago from rehabilitation to punishment. Overcrowding, violence, segregation of difficult or mentally ill prisoners, high rates of disease among prisoners, and inadequate funding for correctional health care: All these factors contribute to dangerous, and sometimes inhumane, circumstances for inmates, staff, and the public. The proposed solutions address the findings: reduce crowding (i.e., set limits for numbers of inmates in a facility), return to a model of rehabilitation, use violence and force only when necessary, upgrade medical care for prisoners, and perhaps extend Medicare and Medicaid benefits to prisoners. The report proposes that failure to address these issues will result in violence, illness, and desperation, which will return to the community when inmates are released—as 95% are (Peirce, 2006). Petersilia (2000) predicts that the increasing numbers of inmates with more complex needs being released without rehabilitation during incarceration increase the likelihood of negative consequences on reentry to the community. These consequences include increases in child abuse and family violence, the spread of infectious diseases, homelessness, and community disorganization.

Reentry is defined as the process of leaving prison and returning to society (Travis, Solomon, & Waul, 2001). Potter (2003), in describing the programs of the HRSA/CDC Corrections Demonstration Projects, 1999–2004, detailed the root of the problems. By the mid-1990s, public health personnel working in areas with high rates of HIV and STDs noted the strong relationships of disease, drug use, and stints in jail among those infected with HIV. This was especially true among injecting drug users. Corrections-based programs were developed that tested models of disease prevention information, early disease detection, appropriate treatment, discharge planning, and community case management. The basic premise of the initiative was that corrections facilities offer a prime opportunity to identify and intervene with individuals who engage in high-risk behavior and who are difficult to track in the community.

Unless HIV-positive inmates who are released back to the community receive adequate care and follow-up, they may pose a threat not only to their own health but also to that of other people in the community. One recent study, for example, found that a majority of HIV-positive prison inmates in Texas do not fill their prescriptions in a timely manner after release (Baillargeon et al., 2009). This study, which is the first to track people living with HIV from prison release to community-based care, followed 2,115 inmates living with HIV in the Texas prison system between 2004 and 2007. Researchers concluded that only a small percentage (30%) of Texas prison inmates receiving ART while incarcerated filled an initial ART prescription within 60 days of their release. The researchers also found that black and Hispanic former inmates were less likely than white former inmates to fill their prescriptions in a timely manner. Because some former inmates may resume high-risk behaviors following their release to the community, those who discontinue their medical regimen may pose a higher risk of transmitting drug-resistant HIV within their communities.

Some of the reentry needs of HIV positive inmates that were identified during these projects include those critical for successful transition in the first 72 hours. These needs can be effectively addressed through collaboration between corrections medical providers and nurses, corrections and community case managers, and other community-based HIV service organizations. These needs include housing, personal identification, certification for benefits, plans for employment and job training, substance abuse treatment, referral for mental health treatment and medications, referral and appointment for HIV treatment and medications, and assessment of medication adherence. Nurses and medical providers in the corrections health care setting, in collaboration with the corrections and community case managers, are quite effective at facilitating these transitions.

CONCLUSION

The number of persons incarcerated in U.S. jails and prisons grew over the past two decades. A disproportionate number of this population is comprised of young persons from ethnic minority communities, many who lacked access to health care prior to incarceration and many of whom are incarcerated for offenses that placed them at risk of acquiring one or more infectious diseases, including HIV/AIDS; thus the prevalence of HIV and other infections in U.S. prisons is much higher than that in the general population. Nursing care of care of incarcerated persons who are HIV positive may include screening and testing, health assessments, administration of medications for HIV and opportunistic infections, symptom management, education about HIV/AIDS, and discharge planning. While prison systems in other parts of the world may offer condoms, clean needles, bleach, and drug substitution treatment, many of these interventions are not available to inmates in U.S. jails and prisons. Incarceration can be an opportunity for both HIV prevention and care, as well as the opportunity to break the cycle of recidivism. Because the majority of incarcerated persons return to the community, prevention activities hold the potential to promote positive results for the health of individuals, families, and communities.

REFERENCES

Allender, J. A., & Spradley, B. W. (2005). Clients in correctional facilities. In J. A. Allender & B.W. Spradley (eds.), Community health nursing: *Promoting and protecting the public's health* (6th ed., pp. 868–881). Philadelphia: Lippincott Williams & Wilkins.

Arriola, K., Braithwaite, R., & Newkirk, C. (2006). At the intersection between poverty, race, and HIV infection: HIV-related services for incarcerated women. *Infectious Diseases in Corrections Report, 9*(6 & 7), 1–8.

Beckwith, C., & Poshkus, M. (2007). HIV behind bars: Meeting the need for HIV testing education, and access to care. *Infectious Diseases in Corrections Report, 9*(17), 1, 3.

Baillargeon, J., Giordano, T., Rich, J., Wu, J., Wells, K., Pollock, B., et al. (2009). Accessing antiretroviral therapy following release from prison. *Journal of the American Medical Association, 301,* 848–857.

Brown, K., & Herbert, E. (2002). Health status report: Infectious diseases in corrections. *HIV Education Prison Project News, 5*(10), 1–7.

Centers for Disease Control and Prevention (CDC). (2001). HIV/AIDS counseling and testing in the criminal justice system (Fact Sheet Series). Retrieved January 28, 2009, from www.cdc.gov/idu/facts/cj-ct.htm.

Centers for Disease Control and Prevention (CDC). (2006). HIV transmission among male inmates in a state prison system: Georgia, 1992–2005. *Morbidity and Mortality Weekly Report, 55,* 421–426.

Estelle v. Gamble, 429 U.S. 97 (1976).

Hammett, T., Harmon, P., & Rhodes, W. (2002). The burden of infectious disease among inmates and releasees from correctional facilities. In *The health status of soon-to-be-released inmates: A report to Congress.* Chicago: National Commission on Correctional Health Care.

Harrison, P., & Beck, A. (2002). Prisoners in 2001. *Bureau of Justice Statistics Bulletin* (Publication No. NCJ 195189). Washington, DC: U.S. Department of Justice, Bureau of Justice Statistics.

Harrison, P., & Beck, A. Prisoners in 2004. (2005). *Bureau of Justice Statistics Bulletin* (Publication No. NCJ 210677). Washington, DC: U.S. Department of Justice, Bureau of Justice Statistics.

Healey, K. M. (1999). Case management in the criminal justice system. *National Institute of Justice Research in Action* (NCJ Publication No. 173409). Washington, DC: U.S. Department of Justice.

Horsburgh, C., Jarvis, J., McArther, T., Ignacio, T., & Stock, P. (1990). Seroconversion to human immunodeficiency virus in prison inmates. *American Journal of Public Health, 80,* 209–210.

Jurgens, R. (2006). From evidence to action on HIV/AIDS in prisons: A report from the XVI International AIDS Conference. *Infectious Diseases in Corrections Report, 9*(9), 1, 3–5.

Kantor, E. (2006). HIV transmission and prevention in prisons. In HIV InSite Knowledge Base. Retrieved February 15, 2007, from http://hivinsite.ucsf.edu/InSite?page=kb-07-04-13#S1X.

Maruschak, L. M. (2004). HIV in prisons and jails, 2002. *Bureau of Justice Statistics Bulletin* (NCJ Publication No. 205333). Washington, DC: U.S. Department of Justice. Retrieved January 29, 2009, from www.ojp.usdoj.gov/bjs/pub/pdf/hivp05.pdf.

Maruschak L. (2005). HIV in Prisons, 2003. *Bureau of Justice Statistics Bulletin* (Publication No. NCJ 210344). Washington, DC: U.S. Department of Justice. Retrieved January 29, 2009, from www.ojp.usdoj.gov/bjs/pub/pdf/hivp03.pdf.

Maruschak L. (2008). HIV in Prisons, 2006. *Bureau of Justice Statistics Bulletin.* Washington, DC: U.S. Department of Justice. Retrieved January 29, 2009, from www.ojp.usdoj.gov/bjs/pub/html/hivp/2006/hivp06.htm.

Panlilio, A. L., Cardo, D. M., Grohskopf, L. A., Heneine, W., & Ross, C. S. (2005, September). Updated U.S. Public Health Service Guidelines for the management of occupational exposures to HIV and recommendations for post-exposure prophylaxis. *Morbidity and Mortality Weekly Report, 54*(RR-9), 1–17. Retrieved January 29, 2009, from www.cdc.gov/mmwr/preview/mmwrhtml/rr5409a1.htm.

Peirce, N. (2006, June 26). Violence, illness, desperation: The jailbreak we won't discuss. *Stateline.org, Where Policy and Politics News Click.* Retrieved February 15, 2007, from www.stateline.org/live/details/story?contentId=122904.

Perry, D. L. (2002, January 31). Criminals should be far down on the transplant list, op-ed. *San Jose Mercury News.* Retrieved January 27, 2009, from www.scu.edu/ethics/publications/submitted/Perry/transplant.html.

Petersilia, J. (2000, November). When prisoners return to the community: Political, economic, and social consequences. Sentencing and Corrections, *Issues for the 21st Century* (Publication No. 9). Washington, DC: U.S. Department of Justice.

Pew Center on the States. (2008). One in 100: Behind bars in America 2008. Retrieved May 8, 2008, from www.pewcenteronthestates.org/report_detail.aspx?id=35904.

Potter, R. H. (2003). Corrections demonstration project fosters collaboration on HIV in the community. *Large Jail Network Exchange 2003.*

Rold, W. (2006, Summer). *30 years after Estelle v Gamble:* A legal retrospective. *CorrectCare, 20*(3), 7, 18.

Sabol, S. J., & Couture, H. (2008, June). Prison inmates at midyear 2007. *Bureau of Justice Statistics Bulletin* (NCJ Publication No. 221944), pp. 1–24.

Sabol, S. J., & Minton, T. D. (2008, June). Jail inmates at midyear 2007. *Bureau of Justice Statistics Bulletin* (NCJ Publication No. 221945), pp. 1–11.

San Francisco Partnership for Incarcerated Parents (2003). *Children of incarcerated parents: A bill of rights.* Stockton, CA: Friends Outside.

Spaulding, A., Arriola, K., Ramos, K., Hammett, T., Kennedy, S., Norton, G., et al. (2007). Enhancing linkages to HIV primary care in jail settings. *Journal of Correctional Health Care, 13*(2), 93–128.

Travis, J., & Waul, M. (2003). *Prisoners once removed: The impact of incarceration and reentry on children, families, and communities.* Washington, DC: The Urban Institute.

Travis, J., Solomon, A., & Waul, M. (2001). *From prison to home: The dimensions and consequences of prisoner reentry.* Washington, DC: The Urban Institute.

U.S. Department of Health and Human Services, Health Resources and Services Administration. (2007). *Opening doors: The HRSA-CDC corrections project for people with HIV/AIDS.* Rockville, MD: Health Resources and Services Administration, HIV/AIDS Bureau. Retrieved January 29, 2009, from ftp.hrsa.gov/hab/opening_doors.pdf.

Vera Institute of Justice. (2006). Confronting confinement: A report of the commission on safety and abuse in America's prisons. Washington, DC: The Vera Institute of Justice. Retrieved January 29, 2009, from www.prisoncommission.org/pdfs/Confronting_Confinement.pdf.

Weinbaum, C., Lyerla, R., & Margolis, H. S. (2003). Prevention and control with epatitis viruses in correctional settings. *Morbidity and Mortality Weekly Report, 52*(RR-1), 1–36.

World Health Organization (WHO). (2007). Interventions to address HIV in prisons: Prevention of sexual transmission (Evidence for Action Technical Papers). Retrieved January 28, 2009, from www.who.int/hiv/idu/oms_ea_sexual_transmission_df.pdf.

Zalumas, J. C. (Project Director). (2005). *Keeping your guard up: Exposure risks for HIV and hepatitis for detention and corrections officers* [Video]. (Available through the CDC, NPIN Web Site: www.cdcnpin.org/scripts/about/train.asp.)

Zalumas, J., & Dawson Rose, C. (2003). HIV and Hepatitis C in incarcerated populations: Fights, bites, searches, and syringes. *Journal of the Association of Nurses in AIDS Care, 14*(5), 108S–115S.

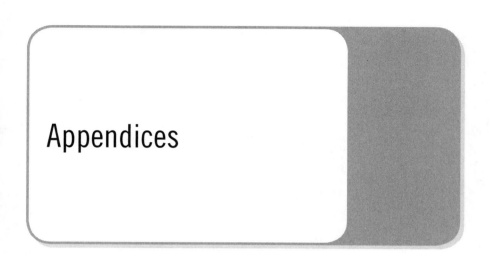

Appendices

Appendix I

Federal and State Resources for HIV/AIDS-Related Information, Guidelines, and Data

BASIC INFORMATION

Basic Information—HIV
www.cdc.gov/hiv/topics/basic/index.htm

Revised Surveillance Case Definitions for HIV Infection Among Adults, Adolescents, and Children Aged <18 Months and for HIV Infection and AIDS Among Children Aged 18 Months to <13 Years— United States, 2008
www.cdc.gov/mmwr/preview/mmwrhtml/rr5710a1.htm?s_cid=rr5710a1_e

AIDS-Defining Conditions
www.cdc.gov/mmwr/preview/mmwrhtml/rr5710a2.htm

Comparison of the Revised World Health Organization and CDC Surveillance Case Definitions and Staging Systems for HIV Infection
www.cdc.gov/mmwr/preview/mmwrhtml/rr5710a3.htm

HIV/AIDS Glossary
www.aidsinfo.nih.gov/Glossary/GlossaryDefaultCenterPage.aspx?MenuItem=AIDSinfoTools

HIV/AIDS Fact Sheets
www.cdc.gov/hiv/topics/surveillance/factsheets.htm

HIV and Mental Health, New York State Department of Health AIDS Institute
www.hivguidelines.org/Content.aspx?PageID=261

HIV and Oral Health, New York State Department
of Health AIDS Institute
www.hivguidelines.org/Content.aspx?PageID=263

HIV and Substance Use, New York State Department of Health AIDS Institute
www.hivguidelines.org/Content.aspx?PageID=262

INTERNATIONAL DIMENSIONS

U.S. President's Emergency Plan for AIDS Relief
www.pepfar.gov/

USAID HIV/AIDS Resources
www.usaid.gov/our_work/global_health/aids/Resources/index.html

PREVENTION

Compendium of HIV Prevention Interventions with
Evidence of Effectiveness
www.cdc.gov/hiv/resources/reports/hiv_compendium/index.htm

CDC HIV Prevention Plan: Extended Through 2010
www.cdc.gov/hiv/resources/reports/psp/pdf/psp.pdf

USPHS/IDSA Guidelines for the Prevention of Opportunistic
Infections in Persons Infected with Human Immunodeficiency Virus
www.aidsinfo.nih.gov/Guidelines/GuidelineDetail.aspx?MenuItem=Gu
idelines&Search=Off&GuidelineID=13&ClassID=4

Prevention and Treatment of Tuberculosis Among Patients Infected
with Human Immunodeficiency Virus: Principles of Therapy and
Revised Recommendations
www.cdc.gov/mmwr/preview/mmwrhtml/00055357.htm

2003–2008 HIV Prevention Community Planning Guidance
www.cdc.gov/hiv/topics/cba/resources/guidelines/hiv-cp/index.htm

HIV Prevention Demonstration Projects
www.cdc.gov/hiv/topics/prev_prog/AHP/AHP-Demonstration.htm

Incorporating HIV Prevention into the Medical Care of Persons Living
with HIV
www.cdc.gov/mmwr/preview/mmwrhtml/rr5212a1.htm

HIV Health Education and Risk Reduction Guidelines
www.cdc.gov/hiv/resources/guidelines/herrg/index.htm

HIV Prevention Case Management Guidance
www.cdc.gov/hiv/topics/prev_prog/CRCS/resources/PCMG/index.htm

HIV Prevention Through Early Detection and Treatment of Other
Sexually Transmitted Diseases—United States Recommendations of
the Advisory Committee for HIV and STD Prevention
www.cdc.gov/mmwr/preview/mmwrhtml/00054174.htm

RESEARCH

Overview of Federal Involvement in HIV/AIDS Research
www.aids.gov/research

HAART Clinical Trials (NIH)
http://clinicaltrials.gov/search/open/intervention=%22Antiretroviral+
Therapy,+Highly+Active%22+OR+HAART

HIV Clinical Trials (NIH)
http://clinicaltrials.gov/search/open/term=HIV+%5BCONDITION%5
D+AND+((anti-hiv+OR+antiretroviral)+AND+medicines)+%5BTREA
TMENT%5D

AIDS Clinical Trials Group (ACTG)
www.actgnetwork.org/login.aspx?ReturnUrl=%2findex.aspx

Centers for AIDS Research (NIH)
www3.niaid.nih.gov/research/cfar

Office of Human Research Protections: HIV/AIDS
www.hhs.gov/ohrp/policy/#hiv

Pediatric AIDS Clinical Trials Group
http://www.niaid.nih.gov/Daids/pdatguide/pactg.htm

Post-Doctoral Research Fellowships for HIV Prevention in Communities of Color
www.cdc.gov/hiv/aboutdhap/orise/index.htm

STATISTICS AND SURVEILLANCE

Basic Statistics (March 2009)
www.cdc.gov/hiv/topics/surveillance/basic.htm

HIV/AIDS Statistics and Surveillance
www.cdc.gov/hiv/topics/surveillance/index.htm

HIV/AIDS Statistics and Surveillance Slide Sets
www.cdc.gov/hiv/topics/surveillance/resources/slides/index.htm

Cases of HIV Infection and AIDS in Urban and Rural Areas of the United States, 2006
www.cdc.gov/hiv/topics/surveillance/resources/reports/2008supp_vol13no2/default.htm

Cases of HIV Infection and AIDS in the United States and Dependent Areas, 2007
www.cdc.gov/hiv/topics/surveillance/resources/reports/2007report/default.htm

TESTING AND COUNSELING

Revised Recommendations for HIV Testing of Adults, Adolescents, and Pregnant Women in Health Care Settings
www.cdc.gov/mmwr/preview/mmwrhtml/rr5514a1.htm

HIV Testing Slide Sets
www.cdc.gov/hiv/topics/testing/slidesets.htm

HIV Testing Consultation Materials (UCSF/AETC National Resource Center)
www.nccc.ucsf.edu/Training/index.html

HIV Partner Counseling and Referral Services—Guidance
www.cdc.gov/hiv/resources/guidelines/pcrs/index.htm

Compendium of State HIV Testing Laws—2009
http://www.nccc.ucsf.edu/StateLaws/Index.html

One Test, Two Lives: Prenatal HIV Screening (CDC)
www.cdc.gov/hiv/topics/perinatal/1test2lives/default.htm

HIV Testing Implementation Guidance for Correctional Settings
www.cdc.gov/hiv/topics/testing/resources/guidelines/correctional-settings/pdf/Correctional_Settings_Guidelines.pdf

Summary of Recommendations for Partner Services Programs for HIV Infection, Syphilis, Gonorrhea, and Chlamydial Infection—Legal and Ethical Concerns
www.cdc.gov/mmwr/preview/mmwrhtml/RR5709a2.htm

TREATMENT AND CARE

Treatment Hotlines
www.cdc.gov/hiv/topics/treatment/index.htm#hotlines

Clinical Guidelines Portal
http://aidsinfo.nih.gov/Guidelines/Default.aspx?MenuItem=Guidelines&Search=On

DHHS Treatment Guidelines for Adults and Adolescents (November 2008)
http://aidsinfo.nih.gov/Guidelines/GuidelineDetail.aspx?MenuItem=Guidelines&Search=Off&GuidelineID=7&ClassID=1

Pediatric Treatment Guidelines (February 2009)
http://aidsinfo.nih.gov/Guidelines/GuidelineDetail.aspx?MenuItem=Guidelines&Search=Off&GuidelineID=8&ClassID=1

U.S. Department of Health and Human Services Perinatal Guidelines (April 2009)
www.aidsinfo.nih.gov/Guidelines/GuidelineDetail.aspx?MenuItem=Guidelines&Search=Off&GuidelineID=9&ClassID=2

DHHS Guidelines for Prevention and Treatment of Opportunistic Infections Among HIV-Exposed and HIV-Infected Children (June 2008)
http://aidsinfo.nih.gov/contentfiles/Pediatric_OI.pdf

Guidelines for Prevention and Treatment of Opportunistic Infections in HIV-Infected Adults and Adolescents (CDC, March 2009)
www.cdc.gov/mmwr/pdf/rr/rr58e324.pdf

Recommended Infection Control Practices for Dentistry (2003)
www.cdc.gov/oralhealth/infectioncontrol/guidelines/index.htm

National Center for HIV/AIDS, Viral Hepatitis, STD, and
TB Prevention, Division of Tuberculosis Elimination
Tuberculosis Guidelines
www.cdc.gov/tb/pubs/mmwr/Maj_guide/default.htm

Sexually Transmitted Disease Treatment Guidelines 2006
www.cdc.gov/std/treatment/2006/rr5511.pdf

Updated U.S. Public Health Service Guidelines for the Management
of Occupational Exposures to HIV and Recommendations for
Postexposure Prophylaxis (2005)
www.cdc.gov/mmwr/preview/mmwrhtml/rr5409a1.htm

Antiretroviral Postexposure Prophylaxis After Sexual, Injection Drug
Use, or Other Nonoccupational Exposure to HIV in the United States
www.cdc.gov/mmwr/preview/mmwrhtml/rr5402a1.htm

Recommendations for Postexposure Interventions to Prevent
Infection with Hepatitis B Virus, Hepatitis C Virus, or Human
Immunodeficiency Virus, and Tetanus in Persons Wounded During
Bombings and Other Mass-Casualty Events—United States, 2008
www.cdc.gov/mmwr/preview/mmwrhtml/rr5706a1.htm?s_
cid=rr5706a1_e

Drugs Used in the Treatment of HIV Infection (FDA)
www.fda.gov/oashi/aids/virals.html

AIDSinfo Drug Data Base
http://aidsinfo.nih.gov/DrugsNew/Default.aspx?MenuItem=Drugs

FDA-Approved HIV/AIDS-Related Drugs
www.aidsinfo.nih.gov/DrugsNew/SearchResults.aspx?MenuItem=
Drugs&DrugName=&DrugClass=All&DrugType=FDA-approved
%20Drugs

Drugs Used in the Treatment of Pediatric HIV Infection (FDA)
www.fda.gov/oashi/aids/pedlbl.html

Drug Dosing Toolkit (VA)
www.hiv.va.gov/vahiv?page=treat-drug-00

Database of Antiretroviral Drug Interactions (UCSF, HIV InSite)
http://hivinsite.ucsf.edu/insite?page=ar-00-02

HIV Drug Interaction (University of Liverpool)
www.hiv-druginteractions.org

HIV Drug–Drug Interactions, New York State Department of Health
www.hivguidelines.org/GuideLine.aspx?guideLineID=12

Drug–Drug Interactions with HIV-Related Medications (AETC)
http://aidsetc.org/aetc?page=cm-312_drug

Drug–Drug, Drug–Food, and Drug–Herb Interactions
(Dalhousie University)
http://dir.pharmacy.dal.ca/drugprobinteraction.php

Recreational Drugs and HIV Antivirals: A Guide to Interactions for
Clinicians (New York/New Jersey AETC)
www.aidsetc.org/pdf/tools/nynj_rec_drug_interactions.pdf

HIV/AIDS Investigational Drugs
www.aidsinfo.nih.gov/DrugsNew/SearchResults.aspx?MenuItem=Drug
s&DrugName=&DrugClass=All&DrugType=Investigational%20Drugs

AIDS Medicines (Medline Plus)
www.nlm.nih.gov/medlineplus/aidsmedicines.html

Alternative and Complementary Therapies
www.aidsinfonet.org/fact_sheets/view/700?lang=eng

HIV-Related Clinical Trials
www.aidsinfo.nih.gov/ClinicalTrials/search.aspx?MenuItem=Clinical
Trials&term=%22February%207,%202009%22:%22March%209,%202
009%22[FIRST-RECEIVED-DATE]AND%20HIV[CONDITION]

HIV Prevention Case Management—Literature Review and Current
Practice
www.cdc.gov/hiv/topics/prev_prog/CRCS/resources/PCML/index.htm

Caring for Someone with AIDS at Home
http://www.cdc.gov/hiv/resources/brochures/careathome/index.htm

HRSA: A Guide to Primary Care for People with HIV/AIDS,
2004 edition
www.hab.hrsa.gov/tools/primarycareguide/index.htm

HRSA: A Guide to the Clinical Care of Women with HIV/AIDS,
2005 edition
http://hab.hrsa.gov/publications/womencare05/

Appendix II

HIV/AIDS and HIV/AIDS-Related Serial Publications

The following serial publications focus on HIV/AIDS or are HIV/AIDS-related. The descriptive information for each publication was extracted from the publication's web page.

Selected Serial Publications with a Professional Readership

African Journal of AIDS Research

The *African Journal of AIDS Research* (AJAR) is a peer-reviewed research journal publishing papers that make an original contribution to the understanding of social dimensions of HIV/AIDS in African contexts. AJAR includes articles from, amongst others, the disciplines of sociology, demography, epidemiology, social geography, economics, psychology, anthropology, philosophy, health communication, media, cultural studies, public health, education, nursing science and social work. Papers relating to impact, care, prevention and social planning, as well as articles covering social theory and the history and politics of HIV/AIDS, will be considered for publication.
www.ajol.info/journal_index.php?jid=46

AIDS Alert

AIDS Alert is the definitive source of AIDS news and advice for health care professionals. It covers up-to-the-minute developments and guidance on

the entire spectrum of AIDS challenges, including treatment, education, precautions, screening, diagnosis and policy.
www.ahcpub.com/products_and_services/?prid=161

AIDS and Behavior

AIDS and Behavior provides an international venue for the scientific exchange of research and scholarly work on the contributing factors, prevention, consequences, social impact, and response to HIV/AIDS. The journal publishes original peer-reviewed papers addressing all areas of AIDS behavioral research including: individual, contextual, social, economic and geographic factors that facilitate HIV transmission; interventions aimed to reduce HIV transmission risks at all levels and in all contexts; mental health aspects of HIV/AIDS; medical and behavioral consequences of HIV infection—including health-related quality of life, coping, treatment and treatment adherence; and the impact of HIV infection on adults children, families, communities and societies. The journal publishes original research articles, brief research reports, and critical literature reviews.
www.springer.com/public+health/journal/10461

AIDS Care: Psychological and Socio-medical Aspects of AIDS/HIV

AIDS Care provides a forum for publishing in one authoritative source research and reports from the many complementary disciplines involved in the AIDS/HIV field. These include, among others: psychology, sociology, epidemiology, social work and anthropology, social aspects of medicine, nursing, education, health education, law, administration, counseling (including various approaches such as behavioral therapy, psychotherapy, family therapy etc.). AIDS and HIV infection, the planning of services, prevention and the fear of AIDS affect many echelons of society ranging from individuals, couples and families through to institutions and communities. A particular aim is to publish work emanating from many centers and in so doing address the global impact of AIDS.
www.tandf.co.uk/journals/carfax/09540121.html

AIDS Education and Prevention

AIDS Education and Prevention is an international journal designed to support the efforts of professionals working to prevent HIV and AIDS.

Keeping readers up-to-date on the latest information in the field, AIDS Education and Prevention publishes scientific articles by leading authorities from many disciplines, such as public health, psychosocial, ethical concerns related to HIV and AIDS, and public policy. In addition to discussing models of AIDS education and prevention, the journal covers research reports on the effectiveness of new strategies and programs, debates about key issues, and reviews of book and video resources.
www.guilford.com/cgibin/cartscript.cgi?page=pr/jnai.htm&dir=periodicals/per_pub&cart_id=

AIDS Patient Care and STDs

Patients with AIDS are living longer than ever before, due to new medications and therapeutic regimens. *AIDS Patient Care and STDs* enables you to keep pace with the latest developments in this rapidly evolving field by providing the latest research and advances in diagnostics and therapeutics designed to prolong the lifespan of patients and improved their quality of life.
www.liebertpub.com/products/product.aspx?pid=1

AIDS Reader

The *AIDS Reader* is designed to provide clinicians with practical, scientifically sound information on the prevention, diagnosis, and treatment of HIV disease. Our goal is to help clinicians improve the quality of life and treatment options for their patients, by helping to bridge the gap between the specialist and the primary care physician.
www.medscape.com/viewpublication/93

AIDS Research and Human Retroviruses

AIDS Research and Human Retroviruses has been the leading scientific journal in the field for over 20 years. This core journal for researchers in HIV, human retroviruses, and their associated diseases provides the broadest coverage from molecular biology to clinical studies and outcomes research.
www.liebertpub.com/products/product.aspx?pid=2

AIDS Research and Therapy

AIDS Research and Therapy is an open access, online journal that publishes peer-reviewed original research articles from scientists working

to prevent the spread of AIDS. *AIDS Research and Therapy* aims to publish articles on basic preclinical, clinical, social, epidemiological and behavioral sciences as well as education research articles that help in abating the spread and burden of AIDS. *AIDS Research and Therapy* publishes articles on novel and developing treatment strategies for AIDS, as well as on the outcomes of established treatment strategies. Original research articles on animal models that form an essential part of the AIDS treatment research are also published. The ultimate goal of the journal's focus is to lead bench research to bedside practice to combat AIDS. AIDS is spreading at alarming rates in several African and Asian countries. Thus, any development that occurs in combating AIDS should be disseminated as rapidly as possible through the world. *AIDS Research and Therapy* is a multidisciplinary journal that aims to keep scientists and clinicians globally abreast of the latest research on HIV-1 and AIDS.
www.aidsrestherapy.com/home

AIDS Research Today

AIDS Research Today is a free monthly online journal that collates and summarizes the latest research about AIDS, including details on testing, treatment, prevention, HIV, life expectancy.
http://aids.researchtoday.net

AIDS Reviews

AIDS Reviews is published quarterly, and covers timely and important topics on the different areas of HIV/AIDS including clinical aspects, therapy, drug resistance, vaccines, virology, evolution, immunology, pathogenesis, diagnostics, epidemiology, opportunistic infections, and prevention.
www.aidsreviews.com

Antiviral Therapy

Antiviral Therapy is the first international journal solely devoted to the clinical development and use of antiviral agents. It publishes original scientific papers in all therapeutic areas, including: results of clinical studies in all phases; viral diagnostics and individualization of antiviral therapy; study design issues in the clinical assessment of antivirals; antiviral drug safety and safety monitoring; mechanisms of resistance to antiviral agents; and pharmacoepidemiology of viral diseases. *Antiviral Therapy* also features review articles, editorials, book reviews and a letters section to provide

a forum for discussion. *Antiviral Therapy* is an official publication of the International Society for Antiviral Research.
www.intmedpress.com/General/showSectionSub.cfm?SectionID =2&SectionSubID=1&SectionSubSubID=1

Bulletin of Experimental Treatments for AIDS

BETA, the *Bulletin of Experimental Treatments for AIDS*, covers new developments in HIV/AIDS prevention, treatment, and research. *BETA* includes in-depth articles on HIV prevention technologies and approaches, as well as HIV treatment and strategies for living well with HIV. It is published biannually in English and Spanish by the San Francisco AIDS Foundation. Contributing writers to *BETA* include well-known HIV/ AIDS researchers, clinicians, and community advocates. Each issue of *BETA* includes News Briefs, Drug Watch, a Women and HIV department, feature articles on a range of topics, and a list of open clinical trials.
www.sfaf.org/beta

Clinical Infectious Diseases

Clinical Infectious Diseases, one of the most heavily cited journals in the fields of infectious diseases and microbiology, publishes articles on diverse topics in infectious diseases, with a focus on clinical practice. Every issue includes special sections focusing on key topics such as HIV/AIDS, antimicrobial resistance, aging and infectious diseases, and biological weapons. Many articles are published with commentaries by prominent researchers, and current trends and best practices are regularly covered in review articles and practice guidelines. *CID* also publishes numerous supplements devoted to single topics in the field.
www.idsociety.org/Content.aspx?id=9464

Current HIV/AIDS Reports

The *Current Reports* journals were developed out of the recognition that specialists have increasing difficulty keeping up to date with the expanding volume of information published in their field. In *Current HIV/AIDS Reports*, we aim to help the reader by providing in a systematic manner: (1) the views of experts on current advances in HIV/AIDS in a clear and readable form; (2) selections of the most important papers from the great wealth of original publications, annotated by experts.
www.current-reports.com/home_journal.cfm?JournalID=HI

Current HIV Research

Current HIV Research aims to cover all the latest and outstanding developments of HIV research. We invite comprehensive review articles and novel, pioneering work in the basic and clinical fields on all areas of HIV research, including virus replication and gene expression, HIV assembly, virus-cell interaction, viral pathogenesis, epidemiology and transmission, anti-retroviral therapy and adherence, drug discovery, the latest developments in HIV/AIDS vaccines and animal models, mechanisms and interactions with AIDS related diseases, social and public health issues related to HIV disease, and prevention of viral infection. Each issue of the journal contains a series of timely in-depth reviews and original research written by leaders in the field covering a range of current topics on HIV research. Periodically, the journal will invite guest editors to devote an issue on a particular area of HIV research of great interest that increases our understanding of the virus and its complex interaction with the host.
www.bentham.org/chivr/index.htm

Current Infectious Diseases Reports

The *Current Reports* journals were developed out of the recognition that specialists have increasing difficulty keeping up to date with the expanding volume of information published in their field. In *Current Infectious Disease Reports,* we aim to help the reader by providing in a systematic manner: (1) the views of experts on current advances in infectious disease in a clear and readable form; (2) selections of the most important papers from the great wealth of original publications, annotated by experts.
http://www.current-reports.com/home_journal.cfm?JournalID=IR

Current Opinion in HIV and AIDS

This reader-friendly, broad-based resource empowers those working in the field of HIV and AIDS to put to good use vital clinical and research advances from throughout the world. The journal provides easy access to the very best thinking of the best minds in this dynamic, burgeoning field. Each bimonthly issue features distinguished guest editors who focus exclusively on topics in their specialty. The journal delivers unvarnished, expert assessments of developments from the previous year—

overviews found nowhere else. Insightful editorials and on-the-mark invited reviews bring readers up to speed on key subjects such as the T-Cell in HIV infection and disease, reservoirs, host factors, HIV vaccines, anti-retro viral therapy and clinical trial design.
www.co-hivandaids.com/pt/re/cohiv/home.htm

Current Opinion in Infectious Diseases

This reader-friendly, bimonthly resource provides a powerful, broad-based perspective on the most important advances from throughout the world. Featuring renowned guest editors and focusing exclusively on two topics, every issue of *Current Opinion in Infectious Diseases* delivers unvarnished, expert assessments of developments from the previous year. Insightful editorials and on-the-mark invited reviews cover key subjects such as HIV infections and AIDS; skin and soft tissue infections; pathogenesis and immune response; antimicrobial agents: parasitic, viral, bacterial, and fungal; tropical and travel-associated diseases; infections of the immunocompromised host; pediatric and neonatal infections—some 12 items, all of major relevance.
www.co-infectiousdiseases.com/pt/re/coinfdis/home.htm

FOCUS: A Guide to AIDS Research and Counseling

FOCUS remains a leading HIV and mental health newsletter. Published 10 times per year, *FOCUS* reviews the counseling aspects of AIDS: how HIV-related counseling is affected by the medical, epidemiological, and social realities of AIDS, as well as the emotional response to the disease. It is written for mental health and health care providers working on the front lines and is of interest to researchers, policy makers, and program administrators.
www.ucsf-ahp.org/HTML2/services_providers_publications_focus.html

HIV/AIDS Policy & Law Review

Providing analysis and summaries of current developments in HIV/AIDS-related policy and law, the *HIV/AIDS Policy & Law Review* promotes education and the exchange of information, ideas, and experiences from an international perspective.
www.aidslaw.ca/EN/publications/HIV_AIDS_Policy_Law_Review/index.htm

HIV Clinical Trials

HIV Clinical Trials is devoted exclusively to keeping you in touch with the latest developments and techniques in HIV/AIDS therapeutics. This is where you'll gain a more complete picture of worldwide developments. *HIV Clinical Trials* coverage includes: the results of therapeutic; diagnostic; or preventive clinical trials; reports of clinical research; meta-analyses; pilot studies; methodological papers; review articles; quality of life and pharmacoeconomic evaluations; controversies; invited editorial comments; book reviews; letters to the editor; and abstracts of conferences.
www.thomasland.com/about-HIVtrials.html

HIV Medicine

HIV Medicine aims to provide an alternative outlet for publication of international research papers in the field of HIV Medicine, embracing clinical, pharmacological, epidemiological, ethical, preclinical and in vitro studies. In addition, the journal will commission reviews and other feature articles. It will focus on evidence-based medicine as the mainstay of successful management of HIV and AIDS.
www.wiley.com/bw/journal.asp?ref=1464-2662

HIV Meds Quarterly

HIV Meds Quarterly provides brief updates and analysis of new findings related to common therapies used by HIV clinicians.
www.aidsetc.org/aidsetc?page=hmq-0902-00

HIV Therapy

HIV Therapy delivers essential information in concise, at-a-glance article formats. Key advances in the field are reported and analyzed by international experts, providing an authoritative but accessible forum for this globally important area of research.
www.futuremedicine.com/toc/hiv/3/2

HIV Treatment Bulletin

HIV Treatment Bulletin is a not-for-profit community publication that aims to provide a review of the most important medical advances related

to clinical management of HIV and its related conditions as well as access to treatments. Comments to articles are compiled from consultant, author and editorial responses.
www.i-base.info/htb/index.html

Infectious Diseases in Corrections Report

A forum for correctional problem solving, *Infectious Diseases in Corrections Report* targets correctional administrators and HIV/AIDS and hepatitis care providers including physicians, nurses, outreach workers, and case managers. Continuing Medical Education credits are provided by Nova Southeastern University Health Professions Division (NSU) to physicians who accurately respond to the questions on the last page of the newsletter.
www.idcronline.org

International Journal of STD & AIDS

This peer-reviewed journal provides a clinically oriented forum for investigating and treating sexually transmissible infections, HIV and AIDS. Contributors from around the world promote activities aimed at research, prevention and control of these infections. The journal contains in-depth editorial reviews, original articles and research, short papers, case reports, audit reports and CPD papers. There is also a lively correspondence column, a book review section, and news from the genitourinary medicine associations.
http://ijsa.rsmjournals.com/

Journal of Acquired Immune Deficiency Syndromes

The *Journal of Acquired Immune Deficiency Syndromes* (JAIDS) is an interdisciplinary journal co-edited by the foremost leaders in clinical virology, molecular biology, and epidemiology. It provides a synthesis of information on HIV and AIDS from all relevant clinical and basic sciences. Under the guidance of an eminent international editorial board, this groundbreaking journal brings together rigorously peer-reviewed original articles, reviews of current research, and results of clinical trials.
www.jaids.com/pt/re/jaids/home.htm

Journal of the Association of Nurses in AIDS Care

The *Journal of the Association of Nurses in AIDS Care* (JANAC) covers the spectrum of nursing issues in HIV/AIDS: education, treatment, prevention, research, practice, clinical issues, awareness, policies and program development. This peer-reviewed journal is a forum for nurses and other health care professionals whose focus is the care and treatment of individuals infected and affected by HIV/AIDS.
www.elsevier.com/wps/find/journaldescription.cws_home/704632/description#description

Journal of HIV/AIDS & Social Services

The *Journal of HIV/AIDS & Social Services* provides a forum in which social workers and other professionals in the field of HIV/AIDS work can access the latest research and techniques in order to provide effective social, educational, and clinical services to all individuals affected by HIV/AIDS. From best practices and advice on case management to evaluations of the impact of various legislation and social policy decisions, this journal will keep you at the forefront of the field! Comprehensive and thorough, this peer-reviewed, refereed journal presents the empirical experiences of others to use as learning tools, state-of-the-art interventions and programs, and practical ideas for working with the various populations infected with and affected by HIV/AIDS.
www.haworthpress.com/store/product.asp?sku=J187

Journal of Immunology

The *Journal of Immunology* (JI) is published by the American Association of Immunologists, Inc. (AAI) twice a month. The JI is the definitive record for research progress in immunology. No other publication even approaches. The JI's comprehensive record of what's new, what's true and what's important in immunology.
www.jimmunol.org/

Journal of Infection

The *Journal of Infection* publishes original papers on all aspects of infection—clinical, microbiological and epidemiological. The Journal seeks to bring together knowledge from all specialties involved in infection

research and clinical practice, and present the best work in the ever-changing field of infection. Each issue brings you Editorials that describe current or controversial topics of interest, high quality Reviews to keep you in touch with the latest developments in specific fields of interest, an Epidemiology section reporting studies in the hospital and the general community, and a lively correspondence section.
www.elsevier.com/wps/find/journaldescription.cws_home/623054/description#description

Journal of Infectious Diseases

Founded in 1904, the *Journal of Infectious Diseases* is the premier publication in the Western Hemisphere for original research on the pathogenesis, diagnosis, and treatment of infectious diseases; on the microbes that cause them; and on disorders of host immune mechanisms. Articles in JID include research results from microbiology, immunology, epidemiology, and related disciplines.
www.journals.uchicago.edu/toc/jid/current

Journal of the International AIDS Society

The *Journal of the International AIDS Society,* an official journal of the Society, provides an open access forum for essential and innovative HIV/AIDS research. Submission of research carried out by investigators in low- and middle-income countries is strongly encouraged. The emerging field of operations research can provide valuable information on various algorithms for monitoring and providing support for comprehensive yet affordable and sustainable treatment, prevention and care programmes for different contexts. Journal of the International AIDS Society will give higher priority to publications in this area of research.
www.jiasociety.org/home

Lancet Infectious Diseases

The journal publishes a range of article types that encompass all aspects of infectious diseases and medicine: Reflection and Reaction, Newsdesk, Media Watch, Reportage, Review, Historical Review, Personal View, Forum, Grand Round, and Clinical Picture. *Lancet Infectious Diseases* does not publish original research.
www.thelancet.com/journals/laninf/issue/current

Morbidity and Mortality Weekly Report

The *Morbidity and Mortality Weekly Report* (MMWR) Series is prepared by the Centers for Disease Control and Prevention (CDC). Often called "the voice of CDC," the MMWR series is the agency's primary vehicle for scientific publication of timely, reliable, authoritative, accurate, objective, and useful public health information and recommendations. MMWR readership predominately consists of physicians, nurses, public health practitioners, epidemiologists and other scientists, researchers, educators, and laboratorians.
www.cdc.gov/mmwr/

Open AIDS Journal

The *Open AIDS Journal* is an Open Access online journal, which publishes research articles and letters in all areas of research on HIV/AIDS. The journal covers recent studies on experimental; clinical; therapeutic; pathogenesis; vaccines; drug resistance; diagnostics and virology on HIV/AIDS. *The Open AIDS Journal,* a peer-reviewed journal, aims to provide the most complete and reliable source of information on current developments in the field. The emphasis will be on publishing quality papers rapidly and freely available to researchers worldwide.
www.bentham.org/open/toaidj/index.htm

Retrovirology

Retrovirology is an Open Access, online journal that publishes stringently peer-reviewed, high-impact articles on basic retrovirus research. Retroviruses are pleiotropically found in animals. Well-described examples include avian, murine and primate retroviruses. Two human retroviruses are especially important pathogens. These are the human immunodeficiency virus, HIV, and the human T-cell leukemia virus, HTLV. HIV causes AIDS while HTLV-I is the etiological agent for adult T-cell leukemia. There is a large amount of basic research being conducted on HIV and HTLV-I spanning gene expression, virus structure-assembly, integration, replication, and pathogenesis. *Retrovirology* intends to cover these areas of human and animal retrovirus research.
www.retrovirology.com

SAHARA—Journal of Social Aspects of HIV/AIDS Research Alliance

SAHARA is a vehicle for facilitating the sharing of research expertise, sharing knowledge, conducting multi-site multi-country research projects that are intervention-based with the explicit aim of generating new social science evidence for prevention, care and impact mitigation of the HIV/AIDS epidemic. SAHARA brings together key partners in the region, including policy makers, programme planners, researchers in universities and fellow science councils, NGOs, community groups, donors and multilateral agencies to participate in a flexible alliance for social aspects.
www.journals.co.za/ej/ejour_m_sahara.html

Sexually Transmitted Diseases

Sexually Transmitted Diseases publishes original, peer-reviewed articles on clinical, laboratory, immunologic, epidemiologic, sociologic, and historical topics pertaining to sexually transmitted diseases and related fields. Reports from the CDC and NIH provide up-to-the-minute information. A highly respected editorial board is composed of prominent scientists who are leaders in this rapidly changing field. Included in each issue are studies and developments from around the world.
www.stdjournal.com/pt/re/std/home.htm

Sexually Transmitted Infections

Sexually Transmitted Infections is the world's longest running international journal on sexual health. It aims to keep practitioner, trainees, up to date in the prevention, diagnosis, and treatment of STI's and HIV. The journal publishes original work and evidenced based reviews, epidemiological, sociological and laboratory aspects of sexual health from around the world.
http://sti.bmj.com

Surveillance Summaries

The *Surveillance Summaries* provide a means for CDC programs to disseminate surveillance findings, permitting detailed interpretation of trends and patterns based on those findings.
www.cdc.gov/mmwr/mmwr_ss.html

Topics in HIV Medicine

Topics in HIV Medicine is an English-language journal covering current issues in HIV medical care. The journal is indexed in Index Medicus/ MEDLINE and PubMed, and is edited by Dr Douglas D. Richman. Topics in HIV Medicine is published 4 to 6 times a year is intended to be a resource for physicians, physician assistants, nursing professionals, and other health care practitioners who are actively involved in HIV and AIDS care. The journal is mailed to approximately 13,000 practitioners nationally and internationally, and features summaries of talks given at IAS–USA CME courses, highlights of scientific meetings, and special review articles on salient topics in the field of HIV/AIDS.
www.iasusa.org/pub

TreatmentUpdate

TreatmentUpdate is CATIE's (Canadian AIDS Treatment Information Exchange) flagship treatment digest on cutting-edge developments in HIV/AIDS research and treatment. (8 issues per year.)
www.catie.ca/eng/Publications/PublicationsIndex.shtml

SERIAL PUBLICATIONS FOR PERSONS LIVING WITH HIV/AIDS

HIV Positive!

The mission of this site is exactly the same as the mission of the print version of *HIV Positive!* magazine: to help you live a long, productive, fantastic life with HIV. We print 160,000 copies bi-monthly and distribute them, free-of-charge, to people living with HIV through AIDS Services Organizations, clinics, testing sites and other helping organizations across America.
www.hivpositivemagazine.com/index.html

HIV Treatment ALERTS

This newsletter is intended for those affected by HIV and their care-givers. It is published twice each year by the Center for AIDS Information and Advocacy.
www.centerforaids.org/publications/alerts.php

Positive Nation

"Tranforming the UK's response to HIV"
www.positivenation.co.uk/index.php

Positively Aware

Positively Aware is devoted to HIV treatment and health. Positively Aware is published bi-monthly by Test Positive Aware Network (TPAN) in Chicago. Founded in 1987, TPAN is Chicago's oldest peer-led AIDS service organization and specializes in peer-led treatment information and support services. The annual HIV Drug Guide provides extensive information on all FDA approved HIV antivirals, plus experimental ones close to approval or wide access. Positively Aware is supported in part by grants from Abbott Virology and GlaxoSmithKline.
http://positivelyaware.com

The Positive Side

The electronic version of CATIE's magazine for people living with HIV. *The Positive Side* touches on all the aspects of your health that need nurturing: physical, mental, emotional, spiritual and sexual. It is chock-full of resources, practical information and useful tips to inform and empower your decisions about maintaining your health and well-being. Many of these pointers come directly from people who are living with HIV. Our main message? There may be some things in life—and living with HIV—that are beyond your control, but there are many things you can do to make the best of living with HIV.
http://www.positiveside.ca/splash.htm

POZ

Working with photographers, writers, designers and doctors, our team chronicles the HIV epidemic, both in the States and overseas. The magazine is published 11 times per year. POZ.com offers daily news updates, treatment information, POZ Personals, POZ Mentor and more.
www.poz.com

Appendix III

Federal, International, and Independent HIV/AIDS-Related Organizations

UNITED STATES GOVERNMENT-AFFILIATED ORGANIZATIONS

AIDS Clinical Trials Group (ACTG)

The ACTG was initially established in 1987 to broaden the scope of the AIDS research effort of the National Institute of Allergy and Infectious Diseases (NIAID). The ACTG established and supports the largest network of expert clinical and translational investigators and therapeutic clinical trials units in the world, including sites in resource-limited countries. These investigators and units serve as the major resource for HIV/AIDS research, treatment, care, training and education in their communities.
www.actgnetwork.org/login.aspx?ReturnUrl=%2findex.aspx

AIDS Drug Assistance Program (ADAP)

The AIDS Drug Assistance Program (ADAP) provides medications for the treatment of HIV disease. Program funds may also be used to purchase health insurance for eligible clients. Amendments to the Ryan White Comprehensive AIDS Resources Emergency (CARE) Act in October 2000 added language allowing ADAP funds to be used for services that enhance access to, adherence to, and monitoring of drug

treatments. The program is funded through Title II of the CARE Act, which provides grants to states and territories.
http://hab.hrsa.gov/programs/adap

AIDS Education and Training Centers (AETC) National Resource Center

The AIDS Education and Training Centers (AETC) Program of the Ryan White CARE Act currently supports a network of 11 regional centers (and more than 130 local performance sites) that conduct targeted, multidisciplinary education and training programs for health care providers treating persons with HIV/AIDS. The AETCs serve all 50 states, the District of Columbia, the Virgin Islands, Puerto Rico, and the six U.S.–affiliated Pacific jurisdictions. The mission of the AETCs is to improve the quality of life of patients living with HIV/AIDS through the provision of high-quality professional education and training. The AETC Program is administered by the Health Resources and Services Administration (HRSA), HIV/AIDS Bureau.
www.aidsetc.org

AIDS.gov

AIDS.gov is a website linking users to multiple sources of HIV/AIDS information offered by the federal government including blogs and podcasts.
www.aids.gov

AIDSinfo

AIDSinfo is a project that offers the latest federally approved information on HIV/AIDS clinical research, treatment and prevention, and medical practice guidelines for people living with HIV/AIDS, their families and friends, health care providers, scientists, and researchers.
www.aidsinfo.nih.gov

AIDS in Prison Project

This project offers a hotline providing information about AIDS in prisons: general HIV/AIDS and hepatitis C information, HIV and infectious disease prevention, referrals for services within correctional facilities, transitional planning for people in prison who are living with HIV

(including assistance finding housing, medical care, and counseling), peer counseling and support, advocacy for people in prison who have special AIDS/HIV-related needs, and medical parole.
www.osborneny.org/aids_in_prison_project.htm

Centers for AIDS Research (NIH)

The Centers for AIDS Research (CFAR) program at the National Institutes of Health provides administrative and shared research support to synergistically enhance and coordinate high-quality AIDS research projects. CFAR accomplishes this through core facilities that provide expertise, resources, and services not otherwise readily obtained through more traditional funding mechanisms.
www3.niaid.nih.gov/research/cfar

Centers for Disease Control and Prevention: HIV/AIDS

The CDC provides leadership in helping control the HIV/AIDS epidemic by working with community, state, national, and international partners in surveillance, research, and prevention and evaluation activities.
www.cdc.gov/hiv/default.htm

Centers for Disease Control and Prevention: HIV/AIDS Workplace Education (BRTA/LRTA)

The Centers for Disease Control and Prevention Business Responds to AIDS and Labor Responds to AIDS programs (BRTA/LRTA) help large and small businesses and labor unions meet the challenges of HIV/AIDS in the workplace and the community. To fulfill its mission of promoting the development of comprehensive workplace HIV/AIDS programs, BRTA/LRTA works in partnership with groups such as businesses and labor unions, trade associations, public health departments, AIDS service organizations, and government agencies. The Business/Labor Responds to AIDS programs have five core components: HIV/AIDS policy development, manager/labor leader training, employee/worker education, employee/worker family education, and HIV-related community service, volunteerism, and philanthropy.
www.hivatwork.org

Centers for Disease Control:
National Prevention Information Network (NPIN)

NPIN is the U.S. reference, referral, and distribution service for information on HIV/AIDS, viral hepatitis, sexually transmitted diseases (STDs), and tuberculosis (TB). NPIN produces, collects, catalogs, processes, stocks, and disseminates materials and information on HIV/AIDS, viral hepatitis, STDs, and TB to organizations and people working in those disease fields in international, national, state, and local settings.
www.cdcnpin.org/scripts/index.asp

Centers for Disease Control and Prevention:
STD Communications Database

The STD Communications Database is a tool to help public health practitioners create specialized STD prevention programs. It provides access to: best practices in communications, audience profile, theoretical approaches, and training decision-support tools.
www.cdc.gov/std/commdata

Department of Defense:
HIV/AIDS Prevention Program (DHAPP)

The DHAPP goal is to reduce the incidence of HIV/AIDS among uniformed personnel in selected African nations and beyond. DHAPP assist in the following areas: developing and implementing military-specific HIV prevention programs; integrating with other U.S. government, nongovernmental organization, and U.N. programs; and supporting the mission of the President's Emergency Plan for AIDS Relief (PEPFAR).
www.med.navy.mil/sites/nhrc/dhapp/Pages/default.aspx

Food and Drug Administration (FDA)—HIV Testing

This resource of the federal government provides information about HIV testing and offers links to other sources of information about HIV testing.
www.fda.gov/oashi/aids/test.html

Health Resources and Services Administration (HRSA): The HIV/AIDS Programs (Caring for the Underserved)

HRSA is the primary federal agency for improving access to health care services for people who are uninsured, isolated, or medically vulnerable. HRSA provides leadership and financial support to health care providers in every state and U.S. territory. HRSA grantees provide health care to uninsured people, people living with HIV/AIDS, and pregnant women, mothers, and children.
www.hab.hrsa.gov

HIV/AIDS Awareness Days

Throughout the year, health departments, community-based organizations, faith organizations, and other groups and individuals participate in annual national and global awareness days to address the HIV/AIDS pandemic. This resource helps to educate, motivate, and mobilize local communities in the response to HIV/AIDS!
www.hhs.gov/aidsawarenessdays

Indian Health Service (USDHHS)

The IHS HIV/AIDS Program is cultivated from a myriad of services, projects, facilities, funding sources, and field expertise. Interagency and community input are gathered for gap analysis, needs assessment, and further strengthening of the program across multiple levels of influence. Given current epidemiological trends and known vulnerabilities to HIV/AIDS in the AI/AN population, it is critical we consider the larger preventive public health and population approaches for effective response. The program is implemented and executed via an integrative and comprehensive approach through collaborations across multihealth sectors, both internal and external to the agency. It attempts to encompass all types of service delivery "systems" including IHS, tribal, and urban facilities.
www.ihs.gov/MedicalPrograms/HIVAIDS

National HIV and STD Testing Resources (CDC)

This resource provides consumer information and links to HIV and STD testing.
www.hivtest.org/index.cfm

National Institutes on Health:
HIV/AIDS and Older People (NIA)

NIA's mission is to improve the health and well-being of older Americans through research and, specifically, to: support and conduct high-quality research, train and develop highly skilled research scientists from all population groups, develop and maintain state-of-the-art resources to accelerate research progress, and disseminate information and communicate with the public and interested groups on health and research advances and on new directions for research.
www.nia.nih.gov/HealthInformation/Publications/hiv-aids.htm

National Institutes of Health (NIH):
Alcohol and HIV/AIDS

The NIH Office of AIDS Research has identified alcohol use, abuse, and dependence as an important factor in the spread of HIV both here and abroad. The goal of this website is to serve as a resource for the many partners involved in developing a robust research program exploring the complex and intertwined issues of alcohol abuse and the HIV/AIDS pandemic.
www.niaaa.nih.gov/ResearchInformation/ExtramuralResearch/NIAAA-ResearchAreas/AlcoholAIDS.htm

National Institute of Allergy and Infectious Disease (NIAID):
Division of Acquired Immunodeficiency Syndrome (DAIDS)

Created to address the HIV/AIDS epidemic with the mission to help ensure an end the HIV/AIDS epidemic by increasing basic knowledge of the pathogenesis and transmission of the human immunodeficiency virus (HIV), supporting the development of therapies for HIV infection and its complications and coinfections, and supporting the development of vaccines and other prevention strategies.
www3.niaid.nih.gov/about/organization/daids

National Institutes of Health: Pediatric, Adolescent & Maternal AIDS (PAMA) Branch

Supports and conducts both domestic and international research into the epidemiology, natural history, pathogenesis, transmission, treatment, and prevention of HIV infection and its complications in infants, children, adolescents, pregnant women, mothers, women of childbearing age, and the family unit as a whole.
www.nichd.nih.gov/about/org/crmc/pama/index.cfm

National Institute of Diabetes and Digestive and Kidney Diseases (NIDDK)

Each of the three divisions in NIDDK supports an AIDS and HIV program. The Division of Digestive Diseases and Nutrition encourages research into the characterization of intestinal injury, mechanisms of maldigestion, and intestinal mucosal functions, as well as hepatic and biliary dysfunction in patients with AIDS or in appropriate animal models. The HIV program in the Division of Kidney, Urologic, and Hematologic Diseases supports basic and clinical studies on renal and genitourinary tract structure and function and hematopoietic function in individuals with HIV infection. The Division of Diabetes, Endocrinology, and Metabolic Diseases is interested in the metabolic complications of HIV infection, which encompass research on the endocrine and body composition abnormalities associated with HIV infection and its treatment.
www2.niddk.nih.gov/Research/ScientificAreas/HIVAIDS

National Institute of Dental and Craniofacial Research (NIDCR)

The mission of the NIDCR is to improve oral, dental, and craniofacial health through research, research training, and the dissemination of health information. We accomplish our mission by: performing and supporting basic and clinical research; conducting and funding research training and career development programs to ensure an adequate number of talented, well-prepared, and diverse investigators; coordinating and assisting relevant research and research-related activities among all sectors of the research community; promoting the timely transfer of knowledge gained from research and its implications for health to the public, health professionals, researchers, and policy makers.
www.nidcr.nih.gov/OralHealth/Topics/HIV

National Institute on Drug Abuse (NIDA)

NIDA's response to the ongoing epidemic of HIV/AIDS is multifaceted. We support research from basic research projects to behavioral HIV prevention research trials. The common thread in this research is to elucidate the pivotal role of drug use and abuse in the transmission and progression of HIV. Research has demonstrated that pharmacological and behavioral drug use treatments are as effective as HIV prevention interventions. Drug treatment programs can also serve an important role by providing current information on HIV/AIDS, counseling and testing services, and other medical and social services.
www.nida.nih.gov/about/organization/arp/index.html

National Institute of Mental Health (NIMH)

The NIMH's Office of AIDS (1) plans, directs, coordinates, and supports biomedical and behavioral research designed to develop a better understanding of the biological and behavioral causes of HIV (AIDS virus) infection and more effective mechanisms for the diagnosis, treatment, and prevention of AIDS; (2) analyzes and evaluates national needs and research opportunities to identify areas warranting either increased or decreased program emphasis; and (3) consults and cooperates with voluntary and professional health organizations, as well as other NIH components and federal agencies, to identify and meet AIDS-related needs.
www.nimh.nih.gov/about/organization/od/office-on-aids-oa.shtml

National Institute of Neurological Disorders and Stroke (NINDS)

NINDS supports research on the neurological consequences of AIDS. The NINDS works closely with its sister agency, the National Institute of Allergy and Infectious Diseases (NIAID), which has primary responsibility for research related to HIV and AIDS.
www.ninds.nih.gov/disorders/aids/aids.htm

National Institutes of Health (USDHHS)

The NIH is the primary federal agency for conducting and supporting medical research. Helping to lead the way toward important medical discoveries that improve people's health and save lives, NIH scientists

investigate ways to prevent disease as well as the causes, treatments, and even cures for common and rare diseases.
www.health.nih.gov/result.asp/15

National Library of Medicine Director of Health Organizations

This site provides a user-friendly means to identify health organizations, including those focused on HIV/AIDS
http://dirline.nlm.nih.gov

National Library of Medicine: Prisoners/Prisons

This website provides specialized information and links to resources on issues and care relative to care of prisoners with HIV.
http://sis.nlm.nih.gov/hiv/prison.html#a0

Office of AIDS Research (OAR)

The NIH represents the largest and most significant public investment in AIDS research in the world. Our response to the epidemic requires a unique and complex multiinstitute, multidisciplinary, global research program. Through its unique comprehensive trans-NIH planning, budgeting, and portfolio assessment processes, OAR is enhancing collaboration and ensuring that research dollars are invested in the highest priority areas of scientific opportunity that will lead to new tools in the global fight against AIDS.
www.oar.nih.gov

Office of Public Health and Environmental Hazards

The office's goal is to improve veterans' health through prevention and treatment, outreach, surveillance, and focusing on special populations, including women veterans, veterans with HIV/AIDS, veterans with hepatitis C, and veterans exposed to hazardous materials during military service. The office also manages VA's medical response to emergencies and protects the safety and health of Veterans Health Administration employees.
www.hiv.va.gov

Office on Women's Health (OWH) (USDHHS)

The office's vision is to ensure that "All women and girls are healthier and have a better sense of well- eing." Its mission is to "provide leadership to promote health equity for women and girls through sex/gender-specific approaches." The strategy OWH uses to achieve its mission and vision is through the development of innovative programs, by educating health professionals, and by motivating behavior change in consumers through the dissemination of health information.
www.womenshealth.gov/HIV

Pediatric AIDS Clinical Trials Group

The Pediatric AIDS Clinical Trials Group (PACTG) is a self-governed organization with its own scientific agenda and process to determine what will be evaluated in its clinical trials. The PACTG is a cooperative clinical trials network funded by the National Institute of Allergy and Infectious Diseases (NIAID) and the Eunice Kennedy Shriver National Institute of Child Health & Human Development (NICHD) to evaluate clinical interventions, including the efficacy of drugs and drug combinations for treating HIV infection and HIV-associated illnesses in infants, children, adolescents, and pregnant women. The PACTG is comprised of a Coordinating and Operations Center, a Statistical and Data Management Center, and 21 Pediatric AIDS Clinical Trials Units throughout the United States.
www.niaid.nih.gov/Daids/pdatguide/pactg.htm

Presidential Advisory Council on HIV/AIDS (PACHA)

The PACHA provides advice, information, and recommendations to the secretary regarding programs and policies intended to promote effective prevention of HIV disease and to advance research on HIV disease and AIDS. The role of the council is solely advisory. The secretary provides the president with copies of all written reports provided to the secretary by the advisory council.
www.pacha.gov

Substance Abuse and Mental Health Service Administration (SAMHSA)

The growing numbers of people living with and affected by HIV/AIDS makes it important to get the latest word out about problems related to

the illness, prevention, and its treatment. Comprehensive HIV prevention and treatment includes a variety of complementary components to help drug-using populations increase their protective behaviors and reduce their risks for HIV/AIDS as well as other blood-borne infections, such as hepatitis C (HCV), and other sexually transmitted diseases (STDs).
www.samhsa.gov/Matrix/matrix_HIV.aspx

U.S. Department of Housing and Urban Development: HIV/AIDS Housing

To address housing needs for low-income persons who are living with HIV/AIDS and their families, HUD manages the Housing Opportunities for Persons with AIDS (HOPWA) program. The HOPWA program is the only federal program dedicated to address the housing needs of persons living with HIV/AIDS and their families.
www.hud.gov/offices/cpd/aidshousing/index.cfm

USAID: HIV/AIDS

USAID programs in global health represent the commitment and determination of the U.S. Government to prevent suffering, save lives, and create a brighter future for families in the developing world. USAID's commitment to improving global health includes confronting global health challenges through improving the quality, availability, and use of essential health services. USAID's objective is to improve global health, including child, maternal, and reproductive health, and to reduce abortion and disease, especially HIV/AIDS, malaria, and tuberculosis.
www.usaid.gov/our_work/global_health/aids

U.S. President's Emergency Plan for AIDS Relief (PEPFAR)

On July 30, 2008, H.R. 5501, the Tom Lantos and Henry J. Hyde United States Global Leadership Against HIV/AIDS, Tuberculosis, and Malaria Reauthorization Act of 2008 was signed into law, authorizing up to $48 billion over the next five years to combat global HIV/AIDS, tuberculosis, and malaria. Through FY2013, PEPFAR plans to work in partnership with host nations to support: treatment for at least 3 million people, prevention of 12 million new infections, and care for 12 million people, including 5 million orphans and vulnerable children To meet these goals and build sustainable local capacity, PEPFAR will

support training of at least 140,000 new health care workers in HIV/
AIDS prevention, treatment and care.
www.pepfar.gov

OTHER HIV/AIDS-RELATED ORGANIZATIONS

Aaron Diamond AIDS Research Center

The Aaron Diamond AIDS Research Center is committed to finding
solutions to end the AIDS epidemic. In the 25 years since HIV was
identified, researchers have learned more about this virus than about
any other in history. We remain optimistic that research will ultimately
succeed in finding a way out of the crisis.
www.adarc.org

AIDS Alliance for Children, Youth, and Families

AIDS Alliance for Children, Youth, & Families is a national nonprofit
membership organization. We were established in 1994 to give voice
to the needs of women, children, youth, and families living with and
affected by HIV and AIDS.
www.aids-alliance.org

AIDS Education Global Information System (AEGiS)

This nonprofit organization was established in response to the growing
HIV/AIDS pandemic to gather and disseminate information. Our
mission is aimed to: facilitate access to current patient/clinician information specific to HIV/AIDS via our website and its specified services and
preserve for future generations a global history of the pandemic with
our historical news, scientific publications, and treatment database.
www.aegis.com

American Academy of HIV Medicine (AAHIVM)

The academy is an independent organization of AAHIVM HIV specialists and others dedicated to promoting excellence in HIV/AIDS
care. Through advocacy and education, the academy is committed to
supporting health care providers in HIV medicine and to ensuring better
care for those living with AIDS and HIV disease.
www.aahivm.org

American Foundation for AIDS Research (amfAR)

Founded in 1985, amfAR is dedicated to ending the global AIDS epidemic through innovative research. With the freedom and flexibility to respond quickly to emerging areas of scientific promise, amfAR plays a catalytic role in accelerating the pace of HIV/AIDS research and achieving real breakthroughs. amfAR-funded research has increased our understanding of HIV and has helped lay the groundwork for major advances in the study and treatment of HIV/AIDS. Since 1985, amfAR has invested nearly $275 million in its mission and has awarded grants to more than 2,000 research teams worldwide.

www.amfar.org

Association of Nurses in AIDS Care (ANAC)

ANAC strives to promote the individual and collective professional development of nurses involved in the delivery of health care to persons infected or affected by the human immunodeficiency virus (HIV) and to promote the health and welfare of infected persons by: creating an effective network among nurses in AIDS care; studying, researching, and exchanging information, experiences, and ideas leading to improved care for persons with AIDS/HIV infection; providing leadership to the nursing community in matters related to HIV/AIDS infection; advocating for HIV-infected persons; and, promoting social awareness concerning issues related to HIV/AIDS. Inherent in these goals is the abiding commitment to the prevention of further HIV infection.

www.nursesinaidscare.org/i4a/pages/index.cfm?pageid=1

AVERTing HIV and AIDS (AVERT)

AVERT is an international HIV and AIDS charity based in the United Kingdom, working to AVERT HIV and AIDS worldwide. AVERT has HIV and AIDS projects in countries where there is a particularly high rate of infection, such as sub-Saharan Africa, or where there is a rapidly increasing rate of infection, such as in India. We also take AIDS education and information to people in almost every country in the world through our website.

www.avert.org

The Body: The Complete HIV/AIDS Resource

The Body's mission is to use the web to lower barriers between patients and clinicians, to demystify HIV/AIDS and its treatment, to improve patients' quality of life, and to foster community through human connection.
www.thebody.com/index.html

Case Center for AIDS Research

The Case Western Reserve University/University Hospitals Center For AIDS Research (Case CFAR) has been continually funded since its initiation in April 1994 as one of 11 such centers of excellence established by the National Institutes of Health. The CFAR has a mandate to coordinate basic and clinical research activities and to promote interdisciplinary research in HIV infection and AIDS. Comprising more than 140 faculty researchers at the Schools of Medicine, Nursing, Arts and Sciences, and Law, the CFAR provides core resources, seminars, lectureships, publications, and developmental funding to promote and strengthen the AIDS research programs at the university and its affiliated institutions. Current key areas of research strength include: (a) international aspects of AIDS; (b) AIDS clinical research; (c) HIV immunology; (d) molecular virology; (e) mycobacterial disease; (f) AIDS-related malignancies; and (g) HIV prevention.
www.clevelandactu.org/CFAR/index.htm

Elizabeth Glaser Pediatric AIDS Foundation

Whether we're working to attract top researchers to the field of pediatric AIDS, creating programs that provide a full continuum of care in developing countries, or collaborating to accelerate clinical discoveries, our programs offer hope for all children and families living with HIV/AIDS.
www.pedaids.org

François-Xavier Bagnoud Center

The François-Xavier Bagnoud Center is committed to improving the health of vulnerable women, children, youth, and families—including those infected/affected by HIV—and to building capacity in the commu-

nities and systems that serve them. The Center provides culturally competent models of clinical care, education, and consultation state-wide, nationally, and globally.
www.fxbcenter.org

Gay Men's Health Crisis

Gay Men's Health Crisis (GMHC) is a not-for-profit, volunteer-supported, and community-based organization committed to national leadership in the fight against AIDS. We provide prevention and care services to more than 15,000 men, women, and families who are living with, or affected by, HIV/AIDS in New York City, and advocate for scientific, evidence-based public health solutions for hundreds of thousands worldwide.
www.gmhc.org

Global Fund to Fight AIDS, Tuberculosis and Malaria

The Global Fund to Fight AIDS, Tuberculosis and Malaria is an international financing institution that invests the world's money to save lives. To date, it has committed US$14.9 billion in 140 countries to support large-scale prevention, treatment, and care programs against the three diseases.
www.theglobalfund.org/en

Global HIV Prevention Working Group

The Global HIV Prevention Working Group (PWG) is an international panel of more than 50 leading public health experts, clinicians, biomedical, and behavioral researchers, advocates, and people affected by HIV/AIDS, convened by the Bill & Melinda Gates Foundation and the Henry J. Kaiser Family Foundation.
www.globalhivprevention.org/index.html

Harvard School of Public Health AIDS Initiative

For almost two decades, HAI has been dedicated to promoting research, education, and leadership to end the AIDS epidemic. As the number of AIDS cases continues to escalate disproportionately in Africa and other resource-scarce settings, HAI has directed its research efforts toward

developing prevention and treatment strategies to stem the epidemic in these regions.
www.aids.harvard.edu

HIV & Hepatitis Resource

The HIV & Hepatitis Resource website is developed by the Mountain Plains AIDS Education and Training Center (MPAETC). Our goal is to help meet the education needs of clinicians through HIV and hepatitis coinfection-specific education materials and resources.
www.mpaetc.org/hep/index.html

HIV InSite

HIV InSite is developed by the Center for HIV Information (CHI) at the University of California San Francisco (UCSF). Within UCSF, HIV InSite is produced in collaboration with the San Francisco Veterans Affairs Medical Center and other components of the University's AIDS Research Institute. Launched in March 1997, HIV InSite's mission is to be a source for comprehensive, in-depth HIV/AIDS information and knowledge. The site has an extensive collection of original material, including the *HIV InSite Knowledge Base,* a complete textbook with extensive references and related links organized by topic. Unlike many commercially oriented sites, HIV InSite's policy is to link to the best of the web, and thousands of links to external websites are incorporated into the site's original content.
http://hivinsite.ucsf.edu/InSite

HIV Medicine Association

The HIV Medicine Association is an organization of medical professionals who practice HIV medicine. We represent the interests of our patients by promoting quality in HIV care and by advocating for policies that ensure a comprehensive and humane response to the AIDS pandemic informed by science and social justice.
www.hivma.org

Infectious Diseases Society of America (IDSA)

The IDSA represents physicians, scientists, and other health care professionals who specialize in infectious diseases. IDSA's purpose is to improve

the health of individuals, communities, and society by promoting excellence in patient care, education, research, public health, and prevention relating to infectious diseases.
www.idsociety.org

International AIDS Society

The International AIDS Society is the world's leading independent association of HIV/AIDS professionals. By convening the world's largest meetings on HIV/AIDS, IAS provides critical platforms for presenting new research, sharing best practice, and advancing the fight against HIV/AIDS. By promoting dialogue, education, and networking, IAS helps close gaps in knowledge and expertise at every level of the response. By providing support services to our members, we help them do what they do best, advancing the state of the art and expanding access to HIV prevention, treatment, and impact mitigation.
www.iasociety.org

International AIDS Vaccine Initiative (IAVI)

IAVI's mission is to ensure the development of safe, effective, accessible, preventive HIV vaccines for use throughout the world. IAVI is a global not-for-profit, public-private partnership working to accelerate the development of a vaccine to prevent HIV infection and AIDS. Founded in 1996, IAVI researches and develops vaccine candidates, conducts policy analyses, and serves as an advocate for the field with offices in Africa, India, and Europe. IAVI supports a comprehensive approach to HIV and AIDS that balances the expansion and strengthening of existing HIV prevention and treatment programs with targeted investments in new AIDS-prevention technologies. As the world's only organization focused solely on the development of an AIDS vaccine, IAVI also works to ensure a future vaccine will be accessible to all who need it.
www.iavi.org

International Association of Physicians in AIDS Care (IAPAC)

IAPAC is a not-for-profit organization that strives to develop partnerships with health care professions, business government, academe, and religious communities. IAPAC accomplishes its mission through a

comprehensive program of education, policy and advocacy, direct technical assistance, and care provision initiatives spearheaded by physician members.
www.iapac.org

International Council of AIDS Service Organizations (ICASO)

Founded in 1991, the International Council of AIDS Service Organizations' (ICASO) mission is to mobilize and support diverse community organizations to build an effective global response to HIV and AIDS. This is done within a vision of a world where people living with and affected by HIV and AIDS can enjoy life free from stigma, discrimination, and persecution and have access to prevention, treatment, and care.
www.icaso.org

International Training and Education Center on HIV (I-TECH)

I-TECH is a global network that supports the development of a skilled health work force and well-organized national health delivery systems to provide effective prevention, care, and treatment of infectious disease in the developing world.
www.go2itech.org

Kaiser Family Foundation

The Kaiser Family Foundation is a source of independent and current information on the epidemic for policy makers, the media, advocates and community members, and individuals and families affected by HIV. Our HIV/AIDS-related work spans all areas of the Foundation, including policy research and analysis, media and public health partnerships, journalist training and education, health and development in South Africa, primarily through loveLife and online news and information resources through Kaiser network, including the Daily HIV/AIDS Report, webcasts, and the HIV/AIDS Issue Spotlight. The Foundation's HIV/AIDS-related activities focus both on the epidemic in the United States and globally.
www.kff.org/hivaids/index.cfm

Latino Commission on AIDS

The Latino Commission on AIDS is a nonprofit membership organization dedicated to fighting the spread of HIV/AIDS in the Latino community. The Commission is dedicated to resolving the HIV crisis in the Latino community, where social stigma, poverty, language barriers, immigration status fears, and access to care deter testing and increase the infection rate. Over 200,000 Latinos in the United States and Puerto Rico are living with HIV/AIDS. The fastest growing ethnic group in the United States, Latinos constitute 14% of the U.S. population but account for over 20% of the AIDS cases.
www.latinoaids.org

Names Project Foundation
(The AIDS Memorial Quilt)

Founded in 1987, the AIDS Memorial Quilt is a poignant memorial, a powerful tool for use in preventing new HIV infections, and the largest ongoing community arts project in the world. Each "block" (or section) of the AIDS Memorial Quilt measures approximately 12 feet square, and a typical block consists of eight individual three-foot by six-foot panels sewn together. Virtually every one of the more than 40,000 colorful panels that make up the Quilt memorializes the life of a person lost to AIDS.
www.aidsquilt.org

National AIDS Treatment Advocacy Project (NATAP)

NATAP is a nonprofit corporation whose mission is to educate individuals about HIV and hepatitis treatments and to advocate on the behalf of all people living with HIV/AIDS and HCV. Our efforts in these areas are conducted on local, national, and international levels.
www.natap.org

National Alliance of State and Territorial
AIDS Directors (NASTAD)

The National Alliance of State and Territorial AIDS Directors (NASTAD) represents the nation's chief state health agency staff who have programmatic responsibility for administering HIV/AIDS health care, prevention, education, and supportive service programs funded by state and federal governments. NASTAD is dedicated to reducing the incidence of HIV/AIDS infection in the United States and its territories, providing comprehensive, compassionate, and high-quality care to all persons living with HIV/AIDS and ensuring responsible public policies. NASTAD provides national leadership to achieve these goals and to educate about and advocate for the necessary federal funding to achieve them, as well as to promote communication between state and local health departments and HIV/AIDS care and treatment programs. NASTAD supports and encourages the use of applied scientific knowledge and input from affected communities to guide the development of effective policies and programs. www.nastad.org

National Association on HIV Over Fifty (NAHOF)

Recognizing that no national mechanism to gather information about HIV issues for people above age 50 exists, the National Association on HIV Over Fifty, Inc. (NAHOF) was founded in 1995 in New York City. NAHOF was formed to provide advocacy, education, communication, and support for HIV-positive older adults, their families, and those who provide care or conduct research on their behalf. www.hivoverfifty.org/index.html

National Association of People with AIDS (NAPWA)

The National Association of People with AIDS was founded in 1983 by members of the Patient Advisory Committee of the Second National AIDS Forum, held in Denver, Colorado, by what is now the National Lesbian and Gay Health Association. Over the years, NAPWA has been a strong and consistent national leader for people with AIDS, ensuring that our voice is always at the table when decisions affecting our lives are being made. NAPWA has withstood financial setbacks and other serious threats to its leadership. www.napwa.org/index.shtml

National HIV/AIDS Clinicians Consultation Center: Telephone Consultation Service

The National HIV Telephone Consultation Service (Warmline) offers physicians and other health care providers up-to-the-minute HIV clinical information and individualized expert case consultation across the

broad range of clinical HIV/AIDS problems. The Warmline is staffed by clinicians experienced in HIV care who can help you provide the best possible care to your HIV-positive patients.
www.nccc.ucsf.edu/Hotlines/Warmline.html

National HIV/AIDS Clinicians Consultation Center: Post-Exposure Prophylaxis Hotline

The National Clinicians' Post-Exposure Prophylaxis Hotline (PEPline) offers treating clinicians up-to-the-minute advice on managing occupational exposures (i. e., needlesticks, splashes, etc.) to HIV, hepatitis, and other blood-borne pathogens.
www.nccc.ucsf.edu/Hotlines/PEPline.html

National HIV/AIDS Clinicians Consultation Center: The National Perinatal HIV Consultation and Referral Service

The Perinatal Hotline is a service of the National HIV/AIDS Clinicians' Consultation Center (NCCC) at San Francisco General Hospital. Free 24-hour clinical consultation and advice are offered on: management of HIV in pregnant women, HIV testing in pregnancy, and care of HIV-exposed infants.
www.nccc.ucsf.edu/Hotlines/Perinatal.html

National Minority AIDS Council

NMAC has advanced its mission through a variety of public policy education programs; national conferences; treatment and research programs and trainings; electronic and printed resource materials; and a website: www.nmac.org. NMAC represents a coalition of 3,000 F/CBOs and AIDS service organizations (ASOs) delivering HIV/AIDS services in communities of color nationwide. NMAC's advocacy efforts are funded through private funders and donors only.
www.nmac.org

National Network of STD/HIV Prevention Training Centers (NNPTC)

NNPTC is a group of regional centers created in partnership with health departments and universities. The PTCs are dedicated to increasing the

knowledge and skills of health professionals in the areas of sexual and reproductive health. The NNPTC provides health professionals with a spectrum of state-of-the-art educational opportunities including experiential learning with an emphasis on prevention.
http://depts.washington.edu/nnptc

Native American AIDS Prevention Center

The National Native American AIDS Prevention Center (NNAAPC) helps organizations that serve Native communities to plan, develop and manage HIV/AIDS prevention, intervention, care, and treatment programs. NNAAPC seeks to address the impact of HIV/AIDS on American Indians, Alaska Natives, and Native Hawaiians through culturally appropriate advocacy, research, education, and policy development in support of healthy Indigenous people.
www.nnaapc.org/index.htm

Phillip T. and Susan M. Ragon Institute at MGH, MIT, and Harvard

The Phillip T. and Susan M. Ragon Institute was officially established in February 2009 at MGH, MIT, and Harvard with a dual mission: to contribute to the accelerated discovery of an HIV/AIDS vaccine and subsequently to establish itself as a world leader in the collaborative study of immunology. Founded with a commitment of $100 million from Mr. and Mrs. Ragon, the institute is structured and positioned to significantly contribute to a global effort to successfully develop an HIV/AIDS vaccine.
www.ragoninstitute.org/index.html

Project Inform

Project Inform represents HIV-positive people in the development of treatments and a cure, supports individuals to make informed choices about their HIV health, advocates for quality health care to respond to HIV and related conditions, and promotes medical strategies that prevent new infections. Working at the local, state, and national levels since 1985, Project Inform lends an independent voice to ensure a thoughtful, compassionate response to the epidemic by government, academia, industry, and the community, and we empower all individuals living with HIV to make fully informed health decisions to build quality of life.
www.projectinform.org

Rural Center for AIDS/STD Prevention (RCAP)

The major focus of the Rural Center for AIDS/STD Prevention (RCAP) is the promotion of HIV/STD prevention in rural America, with the goal of reducing HIV/STD incidence. The RCAP develops and evaluates educational materials and approaches, examines the behavioral and social barriers to HIV/STD prevention that can be applied to prevention programming, and provides prevention resources to professionals and the public.
www.indiana.edu/~aids/whatsnew.html

Sibusiso

Sibusiso is a nonprofit organization dedicated to improve the quality of life for people infected and affected by HIV/AIDS in resource-poor settings. With a vast array of international experience serving the needs of impoverished communities, Sibusiso's dedicated group of volunteers emanate from the medical, pharmaceutical, business, education, human rights, and humanitarian fields.
www.sibusiso.org

Statistical Center for HIV/AIDS Research & Prevention (SCHARP)

The Statistical Center for HIV/AIDS Research & Prevention (SCHARP) is part of the Public Health Sciences Division of the Fred Hutchinson Cancer Research Center in Seattle, Washington. SCHARP provides statistical collaboration to HIV/AIDS researchers around the world and conducts a complementary program of statistical methodology and mathematical modeling research. SCHARP also collects, manages, and analyzes data from clinical trials and epidemiological studies dedicated to the elimination of HIV/AIDS as a threat to human health.
www.scharp.org/index.html

Treatment Action Group

Treatment Action Group is an independent AIDS research and policy think tank fighting for better treatment, a vaccine, and a cure for AIDS. TAG works to ensure that all people with HIV receive life saving treatment, care, and information.
www.aidsinfonyc.org/tag

UNAIDS

UNAIDS, the Joint United Nations Programme on HIV/AIDS, is an innovative joint venture of the U.N. family, bringing together the efforts and resources of ten U.N. system organizations in the AIDS response to help the world prevent new HIV infections, care for people living with HIV, and mitigate the impact of the epidemic.
www.unaids.org/en/default.asp

University of Alabama Center for AIDS Research

The University of Alabama at Birmingham Center for AIDS Research (CFAR), situated in the Medical Center complex of the University, is one of the seven original centers, established in 1988 by the National Institute for Allergy and Infectious Diseases (NIAID), to stimulate research and scientific advancement concerning AIDS and HIV. The CFAR program was expanded in 1998 and currently includes 20 centers funded through a consortium of six National Institutes of Health (NIH). From its inception in 1988 the Birmingham CFAR has played a pivotal role in stimulating and supporting research in both the basic and clinical sciences.
www.uabcfar.org

University of California AIDS Research Institute

The AIDS Research Institute (ARI) coordinates and integrates all AIDS research activities at the University of California, San Francisco. The ARI stimulates innovation and supports interdisciplinary collaboration aimed at all aspects of the epidemic domestically and around the world. Bringing together hundreds of scientists and more than 50 programs from throughout the university and affiliated labs and institutions, and working in close collaboration with affected communities, the ARI is one of the premier AIDS research entities in the world.
http://ari.ucsf.edu

University of California San Diego AIDS Research Institute

The mission of the AIDS Research Institute is to become a regional resource for HIV/AIDS research by coordinating and stimulating collaborative scientific research and exchange within the academic commu-

nity, offering relevant educational and training opportunities in the many areas related to HIV infection, and providing clinical resources and education to the San Diego community. The ARI serves as the nexus for AIDS researchers to share research and ideas and, together, devise new approaches to prevent, diagnose and treat HIV/AIDS.
http://ari.ucsd.edu

University of California San Francisco— Center for AIDS Prevention Studies

The mission of CAPS is to conduct domestic and international research to prevent the acquisition of HIV and to optimize health outcomes among HIV-infected individuals.
www.caps.ucsf.edu

Women, Children, and HIV Web site

The Women, Children, and HIV Web site is the result of collaboration between the François-Xavier Bagnoud (FXB) Center at the University of Medicine and Dentistry of New Jersey (UMDNJ) and the Center for HIV Information (CHI) at the University of California, San Francisco. The goals of this website are to: disseminate state-of-the-art clinical information and training resources on mother-to-child transmission of HIV (MTCT) and related topics, communicate the best practices in preventing mother-to-child transmission of HIV (PMTCT) and caring for infected children, disseminate PMTCT program resource materials, disseminate state-of-the-art clinical information and training resources on perinatally acquired pediatric HIV infection, and implement services responsive to the needs of the CDC Global AIDS Program (CDC/GAP).
http://womenchildrenhiv.org

World Health Organization

As the directing and coordinating authority on international health, the World Health Organization (WHO) takes the lead within the U.N. system on the global health sector response to HIV/AIDS. The WHO HIV/AIDS Program provides evidence-based, technical support to WHO member states to help them scale up treatment, care, and prevention services, as well as maintain and increase access to drugs and diagnostics. This is to ensure a comprehensive and sustainable response to HIV/AIDS.
www.who.int/hiv/en

Index